RADIATION
THERAPY
PLANNING

RADIATION THERAPY PLANNING

SECOND EDITION

Gunilla C. Bentel, R.N., R.T.T.

Clinical Associate
Department of Radiation Oncology
Duke University Medical Center
Durham, North Carolina

McGraw-Hill
Health Professions Division

New York   St. Louis   San Francisco   Auckland   Bogotá   Caracas
Lisbon   London   Madrid   Mexico City   Milan   Montreal
New Delhi   San Juan   Singapore   Sydney   Tokyo   Toronto

McGraw-Hill

A Division of The **McGraw·Hill** Companies

RADIATION THERAPY PLANNING, 2/e

Copyright © 1996, 1992 by The McGraw-Hill Companies, Inc. All rights reserved. Printed in Colombia. Except as permitted under the United States Copyright Act of 1976, no part of this publication may by reproduced or distributed in any form or by any means or stored in a data base or retrieval system, without the prior written permission of the publisher.

Original copyright © 1992 by Macmillan Publishing Company, a division of Macmillan, Inc.

22 23 24 SCI/SCI 19 18

ISBN 0-07-005115-1

This book was set in Times Roman by Progressive Information Technologies.
The editors were Martin J. Wonsiewicz and Muza Navrozov;
the production supervisor was Clare B. Stanley;
the cover was designed by Karen Quigley;
the index was prepared by Mary Kidd.
Worldcolor/Fairfield was printer and binder
This book was printed on acid-free paper.

Library of Congress Cataloging-in-Publication Data

Bentel, Gunilla Carleson.
    Radiation therapy planning: including problems and solutions/
Gunilla C. Bentel.— 2 ed.
      p.   cm.
    Includes bibliographical references and index.
    ISBN 0-07-005115-1 (softcover)
    1. Cancer—Radiotherapy.   2. Cancer—Radiotherapy—Problems,
exercises, etc.   I. Title.
    [DNLM: 1. Neoplasms—radiography.   2. Brachytherapy—methods.
3. Radiotherapy Dosage.   4. Radiometry.   QZ 269 B475r   1996]
RC271.R3B45   1996
616.99′40642—dc20
DNLM/DLC
for Library of Congress   95-16244

To the memory of Dr. Olle Hallberg and Dr. Bengt Mårtensson and to the now retired Dr. Karl-Johan Vikterlöf, my teachers at Örebro Regional Hospital in Örebro, Sweden. It was because of their expertise and enthusiasm and their skill in teaching radiation therapy that I was inspired to choose this exciting and interesting field as my specialty. I have never regretted this choice; instead, I consider working in this field a privilege. Learning never stops, and I have learned new things every day during the 36 years I have worked in radiation therapy.

I would also like to dedicate this edition to the cancer patients, who so bravely face their illness and often suffer, physically and mentally, quietly and alone. Their courage is an inspiration to all of us who strive to cure their ailments. Although we learn how to treat their disease from textbooks, a more important lesson is learned from our patients; to be humble and thankful that we are healthy and able to go to work every day. It is my hope that in some way this text will promote the application of improved techniques for the treatment of cancer.

Disclaimer

Great care has been taken to maintain the accuracy of the information contained in this volume. Treatment plans and dose calculations described in the text are suggested methods only, and no responsibility is accepted for their wrongful application. Consideration must be given to a particular patient's contour or target volume, and to the beam data particular to the individual treatment machine.

All radiation doses stated assume fractionation at 180 to 200 cGy per day in a continuous course of 5 fractions per week, unless otherwise indicated.

Contents

Color Plates appear between pages 532 and 533.

Foreword

Radiation therapy for malignant and benign diseases is technically difficult and potentially dangerous. It is incumbent upon radiation oncologists to optimize the therapeutic ratio of treatment by accurately delivering therapeutic doses of radiation to the target volume while minimizing the dose to uninvolved normal structures. Careful attention to the treatment process, including immobilization, simulation, treatment planning, dose calculation, and treatment implementation serves to achieve these goals. During her thirty-year career in clinical radiation oncology, Gunilla Bentel has diligently and effectively pursued precision treatment planning. She now offers the wisdom acquired by vast experience to the reader. This is an extremely practical book, which includes detailed planning options and recommendations for treatment implementation. In addition, the logic and practical considerations that underlie her recommendations are explained. Numerous illustrations enhance the reader's understanding of the treatment planning process. This book will occupy an honored place on the bookshelf as an excellent educational tool for all the professionals involved in radiation oncology, including physicians, physicists, dosimetrists, radiation therapists, as well as students and residents in these disciplines.

I have had the pleasure and good fortune of working with the author for six years. Her expertise is invaluable in our clinic, and her tireless efforts have served our patients well. The attention to detail that she adheres to in the clinic is evidenced by the excellent job that she has done on this book. Just as I have learned from working with the author, I am confident that readers of this book will benefit from Ms. Bentel's insights.

Lawrence B. Marks, M.D.
Duke University Medical Center

Preface

As new sophisticated technologies are introduced, radiation therapy becomes more complex. The need for a comprehensive text which describes the technical aspects of radiation therapy planning has been met with the development of *Radiation Therapy Planning, Second Edition*. The objectives of this book are to present a practical guide to radiation therapy treatment planning and to contribute to a better understanding and proper application of new technologies.

The first edition, although primarily intended for radiation therapy technologists and dosimetrists, was also well received by physicians, physicists, nurses, and by vendors training their staff in the technical aspects of radiation therapy. The favorable response to the first edition of *Radiation Therapy Planning* was very stimulating and has given me incentive to produce the second edition.

In addition to a substantial expansion, the material which was covered in the first edition has been extensively revised. Nine new chapters have been added, six of them describing typical treatment plans used to treat different anatomic sites as well as patient positioning and immobilization. When radiation treatments are planned, field orientations are often limited by the tolerance of the adjacent normal tissues. It is therefore necessary for the planner to be familiar with the range of doses required in the tumor as well as the dose levels tolerated by the normal tissues. A brief description of some commonly irradiated diseases and doses frequently used is therefore also included.

This edition also includes descriptions of isodose curves, combining isodose curves, and the principles of multiple beam planning. In-depth descriptions of the pretreatment procedures as well as the underlying concepts of three-dimensional treatment planning are also discussed. Presentations regarding treatment documentation, including sections of a treatment chart, treatment uncertainties, the effect of errors in treatment delivery, and quality assurance are included. An effort has been made, particularly in Chapter 7, to offer alternative target localization methods when state-of-the-art equipment is not available.

Acknowledgments

The development of a text this size would not be possible without the assistance of many coworkers. I am indeed fortunate to be associated with the very knowledgeable and experienced staff in the Department of Radiation Oncology at Duke University, who freely offered their advice and answered many questions during the maturation of this book. I truly value their advice and many helpful suggestions.

I am particularly grateful for the immeasurable efforts of Dr. Lawrence B. Marks, who with untiring energy guided me through several chapters. I am also grateful for the support of Dr. Leonard R. Prosnitz (Chairman), Dr. Edward C. Halperin, Dr. A. Joy Hilliard, Dr. Mitchell Anscher, Dr. Gustavo S. Montana, and Dr. David M. Brizel. I am also grateful for the many helpful suggestions and editing skills of Dr. Fearghus O'Foghludha, Professor Emeritus.

This manuscript contains many illustrations which would not have been possible without the expertise of my colleagues in radiation physics. I am indebted to Dr. George W. Sherouse, Dr. David P. Spencer, Dr. Marc R. Sontag, Dr. Sujit Ray, and Dr. Phillip A. Antoine for their help with computer-generated pictures and superb support in many other areas. While the computers did not always cooperate, the expertise and calming words extended by these associates helped me through many terrifying moments.

I would also like to recognize the efforts of all technical staff in the Departments of Radiation Oncology at Duke University and the Memorial Hospital of Martinsville and Henry County, Virginia. During the development of this rather large text, I frequently needed help with many jobs such as procuring suitable radiographs, copying x-rays, and someone to pose for a picture. Willing and capable staff were always available to assist, and to them I am forever grateful. I am particularly indebted to Gail Ellis, Henry Pendleton, Lori Absalom, Kathy Temple, Lisa Asbury, and Denise Torain.

Heartfelt thanks are also extended to Jane Hoppenworth for her help with formatting the text, coordinating copyright permissions, and many other chores. I would also like to acknowledge the assistance of the skillful staff in the Audiovisual Department at Duke University.

Abbreviations

AAPM	American Association of Physicists in Medicine	dps	disintegrations per second
Al	aluminum	DRR	digitally reconstructed radiograph
A/P	area/perimeter	DVH	dose-volume histogram
avg	average	EPID	electronic portal imaging devices
Au	gold		
BEV	beam's-eye view	eq sq	equivalent square
BSF	backscatter factor	FL	field length
Bq	becquerel	FS	field size
CA	central axis	f_{tis}	roentgen to centigray in tissue
$CaCl_2$	calcium chloride		
CaF_2	calcium fluoride	g	gram
CCCT	computer-controlled conformal therapy	GTV	gross tumor volume
		Gy	gray
cGy	centigray	h	hour
cGy/mi	centigray per minute	HBB	half-beam block
cGy/MU	centigray per monitor unit	HVL	half-value layer
Ci	curie	HVT	half-value thickness
cm	centimeter	I	iodine
cm^3	cubic centimeter	ICRU	International Commission on Radiation Units and Measurements
Co	cobalt		
COPD	chronic obstructive pulmonary disease		
		Ir	iridium
Cs	cesium	ISF	inverse square factor
CSI	craniospinal irradiation	J	joule
CT	computed tomography	keV	kiloelectron volt
CTV	clinical target volume	kVp	peak kilovoltage
Cu	copper	LiF	lithium fluoride
%DD	percentage depth dose	LAO	left anterior oblique
D	depth	LPO	left posterior oblique
D_{max}	maximum dose	mCi	millicurie
d_{max}	depth of maximum dose	mm	millimeter

MeV	million electron volt	RTOG	Radiation Therapy Oncology Group
mgh	milligram hour	SAD	source-axis distance
mg Ra eq	milligram radium equivalent	SAR	scatter-air ratio
mg Ra	milligram radium	SFD	source-to-film distance
MLC	multileaf collimator	s	second
MRI	magnetic resonance imaging	SMR	scatter-maximum ratio
MU	monitor unit	Sn	tin
MV	million volts	SPECT	single positron emission tomography
NaCl	sodium chloride		
NIST	National Institute of Standards and Technology	Sr	strontium
		SSD	source-surface distance
		STLI	subtotal lymphoid irradiation
OAR	off-axis ratio		
P	phosphorus	T_{avg}	average life
Pb	lead	TAR	tissue-air ratio
PEL	permissible exposure limit	TBI	total body irradiation
		TD	tumor dose
Pt	platinum	TFD	target-to-film distance
PTV	planning target volume	TLD	thermoluminescent dosimeter
R	roentgen		
Ra	radium	TLI	total lymphoid irradiation
RAO	right anterior oblique	TMR	tissue-maximum ratio
ref	reference	TPR	tissue-phantom ratio
Rn	radon	TTD	target-to-tray distance
RPC	Radiological Physics Center	X_r	exposure rate
		Yt	yttrium
RPO	right posterior oblique		

RADIATION THERAPY PLANNING

Historical Perspective of Radiation Therapy

THE DISCOVERY OF ROENTGEN RAYS AND RADIOACTIVITY

On Friday, November 8, 1895, while passing an electric current through a Hittorf-Crookes high-vacuum tube, Wilhelm Conrad Röntgen* noticed a light coming from a workbench about a yard away. He identified the shining object as a piece of paper painted with barium platinocyanide. Realizing that this light must have been caused by a new kind of rays, he called them x-rays which later became known as *roentgen rays*. He continued the investigation of these rays and found that when he replaced the fluorescent screen with a photographic plate, he could obtain pictures. The most dramatic picture,

taken on December 22, only 6 weeks following the discovery of the invisible rays, showed the bones in his wife's hand. Density variations, depending on the tissues in the path of the rays, were observed, and the value of such radiographic images in the diagnosis of human ailments immediately became evident.

On December 28, 1895, Röntgen delivered a written presentation of his discovery to the Physical-Medical Society of Würzburg. Within a few weeks, this preliminary communication entitled *On a New Kind of Rays* was translated into many languages. On New Year's Day, 1896, he mailed copies of his paper along with some radiographs to several European physicists whom he knew. The news of the discovery spread very quickly and was soon known all over the world.

Only a few weeks after Röntgen's discovery,

* Usually written "Roentgen" in the English-language literature.

Henri Becquerel began investigating the possibility of similar rays being produced by known fluorescent or phosphorescent substances. He observed the darkening of photographic plates (Chap. 3) by uranium salts and realized that these rays were emitted spontaneously and continuously from the uranium; thus, radioactivity was discovered.

Marie Curie, who at this time was studying minerals in Paris, became interested in the phenomenon of radioactivity and chose this subject for her doctoral thesis. Pierre Curie eventually joined his wife in her research, and in July 1898 they discovered polonium; in December of the same year, they reported the discovery of radium.

Both Becquerel and Pierre Curie experienced erythema on the skin of the chest from carrying small samples of radium in their vest pockets. Pierre Curie applied radium to his arm and described in detail the various phases of a moist epidermitis and his recovery from it. He also provided radium to physicians, who tested it on patients.

The news of these discoveries spread quickly, and —having learned that redness of the skin was observed by the users of these rays—several physicians began investigating their effect on malignant tumors; thus, the use of ionizing radiation in the treatment of cancer began.

THERAPEUTIC USES OF X-RAYS AND RADIOACTIVITY

More than any other innovation, the ability to visualize the interior of the living human body painlessly has governed the practice of medicine during the twentieth century. The radiotherapeutic application of these discoveries also had a profound effect on cancer survival rates. This chapter focuses on the therapeutic uses of x-rays and radioactivity.

The discovery of x-rays and radioactivity was promptly followed by their therapeutic application. The first therapeutic use of x-rays is reported to have taken place on January 29, 1896, when a patient with carcinoma of the breast was treated; by 1899, the first cancer, a basal cell epithelioma, had been cured by radiation.

The initial dramatic responses observed in the treatment of skin and other superficial tumors generated the hope that a cure for cancer had finally been found. This hope was soon followed by a wave of disillusionment and pessimism when tumor recurrences and injuries to normal tissues began to appear. The treatments often involved single massive exposures aimed at the eradication of tumors, and the patients who survived the immediate postirradiation period often developed major complications. Because of these disappointing results, the use of x-rays to treat tumors would soon have been abandoned had it not been for laboratory and clinical work by Claude Regaud and Henri Coutard. They found that by administering fractionated doses of radiation (that is, smaller daily doses rather than a large single dose), they could achieve the same tumor response but without serious injury to the adjacent normal tissues.

From the early experience, it was evident that the unique advantage of radium lay in intracavitary and interstitial applications. Here, where the radioactivity was placed directly on or inside the tumor, the radiation did not first have to traverse normal tissue; the short distance and rapid fall-off of dose offered an advantage in this setting. Initially, containers were rather bulky and could be used only for intracavitary gynecologic implants. In 1914, methods were developed for collecting radon (a daughter product of radium) in small glass tubes, which were then placed inside hollow metal seeds. Like radium needles, these could be inserted directly into the tumors. Radium needles and radon seeds were very popular for many years but have more recently been replaced by safer, artificially produced isotopes.

Many of the physical facts of radium were discovered early. The skin burns suffered by Becquerel and Curie served as a warning to other users. The value of filtration and the importance of distance from the source to the treated tissue were soon recognized by the many chemists, physicists, and medical specialists who worked together in the treatment of patients.

Initially, the only countries where radium could be obtained were France and Austria. Later, it was also discovered in Colorado, and in 1911 radium was purified from the Colorado ore. To reduce and purify 1 g of radium, it was necessary to use 500 tons of ore, 10,000 tons of distilled water, 1000 tons of coal, and 500 tons of chemicals. A gram of radium sold for $120,000.

The first use of radium (imported from Europe) in the United States was around 1908. The radium tubes were primarily used in the treatment of gynecologic malignancies, whereas radium solutions were used to treat arthritis and gout. The latter use was discontinued after a few years.

The clinical pioneers in radiation therapy, mostly surgeons and dermatologists, used the "erythema dose," or radiation dose necessary to cause redness of the skin, to estimate the proper length of the treatments.

It was recognized early that accurate dosimetry was fundamental to success in any type of radiation treatment. In radium therapy, this comprised three parts: the accurate measurement of the radium content of the various sources, the determination of the radiation output of each source in terms of an acceptable dose unit, and a knowledge of the distribution of radiation within the tissues under treatment.

Until 1911, there was no satisfactory method to standardize radium. Madame Curie then began to prepare an accurate standard of carefully weighed quantities of pure radium salt. This standard was deposited with the International Bureau of Weights and Measures, at Sèvres near Paris, and continues to serve as the standard for radioactivity.

Madame Curie's standard was used for determining the amount of radioactivity in each source. Output measurements in terms of radiation exposure were very complicated, but following tedious work by many investigators, it was determined that a point source of radium, filtered by 0.5 mm of platinum, delivers what later became known as 8.25 roentgen per hour at 1 cm from the source.

As for the distribution of the sources within the tissues, a dosage system that is still used in many hospitals was begun in 1932 and published in 1939 by Ralston Paterson and Herbert Parker at Christie Hospital in Manchester, England. Their dosage system was developed on the theory that nonuniform spacing of the radioactivity within the tissue could result in a relatively uniform dose distribution. In 1941, Edith Quimby, first at Memorial Hospital and later at the College of Physicians and Surgeons in New York, published a dosage system in which the sources were arranged in a uniform pattern and the resulting dose distribution was nonuniform.

Several other systems for radium distribution (Chap. 15) were worked out both in the United States and in Europe. The Manchester (Paterson and Parker), Paris, and Stockholm techniques are the most notable and are more or less followed by other institutions.

MEASUREMENTS OF QUALITY AND QUANTITY OF RADIATION BEAMS

During the early years of radiology, the methods of measuring the *quality* (or penetrating power) and *quantity* of x-ray beams were unsatisfactory. Direct measurements of radiation quality were made by means of a "penetrometer," which was introduced by Benoist in 1901. This instrument consisted of a thin silver disk surrounded by a ring of aluminum wedges arranged like a stair, with 12 steps of increasing thickness. The aluminum step that matched the silver disk in absorption was fluoroscopically or photographically determined and used to represent the radiation quality in designated units.[1]

Also at the beginning of the century, Holzknecht described a "chromoradiometer," an instrument to measure quantity of dose. It consisted of small disks of a fused mixture of potassium chloride and sodium carbonate. These compounds became discolored when irradiated with x-rays. Holzknecht called the dose producing a minimal degree of discoloration "$_1$H." Doses high enough to produce a skin erythema would be of the order of $_3$H.[1]

Another device, a *radiometer*, was developed in 1904 to measure quantity of dose. This device was used for many years, primarily by dermatologists. A method of measuring dose in calories was also used at the beginning of the century. These methods were unsatisfactory, and during the subsequent 50 years, many efforts were made to develop accurate and reliable methods of determining the amount of dose. From 1914 to 1925, a number of physicists worked on the determination of a unit of dose and built various types of instruments, most notably a primary standard ionization chamber for the determination of the dose unit and a secondary instrument to measure dose on the patient.[1]

In 1928, H. Geiger and W. Mueller constructed an improved detector tube based on a counter built as early as 1906. In various modified forms, both of these instruments were used well into the 1960s.[1]

Antoine Béclère in Paris, Gösta Forssell in Stockholm, J. J. Thomson in Liverpool, and George Pfahler in Boston were among the pioneers who laid the groundwork of radiation therapy. They and many other dedicated scientists soon recognized the need for an internationally accepted unit of dose and a method by which to define the quality of the rays. In 1913, the term *half-value layer,* or HVL (a term now replaced, as in this text, by half-value thickness, or HVT), was suggested as a measure of quality. It was not until 1928 that the roentgen as a unit of measurement for x-rays and gamma rays was internationally accepted, and in 1953, the International Commission on Radiological Units and Measurements (ICRU) recommended the rad as the unit of absorbed dose. The rad has more recently been replaced by the centigray (cGy).

TECHNICAL DEVELOPMENTS

TECHNICAL DEVELOPMENTS: 1920–1940

The equipment used in the treatment of malignant disease during the first years of radiation therapy was primitive and temperamental; it also had very low penetrating power. The use of x-rays was limited by the low kilovoltage available. But as the applicability of roentgen rays expanded, the demand for better equipment increased. During the 1920s, Coolidge invented a vacuum x-ray tube capable of operating at peak kilovoltages (kVp) of 200 to 250. With such machines, more deep-seated tumors could be treated without excessive injury to the overlying skin.

Figure 1.1, copied from Albert Bachem's textbook *Principles of x-ray and Radium Dosage,* depicts the use of water bags as compensators, indicating an understanding of isodose distributions and the composition of tissue-equivalent materials prior to 1920.[2] Improved treatment techniques where multiple beams were aimed at the tumor from different directions (Fig. 1.2), the so-called crossfire techniques, were also used. Other advances during this era were improved design and reliability of treatment machines.

Much had been learned about the need for filtration of the radiation produced by these machines. The concept of the inverse-square law, scattering, and the effect of treatment distance on the percentage depth dose (%DD) were also understood. The treatment times for external beam treatment were expressed in erythema time factors, whereas the standard measure of erythema dose in radium treatment consisted of 100 milligram hours (mgh).[2] The erythema dose as a measure of how much dose to de-

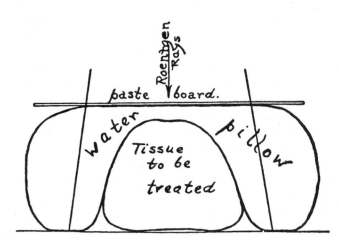

Figure 1.1 The use of water bags as tissue-equivalent material in this illustration, first published in 1923, indicates an early understanding of isodose distributions and the need for compensators.

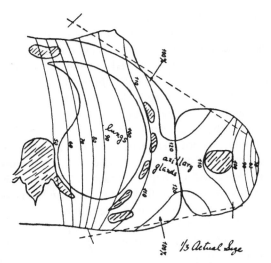

Figure 1.2 A multiple-beam arrangement in the treatment of breast cancer was used in the early days of radiation therapy, as depicted in this illustration from Albert Bachem's textbook, published in 1923.

liver was replaced during this era by the first physical unit, the roentgen.

The discovery of artificial radioactivity in 1934 had a profound impact on the future of brachytherapy; however, the use of radium continued for many years. It was not until World War II that neutron reactors, which are capable of producing artificial radionuclides in large quantities, were developed; isotopes for medical use were thereafter produced on a large scale.

The combination of external beam treatment with intracavitary radium was used during this time period and elaborate systems for calculating the combined dose were devised.

TECHNICAL DEVELOPMENTS: 1940–1960

As cure rates improved and the complication rate declined, radiation therapists were encouraged and looked for machines with even higher energy producing better dose distributions. The first use of "supervoltage" radiation therapy equipment, then considered to be anything operating at greater than 1 million volts (MV), occurred in 1937 at St. Bartholomew's Hospital in London. Clinical experience with this machine clearly showed the advantages

of high-energy beams. Several investigators[3-5] described different methods of accelerating particles, and following this initial work, betatrons and linear accelerators for medical use emerged. Machines using reactor-produced sources of cobalt 60, described in Chaps. 2 and 15, became available at about the same time.

In addition to the improved percentage depth dose with higher-energy beams, a skin-sparing effect was gained, because the high-energy beams deposit the maximum dose at some depth under the skin surface. This skin-sparing effect allowed delivery of high doses even to deep-seated tumors without causing significant skin erythema. Another advantage of the high-energy beams was the more forward direction of radiation scattering and the sharper edges (penumbra) of the radiation beam. As physical improvements to the beam were made, along with advances in the design and versatility of treatment machines, and as simulators became available, the doors on a new era in radiation therapy were opened.

Instruments capable of mapping the isodose distribution in phantoms were developed. A better understanding of the need to concentrate the radiation dose in the tumor while minimizing the dose to the adjacent normal tissues followed. The need for wedges to produce the desired dose distribution was recognized, and a renewed interest in tissue compensators emerged. Treatment-planning computers began to appear on the horizon, and the developments that followed have been overwhelming in terms of treatment techniques and equipment.

During this era, radium continued to be the primary source for temporary intracavitary and interstitial therapy. Radon, encapsulated in gold seeds, was used for permanent interstitial implants. Radon seeds were primarily inserted during surgery in deep-seated pelvic or abdominal tumors, where subsequent removal of the radioactivity was impractical. Gynecologic intracavitary implants continued to be the primary use of radium.

TECHNICAL DEVELOPMENTS: 1960–PRESENT

Modern developments in electronics and computers have led to an unbelievable bonanza of equipment to diagnose and treat patients with cancer, visualize the relationship of the tumor to normal organs, align and position the patient, and measure and calculate dose.

Significant improvements have been made in the design and versatility of treatment machines, simulators, treatment-planning computers, and instruments to measure and map dose. The development and use of computed tomography (CT) and magnetic resonance imaging (MRI) to define the target volume and map the patient's external contour—as well as internal organs and target volumes—have had an unprecedented impact on radiation therapy. The use of CT images as an aid in calculating the effect of tissue inhomogeneities has improved the accuracy with which the dose can be calculated. The precision with which radiation therapy can be delivered has been greatly improved and may have an impact on cancer cure rates. As a result of the ability to better localize and treat the target and thus reduce the radiation dose to adjacent normal tissue, the need for improved positioning and immobilization techniques became evident.

The collimators of radiation therapy machines have traditionally been built to produce only square or rectangular field shapes; other field shapes have had to be formed by the tedious and not very precise addition of lead blocks placed on a tray in the path of the beam. Through the development of customized shielding blocks, the reproducibility of the treatment field and the sparing of adjacent normal tissue have been greatly improved.

Some modern treatment machines are equipped with multileaf collimators. These multileaf collimators, described in Chap. 2, consist of a large number of individually controlled leaves that can be moved into the beam to the desired extent, thus forming the needed field shape.

In the treatment of cylinder-shaped targets, a rotation or arc technique is well suited. However, in the treatment of irregularly shaped targets, where the shape of the target in the "beam's eye view" constantly changes as the machine moves around the patient, the need for "conformal" therapy was recognized. The development of the multileaf collimator, where the shape of the field can be changed to

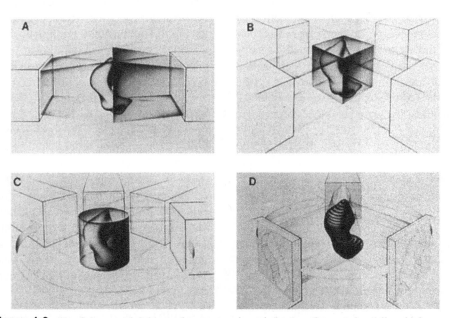

Figure 1.3 Parallel opposed fields used to treat an irregularly shaped target also deliver high doses to a large volume of normal tissue *(A)*. The volume of normal tissue within the high-dose area can be reduced by the use of a four-field technique. *(B)*. A rotational technique will further decrease the volume of normal tissue within the high-dose area *(C)*. By using a conformal therapy technique, the high-dose area can be confined almost exclusively to the target *(D)*. (Courtesy Dr. Alan Lichter, University of Michigan.)

match the shape of the target, has led to very elaborate treatment techniques. Computers can be programmed to drive the leaves of the collimator so that the radiation field always matches the shape of the target as the gantry moves around the patient (Fig. 1.3). This type of conformal therapy, where the field shape and the beam angle change simultaneously, requires very powerful computer systems.

Another, less frequently used treatment technique was developed in the early 1960s and consisted of gravity-oriented shielding blocks (described in Chap. 8). The gravity-oriented shield hangs from the collimator within the beam, so that it always shadows the desired organ (spinal cord, eye, and so on). The shield is formed to the shape of the organ to be shadowed. As the gantry moves, the gravity-oriented shield will always retain the same position and shape with respect to the organ it is shadowing; thus, the organ is shielded regardless of beam direction.

Powerful treatment-planning computers, capable of three-dimensional dose calculations, represent a major contribution to radiation therapy. Traditionally, isodose lines were represented by solid lines indicating a particular dose level. In the modern graphic representation, each isodose level is represented by a color for easier visualization. Internal organs can also be color-coded for easier recognition when viewed in different planes.

Three-dimensional renditions of CT or MRI images give an improved appreciation of the region at hand. Outlining normal organs and the tumor volume permit a beam's eye view of the intended fields with respect to the tumor and the normal anatomy (Fig. 1.4). Field size and beam angle can be changed in real time until the desired placement is obtained.

Along with the improved techniques by which radiation therapy could be delivered came the need for radiographic imaging of treatment fields. Comparison of radiographs taken on the simulation unit and with the treatment beam to verify reproducibility before and at intervals during the course of treatment is common practice. Systems are currently being used by which the treatment field can be viewed in real time on a video monitor at the treatment console. Misalignments can be discovered and corrected when only a fraction of a particular treatment has been delivered.

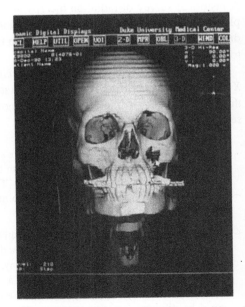
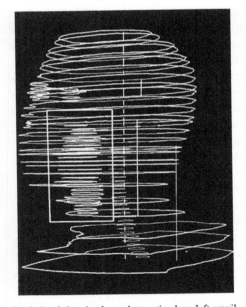

Figure 1.4   *Left:* Three-dimensional rendition of a patient's head showing bone destruction by a left maxillary sinus tumor. *Right:* External contours, spinal cord, eyes, and a tumor outlined on several CT images of another patient; a rectangular field, angled to include the tumor without including the spinal cord, is shown.

Fast neutrons, pi mesons, and heavy ions are also used in radiation therapy. Machines required to generate these particles are very complex and expensive. Their use is therefore limited to only a few institutions around the world.

Along with the tremendous popularity of using artificially developed isotopes came the development of afterloading techniques in brachytherapy. Radium fell out of favor and was largely replaced when other, less hazardous radioactive materials became available. Cobalt 60 and cesium 137 replaced radium in intracavitary gynecologic applications because they have characteristics somewhat similar to radium, and ribbons carrying radioactive seeds replaced radium needles. The most popular isotope for this use is iridium 192. These ribbons, in addition to being safer than radium, also have the advantage that they can be afterloaded through plastic tubes inserted interstitially.

The development of afterloading techniques was a major step in reducing the exposure to a large number of staff. The benefit of inserting empty intracavitary and interstitial source carriers in the operating room was not limited to the reduced exposure of staff; by freeing staff from the pressure of working quickly in order to reduce exposure, it also led to better placement. Radiographic verification of the placement—and often of the dose calculation prior to inserting the radioactive sources—yielded better dose distributions.

More recently, *remote* afterloading equipment for brachytherapy has been developed (Chap. 16). These devices allow afterloading and removal of radioactive sources from the patient via remote control; thus, the exposure to staff is practically eliminated. The sources are removed and deposited in a shielded safe while, for example, nursing care is provided to the patient. After the staff leaves the room, the sources are again loaded into the patient via a pneumatic tube, and treatment is resumed.

Prior to the introduction of treatment-planning computers in radiation therapy, dose calculations were very tedious and time-consuming. Generally, the dose was calculated only at certain points in the vicinity of the implant, using standard dose tables developed by early investigators, most notably Pa-terson and Parker during the 1930s and Quimby during the 1940s. With the use of computers, isodose distributions can quickly be calculated and evaluated, often prior to the insertion of the radioactive sources. Source strengths can thus be selected to yield an acceptable dose distribution.

The diminished use of radium created a need for safe disposal of these highly radioactive sources with a half-life of about 1600 years. Sources that were bought at great expense may years ago are now without value and, because they are still extremely hazardous, can only be disposed of at very high cost if at all.

The benefits of combining external beam treatment with brachytherapy have been known for many years; however, research is still being conducted to improve dose-delivery sequencing. Hyperthermia is a promising new modality, which has been added to both external beam and brachytherapy treatments. Quite promising results have been obtained, and research over the next several years is likely to lead to a better understanding of this treatment modality.

RADIOBIOLOGY

A historical survey of radiation therapy is not complete without some mention of the evolution of radiobiology, although no attempt is made in this text to present a complete history.

The following paragraphs from *Principles of X-ray and Radium Dosage*[2] serve as an example of the understanding of radiobiology held more than seventy years ago:

> "Since tissue congested with blood is more sensitive to radiation, the suggestion has been made to treat the region to be rayed beforehand by diathermy. The congestion produced in this way is supposed to make the tissues more sensitive."

> "The cells of the body are most radio-sensitive at the instant of their division. Hence one method which promises to be successful is to distribute the raying over such a period that all the cells go through a division during this time. Of course, the correct exposure time would be different for various tumors depending on their rapidity of growth."

". . . Roentgen sickness may be due to three causes: 1) poisonous gases in the treatment room, 2) electrostatic charges influencing the cells of the body, and 3) direct poisoning of some organ due to excessive dosage, particularly in the treatment of the stomach, liver, pancreas and suprarenals."

"To avoid roentgen sickness the following must be observed: 1) the production of ozone must be reduced to a minimum; this is best accomplished by installing the rectifier, the spark gap, and the tube in a separate room (couch, cylinder). The treatment room must be well ventilated. A large lead covered tube box with a blower to draw off the air is ideal. 2) Holfelder advises grounding of the patient. If precautions are taken to avoid accidental electric shock, the grounding of the patient is not dangerous and may be beneficial. In the case of the couch, the window and the tube box methods of treatment, it is not necessary. 3) The region rayed should not be too large; a well planned treatment avoids unnecessary exposure. The symptoms may also be mitigated by administering calcium chloride or by injecting it into the veins previous to the treatment. Voltz found a decrease in the chloride contents of the blood after intensive radiation. Pape accordingly increased the chlorine content of the blood by means of 200 cc of physiological NaCl (sodium chloride) and CaCl$_2$ (calcium chloride) solution and avoided roentgen sickness in many cases."

During the first three decades of this century, radiobiologists and radiotherapists worked closely together in an effort to understand the intricate phenomena of the biological effects caused by ionizing radiation.

During the 1920s and 1930s, protracted fractionation methods were formulated and the relative radiosensitivity of different tissues was studied primarily by Claude Regaud and Henri Coutard in France. With the beginning of fractionated radiation therapy, many new biological questions were raised and as improved cancer cure rates were experienced; radiobiologists explored the significance of repair, recovery, reoxygenation, redistribution, and repopulation.[6]

Adverse effects on normal tissue and radiation sickness necessitated fractionation of the dose, and it was found that higher doses could then be delivered.

Careful evaluation of the results of such treatment, along with better understanding of the characteristics of the rays, led to the development of different time-dose fractionation schemes. Much of the current clinical application of radiation therapy has evolved from similar experiments, and further refinements in fractionation schedules continue today.

Recognition of the typical patterns of spread of malignancies occurring in various types of tissues and in various sites and the adaptation of treatment strategies for each disease have required many years of dedicated work by many radiation therapists. Collecting data and sharing it with colleagues has led to the development of the foundations of modern clinical radiation oncology. Similarly, careful recording and evaluation of complications and results have yielded a large base on which radiation tolerance and dose requirements for tumor eradication are built.

RADIATION PROTECTION

As early as March 1896, Thomas Edison, an x-ray pioneer, reported eye irritation and cautioned against the use of x-rays. Clarence M. Dally, his laboratory assistant, developed acute x-ray dermatitis and died later as a result of overexposure. Henri Becquerel and Pierre Curie sustained acute dermatitis on the skin of the chest after carrying small amounts of radium in their vest pockets. The small grains of radium looked totally harmless, and it was only through these events that the injurious effects were first observed. The invisible x-rays were also thought of as being harmless (it was the practice, during the early days, to test the "hardness," or penetrating power, of the rays by placing the hand of the operator between the tube and the fluorescent screen) until the injuries began to appear.

Protracted exposure to x-rays was found to cause pain, swelling, redness, and often also blistering. By the end of 1896, numerous reports had been published about x-ray dermatitis and burns. The delayed effect of x-rays caused much of the injury to occur before the dangers were evident; thus, many of the pioneers sustained radiation injuries. Several cases of radiation-induced cancer were reported during the first 10 years following the discovery of x-rays and radioactivity. There is strong evidence that Madame Curie's long exposure to radium contributed to her illness and death. The early investigators often handled radium directly with their hands; as a result, many of these workers experienced damage to their fingers, including degeneration in some cases.

The need for protective measures was eventually acknowledged, and the use of x-rays was thereafter limited to physicians' offices. During the ensuing years, much effort was put into improving the equipment and techniques to reduce the radiation exposure.

The recognition, as early as 1900, of increased distance, short exposure time, and the use of shielding as measures to help reduce the incidence of radiation injuries led to the development of shielded storage safes and long-handled tools for handling radium. It is interesting to note that the initial development of radiation protection was aimed at protecting the radium itself, a valuable and expensive commodity, rather than protecting human beings from the radium.

Early on, the practice of what was later to be known as radiology was carried out by electricians and photographers as well as by physicians. In 1899, a newspaper reporter recommended state licensing for radiographers, following a lawsuit in which the courts awarded a $10,000 damage judgment on behalf of a plaintiff who allegedly suffered an injury from improper application of diagnostic x-rays.

During the 1920s, methods of measuring dose were developed and quantitative measurements of radiation exposure were introduced. The use of film badges was recommended during the 1920s; during the 1930s, portable survey meters and ionization chambers became standard equipment in most hospitals.

The difference in biological effectiveness of different radiations was recognized and stated in tolerance doses. Tolerance doses gave way to the concept of maximum permissible dose. The whole body maximum permissible exposure, which was set at 30 roentgen (R) per year in 1936, has been reduced a number of times since then and is now 5 rem per year (the unit *rem* is the sum of the products of the ab-

sorbed dose in rad and the quality factor for each radiation producing the exposure). The quality factor was introduced because the biological effectiveness of one radiation may be different from that of another. The rem is the quantity of any radiation that will produce the same biological effect as 1 cGy of cobalt-60 gamma rays, for which the quality factor is 1.0. The change in units to include the quality factor was made necessary by the more complex radiologic environment that came into being after the development of nuclear weapons in the 1940s.

The radiation protection practiced prior to World War II was aimed at protecting the operator of the radiation-producing equipment, while following the war, radiation protection measures also considered the patient. The importance of radiation protection was generally not recognized until the early 1950s, when the long-term biological effects of exposure to small, fractionated doses of radiation over long periods was appreciated. A large proportion of the world's population was exposed to low levels of radiation when the testing of nuclear weapons began; thus, the biological damage became a matter of concern.

With the use of sophisticated diagnostic and therapeutic equipment, medical radiation protection has become very complex, but the basic principles understood at an early stage still apply. The modern era has also brought further increases in regulatory control, such as mandatory licensing of radionuclides and radiation sources, educational requirements for the operators of radiation machines, and the institution of radiation protection programs based on ALARA (*As Low As Reasonably Achievable*). The concept of ALARA is based on the idea that the radiation exposure should *always* be minimal and all reasonable precautions should be exercised even when the exposure is well below the permissible levels.

THE LIFE OF OUR PIONEERS

Following below are short descriptions of some of the pioneers in radiation therapy extracted from a series of articles entitled *Our History and*

Heritage,[7-9] written by Dr. Juan A. del Regato, a pioneer of radiation therapy in the United States.

WILHELM CONRAD RÖNTGEN

Wilhelm Conrad Röntgen was born on March 27, 1845, in Lennep, Germany. His family later moved to Holland, and Röntgen attended primary school there. At age 17, he registered at a private technical school in Utrecht, from which he eventually was expelled because he refused to reveal the name of the artist who drew a disrespectful caricature of one of the teachers on the blackboard; Röntgen was therefore considered to be an accomplice.[7]

Röntgen learned that the Zürich Polytechnikum accepted students without the traditional credentials. He was admitted and eventually received a Ph.D. from the University of Würzburg, where he discovered the invisible rays 25 years later. He left the University of Würzburg in 1872, but he returned in 1888 as chairman of the department of physics and as director of the Physikalische Institut.

Röntgen was very interested in experimental research and, because of his increased academic responsibilities, worked at night in his laboratory. He focused his attention on cathode rays, which had been shown to produce fluorescence, and this led him to discover x-rays.

Many honors were bestowed upon Röntgen during the ensuing years, the highest being the first Nobel Prize for Physics. He refused all suggestions that he profit by his discovery. For example, he turned over the Nobel cash prize to the University of Würzburg. Röntgen died on February 10, 1923, of cancer. His ashes are buried in the Alte Friedhof in Giessen, Germany.

MARIE SKLODOWSKA CURIE

Marie Sklodowska was born on November 7, 1867, in Warsaw. At age 16 she won a gold medal on completion of her secondary education.[8] Marie had to take work as a teacher and at the same time took part clandestinely in the nationalist "free university," reading in Polish to women workers. In 1885, one of her sisters decided to study medicine in Paris. Marie took various jobs to help and support her sister,

thinking that later on she herself would need her help. After a couple of disappointing jobs, she decided to move to Paris.[9]

After 2 years of hard work, Marie finished first in her class at the Sorbonne and then went back to Poland to visit her father. When she returned to Paris, she began to study the magnetic properties of various minerals. During this time, she met Professor Pierre Curie, the chief of laboratories at the Industrial School of Physics and Chemistry. She obtained a master's degree in mathematical sciences and returned to Poland again to visit her father. She returned to Paris and married Pierre in 1895. In December 1898 they discovered radium.

In 1903, Madame Curie presented her thesis at the Sorbonne and obtained her doctorate. Later in the same year, the Swedish Academy of Science announced that the Nobel Prize for Physics had been awarded to Henri Becquerel and Marie and Pierre Curie. Marie was later (1911) to receive the Nobel Prize in Chemistry also. Twenty-four years later, the Curies' daughter Irène and her husband, Frederic Joliot, received the Nobel Prize in Chemistry for the discovery of artificial radioactivity, an unparalleled accomplishment by this scientific family.

Pierre Curie died on April 19, 1906, when he was run over by a horse-drawn wagon as he tried to cross a street in Paris. Marie was promoted to the chair left vacant by her husband. She had dreamed of a special research institution devoted to the study of radioactivity and its medical applications. In 1911, her dream became a reality with the establishment of the Institut de Radium under the auspices of the Pasteur Institute and the University of Paris. It was at the Radium Institute that such pioneers of radiobiology as Henri Coutard, Antoine Lacassagne, Octave Monod, and others, through years of dedicated work, established the foundations of modern clinical radiotherapy.

Marie Curie died in Paris on July 6, 1934, of complications resulting from long exposure to radiation.

ANTOINE BÉCLÈRE

Antoine Béclère was born on March 17, 1856, in Paris. A physician with a keen interest in experimental medicine, he became intrigued with Röntgen's discovery and eventually became one of the world's leading personalities in the unfolding of the medical applications of radium.[10]

His first experiments were in the use of roentgen rays for diagnostic purposes, but he soon became interested in the therapeutic potential of these invisible rays as well. He obtained the necessary equipment for his office and began the practice of ''radiology,'' a word which he coined. His first roentgen tube relied on a hand-cranked electrical generator, but he later used a battery-operated tube.

As was the custom then, the radiologists would check the performance of the roentgen-ray tube by testing their ability to see the bones of their own hands.[10] Béclère soon recognized the adverse effects on the skin of his own hands, and many of his colleagues suffered similar injuries. He therefore advocated measures to protect physicians and patients. He also insisted that the roentgen rays be kept under the control of physicians and not be entrusted to photographers and other laymen.

Béclère developed an increasing interest in radiation therapy and obtained some radium soon after its discovery. He treated some patients using radium and though the radiations had somewhat different depth doses, etc., he observed effects similar to those of roentgen rays.

During the 1920s, Béclère became interested in using roentgen rays in the treatment of deep-seated tumors. For this, he insisted on careful dosimetry and urged the appointment of a commission on measurements and units to establish a common dose unit in radiation therapy to be adopted around the world.

Béclère also foresaw the need for dose fractionation and the necessity of combining external roentgen therapy and intracavitary ''Curie therapy'' in the treatment of gynecologic malignancies.

Having laid much of the groundwork in radiology, Antoine Béclère died unexpectedly of a heart attack on February 24, 1939.

SOME IMPORTANT MILESTONES IN THE HISTORY OF RADIATION THERAPY

What follows below is extracted from *Physical Foundations of Radiology*[11] and represents an abbre-

viated list of achievements by many scientists who have laid the basis of radiation therapy.

1895   November 8: Wilhelm Conrad Röntgen discovered the invisible rays, which he subsequently called x-rays.

1896   January: The first x-ray treatment of a cancer patient was delivered.

Antoine Henri Becquerel discovered radioactivity.

1897   Joseph John Thomson announced the finding of negatively charged particles, which he called electrons.

Ernest Rutherford found two types of radiation from uranium, which he called alpha and beta rays.

1898   December: Marie and Pierre Curie discovered radium.

P. von Villard discovered gamma rays and found them to be similar to x-rays.

1901   Wilhelm Conrad Röntgen was awarded the first Nobel Prize in Physics for his discovery of x-rays.

1902   Guido Holzknecht presented his chromoradiometer, a device built to measure the quantity of radiation administered.

1903   Antoine Henri Becquerel was awarded a Nobel Prize in Physics for the discovery of radioactivity.

Marie and Pierre Curie were awarded a Nobel Prize in Physics for their work on radioactivity.

1906   H. Geiger and Ernest Rutherford developed an instrument to count alpha particles. With the assistance of W. Mueller, this device was later improved to detect and count other types of radiation.

1908   P. von Villard proposed a unit of dose based on ionization of air by x-rays.

1913   The half-value layer was suggested as a term for the expression of the quality of roentgen rays.

1922   Arthur Holly Compton discovered the change in wavelength of scattered x-rays, the ''Compton effect.''

1925   H. Fricke and Otto Glasser developed the thimble ionization chamber.

1928   The Commission on Measures and Units proposed the roentgen as an international unit of dose.

Geiger and Mueller developed an improved Geiger-counter tube on the basis of the Geiger-Rutherford point counter built in 1906.

Glasser, Portmann, and Seitz built the condenser dosimeter for the measurement of x-rays and radiation from radioactive substances. This type of dosimeter has subsequently become known as the Victoreen condenser R-meter.

1932 E. O. Lawrence invented the cyclotron.

Lauriston S. Taylor developed a standard air-ionization chamber to determine the value of the roentgen.

1933 R. J. van de Graaff built electrostatic generators capable of producing up to 12 million volts.

1934 Frederic Joliot and his wife, Irene Joliot-Curie (Marie and Pierre Curie's daughter), produced artificial radioactivity by bombarding aluminum with alpha particles.

1937 The Fifth International Congress of Radiology (Chicago) accepted the roentgen as an international dosage unit for x-rays and gamma radiation.

1939 The treatment of cancer patients with a neutron beam from a cyclotron was begun.

1940 Kerst constructed the betatron, with which electrons were accelerated to energies of 20 million electron volts (MeV) and later to 300 MeV.

1951 The first teletherapy units employing cobalt-60 were used in radiation therapy (Saskatoon, Saskatchewan, and London, Ontario, Canada).

1952 The first electron linear accelerator designed for radiotherapy was installed (Hammersmith Hospital, London, England).

1953 The Seventh International Congress of Radiology (Copenhagen, Denmark) adopted the rad as the unit of absorbed dose of any ionizing radiation.

1960s Treatment-planning computers were developed.

1971 Geoffrey N. Hounsfield invented computed tomography.

PROBLEMS

1.1 X-rays were discovered by
   (a) Henri Coutard
   (b) Wilhelm Conrad Röntgen
   (c) Henri Becquerel
   (d) Marie Curie

1.2 Radioactivity was discovered by
   (a) Wilhem Conrad Röntgen
   (b) Henri Coutard
   (c) Pierre Curie
   (d) Henri Becquerel

1.3 Radium was discovered by
   (a) Wilhelm Conrad Röntgen and Henri Becquerel
   (b) Marie and Pierre Curie
   (c) Henri Coutard and Claude Regaud

1.4 The erythema dose
   (a) Was the dose that was found to cure all cancer
   (b) Was the only measure of dose by which the early pioneer could estimate the necessary length of the treatments
   (c) Was the highest dose that could be given without causing complications

1.5   That one could achieve the same tumor response with less injury to normal tissue by fractionating the dose was discovered by
  (a) Henri Coutard and Claude Regaud
  (b) Marie and Pierre Curie
  (c) Wilhelm Conrad Röntgen and Henri Becquerel

1.6   The Manchester system of radium distribution was developed by
  (a) Edith Quimby
  (b) Wilhelm Conrad Röntgen and Henri Becquerel
  (c) Ralston Paterson and Herbert Parker

1.7   The penetrometer to measure quality of x-rays was introduced by
  (a) Benoist
  (b) Holzknecht
  (c) J. J. Thomson

1.8   The roentgen was internationally accepted as a unit of measurement for x-rays and gamma rays in
  (a) 1953
  (b) 1936
  (c) 1928

1.9   The rad as a unit of absorbed dose was recommended by the ICRU in
  (a) 1936
  (b) 1953
  (c) 1928

1.10   Artificial radioactivity was discovered in
  (a) 1936
  (b) 1953
  (c) 1934
  (d) 1928

1.11   Artificial radioactivity was discovered by
  (a) Irène Curie and Frederic Joliot
  (b) Marie and Pierre Curie
  (c) Ralston Paterson and Herbert Parker

1.12   Which of the following statements is *not* true:
  (a) Becquerel was awarded a Nobel Prize in Physics for the discovery of radioactivity.
  (b) Röntgen was awarded the first Nobel Prize in Physics.
  (c) Marie and Pierre Curie were awarded a Nobel Prize in Physics for their work on radioactivity.
  (d) Holzknecht was awarded the Nobel Prize for his work on his chromoradiometer.

REFERENCES

1. Glasser O: Technical development of radiology. *Am J Roentgenol Radium Ther Nucl Med* 75:7, 1956.
2. Bachem A: *Principles of X-ray and Radium Dosage.* Chicago: Albert Bachem, 1923.
3. Ising G: Principle of method for production of canal rays at high voltages. *Arch Matem Astron Fys* 18:1, 1924.
4. Wideröe R: Über ein neus Prinzip zur Herstellung hoher Spannungen. *Arch Elektrotech* 21:387, 1928.
5. Van de Graaff RJ, Compton KT, Van Atta CL: Electro-

static production of high voltages for nuclear investigators. *Phys Rev* 43:149, 1933.

6. Hall EJ: *Radiobiology for the Radiologist*, 3d ed. Philadelphia: Lippincott, 1988.

7. Del Regato JA: Our history and heritage: Wilhelm Conrad Röntgen. *Int J Radiat Oncol Biol Phys* 1:133, 1975.

8. *Encyclopedia Britannica*, 14th ed, vol 6, p 903.

9. Del Regato JA: Our history and heritage: Marie Sklodowska Curie. *Int J Radiat Oncol Biol Phys* 1:345, 1976.

10. Del Regato JA: Our history and heritage: Antoine Béclère. *Int J Radiat Oncol Biol Phys* 4:1069, 1978.

11. Goodwin PN, Quimby EH, Morgan RH: *Physical Foundations of Radiology*, 4th ed. New York: Harper & Row, 1970.

External Beam Radiation Therapy Equipment

SUPERFICIAL MACHINES

ORTHOVOLTAGE MACHINES

BETATRONS

LINEAR ACCELERATORS

MACHINES USING ISOTOPES
Cobalt-60 Machines
Cesium-137 Machines

MACHINE CONSTRUCTION

SIMULATORS

Prior to 1950, nearly all external beam radiation therapy was carried out using x-rays generated at voltages up to approximately 300 kVp. Following the development of cobalt-60 (^{60}Co) machines in the early 1950s, this type of treatment machine remained the most popular source of radiation for radiotherapy for many years. High-energy betatrons were introduced at approximately the same time as cobalt-60 machines, but their popularity has diminished in recent years and both are now largely replaced by high-energy linear accelerators. Other machines, which are impractical and economically not feasible for installation in the average radiation therapy department, are cyclotrons and gigantic linear accelerators that produce intense beams of neutrons, protons, mesons, and other particles useful in the treatment of malignant tumors.[1-5] This text is intended as a brief overview of the most commonly used equipment only.

SUPERFICIAL MACHINES

Radiation therapy units operating in the approximate range of 50 to 120 kVp are referred to as *superficial machines*. The penetrating ability of x-rays produced at this low voltage is very poor. Addition of filters, typically aluminum (Al), of variable thickness removes the very soft nonpenetrating x-rays and thus hardens the beam. The degree of hardening, or beam quality, depends on the energy at which the beam is generated as well as on the filter thickness and is expressed as the half-value thickness (HVT). The HVT, which is also discussed in Chap. 3, is defined as the thickness of a specified material which, when introduced into the path of the beam, reduces its intensity to half of its original value. Typical HVTs in the superficial range are 1.0 to 8.0 mmAl.

The custom of expressing the *quality* of a beam in terms of HVT of tin (Sn), copper (Cu), and aluminum (Al) is not to be confused with the filters just described, which consist of the same materials.

Superficial beams, as may be deduced from the name, are used in the treatment of superficial lesions. Treatment fields are often defined by a cone attached to the head of the machine near the focal point, with the distal end placed directly on the skin surface. Alternatively, lead shielding can be placed directly on the patient's skin to shield areas surrounding the lesion. Treatment distances are usually in the range of 15 to 20 cm to decrease depth dose. The dose rate is fairly high in superficial treatments due to the short treatment distance. The backscatter (Chap. 3) is relatively high at these low energies and increases rapidly with increased field size. The maximum dose is on the surface and falls off very rapidly with depth, due to the low energy and short source-surface distance (SSD).

ORTHOVOLTAGE MACHINES

X-ray machines operating in the range of 150 to 500 kVp are referred to as *orthovoltage units*. Filters used to harden the beam in these units consist of copper and sometimes tin in addition to aluminum. The aluminum is placed distal to the copper in the path of the beam to remove soft secondary radiation produced when the beam strikes the copper. Copper, on the other hand, is added distal to the tin filter in the path of the beam to remove soft secondary radiation produced when the beam interacts with the tin filter. Various combinations of filters have been designed to achieve HVTs of up to 4 mmCu in the orthovoltage energy range.

Orthovoltage equipment usually operates at SSD of 50 to 70 cm and can be used with or without a cone. Movable lead shields in the head of some of these machines can be used to define the size of square and rectangular radiation fields; but, as with superficial beams, additional beam-defining lead shields can be placed directly on the patient. Quite small thicknesses of lead are needed to reduce the dose by 95 percent in this energy range; the actual thickness depends on the voltage.

The penetrating capability of orthovoltage beams is better than that of superficial beams; thus, the fall-off of dose with depth is less rapid. In a typical orthovoltage beam, the maximum dose occurs at or very close to the skin surface, falling to about 90 percent at approximately 2 cm of depth. A single field would thus not adequately treat a lesion at a greater depth without delivering a prohibitive dose to the overlying skin.

The backscatter is quite large in the orthovoltage range and, as with superficial beams, increases with increased field size. Dose rates from orthovoltage units are relatively low due to the fairly long SSD and also the heavy filtration of the beam.

BETATRONS

The betatron, developed by Kerst in 1941, is a machine in which electrons are accelerated in a circular orbit via a changing magnetic field.[6,7] The electrons can be extracted from this orbit to produce an electron beam used for radiation therapy, or they can be directed to hit a target inside the machine to produce an x-ray beam.

Betatrons were first used for radiation therapy during the 1950s, but they are now largely replaced by linear accelerators. Primarily, low dose rates and very limited field sizes have led to the decline of new betatron installations. Most betatrons are physically very large and require tremendously large treatment rooms. Due to their size, they also have very limited motions, compromising beam direction and flexibility of patient setup.

LINEAR ACCELERATORS

The first linear accelerator was developed by Wideröe in 1928 to accelerate heavy ions.[8] Electron linear accelerators were first developed during the late 1940s and early 1950s by Fry,[9,10] Ginzton,[11] and Chodorow.[12] Various types of modern linear accelerator designs are available. Linear accelerators use high-frequency electromagnetic waves to accelerate charged particles, such as electrons, to high energies through a linear tube. These electrons, as in the betatron, can be extracted from the unit and used for the treatment of shallow lesions, or they can be directed to strike a target to produce high-energy x-rays for treatment of deep-seated tumors.

Figure 2.1 shows a typical medical linear accelerator and treatment couch, and Fig. 2.2 shows a diagram of the major accelerator components. A power supply provides power to the modulator. High-voltage pulses from the modulator are delivered to the magnetron or the klystron and simultaneously to the electron gun. A wave-guide system injects pulsed microwaves from the magnetron or the klystron into the accelerator tube. At precisely the right instant, electrons produced by the electron gun are injected into the accelerator structure. The accelerator structure consists of a copper tube divided by multiple disks of varying diameter and spacing, which is

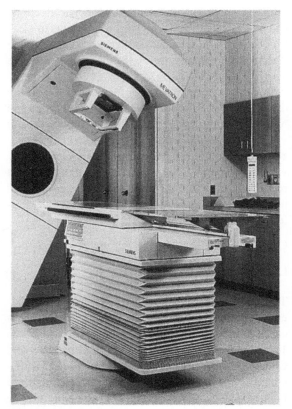

Figure 2.1   Isocentrically mounted medical linear accelerator and treatment couch. (Courtesy Siemens Medical Systems, Inc.)

evacuated to a high vacuum. The electrons, injected at an energy of about 50 keV, interact with the electromagnetic field of the microwaves and gain energy from the electrical field by an acceleration process analogous to that of a surf rider. The spacing between the disks in the wave guide is narrower near the site where the electrons are injected and gradually increases down the guide; this causes the electromagnetic radiation (and the electrons carried along by it) to speed up as it travels along the guide.

In lower-energy machines, as the high-energy electrons emerge from the accelerator structure window, they are allowed to proceed straight on and strike a target, thus producing x-rays. In higher-energy machines, where the accelerator structure is too long and therefore may have to be placed at an angle, the electrons are bent at an appropriate angle (typically 90 or 270°) before striking the target. This is accomplished via a beam transport system consisting of bending magnets, focusing coils, and other components. When the linear accelerator is in the electron mode, the target and the flattening filter are moved aside and the electrons emerge without striking either, striking instead a scattering foil. The very narrow electron beam (about 3 mm in diameter) is spread by the scattering foil, which also causes a fairly uniform electron distribution across the beam.

Since electrons scatter readily in air, the beam collimation must extend as close as possible to the skin surface of the patient. Electron cones of variable sizes attached to the collimator and extending to the patient's skin surface are therefore used to collimate electron beams (Fig. 2.3). Secondary beam shaping can be accomplished by adding lead cutouts at the end of a cone. Due to electron scattering, the dose distribution in electron fields depends strongly on the collimation system and must be determined for each individual setup. The x-ray beam, in both high- and low-energy machines, is defined by a primary collimating system and is intercepted by a flattening filter and multiple ion chambers before exiting the head of the machine through a secondary collimator consisting of movable leaves (Fig. 2.4A).

The flattening filter is placed in the x-ray beam to reduce the intensity of the forward peaked dose in the center of the field. Flattening filters, usually

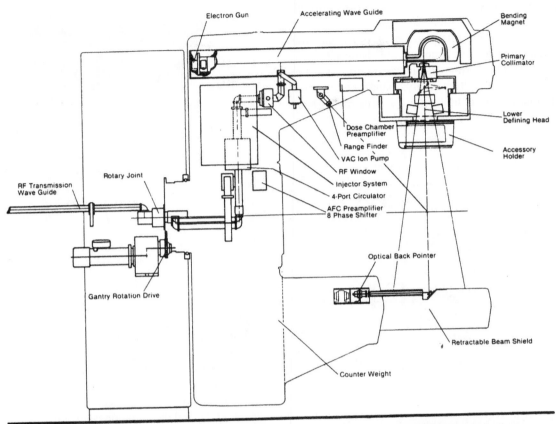

Figure 2.2   Cutaway view of a medical linear accelerator. (Courtesy Siemens Medical Systems, Inc.)

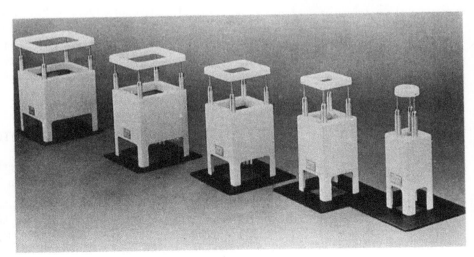

Figure 2.3 Typical electron cones. (Courtesy Siemens Medical Systems, Inc.)

made of lead, are shaped to produce dose uniformity across the radiation field at a specified depth (Fig. 2.4*B*). Flattening filters made of other materials, such as tungsten and uranium, are also used.

A dose-monitoring system, consisting of several ion chambers or, alternatively, a single chamber with multiple plates, is built into the path of the beam.

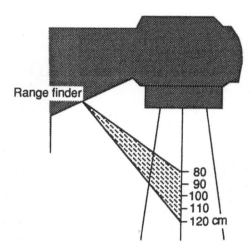

Figure 2.5 A distance scale, projected by a range finder, indicates the treatment distance at the central axis of the beam.

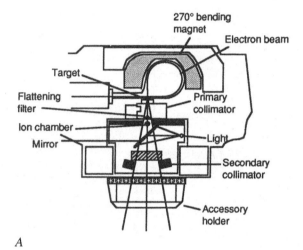

A

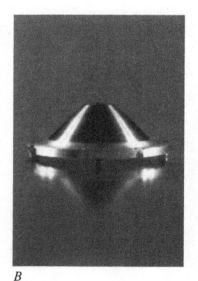

B

Figure 2.4 *A*. Cutaway view of the head of a typical medical linear accelerator. *B*. A flattening filter used in linear accelerators to produce dose uniformity across the radiation field.

This system monitors the dose rate, integrated dose, and beam symmetry.

A light, projected via mirrors in the head of the machine, is arranged to be congruent with the radiation field and is used in the alignment of the radiation beam and the treatment field marked on the patient's skin surface. Frequent checks of the congruency of the light field and the radiation beam are necessary to ensure continuous treatment field alignment.

Another light, projected from some point outside the collimator, casts a scale indicating the treatment distance. The scale is mounted so that the distance from the target is indicated when the scale intersects the central axis of the beam (Fig. 2.5).

A typical linear accelerator installation is shown in Fig. 2.6. For further details on linear accelerators, the reader is directed to a review article and a book by Karzmark[13,14] as well as to other literature.[15–17]

MACHINES USING ISOTOPES

Prior to 1951, machines for external beam irradiation (teletherapy*) employing an isotope were made for

* *Teletherapy* refers to treatments in which the source of radiation is at some distance from the patient. In brachytherapy, on the other hand, the source is very close to the treated tissue (in molds) or may even be embedded in it (interstitial).

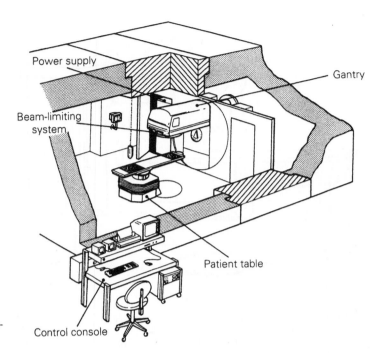

Figure 2.6 A typical linear accelerator installation. (Courtesy General Electric Company.)

use with radium. The prohibitive cost, the "self-filtration" caused by the front layer of the source filtering out radiation from the back portion of the large radium source, and the low dose rates are some of the reasons why teleradium units never gained much popularity.

The development of very strong sources of cobalt-60 in Canada in 1951 led to the introduction of cobalt-60 units for teletherapy.[18] Figure 2.7 shows a diagram of a typical cobalt-60 machine and treatment couch. The cobalt-60 source usually consists of a double-encapsulated cylinder filled with disks or pellets of the isotope (Fig. 2.8). The double steel capsule, which is sealed by welding, is necessary to prevent escape of radioactive material. The cobalt-60 source typically has the shape of a cylinder, with a diameter of from 1 to 1.5 cm. The circular end of the cylinder faces the collimator opening from which the radiation escapes when the machine is in the "on" position.

Unlike linear accelerators or other electrically operated machines, the cobalt-60 source emits radiation constantly; thus, the source must be shielded when the machine is in the "off" position to protect personnel.

Isotope machines consist of a lead-filled container in which the radioactive source is placed near the center (Fig. 2.9). An opening is provided for the radiation beam to exit when the machine is in the "on" position. Various types of mechanisms exist for bringing the source into a position opposite this opening. In one arrangement, the source is mounted on a wheel, itself a good radiation shield, which can be rotated 180° to carry the source between the "on" and "off" positions (Fig. 2.10). In another arrangement, the source is mounted in a drawer and the source slides horizontally between the "on" and "off" positions. Should the power fail while the source is in the "on" position, the source will automatically move to the "off" position via a fail-safe system.

All isotope machines must be equipped with this fail-safe mechanism because, unlike accelerators, these machines are very quiet in their operation and the operator has no audible warning that the source is in the "on" position.

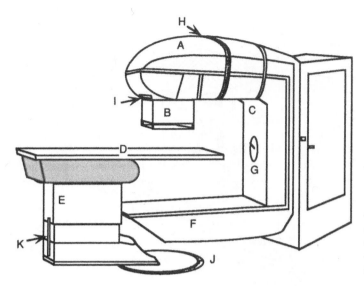

Figure 2.7 Diagram of a typical cobalt-60 machine and treatment couch. Key: A, source head; B, collimator; C, gantry; D, couch top; E, treatment couch; F, beam stopper; G, gantry scale; H, head swivel scale; I, collimator scale; J, couch rotation scale; K, ventrical couch scale.

COBALT-60 MACHINES

Cobalt 60, which is further discussed in Chap. 15, emits two photons per disintegration (1.17 and 1.33 MeV), which are useful in radiation therapy. It decays with time and has a half-life of 5.26 years. The half-life is the time required for an isotope to decay to half of its original strength (Chap. 15). The dose rate is therefore constantly decreasing and an adjustment of treatment times must be made periodically. In the case of cobalt 60, this is typically once a month.

Due to the large size of a cobalt source, the penumbra, or unsharp edge of the beam, is larger than that of the beam from a linear accelerator, which has a very small focal point. The penumbra, which is further discussed in Chap. 3, can be reduced by allowing the beam collimating tunnel to extend further along the path of the beam. This, however, reduces the clearance between the collimator and the patient —a serious disadvantage in isocentrically mounted units. Penumbra can, of course, be reduced by use of a small source; but when the source is small, the activity and hence the dose rate are reduced. Using very high specific-activity cobalt, that is, high activity per cubic centimeter, will help overcome this problem.

CESIUM-137 MACHINES

Another teletherapy isotope machine, first described in 1956, is the cesium-137 unit.[19] Very few cesium machines are still in use. The source head and the mechanism for moving the source to "on" and "off" positions are similar to those of the cobalt machine. The radiation intensity from a cesium

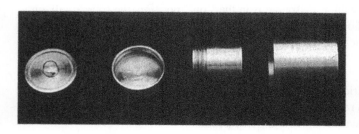

Figure 2.8 Cobalt-60 source capsule. The circular end of the double encapsulated cylinder, which faces the opening, is typically 1 to 1.5 cm in diameter.

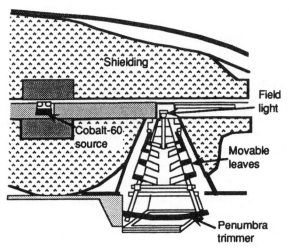

Figure 2.9 Diagram of the head of a typical cobalt-60 machine.

source compared with a cobalt source of equal physical size is relatively low, and sources of sufficient activity to produce a reasonable beam intensity at a long treatment distance are fairly large and cause

very large penumbras. This penumbra can be reduced by using a physically smaller source, but then the activity is low. Consequently, most cesium units have been used at fairly short treatment distances, typically on the order of 20 to 30 cm; this seriously reduces the percentage depth dose that would otherwise be available at the 0.662 MeV photon energy of cesium.

MACHINE CONSTRUCTION

Most modern radiation therapy machines are built to meet the needs of the continually increasing sophistication of treatment techniques in radiation therapy.

Linear accelerators and cobalt machines are compact devices compared with a betatron; they can be rotated 360° around a patient, thus allowing the beam to be directed from any angle toward the tumor site. In some treatments, delivering radiation while the machine continuously rotates around the patient may be superior to multiple stationary fields. The point around which the source of the beam rotates is referred to as the *isocenter*.

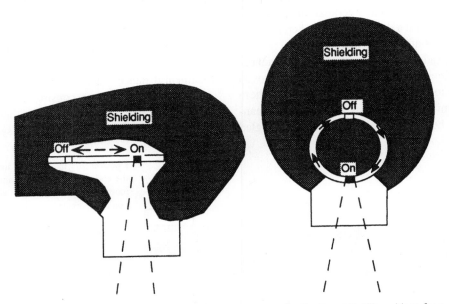

Figure 2.10 Diagram showing two typical arrangements for ''on'' and ''off'' positions for a cobalt-60 source; a sliding drawer mechanism to move the source *(left)*, and a wheel to carry the source from the shielded ''off'' position to its ''on'' position at the collimator port *(right)*.

Adequate distance must be provided between the beam-defining structures and the patient to allow a 360° rotation to take place without colliding with the patient or the treatment couch (Fig. 2.11A).[20] Provision must also be made on the couch to allow a beam of maximum area to enter the patient without interference by attenuating bars or rails on the couch. Most modern treatment couches have removable sections that are replaced by a thin Mylar sheet or tennis-racket-type insert to support the patient. The removable sections, often interchangeable across the couch top, are typically of two different designs. A removable section on each side, with a center spine providing a continuous surface, allows posterior oblique fields to be treated without interference by side rails (Fig. 2.11B). A large removable section across the width of the couch (Fig. 2.11C) allows a large posterior field to be treated. Side rails offer the link necessary to connect the two segments of the couch separated by the opening.

Figure 2.12 shows a typical modern treatment couch with a large removable section to the left and a removable section on each side of the couch to the right. The couch top can then be reversed, so that either end is in to the beam. The pedestal of the couch can be rotated around a vertical line that coincides with the central axis of the beam when the head of the machine is at the "normal" position.

Some older radiation therapy machines are not capable of rotating around the patient but can be moved up and down to adjust the treatment distance. These nonrotating units are usually swivel-mounted, meaning that the head of the machine can be angled around its own horizontal axis, with the beam sweeping across the room (Fig. 2.13).

The head of a treatment machine using isotopes consists of high-density shielding material such as lead or tungsten, inside which the source is housed. Inside the head, there is also a light localization system, a collimator through which the radiation beam exits, and—in the case of a linear accelerator—also the x-ray target, scattering foil, beam-flattening filter, and ion chambers.

The design of the collimating system varies, but basically it consists of a primary fixed collimator located immediately beyond the target in the direction of the beam and secondary movable collimators that shape the beam to square or rectangular fields. The secondary collimators are largely responsible for the sharpness of the edge of the beam and are therefore placed as far down toward the patient as can safely be done without causing secondary electron contamination of the patient's skin or colliding with the patient in the case of rotating equipment. The secondary collimators consist of two pairs of leaves that can be moved in and out from the central axis of the beam to decrease or increase the size of the radiation field. This opening can be totally closed by moving the leaves together or opened to its widest position to provide the maximum radiation field. In most linear accelerators or cobalt-60 machines, the largest field is 30 × 30 to 40 × 40 cm at standard treatment distances such as 80 or 100 cm.

Many collimators are constructed so that these leaves move only in pairs. They can therefore define only square and rectangular fields, symmetrically

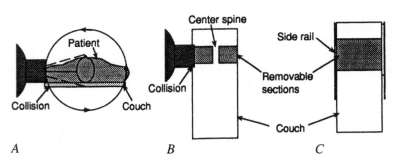

Figure 2.11   *A.* The distance between the end of the collimator and the isocenter must be sufficiently long to allow 360° rotation of the treatment unit. *B.* Some treatment couches have removable sections to facilitate clearance when the machine is rotated 360°. The removable sections must, however, be longer than the largest dimension of the collimator. *C.* A large removable section of the treatment couch, replaced by a Mylar sheet or a tennis-racket-type insert, permits treatment of a posterior field without interference by the couch. However, the side rails may interfere with posterior oblique fields.

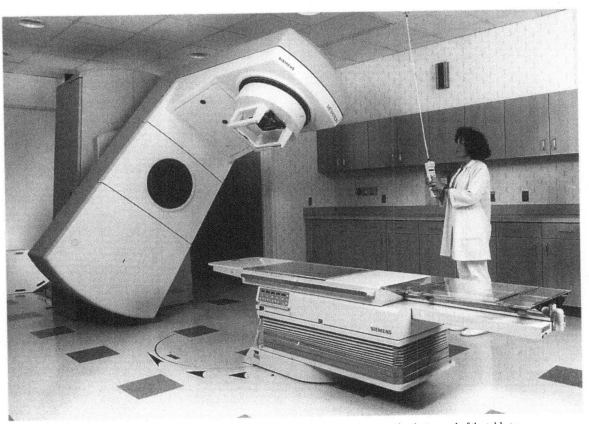

Figure 2.12   A linear accelerator and a modern treatment table. A large section in one end of the table top can be removed *(left)* and two sections, one on each side of a center spine, can be removed in the opposite end *(right)*. The table top can be reversed, allowing either end to be positioned in the beam. The pedestal of the treatment table can be rotated around the central axis of a vertical beam *(arrows)*. (Courtesy Siemens Medical Systems, Inc.)

centered about the central axis of the beam; however, secondary beam-shaping blocks can be inserted in the path of the beam to produce irregularly shaped fields. More modern treatment machines have been built in which each of the four collimator leaves moves independently. This offers the capability of using the collimator leaves to define treatment fields that are asymmetric about the central axis.

Another fairly new device for use in linear accelerators is the multileaf collimator, which is attached to the head of the machine in the path of the beam. Multileaf collimators (Fig. 2.14) consist of a large number (20 to 30) of pairs of narrow rods with motors that drive the rods in or out of the treatment

field, thus creating the desired field shape. The width of these rods varies between manufacturers, but they are usually made to cast a shadow of 0.5 to 1.0 cm at the isocenter (100 cm). The resulting treatment fields thus have jagged edges rather than the smooth, sharp edges achieved with customized beam-shaping blocks.

The capability to change the shape of the field by modifying the distance to which each rod is moved into the beam is particularly useful in moving-beam therapy. The computer-driven rods can be programmed to change the shape of the beam to match the shape of the target as the machine moves around the target, a technique referred to as *dynamic beam*

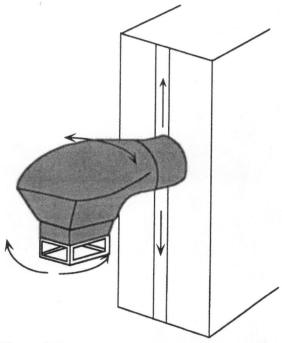

Figure 2.13 Nonrotating machines are often mounted to allow rotation of the head around its own horizontal axis, with the beam sweeping across the room.

meters of depth, thus sparing deeper, normal tissue. Thick surface lesions require treatment with a beam that produces the maximum dose on the surface and maintains a high dose within the first few centimeters and then falls off very rapidly to spare underlying normal tissue. Deep-seated lesions require treatment with a beam that has great penetrating power and provides some sparing of overlying normal tissues. From this, it is obvious that a variety of beam energies is necessary in each modern radiation therapy department.

Other considerations in the selection of equipment are related to the physical capabilities of the machine and the couch and to the dosimetry of the beam.

A. Machine considerations
1. Field size range
2. Maximum wedged field (width and length)
3. Rotational capabilities
4. Clearance of the collimator around the couch and the patient

shaping. Dynamic beam-shaping techniques are very complex but are superior to fixed-beam therapy and conventional moving-beam techniques in terms of normal tissue sparing. Figure 1.3D (Chap. 1) demonstrates the concept of dynamic beam shaping.

The maximum field size which can be treated using a multileaf collimator is usually limited by the weight of this accessory; adding it below the fixed collimator system also reduces the clearance between the head of the treatment machine and the patient, thus increasing the risk of collisions.

Selection of radiation therapy units must be made with clinical needs in mind. A wide range of beam energies is needed to adequately treat tumors at various depths without compromising normal tissue tolerance. Treatment of skin lesions requires a beam that produces the highest dose on the skin surface and then falls off very rapidly within a few milli-

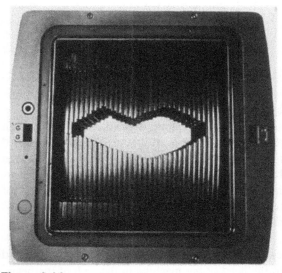

Figure 2.14 A multileaf collimator system with individually driven rods forming the radiation field. (Courtesy Scanditronix, Inc.)

5. Accessories (trays, wedges, electron cones, etc.) and the ease with which they can be inserted, weight, and so on
6. Outer dimensions of the collimator
7. Accuracy of motions (isocenter, angles, field size, distance)

B. Couch considerations
1. Maximum vertical motion
2. Maximum lateral motion
3. Couch rotation capabilities
4. Stability of the couch (no sagging or shaking)
5. Weight tolerance
6. Accuracy of motions and readout of angles

C. Dosimetric considerations
1. Dose rates
2. Depth of maximum dose
3. Energy (single- or dual-photon energy and range of electron energies)
4. Penumbra
5. Beam flatness
6. Surface dose

Other considerations are, of course, cost, reliability, service, and maintenance.

SIMULATORS

A treatment simulator is a machine that is capable of duplicating the geometry and mechanical movements of radiation therapy machines but uses a diagnostic x-ray tube. A simulator is primarily used to localize the target volume and normal tissue with respect to skin marks and to visualize the planned treatment fields with respect to tumor and normal tissue. Following confirmation of correct field location and direction, the fields are marked on the skin surface and shielding blocks are produced to optimize normal tissue sparing.

The use of simulators has improved the precision of radiation therapy because it provides a diagnostic x-ray quality radiograph of the treatment field taken with the precise geometric relationship of the treatment beam.[21]

The range of distances and field sizes of most therapy machines can be reproduced by moving the x-ray tube along an arm that is capable of 360° rotation (Fig. 2.15). The distance from the target to the

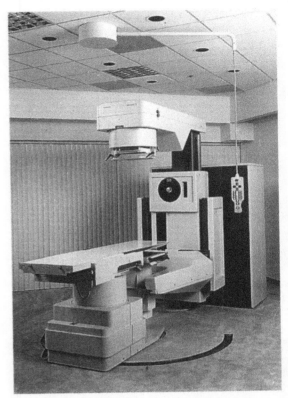

Figure 2.15 A simulator is an x-ray machine designed to simulate the geometry of therapy machines. (Courtesy Siemens Medical Systems, Inc.)

isocenter can therefore easily be changed. Many simulators have fluoroscopic capabilities, providing real-time visualization (before radiographs are taken) of internal organs, of contrast placed in body cavities, and of lead markers on the skin surface. Field-defining wires, built into the path of the beam, can be moved to simulate the planned treatment field. A small circle or a cross hair indicates the central axis of the beam. Some simulators also can provide a grid that projects a centimeter scale at the isocenter (Fig. 2.16). This facilitates easy measurements of real size on the magnified radiograph. Periodic testing of the accuracy of simulators is necessary for continued precision in radiation therapy.[22]

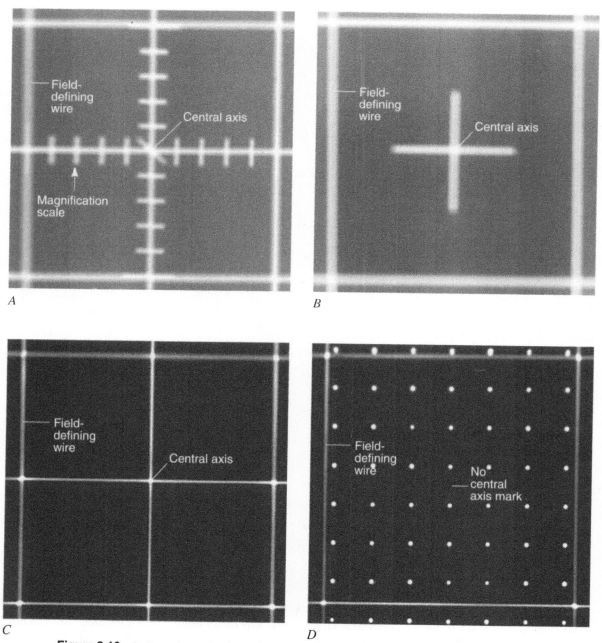

Figure 2.16   Radiographs produced from different simulator units. Radiopaque wires built into the path of the beam indicate the field size and central axis. A grid with known dimensions is useful in calculating the true dimensions of the image. The size of the field (the distance between two opposing field-defining wires) at a known distance can also be used to find the magnification factor.

PROBLEMS

2.1 The use of betatrons in radiation therapy became unpopular primarily because they
(*a*) Were difficult to get
(*b*) Were too expensive
(*c*) Were too large
(*d*) Produced low dose rates and limited field sizes

2.2 Radiation therapy units operating at approximately 50 to 120 kVp are referred to as
(*a*) Linear accelerators
(*b*) Orthovoltage units
(*c*) Superficial units
(*d*) Betatrons

2.3 The half-value thickness (HVT) is
(*a*) The thickness of a given material that causes the beam to be more penetrating
(*b*) The thickness of a given material that, when introduced into the path of the beam, reduces the intensity of the beam to one half its original value
(*c*) The thickness of a filter that hardens the beam and causes it to be reduced to half of its original value
(*d*) The thickness of a filter that determines the quantity of the beam

2.4 Insertion of aluminum, copper, and tin filters into the x-ray beam causes
(*a*) Low-energy x-rays to be absorbed
(*b*) The kVp to increase
(*c*) An unnecessary dose on the skin surface
(*d*) The dose to increase

2.5 Orthovoltage x-ray units usually operate at
(*a*) 15 to 20 cm of source-surface distance (SSD)
(*b*) 20 to 40 cm of source-surface distance (SSD)
(*c*) 50 to 70 cm of source-surface distance (SSD)
(*d*) 80 to 100 cm of source-surface distance (SSD)

2.6 Orthovoltage x-ray units usually operate in the range of
(*a*) 20 to 150 kVp
(*b*) 150 to 500 kVp
(*c*) 200 to 1200 kVp
(*d*) Any kVp below 200 kVp

2.7 Orthovoltage x-ray beams are generally
(*a*) More penetrating than those of linear accelerators
(*b*) More penetrating than superficial beams
(*c*) Equal to superficial beams in penetration

2.8 Linear accelerators were first developed
(*a*) Following World War II
(*b*) During the Depression
(*c*) Following World War I

2.9   Linear accelerators produce high-energy beams
(a) By accelerating charged particles in a linear tube
(b) By accelerating photons in a circular orbit
(c) By accelerating charged particles in a circular orbit

2.10   Because electrons scatter readily in air,
(a) They are removed before they strike the target
(b) Cones extending close to the patient's skin are used
(c) They are bent at 90 to 270° to reduce scattering

2.11   A collimator
(a) Flattens the beam at a specified depth in tissue
(b) Defines the beam
(c) Determines the dose rate

2.12   The photon beam from a linear accelerator is intercepted by
(a) A copper filter that hardens the beam
(b) Ionization chambers and a flattening filter
(c) A scattering foil and an ionization chamber

2.13   A flattening filter
(a) Removes all of the electrons from the beam
(b) Causes the dose rate to be increased
(c) Reduces the dose rate in the center of the unfiltered beam
(d) All of the above

2.14   The first cobalt-60 machine was introduced during
(a) The 1960s
(b) The 1950s
(c) World War II
(d) The 1940s

2.15   The half-life of a cobalt-60 source is
(a) 30.3 years
(b) 1600 years
(c) 5.26 years
(d) 74 days

2.16   The average energy of a cobalt-60 beam is
(a) 0.6 MeV
(b) 1.2 MeV
(c) 2.0 MeV
(d) 4.0 MeV

2.17   The penumbra of a linear accelerator beam is
(a) Smaller than that of a cobalt-60 machine
(b) Larger than that of a cobalt-60 machine
(c) The same as that of a cobalt-60 machine

2.18 The isocenter is
  (a) An imaginary point in the beam where the dose is normalized
  (b) The point on the central axis where the maximum dose occurs
  (c) The point around which the source of the beam rotates

2.19 The secondary collimator of a linear accelerator is largely responsible for
  (a) The sharpness of the beam edges
  (b) The flatness of the beam
  (c) Determining the dose rates

2.20 Simulators are primarily used to
  (a) Localize the target
  (b) Duplicate the geometry of therapy machines
  (c) Duplicate the mechanical movements of the therapy machine
  (d) All of the above

REFERENCES

1. Catterall M, Sutherland I, Bewley DK: First results of a randomized clinical trial of fast neutrons compared with x or gamma rays in treatment of advanced tumours of the head and neck: Report to the Medical Research Council. *Br Med J* 2:653, 1975.
2. Catterall M: Radiology now. Fast neutrons—Clinical requirements. *Br J Radiol* 49:203, 1976.
3. Chen GTY, Singh RP, Castro JR, et al: Treatment planning for heavy ion radiotherapy. *Int J Radiat Oncol Biol Phys* 5:1809, 1979.
4. Saunders WM, Chen GTY, Austin-Seymour M, et al: Precision high dose radiotherapy: II. Helium ion treatment of tumors adjacent to critical central nervous system structures. *Int J Radiat Oncol Biol Phys* 11:1339, 1985.
5. Von Essen CF, Blattman H, Bodendoerfer G, et al. The Piotron: II. Methods and initial results of dynamic pion therapy in phase II studies. *Int J Radiat Oncol Biol Phys* 11:217, 1985
6. Kerst DW: Acceleration of electrons by magnetic induction. *Phys Rev* 60:47, 1941.
7. Kerst DW: The betatron. *Radiology* 40:115, 1943.
8. Wideröe R: Über ein neues Prinzip zur Herstellung hoher Spannungen. *Arch Elektrotech* 21:387, 1928.
9. Fry DW, Harvie RB, Mullett LB, Walkinshaw W: Travelling wave linear accelerator for electrons, *Nature* 160:351, 1947.
10. Fry DW, Harvie RB, Mullett LB, Walkinshaw W: A travelling wave linear accelerator for 4 MeV electrons. *Nature* 162:859, 1948.

11. Ginzton EL, Hansen WW, Kennedy WR: A linear electron accelerator. *Rev Sci Instrum* 19:89, 1948.
12. Chodorow M, Ginzton EL, Hansen WW, et al: Stanford high-energy linear accelerator (Mark III). *Rev Sci Instr* 26:134, 1955.
13. Karzmark C, Pering N: Electron linear accelerators for radiation therapy: History, principles and contemporary developments. *Phys Med Biol* 18:321, 1973.
14. Karzmark CJ, Nunan CS, Tanabe E: *Medical Linear Accelerators.* New York: McGraw-Hill, 1993.
15. Johns HE, Cunningham JR: *The Physics of Radiology,* 4th ed. Springfield, IL: Charles C Thomas, 1983.
16. Khan FM: *The Physics of Radiation Therapy,* 2d ed. Baltimore: Williams & Wilkins, 1994.
17. Sable M, Gunn WG, Penning D, Gardner A: Performance of a new 4 MeV standing wave linear accelerator. *Radiology* 97:169, 1970.
18. Johns HE, Bates LM, Watson TA: 1,000 curie cobalt units for radiation therapy: I. The Saskatchewan cobalt-60 unit *Br J Radiol* 25:296, 1952.
19. Brucer M: An automatic controlled pattern cesium-13 therapy machine. *Am J Radiol* 75:49, 1956.
20. Humm JL: Collision avoidance in computer treatment planning. *Med Phys* 21:1053, 1994
21. Dritschilo A, Sherman D, Emami B, Pi effectiveness of a radiation therapy sim the determination of need. *Int J Ra* 5:243, 1979.
22. McCullough EC, Earle JD: The ing, and quality control of r tors. *Radiology* 131:221, 1

Dose Determination for External Beams

DOSE MEASUREMENTS

When a radiation beam impinges on a patient, the dose delivered to a point within the patient depends on the depth of the calculation point below the surface (depth), the penetrating power of the beam (energy), the type of tissue, that is, muscle, bone, or fat, the beam must penetrate (density), the distance from the radiation source to the skin surface (source-surface distance, or SSD), the size of the field (FS) on the skin surface, and, to some extent, the collimation. The purpose of this section is to give a very brief summary of how these variables are taken into consideration in calculating the dose within the patient.

An essential step in treatment planning is to establish measured data tables for each treatment machine that will be used. Such tables are usually prepared as a result of measurements in dummy patients (phantoms) made of tissue-equivalent material. The phantom material used is often water, which is like soft tissue as far as radiation absorption is concerned. Sheets of various tissue-equivalent plastics are also commonly employed because they are more convenient. The devices called *dosimeters,* used to measure dose distributions within such phantoms, are described briefly below.

Calculation of the dose by the methods in this text with the help of established tables is not enough to ensure that the correct dose is being delivered. First, one must be sure that the machine behavior (radiation output, beam energy, beam flatness, and so on) is the same when the patient is treated as when the data tables were prepared. The constancy of the machine must have been routinely checked; otherwise irreversible harm may be caused either by overdosing, which may lead to tissue damage, or underdosing, which can result in failure to cure, even though all the treatment-planning calculations are quite correct. Routine constancy checking is one of the main responsibilities of the radiation physicist. Second, it is advisable, where possible, to measure the dose actually delivered to the patient by means of dosimeters placed in body cavities or in catheters or needles inserted into the tissues. In this way, errors in the dose calculation itself can be corrected.

PRECISION OF DOSE CALCULATIONS

In this text, many dose calculations are carried to four significant figures; that is, they are expressed in a form such as 223.7 cGy. This may give the false impression that the dose is known with certainty to be 223.7 cGy rather than 223.6 or 223.8 cGy. Similarly, tissue-air ratios (TAR), backscatter factors (BSF), SSD, and so on are frequently given to the same apparent accuracy.

In practice, quantities used in treatment planning and dose calculation are not known to this degree of accuracy; for example, we very rarely know that the percentage depth dose (%DD) is exactly 55.43 percent rather than 55.42 or 55.44 percent. Indeed, unusually careful measurements under very favorable experimental conditions are necessary even to establish the first decimal place value as 55.4 percent. Similarly, the SSD cannot usually be measured to better than, perhaps, 1 mm.

The result of a calculation involving several such uncertainties cannot itself be as accurate as results written with several decimal places might suggest. It is convenient, with a pocket calculator, to carry a large number of decimal places in the calculations, but the treatment planner must cultivate a habit of rounding off the calculated numbers. Hard and fast rules for rounding out numbers are not available; instead, one must use judgment, which comes with experience. For example, in calculating the number of monitor units required to deliver a prescribed dose, whole numbers are given in the calculation because it is not possible to set fractions of a monitor unit on the machine.

DOSE

Before describing the devices that are used to (1) prepare the data tables, (2) check machine behavior, and (3) measure dose within the patient, it is necessary to have a clear idea of what we mean by *dose.* The dose (sometimes called the *absorbed dose*) at a point in an absorber such as tissue is the energy deposited in a small fixed weight of the material surrounding the point in question.

The unit of dose is the *gray* (Gy), which is defined so that 1 Gy equals 1 J/kg. The unit in which the dose is measured is traditionally the *rad*, which is defined as a dose or energy deposition of 100 erg*/g.

$$1 \text{ rad} = 100 \text{ erg/g}$$

One rad is therefore the same as one-hundredth (prefix *centi-*) or a gray, or 1 centigray, usually written cGy:

$$1 \text{ rad} = 1/100 \text{ Gy} = 1 \text{ cGy}$$

We use the gray or centigray as a dose u~ out this text.

Another unit — the roentgen — o~ in radiation therapy, is not emplo~ cept in connection with br~ mainly for historic reasons, ~ as a step in the calculatior~

Central

* The *erg* is a very small am~ one-millionth of a calorie.

METHODS OF DOSE DETERMINATION

The following three devices are most commonly used for dose determination in radiation therapy:

1. Ionization chambers
2. Thermoluminescent dosimeters (TLDs)
3. Photographic film

Although TLDs and photographic films are usually more convenient to use than ionization chambers, it is usually necessary to check their performance by comparing their readings with those of ionization chambers, which must be regarded as the most reliable method of determining dose.

Ionization Chambers. An ionization chamber determines the dose at a point in a rather indirect way. The chamber usually consists of a cylinder (Fig. 3.1), along the center of which runs a rod that is insulated electrically from the cylinder. The chambers used in radiation therapy are usually about as big as a thimble, but they can be made small enough to slide along a catheter or to be inserted in a body cavity. Various other sizes and shapes of ionization chambers are available—for example, a pancake-shaped chamber is often used for surface dose determination (Fig. 3.2).

No electric current will normally flow around the circuit when the terminals of a battery are connected to the outer wall and central rod of the chamber because the air that fills the chamber does not conduct. If the chamber is exposed to x-rays, the air becomes electrified through the breakup, into charged particles, of atoms that are struck by the x-ray photons. These charged particles (which are called *ions,* hence the name *ionization chamber*) drift through the chamber—that is, an electric current flows. The size

of the current, measured by means of a sensitive current-measuring device (Fig. 3.1), tells us how much ionization is produced in the air that fills the chamber. If the chamber is embedded in an absorbing material at the time it is irradiated, knowledge of the amount of ionization produced in the air, together with some other data on the absorbing properties of air and of the surrounding medium, allows us to calculate the energy that would be transferred to the medium—that is, the absorbed dose if the chamber had not been present.

To find the dose in this way from measurements in an air-filled chamber inserted in the absorber, it is first necessary to have the ionization chamber calibrated by the National Institute of Standards and Technology (NIST) or one of its accredited laboratories. Multiplication of the instrument readings with the calibration factor supplied by one of these laboratories and with certain other tabulated numbers gives the absorbed dose at the point where the chamber was placed.

There are requirements both of law and prudence regarding how often a therapeutically used ionization chamber must be calibrated. The qualifications of the expert staff, usually physicists, who make and interpret the measurements are also subject to regulation.

Thermoluminescent Dosimeters. Some crystalline materials retain and store, for very long periods, the energy they absorb when they are exposed to x-rays. The stored energy is released later as visible light; that is, the crystals *luminesce* if they are heated. Because the luminescence is brought about by thermal (heat) influence, the substances are said to be thermoluminescent. The emitted light can be

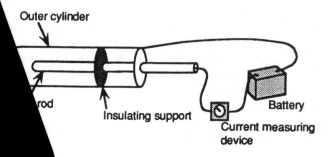

Outer cylinder

rod

Insulating support

Current measuring device

Battery

Figure 3.1 Diagram of an ionization chamber.

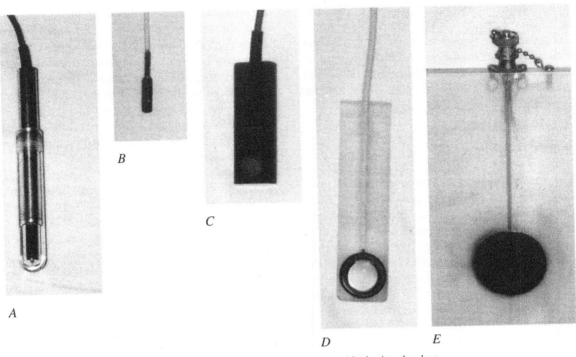

Figure 3.2 Cylindrical and pancake-shaped ionization chambers.

measured and, through previous calibration, expressed in terms of the radiation dose; a thermoluminescent material used in this way is called a *thermoluminescent dosimeter* (TLD). The most commonly used TLD materials are lithium fluoride (LiF) and calcium fluoride (CaF$_2$). Commercial TLD materials are available in many forms and sizes (rods, chips, powder, disks, and so on) that are practical for measuring dose in most clinical situations.

The response of each TLD to radiation is unique, so each one must be calibrated before it can be used for measuring unknown dose. The dose response is established by exposing a given TLD to a known dose of radiation and determining the amount of light produced on later heating. Once the light produced by the known dose of the same kind of radiation has been found, it is a simple matter to measure an unknown dose by measuring the amount of light that the unknown dose produces.

Photographic Film. Radiographic film consists of a transparent base coated with an emulsion containing silver bromide crystals. When the film is exposed to light or radiation, the exposed crystals form an image. When the film is developed, the unaffected granules are removed, leaving only the clear base, while the affected crystals are reduced to silver, which darkens the film. The darkening of the film is directly related to the absorbed radiation.

The variations in darkness of the film can be measured using a densitometer. A densitometer consists of a light source and a light detector that measures the light transmitted through the film. The relative quantity of dose is obtained by subtracting the reading for a sample that is unexposed but developed under the same circumstances as the film used for dosimetry; the net density (difference between the exposed and unexposed) is a measure of the

Film dosimetry is not practical for dose determination because of its sensitivity developing conditions, artifacts on the film, and differences in the emulsion on the film. Dose response of film is very energy-dependent and is therefore not useful in dose determination of orthovoltage radiation. However, it is useful for deducing relative dose distribution, beam-light coincidence, beam flatness, beam symmetry, and so forth.

DEFINITIONS

The process of determining radiation dose is quite complex, and many of the terms used can be difficult to understand. The dose delivery involves two major parts. The first is to determine the output of a machine—that is, the dose delivered at a specified point in the beam, at a specified distance from the target, and in a specified medium. This requires tedious measurements under very specific conditions. The second part is the absorbed dose in the irradiated medium. This requires, for example, knowledge of the composition of the irradiated material, the geometric relationship with the beam, and the size of the irradiated field.

This section provides definition of some terms used in external-beam dose calculations that appear in this text. Definition of terms used in photon and electron beams are described separately.

MAXIMUM ELECTRONIC BUILDUP

Whenever high-energy photon beams strike a medium, secondary electrons are set in motion. These secondary electrons will penetrate the medium to a depth that depends on the photon energy and composition of the medium. Maximum dose is obtained at the depth where electron equilibrium is reached. This maximum depth is referred to as D_{max}.*

The region between the surface and this depth is referred to as the buildup region. The dose in the buildup region rises rapidly as the secondary electrons contribute to the total dose. Therefore, the surface layer receives a smaller dose than layers between the surface and D_{max}. The skin is thus "spared." The skin-sparing effect observed with high-energy beams is reduced or lost when materials such as clothing, treatment couches, positioning devices, and so on are allowed to intercept the beam within a few centimeters of the patient's skin surface. The observed skin-sparing effect is improved with higher energies, and the depth of D_{max} increases with higher energy. The dose at greater depths falls off gradually as the effects of attenuation and increased distance reduce the supply of photons that set the electrons in motion. The %DD falls less rapidly with higher energy, as demonstrated in Fig. 3.3.

Measurement of the exact dose at the surface is technically very difficult because the dose gradient is very steep; therefore, the dose within the instrument used in the dose determination will vary considerably.[1]

HALF-VALUE THICKNESS

A practical way to express the penetration, "quality," or "hardness" of a beam is the half-value thickness (HVT) in a given material. The HVT is the thickness of the material that reduces the intensity of the beam to half its original value. All photon beams can be described in terms of their HVT; however, the quality of high-energy beams is usually described in terms of the accelerating voltage (MV).

The quality of lower-energy beams such as those produced by superficial and orthovoltage equipment depends not only on the peak accelerating voltage (kVp) but also on the filtration used to filter out the nonpenetrating soft x-rays. It is customary to describe the quality of beams in this energy range in terms of their HVT in aluminum, copper, or tin. For example, when we say that the HVT for a given beam is 3 mmCu, we mean that inserting 3 mm of copper in the path of the beam will reduce its intensity to half of its original value. The practice of expressing beam-penetrating power in the same materials as those used to filter out soft, undesirable x-rays stems from the early days of radiation therapy, when these materials were used to determine the penetration of a given peak kilovoltage and filter

---

D_{max} means either the depth (usually written d_{max}) or the dose (usually written D_{max}). The two notations are often used interchangeably, and from the context in which they are used, it should be clear whether depth or dose is intended.

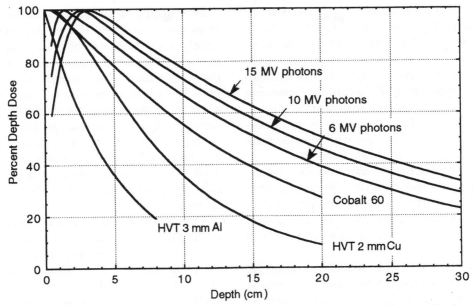

Figure 3.3 Percentage depth dose for 10 × 10 cm beams of different beam energies, plotted as a function of depth in water.

combination; they must not be confused with the filters actually used in the beam.

DOSE RATES

Dose rates and dose distributions from radiation therapy machines are ordinarily measured in the absence of a scattering phantom, sometimes referred to as *in air,* and in tissue-equivalent material. These measurements, or calibrations, are obtained using very carefully measured variables such as the SSD, field size, depth in tissue-equivalent material, and so on. Instruments calibrated against a national standard are used in obtaining these measurements.

It would be impractical to measure the dose at every point within a field at every distance from the source. Measured dose rates plotted at standard distances for multiple field sizes and corresponding isodose curves (see below and Fig. 3.15) for multiple field sizes allow one to calculate the dose to practically any point. Since the dose distributions in tissue from cobalt-60 machines are quite predictable, published tables may be used. Dose distributions from

linear accelerators with the same nominal energy may vary due to differences in flattening filter and collimator design. The percentage depth dose along the central axis may be reproducible from one linear accelerator to another of the same design using the same energy, and published central axis data may therefore be used.

Dose Rates without a Phantom. Dose rates determined without a scattering phantom are measured with a buildup cap of a thickness equal to the depth of D_{max}. These in-air measurements are made on the central axis of the field at the source-axis distan (SAD) for a range of field sizes because the rates vary somewhat with the collimator Special considerations must be made wh dent jaws or multileaf collimators are

Dose Rates in Tissue. Dose ordinarily measured on the cent SSD at the depth of D_{max} in a p depths and positions if require phantom include both the prima due to scatter in the irradiated v

Dependence on Field Size. Dose rates increase with increased field size due to scatter within the irradiated volume from the collimator and other beam-shaping devices.[5] Dose rates increase more rapidly in smaller fields; as the field size becomes larger (approximately 20 × 20 cm), the increase in dose rates stabilizes and they remain practically unchanged (Fig. 3.4). Since the scatter is greatly dependent on the field size, dose rates must be measured for a large number of field sizes.

It is customary to express dose rates for a cobalt-60 machine in cGy/min for a 10 × 10 cm field (dose rate$_{ref}$) at some fixed distance. An area factor is multiplied into the dose calculation for other field sizes to give the correct dose rate for each particular field size.

Linear accelerators can be altered to change the dose rate per time unit so the dose rates are expressed in cGy/monitor unit (MU). A monitor, built into the collimator, indicates a unit on the control console for each measured unit of dose at D_{max}. The monitor unit is often adjusted to be the same as 1 cGy at D_{max} for a given field size (cGy/MU$_{ref}$), usually a 10 × 10 cm field; but since the monitor unit is independent of field size, a cGy/MU factor for a range of field sizes must be measured and tabulated.

Dependence on Distance. The dose rate for a given energy and field size in principle varies inversely with the square of the distance from the source. However, the dependence of dose rates on the inverse square law assumes primary radiation only. The collimator or other scattering devices that add to the scattered radiation in the beam may cause deviation from the inverse square law.

Figure 3.5 demonstrates how the area increases as the distance from the target increases. The same number of interactions takes place in this larger area ($a_1 × b_1$) as in the smaller area ($a × b$) at the shorter distance.

An example of a calculation of the dose rate as a result of increased distance, using the inverse square law, is given below. The dose rate for a 10 × 10 cm cobalt-60 beam at 80.5 cm (SSD + depth of D_{max}) is 117 cGy/min. To find the dose rate at 100.5 cm (SSD + depth of D_{max}) for the same field, but treated at 100-cm SSD, we must find the inverse square factor (ISF).

The inverse square factor is found from

$$ISF = \left(\frac{SSD_1}{SSD_2}\right)^2 \qquad (3.1)$$

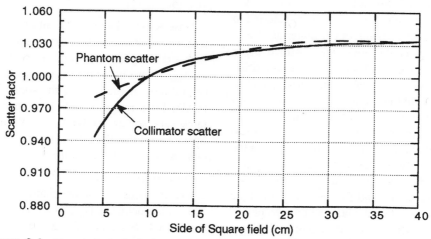

Figure 3.4 Measurement of cGy/MU without a phantom and plotted as a function of field size— collimator and scatter factors relative to a 10 × 10 cm field (6 MV).

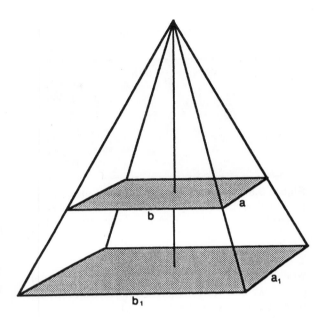

Figure 3.5   The irradiated area becomes larger as the distance from the target increases. The same number of interactions takes place in the larger area ($a_1 \times b_1$) as in the smaller area ($a \times b$).

Therefore

$$\left(\frac{80.5}{100.5}\right)^2 = 0.6416$$

$$117 \times 0.6416 = 75 \text{ cGy/min}$$

One necessary but often omitted step in the calculation of a treatment prescription that includes an inverse square factor is to do the same calculation without the inverse square factor to find the necessary treatment time, or MU, if the treatment was delivered at the "normal" SSD. This is a simple way of verifying that the required treatment time or number of MU is in fact increased when the SSD is longer, or vice versa when the treatment distance is shortened, and that the inverse square equation was not accidentally inverted. Serious accidents can be prevented by careful checks of these calculations.

PERCENTAGE DEPTH DOSE

Percentage depth dose is the absorbed dose at a given depth expressed as a percentage of the absorbed dose at a reference depth on the central axis of the field.

The reference depth is usually taken to be D_{max}, and, in this case, the %DD at point A (Fig. 3.6) is 75 percent.

$$\%DD = \frac{\text{absorbed dose at A}}{\text{absorbed dose at } D_{max}} \times 100\% \quad (3.2)$$

Percentage depth dose is affected by energy, field size, SSD, and the composition of the irradiated medium. Of course the %DD also changes with depth.

Percentage depth dose data are usually tabulated for square or rectangular fields.[6-8] A majority of treatments encountered in clinical practice require other shapes; therefore, a system of equating clinically used fields to fields with tabulated data is required. This is discussed in greater detail in the section on irregular fields in Chap. 5.

Dependence on Field Size and Shape.   For a field of 0×0 cm, the dose at a point in a phantom is effectively due to primary radiation only. This method of considering the primary radiation is feasible in theory only; however, it is a reasonable manner in which to consider the primary dose alone. If the collimator were closed entirely, no radiation

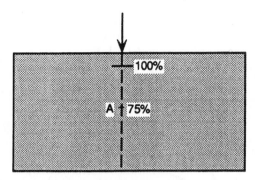

Figure 3.6 Percentage depth dose is the absorbed dose at a given depth expressed as a percentage of the absorbed dose at a reference depth; in this illustration, the reference depth is at D_{max}.

field (100 cm²) symmetrically placed around the calculation point will produce more scatter at this point than a field that is 2 × 50 cm, also 100 cm². This is because the extremes of this field are 25 cm from the calculation point. Large sections of this field are too far from the calculation point to deliver a significant amount of scatter there. This is discussed in more detail in Chap. 5.

Furthermore, higher-energy photons are scattered in a more forward direction than lower-energy photons, thus resulting in less dependence on field size.

Dependence on Energy and Depth. Higher-energy beams have greater penetrating power; thus the %DD at a given depth and the SSD are increased. Figure 3.3 illustrates the %DD along the central axis for a variety of beam energies.

Dependence on Distance. Although the absolute dose rate decreases with increased distance from the source, the percentage depth dose, which is a relative dose with respect to a reference point, *increases* with increased SSD. This is illustrated in Fig. 3.8, where it is shown that for a given field size, the volume within which the same number of interactions takes place is smaller when the distance is

would be delivered; but if the field were *very* small (which we may for convenience show as a 0 × 0 cm field), the dose would effectively be due to primary radiation only. The scattered component of the dose is almost entirely dependent on the size of the radiation field. As the field size is increased, the absorbed dose in a medium is greater due to the increased scatter (Fig. 3.7).

The shape of the field strongly influences the amount of scatter at a given point. A 10 × 10 cm

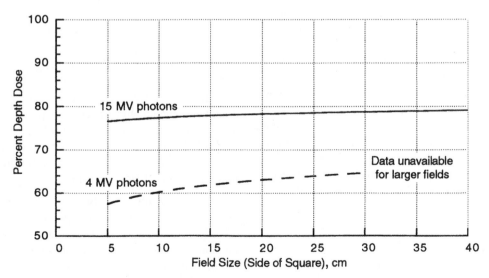

Figure 3.7 Percentage depth dose plotted as a function of field size (10-cm depth) for 4- and 15-MV photon beams. The SSD for the 4-MV photon beam is 80 cm and for the 15-MV photon beam, 100 cm.

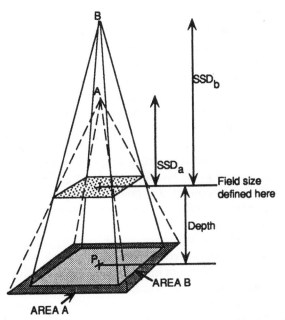

Figure 3.8 The irradiated volume for a given field size is decreased when the SSD is increased.

increased. Grossly simplified, one can say that the interactions are more concentrated when the distance is increased.

The increase of %DD with increased distance can be determined using the Mayneord F factor,[9,10] defined as follows:

$$F \text{ factor} = \frac{[(SSD_2 + D_{max})/(SSD_2 + d)]^2}{[(SSD_1 + D_{max})/(SSD_1 + d)]^2} \quad (3.3)$$

so that

$$\%DD_{SSD_2} = F \times \%DD_{SSD_1}$$

The Mayneord F factor is a reasonably accurate method of calculating the change in %DD for small fields, where the scatter component is small. Significant errors occur when this method is applied under extreme conditions such as low energy, large field, large depth, or large change in SSD.

An example of using the Mayneord F factor in calculating the change in %DD is given below. The %DD for a 10 × 10 cm field at 10-cm depth and an 80-cm SSD (D_{max} at 1.0 cm), using a 4-MV photon beam, is 62.2 percent. Find the %DD dose for the same field size and depth but for a 100-cm SSD.

$$F \text{ factor} = \frac{[(100 + 1)/(100 + 10)]^2}{[(80 + 1)/(80 + 10)]^2}$$

$$= \frac{(101/110)^2}{(81/90)^2}$$

$$= \frac{0.8431}{0.81} = 1.041$$

Thus the %DD is the original 62.2 multiplied by the F factor 1.041:

$$62.2 \times 1.041 = 64.8$$

In making this calculation, caution should be used to prevent any chance of accidentally inverting the equation. One must always remember that as the SSD increases, the %DD will also increase.

Dependence on Composition of the Irradiated Medium. In a patient, the beam may traverse tissues of different density such as lung, bone, fat, muscle, and air. These inhomogeneities affect both the penetration of the beam and the scattering characteristics. The effect of these inhomogeneities on the dose depends on the size of the volume, on the density (g/cm³) of the inhomogeneity, and also on the energy of the beam.

For example, lung tissue, which is largely filled with air, has a much lower density than muscle and thus attenuates the primary photon beam less than an equal thickness of soft tissue. The effect of bone, where the density is higher than in soft tissue, is in the opposite direction.

The density of lung can vary from 0.25 to 1.0 g/cm³, depending on the amount of air in the lung. A value of 0.25 to 0.33 g/cm³ is often used. The density of bone is often quoted as 1.8 g/cm³, but this probably overestimates the attenuation of primary photons. The density of compact bone, for example, is higher than for soft or spongy bone.

The effects of inhomogeneities are in the absorption of the primary beam and in the scatter. For points that lie beyond an inhomogeneity, the dose is primarily affected by the attenuation of the primary beam, while the dose distribution in and near the inhomogeneity is affected more by the scatter. Calculation of dose changes in and beyond an inhomogeneity is very complicated because of variations in density within an inhomogeneity and uncertainties in the three-dimensional shape of the inhomogeneity. Many authors have proposed different methods of calculating the change in dose caused by inhomogeneities.[11-19]

The effect on the dose near the interface between layers of different density is quite complex. For example, there may be loss of electronic equilibrium immediately beyond an air cavity or a layer of low-density material when high-energy beams are used.[20-23]

Figure 3.9 shows a radiation beam traversing water-equivalent phantom (electron density = 1.0), which contains an inhomogeneity shaped like a lung and with a density that is lower than that of water (electron density = 0.25). The primary dose at point A is essentially unchanged because it is located proximal to the lower-density lung; however, the backscattered radiation from the lung is decreased. The effect of the scattered radiation decreases as the photon beam energy increases because more of the scatter is in a forward direction. The primary dose at point B is higher than at the same depth in the absence of the lower-density lung. This is due to the reduced attenuation by the lung. On the other hand, the scattered radiation originating in the lower-density material in the vicinity is reduced and tends to cause lower dose at this point. Depending on the three-dimensional size of the lower-density volume, the reduction in scattered dose could compensate for the increase in the primary dose, causing the dose at B to be unchanged. Point C is inside the water-equivalent volume but immediately outside the low-density volume. The primary dose at this point is higher; however, because it is immediately beyond the proximal boundary of the low-density area, it may suffer loss of electronic equilibrium analogous to that observed in the buildup region near the skin surface. This is particularly evident when high-energy photon beams are used. The primary dose at point D is increased due to the presence of low-density lung "upstream" in the beam; however, the scattered radiation is reduced due to the proximity (in the lateral direction) of the lung tissue. Again, this effect is lower when high-energy photon beams are used, due to the more forward direction of the scatter.

For low-energy x-rays, the absorbed dose within or near the bone may be several times higher than calculated from soft tissue tables. This increased dose is caused by an interaction called photoelectric absorption, which is of major importance only at low energies and in materials of higher atomic number. The complex problem of absorbed dose in bone and the soft tissue–bone interface has been studied in great detail by Spiers.[24,25]

In the past, the difficulties in calculating dose in a beam that transverses an inhomogeneous volume have been related in part to the difficulties of outlining the boundaries of the inhomogeneity and of determining the density within this volume. The use of computed tomography (CT), in which both detailed

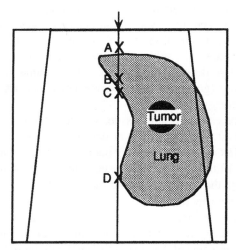

Figure 3.9   A radiation beam traversing a water phantom containing a lower-density lung. The dose along the central axis of the beam is affected by the presence of the inhomogeneity. The dose at A is essentially unchanged. At B, the primary dose is increased while the scattered dose is decreased. The dose at C is affected by the loss of electronic buildup and the proximity of the inhomogeneity. The dose at D is increased due to the presence of the low-density lung; however, the scatter from the lung tissue is decreased.

outlines of inhomogeneities in three dimensions and some information of the physical composition of that volume can be obtained, has greatly enhanced dose-calculation methods when inhomogeneities are present. Algorithms to take into account the three-dimensional shape of inhomogeneities are under way and the accuracy is expected to be improved over current methods. Since the CT numbers and the attenuation coefficients have a linear relationship, it is possible to incorporate a density correction in dose calculations. The validity of using CT information related to the density of an organ is controversial and has been evaluated by several authors.[26-38] Although a gradual change to universal introduction of inhomogeneity correction in reported doses has been proposed,[39,40] generally there is some reluctance to make this change because practically all clinical experience has been gained with dose calculations assuming homogeneity.

TISSUE-AIR RATIO

The concept of tissue-air ratio (TAR) was first introduced for calculation of dose in rotation therapy, where the radiation source moves in a circle around the axis of the gantry rotation (isocenter). The axis is usually placed at or close to the center of the tumor. The SAD and the field size at the distance remain unchanged, while the SSD, the field area on the patient's surface, and the thickness of overlying tissue may vary depending on the patient's surface contour. The TAR concept is practical and is now almost universally used; it can be employed not only in rotation treatments but also for the calculation of dose using stationary fields in both SAD and SSD techniques and for treatments delivered at extended distances using large fields.

Tissue-air ratio is the ratio of the dose at a given point in a medium to the dose at the same point in free space (Fig. 3.10).

$$TAR = \frac{\text{dose in tissue}}{\text{dose in air}} \qquad (3.4)$$

For a given energy, the TAR depends on depth and field size at that depth but is independent of distance.

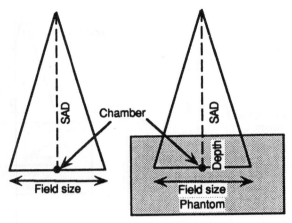

Figure 3.10 Arrangement for determination of tissue-air ratio. Note that the distance to the chamber and the field size are unchanged.

Tissue-air ratio for a *very* small field represented by a 0 × 0 cm field, which is only an abstraction, represents primary dose only, since no scattering material is irradiated. It increases with increasing field size as the scatter from the irradiated volume is added to the primary (0 × 0 cm field).

TISSUE-PHANTOM RATIO

The tissue-phantom ratio (TPR), first introduced by Karzmark in an effort to overcome the limitations of the TAR, is sometimes used instead of TAR in dosimetry of high-energy beams.[41,42] It retains the properties of the TAR but eliminates difficult and unreliable in-air measurements, because the determination of dose in free space would require the use of a buildup cap too large to be fully irradiated when small fields are used.

The TPR is defined as the ratio of dose at a specified point in tissue or in a phantom to the dose at the same distance in the beam at a reference depth, usually 5 cm (Fig. 3.11).

$$TPR = \frac{\text{dose in tissue}}{\text{dose in phantom (ref. depth)}} \qquad (3.5)$$

As with TARs, the dose measurements should be made at the same distance from the source for both

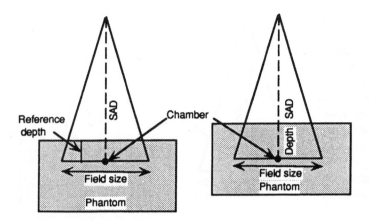

Figure 3.11 Arrangement for determination of tissue-phantom ratio. Note that the distance to the chamber and the field size are unchanged.

determinations, and the field size at the distance of the measuring instrument should also be the same in both cases.

TISSUE-MAXIMUM RATIO

Tissue-maximum ratio (TMR) is a special case of TPR where the reference depth is chosen to be at D_{max}. Tissue-maximum ratio is defined as the ratio of the dose at a specified point in tissue or in a phantom to the dose at the same point when it is at the depth of maximum dose (Fig. 3.12):

$$TMR = \frac{\text{dose in tissue}}{\text{dose in phantom } (D_{max})} \quad (3.6)$$

SCATTER-AIR RATIO

Scatter-air ratio (SAR) is the ratio of the scattered dose at a given point in a medium to the dose in air at the same point. The SAR, like the TAR, is independent of the treatment distance but depends on the energy, field size, and depth (Fig. 3.13).

Since the scattered dose at a given point in the medium is equal to the total dose minus the primary dose at the same point, SARs can be calculated by finding the difference between the TAR for the given field size (primary and scatter are present) and the TAR for a 0×0 cm field (primary only). The TAR for a 0×0 cm field represents the primary component only, since no scattering medium is present.

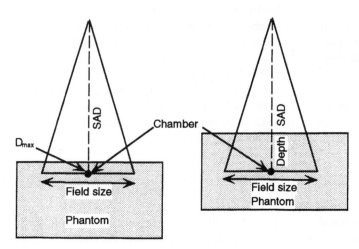

Figure 3.12 Arrangement for determination of tissue-maximum ratio. Note that the distance to the chamber and the field size are unchanged.

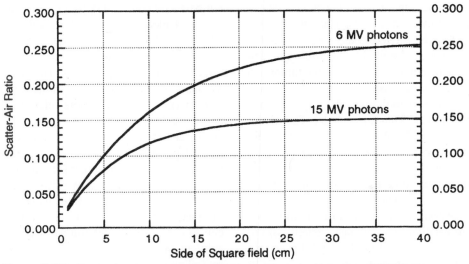

Figure 3.13   Scatter-air ratios as a function of field size (10-cm depth) for 6- and 15-MV photons.

$$SAR(D,fs) = TAR(D,fs) - TAR(D,0) \quad (3.7)$$

where D is depth and fs is field size.

Scatter-air ratios are primarily used for the purpose of calculating scattered dose in a medium. Considering the primary and the scattered doses separately is particularly useful in dose calculation for irregularly shaped fields, discussed in Chap. 5.

SCATTER-MAXIMUM RATIO

Scatter-maximum ratio (SMR) is really just a variation of SAR and, like SAR, is mainly used in calculation of scattered dose in a phantom or tissue. It is defined as the ratio of the scattered dose at a designated point in a phantom to the effective primary dose at the same point at the reference depth of maximum dose. It differs from SAR in that the reference point is different, just as TAR and TMR have different reference points.

BACKSCATTER FACTOR

The backscatter factor (BSF) is defined as the ratio of dose on the central axis at D_{max} to the dose at the same point in air (or free space). The BSF is independent of SSD but depends on the energy and the field size. Backscatter factors and TARs at D_{max} are the same.

The BSF is very high for beam energies having a HVT of 0.6 to 0.8 mmCu and can be as high as 1.5 for large fields at these HVTs.[6-8] For megavoltage beams, where the scatter travels in a more forward direction, the BSF is much lower; in beams generated above 8 to 10 MV, the scatter at D_{max} is very small (less than 5% in a 10 × 10 cm field).

COLLIMATOR SCATTER FACTOR

Output measured without a scattering phantom, sometimes referred to as *in-air,* increases with increased field size. The increase is due to increased photon scattering from the collimator because the surface area of the beam-defining tunnel exposed to the radiation increases as the collimator opening is enlarged (Fig. 3.4).

FIXED SOURCE-AXIS DISTANCE VERSUS FIXED SOURCE-SURFACE DISTANCE TECHNIQUE

A fixed source-axis distance (SAD) technique is also known as an *isocentric* technique. In this technique, the axis of machine rotation (the isocenter) is placed in the target volume (Fig. 3.14A). The gantry of the machine can then be rotated to any angle while the target remains within the field boundaries. One can either make the machine rotate around the tumor in a complete circle (rotation therapy), or a partial circle (arc therapy), or treat multiple stationary fields directed at the target from any angle. The tissue surrounding the target volume, outside of the field boundaries, lies in the beam only during a small fraction of the moving beam treatment, while in a stationary technique some tissue between the fields is almost totally spared. The precise dose distribution depends on several factors such as the rotation pattern (arc, full rotation, or stationary), energy of the beam, field size, number of fields, depth of the isocenter, and weighting of the beam.

The dose in this technique is usually normalized at the isocenter. Either TARs and dose rates in air or TPRs and TMRs are used in calculating the dose. Since TAR and TPR are practically independent of distance (see previous definitions), the precision in measuring the SSD is not as important as in an SSD technique where the %DD, the dose rates in air, and the TMR will vary with the distance. In an isocentric technique, small errors in the dose due to small errors in the treatment distance are reduced if an opposing field is used, because there the distance error will be in the opposite direction, thus practically eliminating an error in the dose.

In a fixed-SSD technique, small errors in SSD are not balanced out in an opposing field, as they are in the SAD method, because the patient is moved to adjust the SSD in this technique. The error in dose could in fact be doubled if the distance error is in the same direction in both fields. The only references available in setting up this treatment technique are skin marks. These unreliable references can cause considerable error in field placement. Small errors in angle can also cause geometric misses of the target, since the axis of rotation is now placed at considerable distance from the target (Fig. 3.14B). In principle, this can be corrected by shifting the patient laterally and, on a curved surface, also higher or lower. In practice, however, the correct shift is often difficult to achieve. Another source of error is the difficulty in precisely setting the SSD when the field central axis is on a very steep-sloping surface or on the posterior surface of a supine patient.

The isocentric, or SAD, technique is obviously superior to an SSD technique. However, some therapy units do not have a rotating gantry, thus precluding isocentric techniques (Fig. 2.13 in Chap. 2).

ISODOSE DISTRIBUTION

It is not sufficient to have information about the dose at various depths along the central axis only. In addition, the dose distribution must be known for a large number of field sizes and for different treatment conditions. Dose distributions are usually measured in a phantom for a large number of field sizes and are

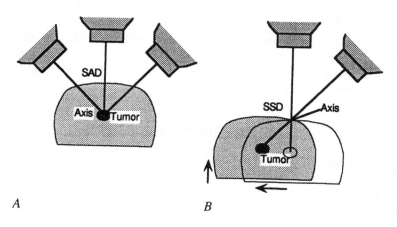

A

B

Figure 3.14 In an isocentric technique (*A*), the beam is constantly aimed at the tumor (axis), while in a fixed SSD technique (*B*), the axis of rotation is placed on the patient's skin surface away from the tumor. To avoid missing the tumor, the patient must be moved laterally and, to adjust the SSD, up or down as well.

plotted in terms of *isodose curves.* An isodose curve is one passing through points of equal dose and representing percentage of dose at a reference point.

ISODOSE CHARTS

Isodose charts consist of a number of isodose curves usually depicted in 10 percent increments. Dose at other points can be found by interpolating between the lines. Figure 3.15 shows isodose distributions produced of different energy beams. Not only are the %DD along the central axis different for the various beam energies, but the shapes of the isodose curves are also quite different.

Field Size. The geometric field size is usually

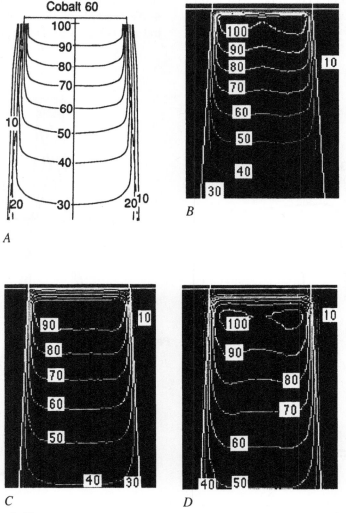

Figure 3.15 Comparison of isodose charts from various beams energies where the dose is normalized to 100 percent at D_{max}. *A.* Isodose distribution from a cobalt-60 beam. *B.* A 4-MV photon beam. *C.* A 6-MV photon beam. *D.* A 15-MV photon beam. The SSD is 80 cm in the cobalt-60 and 4-MV photon beams and 100 cm in the 6- and 15-MV photon beams.

defined by the intersection of the 50 percent isodose line and the surface (Fig. 3.16A). The light source, which coincides with the beam, is aligned to match the 50 percent isodose line in the majority of treatment units.

Penumbra.   Penumbra is the region near the edge of the field margin where the dose falls rapidly. The width of the penumbra depends on the size of the radiation source, the distance from the source to the distal part of the collimator, and the SSD (Fig. 3.16B). The penumbra of a cobalt-60 beam is relatively wide compared with that of a linear accelerator. This is primarily due to the larger radiation source in the cobalt-60 machine but also to the target-collimator distance, the SSD, and the scattered dose. Knowledge of the field size and the characteristics of the penumbra is of particular importance in finding the field separation that will result in optimal dose uniformity across adjoining fields.

Beam Flatness.   Isodose charts reveal information regarding the dose away from the central axis. In Fig. 3.15, it is evident that, in the isodose chart for a cobalt-60 machine, the dose decreases away from the central axis while the isodose distribution for the 4-MV beam shows that the dose away from the central axis is increased. This is particularly evident near

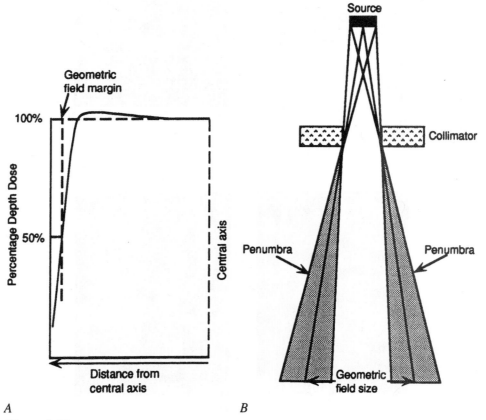

A   *B*

Figure 3.16   The geometric field size is usually defined by the intersection of the 50 percent isodose line and the surface (*A*). The geometric field is defined by the light field, here shown by the solid lines (*B*). The penumbra is the region on either side of the light field, where the dose falls from 90 to 10 percent (*shaded areas*).

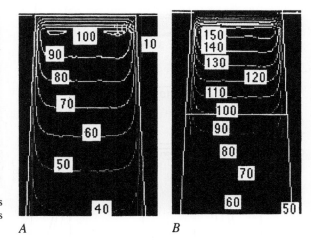

Figure 3.17   An isodose distribution with fixed SSD (*A*) is normalized to 100 percent at D_{max}. In a fixed SAD (*B*), the dose is normalized to 100 percent at the isocenter.

A   *B*

the surface and is a result of overflattening of the beam at shallow depths, which is necessary in order to flatten the isodose curves at greater depths. Without a beam-flattening filter, the dose from a linear accelerator on the central axis would be much higher than away from the central axis. The flattening filter reduces the dose along the central axis and produces a flat beam at a specified depth, usually 10 cm.

Dose Normalization.   In isodose charts for a fixed-SSD treatment technique, the reference point customarily is at D_{max}. The dose at this point is usually fixed at 100 percent (normalized to 100 percent). In an isodose chart for an isocentric technique (fixed SAD), the reference point is at the isocenter.

Two methods of normalizing the dose are shown in Fig. 3.17. It is quite easy to determine the dose at any given point in tissue if the dose at the normalization point is known. For example, if 100 cGy is delivered at D_{max} in field *A* in Fig. 3.17, it is clear that 50 cGy is delivered at any given point along the 50 percent isodose line.

DOSE PROFILES

Dose variation across a field at a given depth can be ascertained from the corresponding isodose curves and is best represented by a dose profile (Fig. 3.18). The dose profile displays relative doses across a field

or across a treatment plan consisting of multiple beams.

BEAM'S-EYE VIEW

Another method of depicting dose variations within a field at a given depth is in the "beam's-eye view" shown in Fig. 3.19. These isodose curves are shown in a plane perpendicular to the central axis of the beam. Although unconventional, this representation of the dose distribution is sometimes useful, particularly in three-dimensional treatment planning.

WEDGES

Frequently, beam-modifying absorbers (sometimes called *filters*) are inserted in the path of a beam. The most commonly used beam-modifying filter is a wedge-shaped piece of dense material, usually lead, which attenuates the beam progressively across the field (Fig. 3.20). The thinner side of the wedge attenuates the beam less than the thicker side, resulting in tilted isodose curves, as shown in Fig. 3.21. The degree of the resulting tilt depends on the shape and composition of the wedge.

Wedge angle refers to the angle through which an isodose curve is tilted at the central axis of the beam at a specified depth. The specification of a depth is critical because the degree of tilt changes with depth.

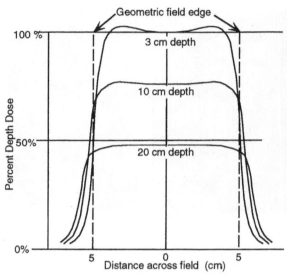

Figure 3.18   Dose profiles plotted across a field at D_{max}, 10-cm depth, and at 20-cm depth. The dose is normalized to 100 percent on the central axis at D_{max}. The beam is flatter at a greater depth than at D_{max}.

The tilt decreases at greater depth because of the increased effect of scattered radiation. While there is no general agreement as to the reference depth, some choose to define the wedge angle at the intersection of the central axis of the beam and the 50 percent isodose curve. This becomes quite impractical

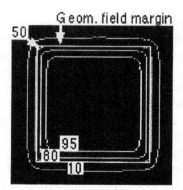

Figure 3.19   Beam's-eye view of the isodose distribution of a 6-MV photon beam at the depth of D_{max}. The hatched lines indicate the geometric field margins.

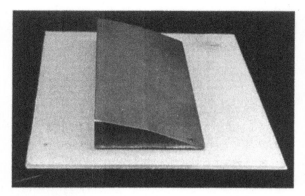

Figure 3.20   A typical 45° wedge.

when high-energy beams are used and also because different methods of dose normalization are practiced.

It should be noted that *wedge angle* refers to the tilt of the isodose curve, *not* the angle of the actual wedge filter. A wedge that will produce a 45° tilt (wedge angle), for example, is often spoken of as a ''45° wedge,'' though, as just explained, the wedge material itself may have quite a different slope.

Wedge filters producing 15°, 30°, 45°, and 60° isodose curves are usually available from the manufacturer of radiation therapy machines. Other angles of isodose tilt can be attained by combining open (unwedged) beams with wedged beams.[43,44]

The wedge progressively attenuates the beam across the entire field, thus also decreasing the dose rate at the central axis. A wedge transmission factor must therefore be included in the dose calculation. The wedge transmission factor expresses the ratio of the dose rates on the central axis with and without the wedge. Some commercial isodose charts are normalized with the wedge transmission factor included. In such an isodose chart, the isodose line at D_{max} along the central axis represents the wedge transmission factor and the other isodose lines also reflect the attenuation caused by the wedge. No transmission factor should be included in the dose calculation when such prenormalized isodose charts are used.

A universal wedge is a wedge of a given angle that is fixed in the beam and serves all beam widths up to

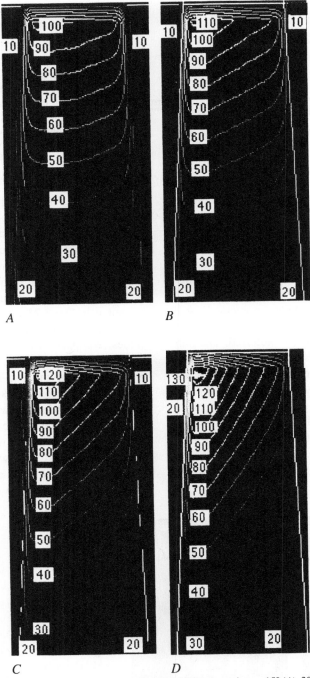

Figure 3.21   The effect of inserting wedges in a 6-MV photon beam; 15° (*A*), 30° (*B*), 45° (*C*), 60° tilt (*D*).

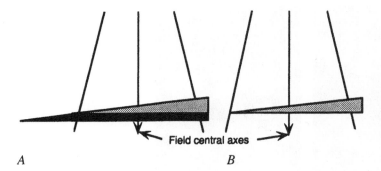

Field central axes

A   *B*

Figure 3.22 *A.* A universal wedge, where the center of the wedge is fixed in the center of the beam; the field can be opened to practically any width. An unused segment of the wedge *(darker shading)* only reduces the dose rate. *B.* An individualized wedge where the thin edge of the wedge is always aligned with the field margin.

a designated limit. As illustrated in Fig. 3.22, when a small field is used, only a small thickness of the wedge is needed to produce the isodose tilt. The remainder of the wedge thickness attenuates the beam the same amount across the field, thus unnecessarily reducing the dose rate. For cobalt-60 units, where dose rates are already relatively low, a universal wedge system would be quite impractical, as it would further reduce the dose rate. An individualized wedge system is therefore preferred. The individualized system consists of multiple wedges for each isodose tilt. Each wedge is designed for a particular field width and is mounted so that the thin edge of the wedge coincides with the edge of the light field. The beam will, therefore, pass through minimal thickness of wedge material and thus minimally reduce the dose rate.

Wedges inserted in the beam will only reshape already existing isodose curves. Isodose curves from linear accelerators usually show higher dose away from the central axis, especially at shallow depths. A wedge inserted in such a beam will only decrease the already higher dose under the thick section of the wedge. Under the thin section of the wedge, the dose is further increased, resulting in isodose curves shaped as in Fig. 3.23.

Dynamic Wedging. With modern treatment machines, equipped with independently moving collimator leaves (Chap. 2), a wedge effect can be produced by driving one of the collimator leaves across the field, thus gradually increasing the field size. The side of the field where the starting position of the moving leaf is located will thus receive a higher dose than the side where its final position is located. The speed with which the collimator leaf moves will determine the angle of the sloping iso-

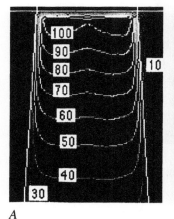
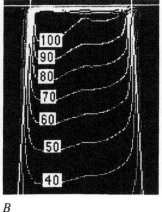

A   *B*

Figure 3.23 An isodose curve from an unwedged 4-MV photon beam (*A*) and a 4-MV photon beam with a 15° wedge inserted (*B*). The isodose curve under the thick part of the wedge is now fairly flat (reduced from being overflattened in the unwedged beam), while under the thin segment, the dose with respect to the central-axis dose is increased.

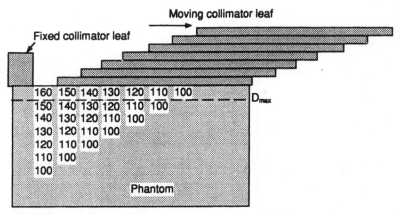

Figure 3.24 Dynamic wedging is accomplished by having an independently moving collimator leaf move across the field during the treatment. While the collimator leaf moves continuously across the beam, the leaf position is shown in this illustration in steps, where 10 cGy is delivered. The hatched line represent the depth of D_{max}. The dose at D_{max} on the right in the phantom is 0 because this point is fully shielded during this treatment. At the next step, 100 cGy is delivered at D_{max} because this point is shielded during only part of the treatment. The dose at D_{max} progressively increases toward the left, where shielding was provided during progressively shorter times. As the D_{max} dose increases, so does the dose at depth; if the points receiving 100 cGy in this case are connected, a sloping isodose curve results.

dose curve. This technique is referred to as dynamic wedging and is best explained by Fig. 3.24.

ELECTRON BEAMS

DOSE RATES

Dose rates and isodose distributions from electron beams are quite different from those of photon beams and are therefore discussed separately. Electron dose rates can vary considerably with field size and energy and from one linear accelerator to another, even when it is the same model. Extensive calibration must therefore be made for every electron energy and with each electron cone and field size. It is customary to fix the cGy/MU to 1.0 for a 10×10 cm cone at D_{max}; the cGy/MU for other cones and field sizes are expressed as an output factor. Shaping of electron beams with secondary blocks also changes the dose rates and distributions, requiring careful measurements of each field.[45–53] Frequent constancy checks of electron dose rates are essential.

PERCENTAGE DEPTH DOSE

The dose distribution from electron beams is characterized by relative uniformity within the first few centimeters in tissue, followed by a very rapid fall-off of dose. The depth at which the rapid fall-off of dose sets in depends on the electron energy. As a guideline for selecting the appropriate electron energy for a given tumor, one can say that the electron energy in MeV should be three times the maximum depth of the tumor; that is, for a 3-cm treatment depth, a 9-MeV electron beam should be used. The isodose distribution varies with beam collimation, field size, cone design, and so on. Typical depth dose curves for clinically useful electron energies are shown in Fig. 3.25.

Some skin sparing is afforded with electron beams, especially with lower energies. The peak dose (D_{max}) is relatively broad, particularly with the higher-energy electron beams.

ISODOSE CHARTS

Isodose curves for electron beams can vary from machine to machine due to differences in the design

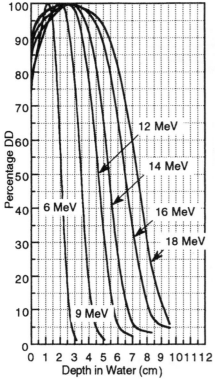

Figure 3.25 Typical depth dose curves for several electron beam energies (15 × 15 cm cone).

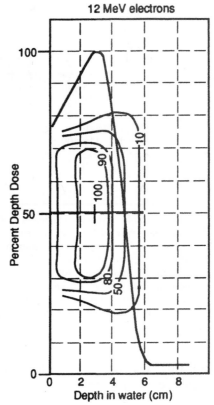

Figure 3.26 Typical electron isodose curve.

of the machine, collimating system, and cones. A library of isodose curves for each energy and cone or field size should therefore be obtained for each machine. The converging of the 90 and 80 percent isodose lines and the bulging out of the 50 and 20 percent isodose curves near the field edges is of considerable importance in treatment planning (Fig. 3.26). Matching isodose curves of adjacent fields is practically impossible without causing "hot" or "cold" spots. Field margins must also be selected so that the target volume lies within the converging 90 percent line (Fig. 3.27).

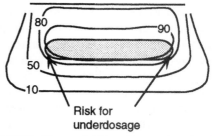

Figure 3.27 Electron field margins must be selected so that underdosage does not occur due to the convergence of the 90 percent isodose line.

PROBLEMS

3.1 1 Gy is the same as
   (*a*) 1 rad
   (*b*) 10 cGy
   (*c*) 100 cGy
   (*d*) 1 erg

3.2 Radiation dose is often determined using the following methods:
   (*a*) TLD
       Photodynamic therapy
       Ionization chambers
   (*b*) Photographic film
       TLD
       Ionization chambers
   (*c*) Ionization chambers
       TLD
       Film badges

3.3 The point of maximum electron equilibrium is referred to as
   (*a*) TAD
   (*b*) SFD
   (*c*) MEE
   (*d*) D_{max}

3.4 A HVT is a way of expressing
   (*a*) The filtration of a beam
   (*b*) The dose
   (*c*) The quality of the beam
   (*d*) The TAR

3.5 Dose rates in air express
   (*a*) The dose measured for a 10×10 cm field at a 10-cm depth in a phantom
   (*b*) The dose measured without a phantom and with a buildup cap at a given distance
   (*c*) The dose measured without a phantom and without a buildup cap at a given distance
   (*d*) The dose measured without a buildup cap for a 10×10 cm field at a given distance

3.6 Dose rates
   (*a*) Decrease with increased field size and increase with increased distance
   (*b*) Increase with increased field size and decrease with decreased distance
   (*c*) Increase with increased field size and decrease with increased distance

3.7 Increasing the distance from 80 to 90 cm causes the dose rate to change by
   (*a*) 0.8095
   (*b*) 0.8111
   (*c*) 0.6400
   (*d*) 0.7901

3.8 Percentage depth dose is dependent on
  (a) SSD
    Distance
    Treatment time
  (b) Distance
    Field size
    cGy/MU
  (c) Field size
    Distance
    Energy
  (d) Energy
    Tissue density
    Treatment time

3.9 The correct match is represented by which option (1, 2, 3, or 4) below?
  (a) The ratio of dose at a specified point in tissue or in a phantom to the dose at the same distance in the beam at a reference depth
  (b) The ratio of the dose at a specified point in tissue or in a phantom to the dose at the same point when it is at the depth of maximum dose
  (c) The ratio of the dose at a specified point in a medium to the dose at the same point in free space

	1.	2.	3.	4.
(a)	TAR	TPR	TMR	TPR
(b)	TPR	TMR	TPR	TAR
(c)	TMR	TAR	TAR	TMR

3.10 The TAR at 5-cm depth for a 10×10 cm field minus the TAR at 5-cm depth for a 0×0 cm field gives the
  (a) TMR
  (b) SAR
  (c) TPR
  (d) SMR

3.11 In a fixed SSD technique, the dose is routinely normalized
  (a) At the isocenter
  (b) At tumor depth
  (c) At D_{max}
  (d) On the surface

3.12 In an isocentric treatment technique, the dose is routinely normalized
  (a) At the isocenter
  (b) At the tumor depth
  (c) At D_{max}
  (d) On the surface

3.13 The width of the penumbra *increases* with
  (a) Decreased SSD
    Decreased source-collimator distance
    Decreased field size
  (b) Decreased SSD
    Increased source-collimator distance
    Increased source size

(*c*) Increased SSD
Decreased source-collimator distance
Increased source size
(*d*) Increased SSD
Increased source-collimator distance
Decreased source size

3.14 Wedge angle refers to
(*a*) The angle of the actual wedge filter
(*b*) The angle at which an isodose curve at a specified depth is tilted as a result of the wedge being inserted in the beam
(*c*) The angle at which an isodose curve at a specified depth is tilted with respect to the central axis of the beam

3.15 A guide for determining the needed electron beam energy (in MeV) is to
(*a*) Divide the maximum tumor depth in centimeters by 3
(*b*) Divide the 80 percent isodose line by 10 and then by the maximum tumor depth in centimeters
(*c*) Multiply the maximum tumor depth in centimeters by 5 and then divide by 3
(*d*) Multiply the maximum tumor depth in centimeters by 3

3.16 In a typical electron beam, which of the following statements is true?
(*a*) All of the isodose curves in the penumbra region bulge out, causing great difficulties in matching adjacent electron fields uniformly.
(*b*) Only the 50 to 90 percent isodose lines bulge out in the penumbra region, causing great difficulties in matching adjacent electron fields uniformly.
(*c*) Only the 10 to 50% isodose lines bulge out in the penumbra region, causing great difficulties in matching adjacent electron fields uniformly.
(*d*) All of the isodose lines converge in the penumbra region, causing great difficulties in matching adjacent electron fields uniformly.

REFERENCES

1. Gerbi BJ, Khan FM: Measurement of dose in the buildup region using fixed-separation plane-parallel ionization chambers. *Med Phys* 17:1, 1990.
2. Khan FM, Gerbi BJ, Deibel FC: Dosimetry of asymmetric x-ray collimators. *Med Phys* 13:936, 1986.
3. Khan FM: Dosimetry of wedged fields with asymmetric collimation. *Med Phys* 20:1447, 1993.
4. Loshek DD, Parker TT: Dose calculation in static or dynamic off-axis fields. *Med Phys* 21:401, 1994.
5. Meli J: Output factors and dose calculations for blocked x-ray fields. *Med Phys* 13:405, 1986.
6. British Institute of Radiology, London UK: Central axis depth dose data for use in ratiotherapy. *Br J Radiol Suppl* 11, 1972.
7. British Institute of Radiology, London UK: Central axis depth dose Data for use in radiotherapy. *Br J Radiol* suppl 17, 1983.
8. Johns HE, Cunningham JR: *The Physics of Radiology*, 4th ed. Springfield, IL: Charles C Thomas, 1983.
9. British Institute of Radiology, London UK: Depth dose tables for use in radiotherapy. *Br J Radiol* suppl 10, 1961.
10. Mayneord WV, Lamerton LF: A survey of depth dose data. *Br J Radiol* 14:255, 1941.
11. Batho HF: Lung corrections in cobalt-60 beam therapy. *J Can Assoc Radiol* 15:79, 1964.
12. Greene D, Stewart JR: Isodose curves in non-uniform phantoms. *Br J Radiol* 38:378, 1965.
13. Jette D, Bielajew A: Electron dose calculation using multiple-scattering theory: Second-order multiple-scattering theory. *Med Phys* 16:5, 1989.
14. Jette D, Lanzi LH, Pagnamenta A, et al: Electron dose calculation using multiple-scattering theory: Thin planar inhomogeneities. *Med Phys* 16:5, 1989.
15. McDonald SC, Keller BE, Rubin P: Method for calculating dose when lung tissue lies in the treatment field. *Med Phys* 3:210, 1976.

16. Sontag MR, Cunningham JR: Corrections to absorbed dose calculations for tissue inhomogeneities. *Med Phys* 4:431, 1977.

17. Sontag MR, Cunningham JR: The equivalent tissue-air ratio method for making absorbed dose calculations in heterogeneous medium. *Radiology* 129:787, 1978.

18. Sundblom L: Dose planning for irradiation of thorax with cobalt in fixed beam therapy. *Acta Oncol* 3:342, 1965.

19. Young MEJ, Gaylord JD: Experimental test of corrections for tissue inhomogeneities in radiotherapy. *Br J Radiol* 43:349, 1970.

20. Epp ER, Lougheed MN, McKay JW: Ionization build-up in upper respiratory air passages during teletherapy units with cobalt-60 radiation. *Br J Radiol* 31:361, 1958.

21. Epp ER, Boyer AL, Doppke KP: Underdosing of lesions resulting from lack of electronic equilibrium in upper respiratory air cavities irradiated by 10 MV x-ray beams. *Int J Radiat Oncol Biol Phys* 2:613, 1977.

22. Gillin MT, Kline RW, Cox JD. Heterogeneity measurements and calculations in the absence of complete build-up (abstr). *23rd Annual American Society of Therapeutic Radiologists Meeting;* 1981.

23. Nilsson B, Schnell PO: Build-up studies at air cavities measured with thin thermoluminescent dosimeters. *Acta Radiol (Ther)* 15:427, 1976.

24. Spiers FW: Effective atomic number and energy absorption in tissues. *Br J Radiol* 19:52, 1946.

25. Spiers FW: Dosage in irradiated soft tissue and bone. *Br J Radiol* 24:365, 1951.

26. Badcock PC: Has CT scanning a role to play in radiotherapy planning? Computer dose calculations. *Br J Radiol* 55:434, 1982.

27. Cassell KJ, Hobday PA, Parker RP: The implementation of a generalized Batho inhomogeneity correction for radiotherapy planning with direct use of CT numbers. *Phys Med Biol* 26:825, 1981.

28. Fullerton GD, Sewchand W, Payne JT, Levitt SH: CT determination of parameters for inhomogeneity corrections in radiation therapy of the esophagus. *Radiology* 124:167, 1978.

29. Giese RA, McCullough EC: The use of CT scanners in megavoltage photon-beam therapy planning. *Radiology* 124:133, 1977.

30. Hogstrom KR, Mills MD, Almond PR: Electron beam dose calculations. *Phys Med Biol* 26:445, 1981.

31. Mira JG, Fullerton GD, Ezekiel J, Potter JL: Evaluation of computed tomography numbers for treatment planning of lung cancer. *Int J Radiat Oncol Biol Phys* 8:1625, 1982.

32. Mohan R, Chui C, Miller D, Laughlin JS: Use of computerized tomography in dose calculations for radiation treatment planning. *CT* 5:273, 1981.

33. Parker RP, Hobday PA, Cassell KJ: The direct use of CT numbers in radiotherapy dosage calculations for inhomogeneous media. *Phys Med Biol* 24:802, 1979.

34. Sontag MR, Battista JJ, Bronskill MJ, Cunningham JR: Implications of computed tomography for inhomogeneity corrections in photon beam dose calculations. *Radiology* 124:143, 1977.

35. Van Dyk J, Battista JJ, Rider WD: Half-body radiotherapy: The use of computed tomography to determine the dose to lung. *Int J Radiat Oncol Biol Phys* 6:463, 1980.

36. Van Dyk J, Keane JJ, Rider WD: Lung density as measured by computed tomography: Implications for radiotherapy. *Int J Radiat Oncol Biol Phys* 8:1363, 1982.

37. Van Dyk J: Lung dose calculations using computerized tomography: Is there a need for pixel based procedures? *Int J Radiat Oncol Biol Phys* 9:1035, 1983.

38. Wong JW, Henkelman RM: A new approach to CT pixel-based photon dose calculations in heterogeneous media. *Med Phys* 10:199, 1983.

39. Orton CG, Mondalek PM, Spicka JT, et al. Lung corrections in photon beam treatment planning: Are we ready? *Int J Radiat Oncol Biol Phys* 10:2191, 1984.

40. Orton CG, Herskovic A: A proposal for universal introduction of lung corrections. *Int J Radiat Oncol Biol Phys* 10:2383, 1984.

41. Holt JG, Laughlin JS, Moroney JP: The extension of the concept of tissue air ratios to high energy x-ray beams. *Radiology* 96:437, 1970.

42. Karzmark CJ, Dewbert A, Loevinger R: Tissue-phantom ratios—An aid to treatment planning. *Br J Radiol* 38:158, 1965.

43. Tatcher M: A method for varying the effective angle of wedge filters. *Radiology* 97:132, 1970.

44. Zwicker RD, Shahabi S, Wu A, Sternick ES: Effective wedge angles for 6-MV wedges. *Med Phys* 12:347, 1985.

45. Dutreix J, Dutreix A: Film dosimetry of high energy electrons. *Ann NY Acad Sci* 161:33, 1969.

46. Hettinger G, Svensson H: Photographic film for determination of isodose from betatron electron radiation. *Acta Radiol* 5:74, 1967.

47. Khan FM, Moore VC, Levitt SH: Field shaping in electron beam therapy. *Br J Radiol* 49:883, 1976.

48. Khan FM: *The Physics of Radiation Therapy,* 2d ed. Baltimore: Williams & Wilkins, 1994.

49. Khan FM, Doppke KP, Hogstrom KR, et al: Clinical electron-beam dosimetry: Report of American Association of Physicists in Medicine Radiation Therapy Committee Task Group No. 25. *Med Phys* 18:73, 1991.

50. Loevinger R, Karzmark CJ, Weissbluth M: Radiation dosimetry with high energy electrons. *Radiology* 77:906, 1961.

51. McGinley PH, McLaren JR, Barnett BR: Small electron beams in radiation therapy. *Radiology* 131:231, 1979.

52. Niroomand-Rad A, Gillin MT, Kline RW, Grimm DF: Film dosimetry of small electron beams for routine radiotherapy planning. *Med Phys* 13:416, 1986.

53. Orton CG, Bagne F: *Practical Aspects of Electron Beam Treatment Planning.* New York: American Institute of Physics, 1978.

4

Dose Calculation for External Beams—Part I

The dose calculations in this chapter are explained with the assumption that the reader has read and fully understood Chap. 3.

Some of the factors used in the dose calculations in this chapter may be eliminated depending on how the available data are presented. For example, it is customary to present the dose rate for a cobalt-60 unit for a 10×10 cm field and then have a table of area factors for other field sizes. An area factor is the ratio of the dose rate for a given field size to that of a reference field size, usually 10×10 cm. The dose rate for a reference field multiplied by the area factor for the treated field gives the dose rate for the treated field. On the other hand, the dose rates may have been measured and tabulated for a large number of field sizes, which eliminates the need for an area factor. Likewise, the cGy/MU may have been set so that 1 cGy is the same as 1 MU for a reference field, which again, is usually a 10×10 cm field.

The results of a survey including 94 institutions showed that the methods of calculating treatment time and MU settings varied widely among the participants.[1] The terminology describing the various factors used in the calculation also differed among the institutions. It would be impossible to illustrate the many different methods that could be used to calculate treatment time and MU settings in this short description, however, with an understanding of the underlying concept, readers can later choose to use the method of their own institution.

In this text, the reference dose rate and cGy/MU (dose rate$_{ref}$ or cGy/MU$_{ref}$) are for a 10×10 cm field.

The two most commonly used techniques in treating patients are with a fixed source-surface distance (SSD) or a fixed source-axis distance (SAD). The SSD method requires moving the patient between treatment of each field to adjust the SSD so that it is the same for every field—with obvious inconvenience, delay, and lack of precision. The methods used in calculating dose in the patient are different in these two techniques. Percentage depth dose (%DD), which requires that the SSD be constant, is used in the SSD technique, while tissue-air ratio (TAR), tissue-phantom ratio (TPR), or tissue-maximum ratio (TMR), which require a fixed SAD, is used in the SAD technique. The text that follows below gives examples of dose calculation on the central axis for square fields using both methods.*

FIXED SOURCE-SURFACE DISTANCE TECHNIQUE

The technique using fixed SSD and %DD is practical when single fields are used. Single fields are not recommended for deep-seated lesions because of the fall-off of dose with depth and the resulting dose gradient through the tissues. Whether one can use a single-field or multiple fields to treat a tumor must be determined for each situation. The criteria are

1. Depth of maximum dose (surface or D$_{max}$)
2. Dose gradient throughout the tumor
3. Availability of other alternatives

In this section, typical dose calculations are shown using a fixed SSD and a variety of beam energies.

* Data tables used in the dose calculations are labeled A.1 to A.8 and can be found in the Appendix.

DOSE CALCULATION AT DEPTH OF MAXIMUM DOSE

Treatment of shallow lesions through a single field is sometimes desirable. The dose is then prescribed either at D$_{max}$ or at an appropriate depth. Shallow lesions are best treated using beams of low penetrating power such as superficial, lower orthovoltage, or electron beams. Single-field treatment, using higher-energy beams, is considered in this text only for the purpose of dose calculation.

In the majority of instances, dose calculation consists of finding the required treatment time or the number of monitor units needed to deliver the prescribed treatment. However, in some instances it is necessary to find what dose was delivered during a certain period of time or while a certain number of monitor units were given. This could happen, for example, when the treatment was interrupted prior to completion, either because the patient became ill or because the machine failed. In these situations, it is necessary to determine what dose was in fact delivered. In the next few examples, we will calculate *both* the required treatment time, or MU, and what dose was delivered during the treatment.

Superficial Beams. Consider the treatment of a 5×5 cm field using a beam with a half-value thickness (HVT) of 2 mmCu. The SSD is 50 cm and the dose rate without the patient present, sometimes referred to as *in air*, is 68 cGy/min at 50-cm distance. The backscatter factor is 1.145.

To find the treatment time for the prescribed dose:

$$\text{Time} = \frac{\text{prescribed dose}}{\text{dose rate in air} \times \text{backscatter}} \quad (4.1)$$

The prescription is for 200 cGy at D$_{max}$, which in this case is the surface. The treatment time is found from

$$\frac{200}{68 \times 1.145} = 2.57 \text{ min (2 min, 34 s)}$$

The dose rate at the surface in the above expression is found as follows:

Dose rate at the surface =

time $\times$ dose rate in air $\times$ backscatter factor   (4.2)

1 min $\times$ 68 $\times$ 1.145 cGy = 77.9 cGy/min

Electron Beams.   Consider the same treatment as in the above example, but this time using a 6-MeV electron beam. The SSD is 95 cm and the dose rate$_{ref}$ for a 10 $\times$ 10 cm field is 1.0; for a 5 $\times$ 5 cm field, it is 0.643. The prescription is 200 cGy at D_{max}, which is at 1.5-cm of depth for the 6-MeV electron beam.

To find the MU necessary to deliver the prescribed dose at D_{max}:

$$MU = \frac{\text{prescribed dose}}{\text{cGy/MU (field}_{ref}) \times \text{cGy/MU (tx. field)}} \quad (4.3)$$

where tx.field = treatment field.

To deliver 200 cGy at D_{max}, the required MU would therefore be

$$\frac{200}{1.0 \times 0.643} = 311 \text{ MU}$$

The cGy/MU at D_{max} in the above expression is found from

$$cGy/MU = MU \times cGy/MU \text{ (field}_{ref})$$
$$\times cGy/MU \text{ (tx. field)} \quad (4.4)$$

1 MU $\times$ 0.643 cGy = 0.643 cGy/MU at D_{max}

Cobalt-60 Beams.   Consider the same treatment as in the previous examples but using a cobalt-60 unit at 80-cm SSD. The dose rate$_{ref}$ at D_{max} is 114 cGy/min for a 10 $\times$ 10 cm field. The area factor for a 5 $\times$ 5 cm field is 0.92.

To find the treatment time necessary to deliver the prescribed dose at D_{max}:

$$Time = \frac{\text{prescribed dose}}{\text{dose rate}_{ref} \times \text{area factor}} \quad (4.5)$$

To deliver 200 cGy at D_{max}, which for cobalt 60 is at 0.5-cm depth, the treatment time would be

$$\frac{200}{114 \times 0.92} = 1.91 \text{ min (1 min, 55 s)}$$

The dose rate at D_{max} in the above expression is found as follows:

$$\text{Dose rate at } D_{max} = \text{time} \times \text{dose rate}_{ref}$$
$$\times \text{area factor} \quad (4.6)$$

1.0 min $\times$ 114 $\times$ 0.92 = 104.9 cGy/min

Linear Accelerator Beams.   Consider the same treatment as in the previous examples but using a 4-MV photon beam at 80-cm SSD. The dose rate$_{ref}$ is 1.0 cGy/MU for a 10 $\times$ 10 cm field. The cGy/MU factor for a 5 $\times$ 5 cm field is 0.945.

To find the MU necessary to deliver prescribed D_{max} dose:

$$MU = \frac{\text{prescribed dose}}{\text{cGy/MU}} \quad (4.7)$$

To deliver 200 cGy at D_{max}, which for 4 MV is at 1-cm depth, the number of MU would be

$$\frac{200}{0.945} = 212 \text{ MU}$$

The dose rate at D_{max} in the above expression was found as follows:

$$\text{Dose rate at } D_{max} = MU \times cGy/MU \quad (4.8)$$

1 MU $\times$ 0.945 = 0.945 cGy/MU

DOSE CALCULATION AT A DEPTH FOR A SINGLE FIELD

In the following examples, the dose prescribed for treatment of a tumor at 5-cm depth is calculated using the same variables as in the previous section except that the field size is increased to 8 $\times$ 8 cm.

Superficial Beams.   Using a beam with a HVT of 2 mmCu, 50-cm SSD, and an 8 $\times$ 8 cm field, the dose rate without the patient present is 68 cGy/min. Note that the dose rate without the patient present is the same as for the 5 $\times$ 5 cm field used in an earlier example. The backscatter factor, however, is 1.250, which is considerably higher than for the 5 $\times$ 5 cm field. The %DD at 5-cm depth for an 8 $\times$ 8 cm field at 50-cm SSD is 64.9 percent. For each 100 cGy delivered at D_{max}, the dose at 5-cm depth is 64.9 cGy.

The treatment time necessary to deliver the prescribed dose is found from

$$\text{Time} = \frac{\text{prescribed dose}}{\text{dose rate in air} \times \text{BSF} \times \%\text{DD}} \quad (4.9)$$

To deliver 200 cGy at 5-cm depth, the treatment time would be

$$\frac{200 \times 100}{68 \times 1.250 \times 64.9} = 3.63 \text{ min (3 min, 38 s)}$$

As a check, we note that the dose delivered at a depth in the above example is

$$\text{Depth dose} = \text{time} \times \text{dose rate in air}$$
$$\times \text{BSF} \times \%\text{DD} \quad (4.10)$$

$$3.63 \text{ min} \times 68 \times 1.250 \times 64.9/100 = 200 \text{ cGy}$$

which is correct.

Electron Beams.   In this example, a 14-MeV electron beam is used. The SSD is 95 cm and the field size is 8 × 8 cm. The dose rate$_{ref}$ is 0.953 cGy/MU for a 10 × 10 cm field. The area factor for an 8 × 8 cm field is 0.995 and the percentage depth dose at 5-cm depth is 80 percent. (Note that the cGy/MU for the 14-MeV electron beam is different from that of the 6-MeV electron beam used in an earlier example; the area factors vary with field size, cones, and energies.)

The MU necessary to deliver the prescribed dose at depth is found as follows:

$$\text{MU} = \frac{\text{prescribed dose}}{\text{cGy/MU} \times \text{area factor} \times \%\text{DD}} \quad (4.11)$$

To deliver 200 cGy at 5-cm depth (80 percent isodose line), the number of MU would be

$$\frac{200 \times 100}{0.953 \times 0.995 \times 80} = 264 \text{ MU}$$

The dose delivered at a depth in the above example is found from

$$\text{Depth dose} = \text{MU} \times \text{cGy/MU}$$
$$\times \text{area factor} \times \%\text{DD} \quad (4.12)$$

or

$$264 \text{ MU} \times 0.953 \times 0.995 \times (80/100) = 200 \text{ cGy}$$

Cobalt-60 Beams.   Using a cobalt-60 unit at 80-cm SSD and an 8 × 8 cm field, 200 cGy is to be delivered at 5-cm depth. The dose rate$_{ref}$ for a 10 × 10 cm field is 114 cGy/min. The area factor is 0.985 for a 8 × 8 cm field and the percentage depth dose from Table A.1 is 77.4 percent. (Note that the dose rate is unchanged from the example of the previous cobalt-60 beam calculation, but the area factor for this larger field is increased.)

The treatment time necessary to deliver the prescribed dose at a depth is found from

$$\text{Time} = \frac{\text{prescribed dose}}{\text{dose rate}_{ref} \times \text{area factor} \times \%\text{DD}} \quad (4.13)$$

To deliver 200 cGy, the treatment time would be

$$\frac{200 \times 100}{114 \times 0.985 \times 77.4} = 2.30 \text{ min} \quad (2 \text{ min, } 18 \text{ s})$$

The dose delivered at a depth in the above example is found from

$$\text{Dose} = \text{time} \times \text{dose rate}_{ref} \times \text{area factor} \times \%\text{DD} \quad (4.14)$$

$$2.30 \times 114 \times 0.985 \times (77.4/100) = 200 \text{ cGy}$$

Linear Accelerator Beams.   Using a 4-MV photon beam at 80-cm SSD and an 8 × 8 cm field, 200 cGy is to be delivered at 5-cm depth. The cGy/MU$_{ref}$ is 1.0 for a 10 × 10 cm field and 0.99 for an 8 × 8 cm field. From Table A.2, the %DD is 81.8.

The MU necessary to deliver the prescribed dose at a depth is found from

$$\text{MU} = \frac{\text{prescribed dose}}{\text{cGy/MU} \times \%\text{DD}} \quad (4.15)$$

To deliver 200 cGy, the required number of MU would be

$$\frac{200 \times 100}{0.99 \times 81.8} = 247 \text{ MU}$$

The dose delivered at a depth in the above example is found from

$$\text{Depth dose} = \text{MU} \times \text{cGy/MU} \times \%\text{DD} \quad (4.16)$$

$$247 \text{ MU} \times 0.99 \times (81.8/100) = 200 \text{ cGy}$$

DOSE CALCULATION FOR PARALLEL OPPOSED BEAMS WITH EQUAL WEIGHTING

Parallel opposed beams are the most commonly used field arrangement. This technique is best suited for situations where reasonable dose uniformity throughout the target volume is desired. This section deals with the dose calculation of this and other multiple field techniques. Superficial and electron beams are not suited for multiple-field arrangements, so the dose calculations in this section are limited to those of cobalt-60 beams and linear accelerators.

Equal weighting implies equal dose somewhere. In a fixed-SSD technique, it is customary to normalize the entrance dose of each field at D_{max} to 100% and to apply the weighting factor of each beam at this point. Weighting factors are usually expressed as ratios of the normalized dose at D_{max} from each field. Therefore, in an equally weighted parallel opposed field arrangement using a fixed-SSD technique, the weighting would be 1 to 1 (Fig. 4.1).

Cobalt-60 Beams.   In this example, it is assumed that 200 cGy is prescribed at middepth of a 20-cm-thick patient. Two equally weighted, parallel opposed 15 × 15 cm fields are used at 80-cm SSD. The dose rate$_{ref}$ for a 10 × 10 cm field is 114 cGy/min. The area factor for a 15 × 15 cm field is 1.04 and the %DD at 10-cm depth from Table A.1 is 58.3.

The treatment time is found from

$$\text{Time} = \frac{\text{prescribed dose}}{\text{dose rate}_{ref} \times \text{area factor} \times \%\text{DD}} \quad (4.17)$$

In this example, each field must deliver an equal D_{max} dose. The tumor dose (TD) and the D_{max} dose will be the same for both fields, since all variables are identical.

The treatment time necessary to deliver 100 cGy at 10-cm depth is

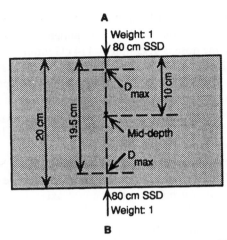

Figure 4.1   Parallel opposed beams using 80-cm SSD and weighted equally.

$$\frac{100 \times 100}{114 \times 1.04 \times 58.3} = 1.45 \text{ min} \quad (1 \text{ min, } 27 \text{ s})$$

The D_{max} dose is found from

$$\text{Dose} = \text{time} \times \text{dose rate}_{ref} \times \text{area factor} \quad (4.18)$$

so

$$1.45 \times 114 \times 1.04 = 172 \text{ cGy per field}$$

Linear Accelerator Beams.   Using the same example as above but with 4-MV photon beams, the calculation is very similar. The cGy/MU for a 15 × 15 cm field is 1.03 and the %DD from Table A.2 is 62.4.

The MU necessary to deliver 100 cGy at 10-cm depth is

$$\frac{100 \times 100}{1.03 \times 62.4} = 156 \text{ MU}$$

CALCULATING ENTRANCE DOSE AND EXIT DOSE FROM PARALLEL OPPOSED BEAMS WITH EQUAL WEIGHTING

Using the same treatment variables as in the previous cobalt-60 example, the total dose (entrance and exit) at the depth of D_{max} is calculated as follows.

Field A (Fig. 4.1) delivers 100 percent at D_{max}. Therefore, in the cobalt-60 treatment, using Eq. (4.18), the dose is 1.45 min $\times$ 114 cGy/min $\times$ 1.04, or 172 cGy. The %DD at 19.5-cm depth (the patient's thickness minus 0.5 cm, which is the depth of maximum dose for cobalt 60) from field B is only 31.3 percent of the D_{max} dose (Table A.1). Using Eq. (4.18), the exit dose from field B is 1.45 $\times$ 114 $\times$ 1.04 $\times$ 31.3%, which is 54 cGy.

The total dose at D_{max} is therefore 172 + 54 = 226 cGy. The dose can, in a similar manner, be calculated at any point on the central axis of parallel opposed fields.

Dose Ratios. In the previous example, it was found that the maximum dose was 226 cGy, while the midplane dose was 200 cGy.

The ratio of these two doses is found by

$$\text{Dose ratio} = \frac{\text{maximum dose}}{\text{midplane dose}} \quad (4.19)$$

so the ratio of the entrance-exit dose and the midplane dose in the previous example is

$$\frac{226}{200} = 1.13$$

Multiplying the midplane dose by the ratio yields the maximum dose. If 4000 cGy is delivered at the midplane in the patient, the maximum dose is

$$4000 \times 1.13 = 4520 \text{ cGy}$$

DOSE CALCULATION FOR PARALLEL OPPOSED BEAMS WITH UNEQUAL WEIGHTING

Unequal weighting in a fixed-SSD technique implies that a different dose is delivered at D_{max} of each field.

The result is a higher dose in the tissue near the entrance of the favored field and a lower dose in the tissue near the entrance of the opposing field.

In the following example, a patient is treated for a parotid tumor using parallel opposed 10 $\times$ 10 cm fields and 80-cm SSD. The patient's thickness is 14 cm and the fields are weighted 2 to 1 favoring the right side. In this treatment, 4-MV photon beams are used, and the prescription is 200 cGy per fraction calculated at the patient's midline (Fig. 4.2).

The cGy/MU is 1.0 and the %DD at 7-cm depth from Table A.2 is 73.0 percent. Since the fields are identical and the dose is prescribed at the midline, the total MU required to deliver 200 cGy is found using Eq. (4.15).

$$\frac{200 \times 100}{1.0 \times 73.0} = 274 \text{ MU}$$

Two-thirds of this dose is to be delivered from the patient's right side and one-third from the left side; therefore

$$\text{Right side: } \frac{2 \times 274}{3} = 183 \text{ MU}$$

$$\text{Left side: } \frac{1 \times 274}{3} = 91 \text{ MU}$$

In the following example, the same treatment is given, but the dose is prescribed at 5-cm depth from the patient's right side (Fig. 4.2).

Using Table A.2, the %DD from the patient's right side, at 5-cm depth, is 82.4 percent; from the left side, at 9-cm depth, it is 64.3 percent.

Since the D_{max} dose is weighted 2 to 1 and the tumor dose from each field is unknown, the com-

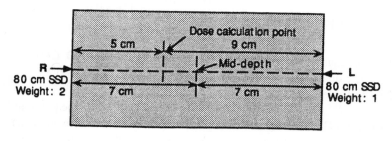

Figure 4.2 Parallel opposed beams using 80-cm SSD and weighted 2 to 1, favoring the right side.

bined MU required to deliver 200 cGy must be calculated first. The average %DD is found from

$$\frac{(82.4 \times 2) + 64.3}{3} = 76.4$$

The %DD from the right side is multiplied by 2, since the weighting from this side is such that the D_{max} dose is 200 percent.

The combined D_{max} dose is found from

$$D_{max} = \frac{\text{prescribed dose}}{\text{cGy/MU} \times \text{average \%DD}} \quad (4.20)$$

so

$$\frac{200 \times 100}{1.0 \times 76.4} = 264 \text{ MU}$$

(cGy equals MU in this example, since the cGy/MU is 1.0.)

Two-thirds of this dose is delivered from the patient's right side and one-third from the left side:

Right side: $\dfrac{2 \times 262}{3} = 175$ MU (cGy at D_{max})

Left side: $\dfrac{1 \times 262}{3} = 87$ MU (cGy at D_{max})

The tumor dose delivered from each side is found as follows:

$$\text{Tumor dose} = \text{MU} \times \text{cGy/MU} \times \text{\%DD} \quad (4.21)$$

so the tumor dose from the patient's right side is

$$175 \text{ MU} \times 1.0 \times 82.4\% = 144 \text{ cGy}$$

and the tumor dose from the patient's left side is

$$87 \text{ MU} \times 1.0 \times 64.3\% = 56 \text{ cGy}$$

CALCULATING ENTRANCE DOSE AND EXIT DOSE FROM PARALLEL OPPOSED BEAMS WITH UNEQUAL WEIGHTING

In an unequally weighted parallel opposed field arrangement, the dose at the depth of D_{max} of each field is different.

Using the parameters in the previous example, the dose at D_{max} of each field is found as follows.

The right field (R) is weighted by a factor of 2, and the left field (L) is weighted by 1. The dose at D_{max} of field R is found from

Entrance dose + exit dose
$$= (\text{MU}_R \times \text{cGy/MU}_R \times \text{\%DD}_R)$$
$$+ (\text{MU}_L \times \text{cGy/MU}_L \times \text{\%DD}_L) \quad (4.22)$$

Via field R, 175 MU is delivered; the cGy/MU is 1.0 and the %DD is 100. The %DD at 13-cm depth from L (patient's thickness minus depth of D_{max}) is 49.8 percent (Table A.2). Via field L, 87 MU is delivered, and the cGy/MU is 1.0. Using Eq. (4.22), the dose at D_{max} of field R is

$$(175 \times 1.0 \times 100/100) + (87 \times 1.0 \times 49.8/100)$$
$$= 218 \text{ cGy}$$

The dose at D_{max} of field L is found by

Entrance dose + exit dose
$$= (\text{MU}_L \times \text{cGy/MU}_L \times \text{\%DD}_L)$$
$$+ (\text{MU}_R \times \text{cGy/MU}_R \times \text{\%DD}_R) \quad (4.23)$$

The dose at D_{max} of field L is therefore

$$(87 \times 1.0 \times 100/100)$$
$$+ (175 \times 1.0 \times 49.8/100) = 174 \text{ cGy}$$

This shows a gradient of dose throughout the volume from a maximum of 218 cGy on the patient's right side to 174 cGy on the left side.

DOSE CALCULATION FOR MULTIPLE BEAMS WITH EQUAL WEIGHTING

Many treatment plans utilize multiple fields directed at a common target. Although such treatment plans are best delivered via isocentric techniques, for the purpose of this exercise, it is assumed to be delivered via a fixed-SSD technique.

Composite isodose distributions are calculated and the dose is usually prescribed at an isodose line that encompasses the target volume. In this example, it is assumed that four equally weighted fields are used. Each field is 10×15 cm, the SSD is 80 cm, and a cobalt-60 unit is used to deliver the treatment. The dose rate$_{ref}$ at D_{max} for a 10×10 cm field is 114 cGy/min and the area factor is 1.035. The prescribed dose is 200 cGy at the 190 percent line (Fig. 4.3). Since the D_{max} dose is the same for all four fields and the combined %DD (190 percent) is the result of four 100 percent D_{max} doses, it is acceptable to assume that one-fourth of 190 percent (47.5 percent) is delivered from each field. That, of course, is not true for all points along this isodose line.

The average %DD in a multiple-field treatment plan can be found from

$$\frac{\text{Total \%DD (isodose line)}}{\text{Number of 100\% } D_{max} \text{ doses}} \quad (4.24)$$

The required treatment time per field can be found from one of two methods:

Treatment time per field

$$= \frac{\text{prescribed dose}}{\text{\% isodose line} \times \text{dose rate} \times \text{area factor}} \quad (4.25)$$

$$\frac{200 \times 100}{190 \times 114 \times 1.035} = 0.89 \text{ min/field (53 s)}$$

or

Treatment time per field

$$= \frac{\text{prescribed dose per field}}{\text{average \%DD} \times \text{dose rate} \times \text{area factor}} \quad (4.26)$$

$$\frac{50 \times 100}{47.5 \times 114 \times 1.035} = 0.89 \text{ min/field (53 s)}$$

The D_{max} dose per field is found from either

$$D_{max} \text{ dose} = \frac{\text{total prescribed dose}}{\text{isodose line}}$$

or

$$\quad (4.27)$$

$$\frac{\text{dose per field}}{\text{average \%DD}}$$

so

$$\frac{200 \times 100}{190} = 105 \text{ cGy} \quad \text{or} \quad \frac{50 \times 100}{47.5} = 105 \text{ cGy}$$

DOSE CALCULATION FOR MULTIPLE BEAMS WITH UNEQUAL WEIGHTING

In the next variation of the previous example, the same treatment is delivered, but it is assumed that two fields are weighted twice as heavily as the other two. The prescribed dose is 200 cGy at the 205 percent line (Fig. 4.3). The total D_{max} dose for all fields combined is still 400 percent, but it is now distributed so that two fields are given one-third each and the other two one-sixth each of the combined D_{max} dose.

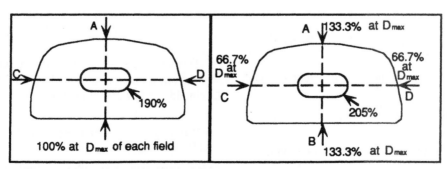

Figure 4.3 Four equally weighted beams normalized to 100% at D_{max} of each field *(left)* result in a total %DD of 190 percent, as indicated. The same field arrangement is used *(right)*, but here two of the fields are weighted twice as heavily as the other two. The total %DD is 205 percent, as indicated.

Table 4.1   Setup Parameters for 3-Field Pancreas Treatment

Field	Anterior	Right Lateral	Left Lateral
SSD	80 cm	80 cm	80 cm
Beam energy	4 MV	4 MV	4 MV
Field size	12 × 8 cm	8 × 8 cm	8 × 8 cm
Equivalent square field	9.5 cm²	8 cm²	8 cm²
Isodose line	230%	230%	230%
Weighting factor	2.0	1.0	1.0
Tray factor	0.96	1.0	1.0
Wedge factor	1.0	0.71	0.71
cGy/MU	0.995	0.98	0.98

The combined D_{max} dose required for this treatment is found from

$$\text{Total } D_{max} \text{ dose} = \frac{\text{prescribed dose}}{\text{average \%DD}} \quad (4.28)$$

The average %DD is found from

$$\text{Average \%DD} = \frac{\text{isodose line}}{\text{number of 100\% } D_{max} \text{ doses}} \quad (4.29)$$

so

$$\frac{205}{4} = 51.3\%$$

and the combined D_{max} dose is

$$\frac{200 \times 100}{51.3} = 390 \text{ cGy}$$

$$\text{Two fields will receive } \frac{1 \times 390}{3} = 130 \text{ cGy each}$$

$$\text{Two fields will receive } \frac{1 \times 390}{6} = 65 \text{ cGy each}$$

In this particular example, the total %DD is higher than in the plan using equal weighting because the two fields with the heavier weighting deliver a higher %DD than the other two fields.

In the following example, a slightly different approach is used. A patient is treated for carcinoma of the pancreas using a three-field technique (Table 4.1). The anterior field is 12 × 8 cm with a small corner of the field blocked out. The right and left lateral fields are 8 × 8 cm and a 30° wedge is used in each field. All fields are treated at 80-cm SSD using a 4-MV photon beam. The anterior field is weighted by a factor of 2 and each lateral field by a factor of 1 (Fig. 4.4).

The prescribed dose is 200 cGy along the 230 percent isodose line. The treatment plan was calculated by entering 200% at D_{max} of the anterior field and 100% for each of the lateral fields. The average %DD is therefore 230/4 or 57.5 percent of each 100 percent D_{max} entrance dose. The combined D_{max} dose is therefore

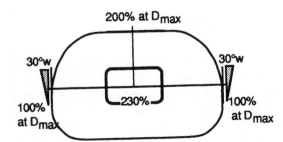

Figure 4.4 A three-field technique with anterior field weighted twice as heavily as each lateral field. The combined %DD is 230 percent, which results from a total D_{max} dose of 400 percent.

$$\text{Combined } D_{max} \text{ dose} = \frac{\text{prescribed dose}}{\text{average \%DD}}$$

$$\frac{200 \times 100}{57.5} = 348 \text{ cGy}$$ (4.30)

Two-fourths or one-half of this dose is to be delivered via the anterior field,

or $$\frac{1 \times 348}{2} = 174 \text{ cGy}$$

One-fourth of the dose at D_{max} is to be delivered via each of the lateral fields:

$$\frac{1 \times 348}{4} = 87 \text{ cGy}$$

The MU per field necessary to deliver the prescribed dose using correct weighting is found by

$$\text{MU} = \frac{\text{dose rate at } D_{max}}{\text{cGy/MU} \times \text{tray factor} \times \text{wedge factor}}$$ (4.31)

The number of MU from the anterior field is therefore

$$\frac{174}{0.995 \times 0.96 \times 1.0} = 182 \text{ MU}$$

This field has no wedge, so the wedge factor is 1.0 and could be omitted.

The number of MU needed for each of the lateral fields is therefore

$$\frac{87}{0.98 \times 1.0 \times 0.71} = 125 \text{ MU}$$

These fields had no block-supporting tray, so the tray factor is 1.0 and could also be omitted. Transmission factors for beam attenuators that intercept only a portion of a field (bars on the treatment couch and so on) should be used with caution. Tissue under the section of the field that is not intercepted by the attenuator will receive a higher dose, which could result in irreversible injury.

The method used in accomplishing desired weighting becomes very important in calculation of the average %DD at the prescribed isodose line. The average %DD is found by dividing the %DD of the isodose line by the number of 100% D_{max} doses and not by the number of fields.

In the first example of the two plans with unequal weighting, the isodose distribution was for four fields calculated with a combined D_{max} dose of 400 percent. Two fields were weighted twice as heavily as the other two, meaning that of the 400 percent, two-sixths or one-third (133 percent) was given via each of the two favored fields, and one-sixth (66.6 percent) was delivered via each of the other two fields. In the second example, the isodose distribution was calculated using three fields with a combined D_{max} dose of 400 percent. One field was weighted twice as heavily as each of the other two fields. In this case the anterior field received one-half of 400 percent or 200 percent and the other two fields were given 100 percent each. In the second case, the same isodose distribution would be achieved if the anterior field was given a D_{max} dose of 100 percent and the lateral fields 50 percent each. Each isodose line would be reduced by one-half because the total weighted %DD at D_{max} was reduced by one-half, from 400 to 200 percent. In this case, the dose would be prescribed to the 115 percent isodose line and, from Eq. (4.24), the average %DD would be 115/2, or 57.5 percent. Other differences between the two examples are the slight variation in field sizes in the second example and the addition of beam attenuators such as a block-supporting tray and wedges.

DOSE CALCULATION FOR TREATMENTS AT AN EXTENDED DISTANCE

In this example, it is assumed that a single field is used to treat a 6 × 40 cm field at 100-cm SSD. The prescribed dose is 200 cGy at D_{max} using a cobalt-60 unit. The dose rate$_{ref}$ for a 10 × 10 cm field is 114 cGy at 80-cm SSD. The area factor for a 6 × 40 cm field is 1.03. The dose decreases inversely with the square of the distance, so it is necessary to find the inverse square factor (ISF) of the distance at which the equipment was calibrated (80 cm plus the reference depth) and the distance at which the treatment is given (SSD plus reference depth). In this example, the calibration was at 80.5 cm from the source and the dose is to be calculated at D_{max}, which is 100.5 cm from the source.

Using Eq. (3.1), the ISF is found by

$$\left(\frac{80.5}{100.5}\right)^2 = 0.6416$$

To find the treatment time necessary to deliver the prescribed dose at an extended distance:

$$\text{Time} = \frac{\text{prescribed dose}}{\text{dose rate} \times \text{area factor} \times \text{ISF}} \quad (4.32)$$

So to deliver 200 cGy at D_{max} using 100-cm SSD, the treatment time would be

$$\frac{200}{114 \times 1.03 \times 0.6416} = 2.65 \text{ min (2 min, 39 s)}$$

To verify that the inverse square factor was applied correctly, we will do the same calculation, but now *without* the inverse square factor, to make sure that the treatment time just calculated for the larger SSD is in fact longer than at the "normal" SSD. Therefore, to deliver the same treatment at the "normal" SSD, the treatment time is

$$\frac{200}{114 \times 1.03} = 1.70 \quad (1 \text{ min, 42 s})$$

which is shorter, as we expected.

The preceding section can be summarized in one large calculation formula as follows:

MU (time)

$$= \frac{\text{prescribed dose}}{(\%\text{DD}/100) \times [\text{cGy/MU(dose rate}_{\text{ref}})]}$$

$$\times \frac{1}{\text{tray factor} \times \text{wedge factor} \times \text{ISF}} \quad (4.33)$$

FIXED SOURCE-AXIS DISTANCE TECHNIQUE

Dose calculations for treatments using a fixed SAD (often referred to as *SAD treatments*) are primarily used for isocentric treatment techniques but are also well suited for dose calculations at extended distances, since TARs, TPRs, and TMRs are independent of distance. An isocentric technique is impractical when a single field is used, so this section is limited to dose calculations for parallel opposed fields (which can often be carried out very conveniently by SAD methods) and for multiple-field arrangements (which are particularly suited for the SAD method).

DOSE CALCULATION FOR PARALLEL OPPOSED BEAMS WITH EQUAL WEIGHTING

Parallel opposed fields are best treated using an isocentric technique. Since the dose throughout the volume is relatively uniform, it is customary to place the isocenter at middepth between the two entry points. This requires measurement of the patient's thickness, or diameter, in the direction of the beam at the central axis. The isocenter is then set by subtracting one-half of the patient's diameter from the SAD. In a patient who is 22 cm in diameter, using a therapy machine with a 100-cm SAD, the SSD would be (100 cm − 11 cm) = 89 cm. Rotating the gantry 180° would result in 89-cm SSD for the opposing field as well.

Cobalt-60 Beams. In this example, we assume a treatment delivered via equally weighted parallel opposed fields using a cobalt-60 machine. The fields are 17 × 17 cm and the patient's diameter is 18 cm. The dose rate$_{\text{ref}}$ without the patient present for a 10 × 10 cm field is 109 cGy/min. The area factor for a 17 × 17 cm field is 1.056. The TAR at 9-cm depth is 0.799 (Table A.3). The prescription is for 200 cGy to be delivered at middepth.

The treatment time is found from

$$\text{Time} = \frac{\text{prescribed dose}}{\text{dose rate}_{\text{ref}} \times \text{area factor} \times \text{TAR}} \quad (4.34)$$

Since these fields are identical and equally weighted, the calculation for the two fields is the same. The treatment time necessary to deliver 100 cGy at 9-cm depth is

$$\frac{100}{109 \times 1.056 \times 0.799} = 1.09 \text{ min (1 min, 5 s)}$$

Linear Accelerator Beams. In this example, we assume that a treatment is delivered via equally weighted parallel opposed beams using a 10-MV photon beam. The patient is 24 cm in diameter, the SAD is 100 cm, and the fields are 17 × 17 cm (Fig. 4.5). The cGy/MU at D_{max} is 1.03 and the TMR from Table A.5 at 12-cm depth is 0.813.

The number of MU is found from

$$\text{MU} = \frac{\text{prescribed dose}}{\text{cGy/MU} \times \text{TAR}} \quad (4.35)$$

To deliver 100 cGy at 12-cm depth,

$$\frac{100}{1.03 \times 0.813} = 119 \text{ MU}$$

CALCULATING ENTRANCE DOSE AND EXIT DOSE FROM PARALLEL OPPOSED BEAMS WITH EQUAL WEIGHTING

Using the parameters in the previous example, the entrance and exit doses are calculated as follows.

Field A (Fig. 4.5) delivers 100 cGy at the iso-center (12-cm depth). The TMR at D_{max} (2.5-cm depth) is 1.0. The distance at this point is 100 cm minus 9.5 cm (Fig. 4.5), or 90.5 cm. The dose is higher at this point by the ISF at this distance. Using Eq. (3.1), the ISF is

$$\left(\frac{100}{90.5}\right)^2 = 1.2210$$

(Note that the reference point in this calculation is at the isocenter, while in a fixed-SSD technique the reference point typically is at D_{max}.)

The dose at a point on the central axis is found from

Dose = MU × cGy/MU × TMR (TAR or TPR) × ISF

$$(4.36)$$

The dose at D_{max} of field A is then

119 MU × 1.03 × 1.0 × 1.2210 = 150 cGy

The cGy/MU at this distance would be slightly less than 1.03 because the field is smaller, but the shorter distance to the collimator causes somewhat more scatter at this point. In this example, we assumed that these factors cancel and that the cGy/MU is the same at 90.5 and at 100 cm except for the effect of the ISF. The dose at the same point from field B is found from Eq. (4.36).

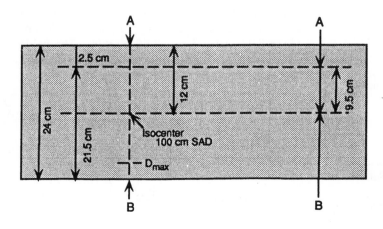

Figure 4.5 Parallel opposed fields using an isocentric technique. The dose is calculated at the isocenter (100-cm SAD) and at D_{max}.

The TMR for field B is 0.616 at 21.5-cm depth (Table A.5).

The distance from field B to this point is 9.5 cm longer than to the isocenter, so it is 109.5 cm (i.e., 100 + 9.5).

Using Eq. (3.1), the inverse square factor for field B is

$$\left(\frac{100}{109.5}\right)^2 = 0.834$$

Using Eq. (4.36), the dose delivered from field B is

$$119 \times 1.03 \times 0.616 \times 0.834 = 63 \text{ cGy}$$

The dose at D_{max} is 150 cGy from field A and 63 cGy from field B, which gives a total dose of 213 cGy, a 6.5 percent higher dose than at middepth.

CALCULATING DOSE FROM PARALLEL OPPOSED BEAMS WITH UNEQUAL WEIGHTING

In an isocentric technique, it is customary to normalize the dose at the isocenter and weight the beam at this point. In this example, where two parallel opposed 4-MV fields are used to treat a right parotid tumor (Fig. 4.6), it is assumed that the isocenter is in the patient's midline. The SAD is 80 cm, and the fields are 9 × 14 cm. The beams are weighted 2 to 1 from the patient's right, meaning that two-thirds of the prescribed dose at the isocenter is delivered via the right field and one-third via the left field. The patient's diameter is 13 cm and the cGy/MU at 80-cm distance is 1.01, without the patient present. From Table A.4, the TAR at 6.5-cm depth is 0.892. The prescription is for 180 cGy to be delivered at the isocenter (Fig. 4.6A).

The MU necessary to deliver this treatment can be found from

$$MU = \frac{\text{fraction of prescribed dose}}{\text{cGy/MU} \times \text{TAR}} \quad (4.37)$$

Since the dose at the isocenter is different for these two fields, they are calculated separately. The MU to be set for the right field would be

$$\frac{2 \times 180}{3 \times 1.01 \times 0.892} = 133 \text{ MU}$$

The MU to be set for the left field would be

$$\frac{1 \times 180}{3 \times 1.01 \times 0.738} = 80 \text{ MU}$$

In the following example, the same treatment is to be delivered, but the isocenter is moved to 4-cm depth from the right side (Fig. 4.6B). The weighting, the field size, and the SAD remain unchanged. The TAR from Table A.4 at 4-cm depth is 0.977 and at 11-cm depth, 0.738. The cGy/MU is 1.01.

The MU necessary to deliver two-thirds of the

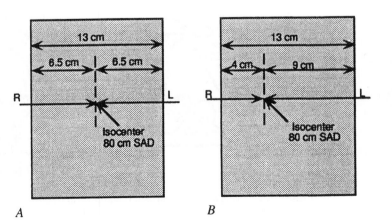

Figure 4.6 Parallel opposed fields using an isocentric technique with the isocenter in the midplane of the patient (A) and at 4-cm depth in tissue (B). The beams are weighted 2 to 1, favoring the right field in both arrangements.

prescribed dose (180 cGy) through the patient's right field at the isocenter is, using Eq. (4.37),

$$\frac{2 \times 180}{3 \times 1.01 \times 0.977} = 122 \text{ MU}$$

The MU necessary to deliver one-third of the prescribed dose through the left field is

$$\frac{1 \times 180}{3 \times 1.01 \times 0.738} = 80 \text{ MU}$$

The calculated number of MU decreased from the right side and increased from the left side when compared with the previous example. Shifting the isocenter farther away from the midplane and suitably weighting the beams could result in the same MU from both fields.

In the next example, a tumor in the posterior aspect of the right lung is treated via parallel opposed oblique fields using 4-MV photon beams (Fig. 4.7). The fields are 10×10 cm, and the SAD is 80 cm. The depth from the anterior skin surface to the isocenter is 23 cm; from the posterior skin surface, it is 7 cm. The TAR at 23-cm depth is 0.410; at 7-cm depth, it is 0.866 (Table A.4). The fields are weighted 2 to 1 favoring the right posterior oblique (RPO) field. The cGy/MU is 1.0. The prescribed dose is 300 cGy at the isocenter.

The MU necessary to deliver two-thirds of the prescribed dose from the right posterior oblique field using Eq. (4.37) is

$$\frac{2 \times 300}{3 \times 1.0 \times 0.866} = 231 \text{ MU}$$

The MU necessary to deliver one-third of the prescribed dose from the left anterior oblique (LAO) field is

$$\frac{1 \times 300}{3 \times 1.0 \times 0.410} = 244 \text{ MU}$$

In this situation, the field with the lower weighting requires a larger number of MU than the field with the higher weighting, due to the greater depth of the isocenter.

CALCULATING ENTRANCE DOSE AND EXIT DOSE FOR PARALLEL OPPOSED BEAMS WITH UNEQUAL WEIGHTING

The entrance and exit doses at D_{max} of each field are calculated as outlined below.

Dose at Depth of Maximum Dose, RPO Field

Entrance Dose. The entrance dose of the RPO field is found by using Eq. (4.36). The MU delivered via the RPO field is 231. The TAR at D_{max} is 1.0 and,

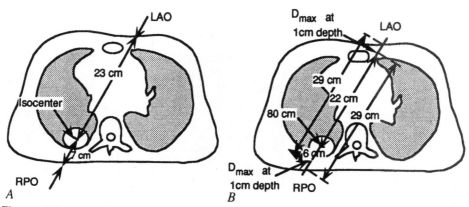

Figure 4.7 Oblique parallel opposed beams used in treatment of a posterior lung lesion. The dose is calculated at the isocenter *(A)* and at D_{max} of each field *(B)*.

using Eq. (3.1), the ISF is

$$\left(\frac{80}{80-6}\right)^2 = 1.1687$$

The entrance dose of the RPO field is therefore

$$231\ \text{MU} \times 1.0 \times 1.1687 = 270\ \text{cGy}$$

Exit Dose. The exit dose of the LAO field is found by using Eq. (4.36). The MU delivered via the LAO field is 244, the TAR at 29 cm (Fig. 4.7B) is 0.305, and the ISF is

$$\left(\frac{80}{80+6}\right)^2 = 0.8653$$

The exit dose from the LAO field at D_{max} of the RPO field is therefore

$$244\ \text{MU} \times 1.0 \times 0.305 \times 0.8653 = 64\ \text{cGy}$$

The total dose at D_{max} of the RPO field is then 270 cGy plus 64 cGy, which is 334 cGy.

Dose at Depth of Maximum Dose, LAO Field

Entrance Dose. The entrance dose of the LAO field is found from Eq. (4.36). The MU delivered via the LAO field is 244, the TAR at D_{max} is 1.0, and using Eq. (3.1), the ISF (Fig. 4.7B) is

$$\left(\frac{80}{80-22}\right)^2 = 1.9025$$

Using Eq. (4.36), the entrance dose at D_{max} of the LAO field is

$$244 \times 1.0 \times 1.0 \times 1.9025 = 464\ \text{cGy}$$

Exit Dose. The exit dose of the RPO field is also found from Eq. (4.36). The MU delivered via the RPO field is 231, the TAR at 29-cm depth (Fig. 4.7B) is 0.305, and the ISF is

$$\left(\frac{80}{80+22}\right)^2 = 0.6151$$

Using Eq. (4.36), the exit dose of the LAO field is

$$231 \times 1.0 \times 0.305 \times 0.6151 = 43\ \text{cGy}$$

The total dose at D_{max} of the LAO field is therefore 507 cGy (i.e., 464 cGy + 43 cGy).

The doses delivered by each field at each point are as shown in Table 4.2.

It is obvious from this example that when the isocenter is offset away from middepth, the weighting factor must be carefully selected to avoid very high doses in either D_{max} region. In this example, equal weighting would further increase the dose at D_{max} in the anterior oblique field and decrease the dose at D_{max} of the posterior oblique field. Increasing the weighting factor on the posterior oblique field would reduce the difference.

A general rule for selecting the weighting factor is to find the ratio of the TAR of each field and apply a similar ratio to the weighting factor. To achieve optimal dose uniformity between the two entrance points, the field with the highest TAR should be favored.

DOSE CALCULATION FOR MULTIPLE BEAMS WITH EQUAL WEIGHTING

Treatment plans consisting of multiple fields are best delivered using an isocentric technique. The dose is

Table 4.2 Dose Summary for Opposed Oblique Fields in Lung Treatment

Dose Calculation Point	RPO Field, cGy 231 MU	LAO Field, cGy 244 MU	Total Dose, cGy
Isocenter	200	100	300
D_{max}, RPO	270	64	334
D_{max}, LAO	43	464	507

customarily normalized at the isocenter, and the dose is prescribed to an isodose line encompassing the target volume.

In this example, a patient is treated via a four-field technique using a 4-MV linear accelerator. The isocenter is at 80 cm and each field is 10×15 cm. The prescribed dose is 200 cGy at the 95 percent isodose line (Fig. 4.8). The cGy/MU is 1.025 for each field and the dose is normalized to 100 percent at the isocenter. The TAR for fields A and B is 0.793; for fields C and D, it is 0.645.

The MU necessary to deliver this treatment is found from

$$MU = \frac{\text{prescribed dose per field}}{\text{cGy/MU} \times \text{TAR} \times \text{isodose line}/100} \quad (4.38)$$

Using Eq. (4.38), the MU necessary to deliver the prescribed dose from fields A and B is

$$\frac{50}{1.025 \times 0.793 \times 0.95} = 65 \text{ MU per field}$$

and the MU necessary to deliver the prescribed dose from fields C and D is

$$\frac{50}{1.025 \times 0.645 \times 0.95} = 80 \text{ MU per field}$$

The difference in the number of MU is due to the difference in the TAR. All other factors are the same for all fields.

DOSE CALCULATION FOR MULTIPLE BEAMS WITH UNEQUAL WEIGHTING

In this example, the same field arrangement is assumed, but fields A and B are weighted by a factor of 2 and fields C and D are weighted by a factor of 1 (Fig. 4.8). In this plan, the dose is normalized to 100 percent at the isocenter. Fields A and B are weighted by a factor of 0.333 (one-third) and fields C and D by 0.167 (one-sixth). One-third of 200 cGy is delivered at the isocenter from each of fields A and B and one-sixth of the prescribed dose is delivered via each of fields C and D.

The MU necessary for each field to deliver the prescribed dose is found from

$$MU = \frac{\text{fraction of the prescribed dose}}{\text{cGy/MU} \times \text{TAR} \times \text{isodose line}/100} \quad (4.39)$$

Using Eq. (4.39), the MU necessary from each of fields A and B is

$$\frac{1 \times 200}{3 \times 1.025 \times 0.793 \times 0.95} = 86 \text{ MU per field}$$

and the MU necessary from each of fields C and D is

$$\frac{1 \times 200}{6 \times 1.025 \times 0.645 \times 0.95} = 53 \text{ MU per field}$$

The effect of beam attenuators is calculated precisely as in other techniques and is therefore not included here.

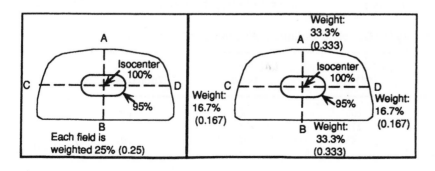

Figure 4.8 Isocentric four-field technique using equal weighting *(left)* and weighted 2 to 1 *(right)*.

The calculation formula for an SAD technique is very similar to that of a fixed-SSD technique and is summarized as follows:

MU (time)

$$= \frac{\text{prescribed dose}}{(\text{TAR, TPR, or TMR}) \, (\text{isodose}/100)(\text{cGy/MU})} \qquad (4.40)$$

$$\times \frac{1}{\text{dose rate}_{\text{ref}} \times \text{area factor} \times \text{tray factor} \times \text{wedge factor}}$$

DOSE CALCULATION FOR TREATMENTS AT AN EXTENDED DISTANCE

In some situations, it is necessary to treat patients at extended distances in order to accommodate large fields. It is then somewhat uncertain how the dose is affected. The dose can, for example, change due to the increased distance between the collimator and the calculation point and also because of scatter from the floor and walls of the treatment room. Actual measurements of dose under these conditions are highly recommended. If time and conditions do not permit actual measurements to be made prior to treatment, it is possible to calculate the dose with reasonable confidence using TAR or TMR methods.

In this example, the lower half-body of a patient is to be treated at 142-cm SSD (Fig. 4.9). The patient's thickness is 16 cm and the maximum collimator opening is used. The treatment is delivered using a cobalt-60 unit with a dose rate$_{\text{ref}}$ of 109 cGy/min at 80-cm distance when the patient is not present. The area factor for the maximum collimator opening is 1.07. The maximum field size for which TAR is available at this energy is 35 × 35 cm (Table A.3).

Though the maximum collimator opening on this machine produces a field size at 150 cm which is much greater than 35 × 35 cm, it is reasonable to use the 35 × 35 cm TAR value (0.935 at 8-cm depth) because the beam flashes over the sides of the patient and the irradiated area is therefore elongated. In any event, the TAR varies very slowly with area when the field is large (as do area factors, cGy/MU, and %DD), particularly at higher energies. For example, the TAR for cobalt 60 (8-cm depth) increases only 6.5 percent, from 0.852 to 0.907 (Table A.3), when the field area is more than doubled from 20 ×

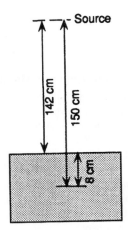

Figure 4.9   Diagram of treatment at an extended distance.

20 cm to 30 × 30 cm; the same field change for 10-MV photons (Table A.5) gives less than 1 percent increase in TAR (0.906 to 0.910). The exact field size chosen in our present problem is therefore not critical.

The treatment time necessary to deliver the prescribed treatment can be found from

Time

$$= \frac{\text{prescribed dose}}{\text{dose rate}_{\text{ref}} \times \text{area factor} \times \text{TAR} \times \text{ISF}} \qquad (4.41)$$

The treatment time necessary to deliver 300 cGy per field can be found from

$$\frac{300}{109 \times 1.07 \times 0.935 \times 0.2844}$$
$$= 9.67 \text{ min} \quad (9 \text{ min, } 40 \text{ s})$$

where 0.2844 is the ISF for a point 8 cm beyond the new SSD of 142 cm—that is, for a point 150 cm from the source:

$$\left(\frac{80}{150}\right)^2 = 0.2844$$

PROBLEMS

SSD TECHNIQUE

Dose Calculation at Depth of Maximum Dose

4.1   *Superficial beam.* A skin lesion is to be treated using a superficial beam. The prescription is for 300 cGy per fraction. The field size is 7×8 cm and the SSD is 50 cm. The HVT is 2.5 mmCu and the backscatter factor is 1.123. The dose rate at 50 cm SSD without the patient present is 57 cGy/min. What is the required treatment time? (Give the answer in minutes and seconds.)

4.2   *Electron beam.* An 8-MeV electron beam is used to deliver 300 cGy at D_{max}. The field size is 8×8 cm and the SSD is 100 cm. The dose rate$_{ref}$ is 1.0 cGy/MU for a 10×10 cm field. The cGy/MU for an 8×8 cm field is 0.872. What MU setting should be used to deliver this treatment?

4.3   *Cobalt-60 beam.* A cobalt-60 beam is used to deliver 200 cGy at D_{max}. The field size is 10×12 cm and the SSD is 80 cm. The dose rate$_{ref}$ for a 10×10 cm field at D_{max} is 112.7 cGy/min. The area factor for a 10×12 cm field is 1.02. What treatment time is needed to deliver this treatment? (Give the answer in minutes and seconds.)

4.4   *Linear accelerator.* A 4-MV photon beam is used to deliver 200 cGy at D_{max}. The field size is 15×15 cm and the SSD is 80 cm. The dose rate$_{ref}$ is 1 cGy/MU for a 10×10 cm field. The cGy/MU for a 15×15 cm field is 1.037. What MU setting should be used to deliver this treatment?

DOSE CALCULATION AT DEPTH FOR A SINGLE BEAM

4.5   *Superficial beam.* A dose of 350 cGy is prescribed at 3-cm depth. The field size is 3×4 cm and the SSD is 50 cm. A 3-mmCu HVT beam is used and the dose rate in the absence of the patient at 50 cm is 63.4 cGy/min. The backscatter factor is 1.094, and the %DD at 3-cm depth is 78 percent. What is the treatment time necessary to deliver this treatment? (Give the answer in minutes and seconds.)

4.6   *Electron beam.* A dose of 250 cGy is prescribed at 3.5-cm depth using a 14-MeV electron beam. The field size is 6×8 cm and the SSD is 100 cm. The dose rate$_{ref}$ is 1.0 for a 10×10 cm field and 0.898 for a 6×8 cm field. The %DD at 3.5 cm is 92 percent. How many MU should be set to deliver this treatment?

4.7   *Cobalt-60 beam.* A dose of 180 cGy is prescribed at 4.5-cm depth using a cobalt-60 beam. The field size is 8×8 cm and the SSD is 80 cm. The dose rate$_{ref}$ at D_{max} for a 10×10 cm field is 109.3 cGy/min. The area factor for an 8×8 cm field is 0.973. What is the treatment time required to deliver this treatment? (Give the answer in minutes and seconds.) Use Table A.1 for %DD.

4.8   *Linear accelerator.* A dose of 100 cGy is prescribed at 5-cm depth to be delivered using a 4-MV photon beam. The field size is 12×12 cm and the SSD is 80 cm. The cGy/MU$_{ref}$ is 1.0 for a 10×10 cm field and it is 1.027 for a 12×12 cm field. What MU setting should be used to deliver this treatment? Use Table A.2 for %DD.

DOSE CALCULATION FOR PARALLEL OPPOSED FIELDS

4.9 *Cobalt-60 beam.* A dose of 180 cGy is prescribed in the midplane of the brain. Parallel opposed lateral cobalt-60 fields are used. The lateral diameter of the head is 14 cm. The field size is 17 × 23 cm and the SSD is 80 cm. The dose rate$_{ref}$ for a 10 × 10 cm field is 107.3 cGy/min and the area factor is 1.047. What treatment time is required per field to deliver this treatment? (Give the answer in minutes and seconds.) Use Table A.1 for %DD.

4.10 *Linear accelerator.* A dose of 200 cGy is prescribed at the midplane of the lung. Parallel opposed anterior and posterior 4-MV photon beams are to be used. The field size is 13 × 13 cm and the SSD is 80 cm. The AP diameter of the patient's chest is 21 cm. The cGy/MU$_{ref}$ is 1.0 for a 10 × 10 cm field; for a 13 × 13 cm field, it is 1.022. What MU setting per field is necessary to deliver this treatment? Use Table A.2 for %DD.

CALCULATING ENTRANCE DOSE AND EXIT DOSE FROM PARALLEL OPPOSED EQUALLY WEIGHTED BEAMS

4.11 Giving 120 MU through each field in the treatment delivered in Problem 10, what will the dose be at (*a*) middepth and at (*b*) D$_{max}$ of either of the two parallel opposed fields? Use Table A.2 for %DD.

4.12 Giving 120 MU through field 1 and 240 MU through field 2 in the treatment in Problem 10, what will the total dose be at (*a*) midplane, (*b*) D$_{max}$ of field 1, and (*c*) D$_{max}$ of field 2?

4.13 A dose of 150 cGy is prescribed at 3-cm depth from the right side of the brain. Parallel opposed cobalt-60 fields are used. The field size is 8 × 8 cm and the SSD is 80 cm. The fields are weighted 2 to 1 favoring the patient's right side. The lateral diameter of the head is 15 cm. The dose rate$_{ref}$ for a 10 × 10 cm field is 105.6 cGy/min and the area factor for an 8 × 8 cm field is 0.985. What will the treatment time be for (*a*) the right field and (*b*) the left field? (Give the answers in minutes and seconds.) Use Table A.1 for %DD.

4.14 A three-field treatment plan is used to treat a brain tumor. Each field is 6 × 6 cm, and the SSD is 80 cm. A 4-MV photon beam is used for all fields. 180 cGy is prescribed to the 206 percent isodose line. The fields are equally weighted. The cGy/MU$_{ref}$ for a 10 × 10 cm field is 1.0; for a 6 × 6 cm field, it is 0.956. A 30° wedge is used in two of the three fields. The wedge factor is 0.81. What MU setting should be used in (*a*) the unwedged field, and (*b*) the two wedged fields?

4.15 A dose of 200 cGy is prescribed at D$_{max}$ in a spine field that is 6 × 30 cm at 80-cm SSD. The cGy/MU$_{ref}$ for a 10 × 10 cm field is 1.0 at D$_{max}$ (81 cm); for a 6 × 30 cm field, it is 1.026 at D$_{max}$ (81 cm). Due to the length of the field, the treatment must be delivered at 90-cm SSD. What MU setting is necessary in order to deliver this treatment?

SAD TECHNIQUE

4.16 *Cobalt-60 beam.* A dose of 190 cGy is prescribed at the midplane of the arm. Parallel opposed cobalt-60 beams are used. The field size is 6 × 12 cm, and the SAD is 80 cm. The dose rate$_{ref}$ is 112.6 cGy/min at 80 cm for a 10 × 10 cm field, and the area factor for a

6×12 cm field is 0.995. The arm is 9 cm in diameter. The isocenter is at middepth in the arm. What is the required treatment time for each field? (Give the answer in minutes and seconds.) Use Table A.3 for TAR.

4.17 *Linear accelerator.* A dose of 200 cGy is prescribed at the midplane of the pelvis. Parallel opposed 10-MV photon beams are used. The field size is 17×17 cm, and the SAD is 100 cm. The cGy/MU$_{ref}$ is 1.0 for a 10×10 cm field and 1.085 for a 17×17 cm field. The pelvis is 25 cm in diameter. The isocenter is at the middepth of the pelvis. What MU setting should be used for each field in order to deliver this treatment? Use Table A.5 for TAR.

4.18 From the treatment delivered in Problem 17, find the maximum entrance and exit doses.

4.19 A dose of 180 cGy is prescribed to the 95 percent isodose line in a four-field isocentric treatment plan. All fields are equally weighted, and 4-MV photon beams are used. The field sizes are 8×8 cm, and the SAD is 80 cm. The cGy/MU$_{ref}$ is 1.0 for a 10×10 cm field and 0.98 for 8×8 cm field. The depth of the isocenter is 10 cm for fields A and B and 16 cm for fields C and D. What is the MU setting required for each field? Use Table A.4 for TAR.

4.20 A dose of 200 cGy is prescribed to the 98 percent isodose line in a treatment plan using parallel opposed isocentric fields. The field sizes are 9×10 cm, and the SAD is 100 cm. A 10-MV photon beam is used. Field A is weighted twice as much as field B. The isocenter is at 5-cm depth in field A and at 15-cm depth in field B. The cGy/MU$_{ref}$ for a 10×10 cm field is 1.0; for a 9×10 cm field, it is 0.995. What is the MU needed for each field to deliver the treatment, and what is the D_{max} dose (entrance and exit) of field A and of field B? Use Table A.4.

REFERENCE

1. Bjärngard BE, Bar-Deroma R, Corrao A: A survey of methods to calculate monitor settings. *Int J Radiat Oncol Biol Phys* 28:749, 1994.

5

Dose Calculation for External Beams—Part II

In Chap. 4, dose calculations on the central axis for square fields were explained. In this chapter, dose calculations on and off the central axis and for rectangular and irregularly shaped fields will be explained. As was evident in Chap. 4, tabulated values are usually available only for square fields. In clinical practice, the problem of finding data for rectangular and irregular fields arises. In this chapter, some methods to solve these problems are shown.

THE CONCEPT OF EQUIVALENT SQUARE FIELDS

In a *very* small field (which we can represent as a 0×0 cm field, although that is only an abstraction, as was previously explained), the dose is effectively due to primary radiation only. As the field size is increased, the scattered radiation resulting from photons interacting with the medium causes the absorbed dose to increase. The amount of scattered radiation is greater at a larger depth than at D_{max}, causing the percentage depth dose to increase with larger field sizes. Since the higher-energy photons are scattered more predominantly in a forward direction, the percentage depth dose increases with increased area and is less pronounced for the higher-energy beams than for the lower-energy beams (Chap. 3, Fig. 3.7).

EQUIVALENT SQUARE METHOD

The shape of the field, not just its area in square centimeters, also affects the percentage depth dose (%DD). In the two fields shown in Fig. 5.1, for example, the total area is the same. However, the %DD

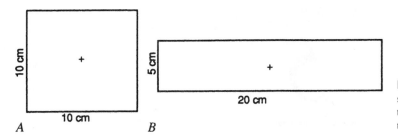

Figure 5.1 The areas in A and B are the same, but the field in B contributes less scatter than A at the calculation point ($+$) because of the elongated shape.

in field B is smaller than in field A because radiation scattered from the distal portions of field B is less likely to reach the center of the field where the %DD is observed than is the scattered radiation from field A, where the area is symmetrically arranged around the calculation point.

Several authors[1-4] have shown that %DD data for rectangular fields can be approximated by an equivalent square method.

Using Table A.6, a 6 × 20 cm field is equivalent to a 9 × 9 cm field. The %DD for a 9 × 9 cm field could therefore be used in calculating dose for the 6 × 20 cm field.

AREA/PERIMETER METHOD

Another method, developed by Sterling,[5] is to equate a rectangular field with a square field if they have the same area/perimeter (A/P).

Since the area (A) of the rectangular field is a × b and its perimeter (P) is 2a + 2b (two sides plus two ends), we have

$$A/P = \frac{a \times b}{2(a + b)} \qquad (5.1)$$

where a is the field width and b is the field length.

Consider for example a 6 × 20 cm field

$$A/P = \frac{6 \times 20}{2(6 + 20)}$$

so

$$\frac{120}{52} = 2.3$$

To find the A/P for a square field, where a = b, we have

$$A/P = \frac{a^2}{4^a} = \frac{a}{4} \qquad (5.2)$$

In a square field of side 9 cm, for example,

$$A/P = \frac{9}{4} = 2.25$$

We found, then, that A/P for a 6 × 20 cm field and for a 9 × 9 cm square field are very nearly the same, so tabulated data for a 9 × 9 cm field (equivalent field) can therefore be used to find the values for a 6 × 20 cm field.

Although this method is widely used in clinical practice, caution must be used in applying it.

CLARKSON'S METHOD

Tabulated data customarily refer to the central axis of square fields, and—as we have just seen—can also be applied to rectangular fields but cannot be used to estimate the dose on the central axis of an irregularly shaped field (Fig. 5.2) or at points away from the central axis of any field. For these situations, the dose may be estimated by finding the primary and scatter components of the dose separately and adding them together, a method originally introduced by Clarkson.[6] This method is best accomplished using TAR and SAR tables or TMR and SMR tables.*

* Data tables used in the dose calculations in this chapter are labeled A.1 to A.8 and can be found in the Appendix.

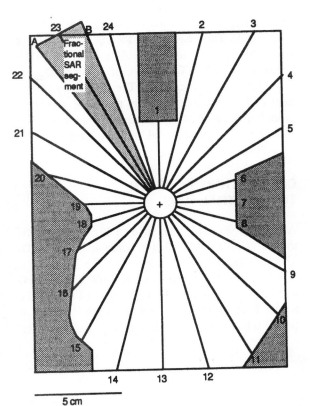

Figure 5.2 An irregularly shaped field illustrating the calculation point (+) and 24 radii used in calculating the SAR (Table 5.1). A small triangle of the field lies outside SAR segment 23 at A. This is, however, offset by a small triangle outside the field, which is included in the SAR segment at B.

The TAR or TMR for a 0×0 cm field represents the primary component of a beam. The TAR or TMR for a given field size includes both the primary and the scattered dose. The difference between the two represents the scatter component or scatter-air ratio in the case of TAR and scatter-maximum ratio (SMR) in the case of TMR. Both SAR and SMR have been previously defined in Chap. 3.

Scatter-air ratio and SMR tables published in the literature are usually tabulated for circular fields only. It is, however, possible to find the equivalent square field from these tables.

Using Table A.3, it is found that the TAR for a 10×10 cm cobalt-60 field at 10-cm depth is 0.701 and the TAR at the same depth for a 0×0 cm field

is 0.534. The scatter component is therefore found from

$$0.701 - 0.534 = 0.167$$

From Table A.7 it is found that a circular field with a radius of 5.65 (100 cm²) at a depth of 10 cm has an interpolated SAR value of 0.174. The difference is a result of the fact that the tabulated values for SARs and SMRs for circular fields correspond to square or rectangular fields having the same scatter rather than the same area.

FRACTIONAL SARs AND SMRs

The scatter of any field can be estimated by using segments of circular fields. If a circular field is di-

Table 5.1 Scatter-Air Ratio Calculation at the Central Axis of the Field in Fig. 5.2 (^{60}Co)

Radius No.	Length, cm	Fractional SAR
1	4.7	0.0013
2	10.5	0.0025
3	11.5	0.0027
4	10.5	0.0025
5	8.5	0.0022
6	4.5	0.0012
7	4.5	0.0012
8	4.7	0.0013
9	8.5	0.0022
10	10.0	0.0024
11	10.5	0.0025
12	10.5	0.0025
13	10.0	0.0024
14	10.5	0.0025
15	9.5	0.0023
16	7.5	0.0019
17	5.5	0.0015
18	4.0	0.0011
19	4.5	0.0012
20	6.5	0.0017
21	8.5	0.0022
22	10.5	0.0025
23	11.5	0.0027
24	10.5	0.0025
		SAR = 0.0490

vided into 15° segments (a convenient choice, since 15° into 360° equals a whole number, or 24), the SAR due to one such segment is one twenty-fourth of the SAR due to the whole circle. In this method, radii separated by 15°, that is, 24 segments, are measured from the calculation point to the field margins. The SARs or SMRs for each radius are found and are then divided by 24 to give the fractional value. The fractional SARs to SMRs for the 24 segments are summed and are then added to the TAR or TMR for a 0×0 cm field (TAR_0 or TMR_0) at the same depth. The sum gives the TAR or TMR value for the calculated field. An alternate method is to find the SAR for each radius, then divide by the number of radii to find the average SAR. The result will be the same as in the method just described.

The fractional SARs or SMRs can also be used to estimate the equivalent square of a rectangular or irregularly shaped field. For example, Table 5.1 shows that the field in Fig. 5.2 yields an SAR of 0.049 at D_{max} using a cobalt-60 beam and 80-cm SSD (Table A.3). The TAR at D_{max} for a 0×0 cm field is 1.0. Adding 0.049 to 1.0 yields a TAR of 1.049. From Table A.3 a TAR value of 1.049 at D_{max} is given for a 15×15 cm field. The irregularly shaped field in Fig. 5.2 therefore has the same scattering properties as a 15×15 cm square field and %DD and TAR tables for this field may be used.

CALCULATING DOSE ON THE CENTRAL AXIS

As another example, the field in Fig. 5.3 is to be treated using a 4-MV photon beam at 80-cm SAD. The prescription is for 100 cGy. The TAR for a 0×0 cm field at 8-cm depth is 0.690 (Table A.4) and the SAR, using Table A.8, is 0.191 (Table 5.2), so the TAR for this field at 8-cm depth is (0.690 + 0.191) 0.881. The cGy/MU for this field is 1.03.

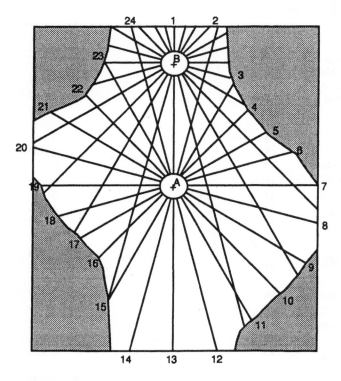

Figure 5.3 An irregularly shaped field indicating two calculation points: the central axis (A) and an off-axis point (B) with 24 radii used in calculating the SAR (Table 5.2).

Table 5.2   Scatter-Air Ratio Calculation for the Field in Fig. 5.3 (4-MV Photons)

	Point A			Point B			
Radius No.	Length, cm	Fractional SAR, D = 8 cm	Radius No.	Length, cm	Fractional SAR, D = 8 cm	Fractional SAR, D = 7 cm	Fractional SAR, D = 5 cm
1	8.5	0.0086	1	2.0	0.0029	0.0028	0.0026
2	9.0	0.0089	2	2.0	0.0029	0.0028	0.0026
3	6.0	0.0071	3	2.0	0.0029	0.0028	0.0026
4	5.5	0.0067	4	3.0	0.0042	0.0041	0.0037
5	6.0	0.0071	5	3.0	0.0042	0.0041	0.0037
6	7.0	0.0078	6	2.5	0.0036	0.0035	0.0032
7	7.5	0.0081	7	2.5	0.0036	0.0035	0.0032
8	7.5	0.0081	8	2.5	0.0036	0.0035	0.0032
9	8.0	0.0084	9	3.0	0.0042	0.0041	0.0037
10	8.0	0.0084	10	10.0	0.0093	0.0088	0.0075
11	8.5	0.0086	11	13.0	0.0100	0.0095	0.0080
12	9.0	0.0089	12	15.0	0.0105	0.0099	0.0083
13	8.5	0.0086	13	15.0	0.0105	0.0099	0.0083
14	9.0	0.0089	14	13.0	0.0100	0.0095	0.0080
15	7.0	0.0078	15	10.5	0.0094	0.0089	0.0076
16	5.5	0.0067	16	10.0	0.0093	0.0088	0.0075
17	5.5	0.0067	17	8.5	0.0086	0.0083	0.0070
18	6.0	0.0071	18	4.5	0.0058	0.0056	0.0049
19	7.0	0.0078	19	3.5	0.0048	0.0046	0.0042
20	8.0	0.0084	20	3.5	0.0048	0.0046	0.0042
21	8.0	0.0084	21	3.5	0.0048	0.0046	0.0042
22	7.0	0.0078	22	3.0	0.0042	0.0041	0.0037
23	7.5	0.0081	23	2.0	0.0029	0.0028	0.0026
24	8.0	0.0084	24	2.0	0.0029	0.0028	0.0026
		SAR = 0.1914			SAR = 0.1399	0.1339	0.1171

The MU required to deliver this treatment is found from

$$MU = \frac{\text{prescribed dose}}{(TAR_0 + SAR) \times \text{cGy/MU} \times \text{tray factor}}$$

$$(5.3)$$

So, for this treatment, the required MU is

$$\frac{100}{(0.690 + 0.191) \times 1.03 \times 0.96} = 115 \text{ MU}$$

CALCULATING DOSE AT AN OFF-AXIS POINT

To estimate the dose at points away from the central axis, the method used is similar to the one described above for a central axis point calculation—the exception being the need for the application of an off-axis ratio

OFF-AXIS RATIO

Flattening filters are used in the beam of linear accelerators to flatten the isodose curves across a field at a specified depth. This, however, frequently causes the dose to be higher away from the central axis, particularly at shallow depths (see Fig. 5.4 and Chap. 3, Fig. 3.15). Isodose charts for cobalt-60 beams, on the other hand, demonstrate a lower dose in the periphery of the field. Such nonuniformity of dose across a beam must be considered in dose calculations away from the central axis of the beam. To estimate the dose at such points, the variation of dose across the beam or the off-axis ratio (OAR) at appropriate depth must be known.

The OAR is defined as

$$\text{OAR} = \frac{\%\text{DD at the off-axis point}}{\%\text{DD on the central axis}} \quad (5.4)$$

The most practical method to estimate the OAR is to find the %DD along the central axis at the depth under consideration and the %DD off the central axis of the beam at the same depth and at the appropriate distance away from the central axis, using an isodose chart measured for the actual beam and for appropriate field size.

For example, the %DD in Fig. 5.4 at the off-axis point is 74, and at the same depth along the central axis, it is 71. The OAR is therefore 74/71 = 1.042, that is, the dose at the off-axis point is 4.2% higher than the dose at the same depth on the central axis. Few departments have isodose charts plotted for every field size and distance, so some assumptions must be made. For example, to find the OAR for an

SAD technique using an isodose chart plotted for an SSD technique, the assumption is made that the shape of the individual isodose curves does not change very much with distance. Interpolation between individual isodose lines and for different field sizes also causes uncertainties in the estimation of the OAR. More elaborate methods of calculating the OAR have been described.[7]

CALCULATING DOSE AT AN OFF-AXIS POINT WITH A FLAT SURFACE

The dose at an off-axis point is best estimated by considering the primary dose and the scatter separately. The SAR is determined as previously described, but the axis from which the radii originate is placed at the off-axis calculation point (Fig. 5.3). In this example, the SAR for a 4-MV photon beam at B is found by using Table A.8 and is 0.140 at 8-cm depth (Table 5.2). The TAR_0 value at 8-cm depth from Table A.4 is 0.690, so the TAR at this point is $0.690 + 0.140 = 0.830$. Using an isodose chart for a 17×17 cm field at 80-cm SSD, the %DD at a point 6.5 cm from the central axis at 8-cm depth is 74 and on the central axis it is 71, so the OAR is 74/71 = 1.042 (Fig. 5.4). As we calculated earlier, the field in Fig. 5.3 is given 115 MU, which delivers 100 cGy at 8-cm depth on the central axis. The dose at the off-axis point is found from

$$\text{Dose} = \text{MU} \times \text{cGy/MU} \times (\text{TAR}_0 + \text{SAR})$$
$$\times \text{OAR} \times \text{tray factor} \quad (5.5)$$

so in this field, the dose at 8-cm depth, assuming that the patient's skin surface is flat (Fig. 5.5), is

$$115 \times 1.03 \times (0.690 + 0.140)$$
$$\times 1.042 \times 0.96 = 98 \text{ cGy}$$

The dose at the off-axis point and at the central axis are practically the same. The higher dose due to the overflattening of the beam is offset by less scatter at the off-axis point.

Calculating Dose at an Off-Axis Point When the Surface Is Not Flat. In the previous example, the surface of the patient was assumed to be flat; that

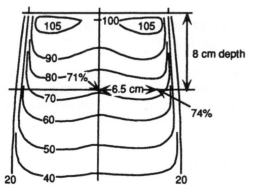

Figure 5.4 The %DD is found on the central axis (71%) and at the off-axis point at the same depth (74%).

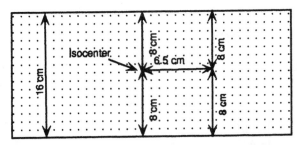

Figure 5.5 An illustration of the geometry of off-axis point calculation using a flat contour.

is, the SSD is the same at the central axis and at the off-axis point. In the following example, the same field is treated as in the previous example, but the patient's irregular surface results in a 3-cm vertical air gap (Fig. 5.6).

In this isocentric treatment, the SAD is, of course, the same at B (Fig. 5.6); however, the depth is reduced from 8 cm to 5 cm. The TAR_0 value at 5 cm-depth using a 4-MV photon beam is 0.835 (Table A.4) and the SAR at the same depth is 0.117 (Table 5.2). Using the same treatment as in the previous example but with an OAR of 1.0595 (89/84) at 5-cm depth, the dose in B is found using Eq. (5.5), so

$$115 \times 1.03 \times (0.835 + 0.117)$$
$$\times 1.0595 \times 0.96 = 115 \text{ cGy}$$

The dose at B in this example is considerably higher than in the previous example when the overlying surface was flat. This is primarily due to a de-

creased amount of attenuating tissue overlying the calculation point in B (Fig. 5.6).

Calculating Dose at an Off-Axis Point at a Different Depth—SAD Technique. In an isocentric treatment technique, it is not necessary to know what the SSD is, since TARs, TPRs, SARs, and SMRs are independent of distance. It is, however, necessary to know the relationship between the dose-calculation point and the isocenter. This is because dose rates, cGy/MU, and so on are customarily specified on the central axis of the beam. Figure 5.6 demonstrates the relationship of the dose-calculation point to the isocenter. In the next example, the dose from parallel opposed anterior and posterior fields using an isocentric technique is calculated to the spinal cord (Fig. 5.7).

In this example, the spinal cord is at 7-cm depth from the anterior surface and at 5-cm depth from the posterior surface. The treatment field in Fig. 5.3 is used again with an identical opposed field. The patient's thickness at the central axis (Fig. 5.3A) is 16 cm and at the off-axis point (Fig. 5.3B) the thickness is (7 + 5) 12 cm. Vertical air gaps are present in both fields (Fig. 5.7), that is, the patient's surface is not flat. The dose-calculation point lies 2-cm posterior of the isocenter; thus, an inverse square factor must be included in the calculation (Chap. 3).

The inverse square factor for the anterior field is $(80/82)^2$ or 0.9518 and for the posterior field is $(80/78)^2$ or 1.0519.

The TAR_0 at 7-cm depth is 0.734 (Table A.4) and the SAR is 0.134 (Table 5.2). The OAR at 7-cm depth is 1.053 (79.5/75.5).

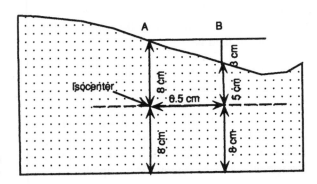

Figure 5.6 Diagram of the geometry when calculating dose on a slanting surface.

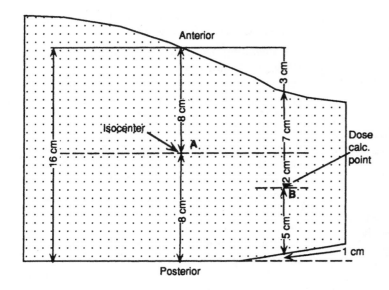

Figure 5.7 An illustration of the geometry of an off-axis calculation at a depth different from the isocenter. The sum of the SSD and the patient's thickness is the same on the central axis and along a vertical axis through point B.

The dose to the spinal cord from the anterior field is found from

$$\text{Dose} = \text{MU} \times \text{cGy/MU} \times (\text{TAR}_0 + \text{SAR}) \times \text{OAR} \times \text{tray factor} \times \text{ISF} \quad (5.6)$$

that is,

$$115 \times 1.03 \times (0.734 + 0.134) \times 1.053 \times 0.96 \times 0.9518 = 99 \text{ cGy}$$

The TAR_0 at 5-cm depth is 0.835 (Table A.4) and the SAR is 0.117 (Table 5.2). The OAR at 5-cm depth is 1.0595.

Using Eq. (5.6), the dose to the spinal cord from the posterior field is

$$115 \times 1.03 \times (0.835 + 0.117) \times 1.0595 \times 0.96 \times 1.0519 = 121 \text{ cGy}$$

In this example, the OAR was estimated at the depth of the off-axis point, and the assumption was made that the change in OAR, caused by the slant of the patient's surface contour, is negligible.

Calculating Dose at an Off-Axis Point at a Different Depth—SSD Technique. In an SSD technique, it is necessary to know the actual SSD at the dose-calculation point, since the %DD used in this dose-calculation method is expressed as a percentage of the dose at D_{max} and depends on the distance.

To illustrate this point, the next example deals with a fixed-SSD technique in the treatment of a lung tumor via parallel opposed fields. The spinal-cord dose is to be calculated at a point 6 cm from the central axis using a cobalt-60 beam at 80-cm SSD (Fig. 5.8). The patient's thickness at the central axis is 18 cm. The treatment time is 1.22 min/field, the dose rate is 114 cGy/min, and the area factor is 1.032 for each field. No beam-shaping block is used, thus no transmission factor for block-supporting tray is included in the calculation. The spinal cord is at 7-cm depth from the anterior surface and the vertical air gap at this point is 4 cm. The OAR is 0.953 and the SAR for this field is found to be the same as for a 12 × 12 cm field. The %DD at 7-cm depth is 69.7 (Table A.1). The dose at an off-axis point using a fixed-SSD technique is found from

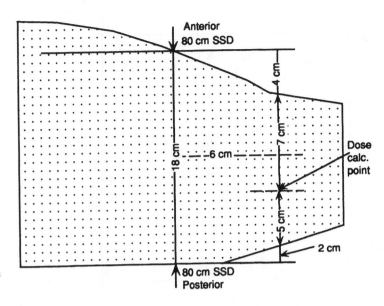

Figure 5.8 Diagram of off-axis calculation point in a SSD treatment technique.

$$\text{Dose} = \text{time (or MU)} \times \text{dose rate}_{(ref)}$$
$$\times \text{area factor} \times \%DD \times OAR \times ISF \quad (5.7)$$

The inverse square factor from Eq. (3.1) is $(80.5/84.5)^2 = 0.9076$.

Using Eq. (5.7), the dose to the spinal cord from the anterior field is

$$1.22 \times 114 \times 1.032 \times (69.7/100)$$
$$\times 0.953 \times 0.9076 = 86.5 \text{ cGy}$$

The spinal cord is at 5-cm depth from the posterior surface and the vertical air gap is 2 cm.

The inverse square factor from Eq. (3.1) is $(80.5/82.5)^2 = 0.9521$.

The OAR is assumed to be the same as for the anterior field (0.953). The %DD at 5-cm depth is 79.2 (Table A.1).

Using Eq. (5.7), the spinal cord dose from the posterior field is

$$1.22 \times 114 \times 1.032 \times (79.2/100)$$
$$\times 0.953 \times 0.9521 = 103 \text{ cGy}$$

Note in Fig. 5.8 that the sum of the patient's thickness and the SSDs at the central axis and at the off-

axis point are the same. The anterior and posterior SSD at the central axis is 80 cm and the patient's thickness is 18 cm. The sum is 178 cm. At the off-axis point, the anterior SSD is 80 + 4 cm and the posterior SSD is 80 + 2 cm. The patient's thickness is 7 + 5 cm. The fact that the sum (84 + 82 + 12 cm) is also 178 cm is a simple check on the accuracy of the measurements.

In the preceding off-axis calculations, a vertical air gap was present. In some situations, the patient's contour may cause the SSD to be shorter than at the central axis. The dose-calculation procedure remains unchanged in that situation.

CALCULATING SARs WHEN THE RADII ARE INTERCEPTED BY A BLOCKED AREA

In many irregularly shaped fields, a radius from the calculation point to the extreme field margins may pass across a blocked area. This is a special situation that must be considered in a special way. Consider the field in Fig. 5.9, where radii numbers 16 to 21 pass through and extend beyond the blocked area. In this situation, the SAR value for the entire length (A

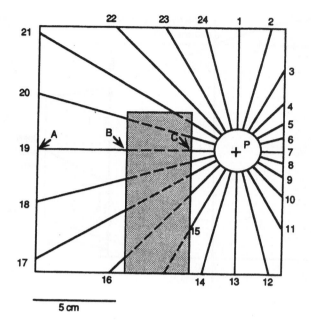

5 cm

Figure 5.9 An irregular shaped field where several radii extend beyond a blocked area *(shaded)*. The SAR was calculated at P.

Table 5.3   Scatter-Air Ratio Calculation for the Field in Fig. 5.9 (4-MV Photons)

Radius No.	Length, cm	Fractional SAR
1	7.5	0.0020
2	7.5	0.0020
3	5.5	0.0015
4	4.0	0.0011
5	3.0	0.0008
6	3.0	0.0008
7	3.0	0.0008
8	3.0	0.0008
9	3.0	0.0008
10	4.0	0.0011
11	5.0	0.0014
12	8.0	0.0022
13	7.5	0.0020
14	8.0	0.0022
15	5.5	0.0015
16	10.5; 9.5; 4.0	$0.0027 - 0.0025 + 0.0011 = 0.0013$
17	14.0; 8.0; 3.0	$0.0030 - 0.0022 + 0.0008 = 0.0016$
18	13.0; 7.0; 3.0	$0.0029 - 0.0019 + 0.0008 = 0.0018$
19	12.0; 6.5; 3.0	$0.0028 - 0.0018 + 0.0008 = 0.0018$
20	12.5; 7.0; 3.0	$0.0029 - 0.0020 + 0.0008 = 0.0017$
21	14.0; 5.0; 3.0	$0.0030 - 0.0014 + 0.0008 = 0.0024$
22	11.0	0.0028
23	9.0	0.0024
24	8.0	0.0022
		SAR = 0.0390

to P) of the radius is first found. Then the SAR value for the part of the radius to the far edge of the block is subtracted (B to P) and the SAR value for the part to the near edge of block (C to P) is added. Table 5.3 shows how the SAR is calculated using 4-MV photon data (Table A.8) for the field in Fig. 5.9.

This method assumes that no primary dose is transmitted through the block and that no scatter is produced by the tissue under the block. In a typical situation, a small amount of primary dose is in fact transmitted, giving rise to some scattered dose under the block.

CALCULATING DOSE UNDER A BLOCK

In some situations, calculation of the dose under a block or outside a field is necessary. Although shielding blocks are intended to reduce the dose to underlying organs, some transmission is unavoidable. This primary dose plus the scattered radiation from the surrounding irradiated volume are the two components that contribute dose under a block. Dose outside the field consists of scatter only.

Figure 5.10 illustrates a large abdominal field

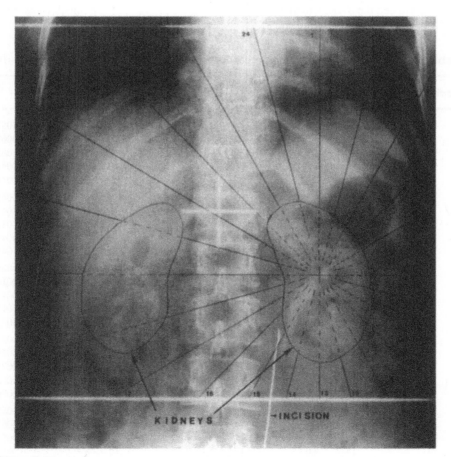

Figure 5.10   Simulation film of an upper-abdominal field; 5-HVT shielding blocks over the contrast-enhanced kidneys. Since radiographs are enlarged images of the patient, all measurements must be reduced to actual size.

treated via a 4-MV photon beam and with a 5-HVT shielding block over each kidney. The dose to the left kidney was calculated at 9-cm depth. As in the equivalent square field calculation, 24 radii separated by 15° were drawn from the dose calculation point under the block to the periphery of the field. Since the calculation point is under a block, all radii pass through a blocked segment. The fractional SARs are found by using the same method as described previously. For example, the entire length of radius 20 in Fig. 5.10 is 18 cm and the fractional SAR (0.278/24) is 0.0116 (Table A.8). The distance from the calculation point to the far edge of the right kidney block is 11 cm and the fractional SAR (0.239/24) 0.0100 is subtracted. The distance from the calculation point to the near edge of the right kidney block is 7.5 cm and the SAR, which is added,

is (0.200/24) 0.0083. The distance from the calculation point to the edge of the left kidney block is 2 cm and the fractional SAR, which is subtracted, is (0.069/24) 0.029, leaving a total SAR value for this radius of (0.0116 − 0.0100 + 0.0083 − 0.0029) 0.0070. The fractional SARs for each radius are similarly found and are then added together to give the SAR of the field under consideration. The SAR at the calculation point in Fig. 5.10 was found to be 0.119 (Table 5.4).

The primary dose delivered to a point under the block is found from

$$\begin{aligned} \text{Primary dose} = &\ \text{MU} \times \text{cGy/MU} \times \text{OAR} \\ &\ \times \text{TAR}_0 \times \text{tray factor} \\ &\ \times \text{block trans. factor} \end{aligned} \quad (5.8)$$

Table 5.4   Scatter-Air Ratio Calculation for the Field in Fig. 5.10 (4-MV Photons)

Radius No.	Length, cm				Fractional SAR
1	13.0;	3.5			0.0105 − 0.0048 = 0.0057
2	13.5;	3.0			0.0106 − 0.0043 = 0.0063
3	13.0;	3.0			0.0105 − 0.0043 = 0.0062
4	9.0;	3.0			0.0092 − 0.0043 = 0.0049
5	7.5;	2.5			0.0083 − 0.0035 = 0.0048
6	6.5;	2.5			0.0076 − 0.0035 = 0.0041
7	6.5;	2.5			0.0076 − 0.0035 = 0.0041
8	6.5;	3.0			0.0076 − 0.0043 = 0.0034
9	7.5;	3.0			0.0083 − 0.0043 = 0.0040
10	9.0;	3.5			0.0092 − 0.0048 = 0.0044
11	7.5;	4.0			0.0083 − 0.0055 = 0.0028
12	6.5;	4.5			0.0076 − 0.0060 = 0.0016
13	6.5;	4.5			0.0076 − 0.0060 = 0.0016
14	6.5;	4.5			0.0076 − 0.0060 = 0.0016
15	7.5;	3.5			0.0083 − 0.0048 = 0.0035
16	9.0;	2.5			0.0092 − 0.0035 = 0.0057
17	12.5;	2.0			0.0104 − 0.0029 = 0.0075
18	18.0;	12.0;	8.5;	2.0	0.0116 − 0.0102 + 0.0089 − 0.0029 = 0.0074
19	17.5;	12.5;	8.0;	2.0	0.0115 − 0.0104 + 0.0086 − 0.0029 = 0.0068
20	18.0;	11.0;	7.5;	2.0	0.0116 − 0.0100 + 0.0083 − 0.0029 = 0.0070
21	20.0;	2.5			0.0118 − 0.0036 = 0.0082
22	19.0;	4.0			0.0117 − 0.0055 = 0.0062
23	15.5;	4.0			0.0112 − 0.0055 = 0.0057
24	14.0;	4.0			0.0108 − 0.0055 = 0.0053
					SAR = 0.1188

The patient received 94 MU, the cGy/MU was 1.06, and the off-axis ratio was 1.05. The TAR for a 0×0 cm field at 9-cm depth from Table A.4 is 0.655. The transmission through the shielding block is assumed to be 3 percent and through the block-supporting tray 96 percent.

Using Eq. (5.8), the primary dose is therefore

$$94 \times 1.06 \times 1.05 \times 0.655 \times 0.96 \times 0.03 = 1.97 \text{ cGy}$$

The scatter at the same point is found from

$$\text{Scatter} = \text{MU} \times \text{cGy/MU} \times \text{tray factor} \times \text{SAR} \qquad (5.9)$$

In this patient, therefore, the scatter is

$$94 \times 1.06 \times 0.96 \times 0.119 = 11.38 \text{ cGy}$$

The total dose at the center of the left kidney during the treatment of this field is the sum of the primary (1.97) and scatter (11.38) contributions—that is,

$$1.97 + 11.38 = 13.35 \text{ cGy}$$

The dose delivered at the patient's midplane on the central axis of each field is 85 cGy.

It should, however, be emphasized that the point in the left kidney selected for this dose calculation is farther from the irradiated volume than other segments of the kidney and thus receives a lower dose.

CALCULATING DOSE OUTSIDE THE COLLIMATED FIELD

In some patients it might be necessary to calculate the dose at some point outside the collimated field —i.e., not under a block but outside the field as it is defined by the collimator. At points outside the field, there is no primary radiation dose; however, the scattered dose must be considered. The amount of dose depends on the beam energy, the size of the irradiated field, and the proximity of the calculation point to the irradiated field. Figure 5.11 shows a typical paraaortic/splenic pedicle field and the dose in the ovary is to be calculated. A 4-MV photon beam is used, and it is estimated that the ovary lies at 9-cm depth.

Radii are drawn from the calculation point (ovary) to the far edge of the irradiated field at 15° intervals, as explained in previous sections. In this illustration, only 5 radii traverse the field, and only those need to be considered in the calculation. The fractional SAR value for the entire length of the radius (P to A) is first found using Table A.8 and dividing the value by 24 (the number of radii in the circle at every 15°). The fractional SAR value for the part of the radius to the near edge of the irradiated area (P to B) is similarly found and is subtracted from the fractional SAR for the entire length. The SAR for this field is then found by adding together the fractional SARs for all radii, in this case only five. The SAR at the calculation point in Fig. 5.11 was found to be 0.0076 (Table 5.5).

In the situation under consideration, there is no primary dose, since the calculation point is outside the collimated field and not under a block, as in the previous section. The scattered dose in the ovary is found from

$$\text{Scatter} = \text{MU} \times \text{cGy/MU} \times \text{tray factor} \times \text{SAR} \qquad (5.10)$$

This patient received 100 MU/field/treatment, the cGy/MU was 1.023, and the tray factor was 0.96. Therefore, the dose to the ovary was

$$100 \times 1.023 \times 0.96 \times 0.0076 = 0.75 \text{ cGy/field/treatment}$$

In this example, it is assumed that the tissues under the blocked area within the field do not give rise to any scattered dose; however, since the block transmits approximately 3 percent, there is a very small amount of scattered dose observed at the calculation point.

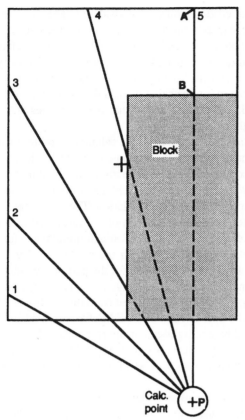

Figure 5.11 A typical paraaortic/splenic pedicle field in which the dose in the ovary (P) is calculated.

CALCULATING DOSE FOR A ROTATION THERAPY TREATMENT

In rotation therapy techniques, the axis of rotation is placed in the tumor and the therapy unit moves around the patient. The dose calculation method is the same whether the treatment machine makes a complete circle around the patient or a partial circle (arc). The SAD remains constant, but the thickness of tissue that lies between the source and the isocenter varies as the patient's contour changes. For the purpose of dose calculation, the treatment can be considered as multiple stationary isocentric fields. In this example, radii are drawn in 15° intervals from the isocenter to the patient's external surface and the fractional TAR values are added (Fig. 5.12). For the purpose of calculating the dose, this TAR is then considered as in a stationary isocentric treatment.

The prescription is for 200 cGy to be delivered at the isocenter while the machine rotates 360° around the patient. The field size is 8 × 8 cm and the cGy/MU is 0.98.

The TAR (Table 5.6) for a 8 × 8 cm 4-MV photon beam used in the rotation treatment illustrated in Fig. 5.12 is found to be 0.624 from interpolated values in Table A.4. Using Eq. (4.34), the required number of MU is therefore

$$\frac{200}{0.98 \times 0.624} = 327 \text{ MU}$$

Table 5.5   Scatter-Air Ratio Calculation for the Field in Fig. 5.11 (4-MV Photons)

Radius No.	Length, cm (Inside)	Fractional SAR	Length, cm (Outside)	Subtr. Fractional SAR	SAR
1	14.0	0.0108	10.6	0.0098	0.0010
2	17.4	0.0116	7.7	0.0085	0.0031
3	24.0	0.0122	8.4	0.0089	0.0033
4	26.6	0.0124	16.4	0.0118	0.0006
5	26.0	0.0124	20.0	0.0118	0.0006
				SAR =	**0.0076**

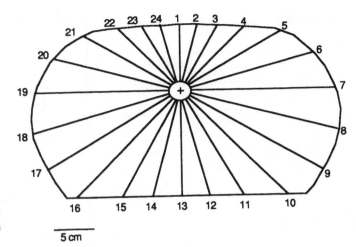

Figure 5.12   In a rotation treatment, the fractional TARs are found for each radius (TAR/24) and are then added together.

5 cm

The speed (degrees/MU) with which the machine must rotate is determined by dividing the number of degrees in the rotation by the number of MU. In this treatment, the machine must complete 360° while delivering 327 MU in order to deliver the prescribed dose at the isocenter. When a cobalt-60 machine is used for the rotation, the degrees per minute is found by dividing the number of degrees by the number of minutes needed to deliver the prescribed dose.

The degrees/MU can be found from

$$\frac{\text{degrees}}{\text{MU}} \qquad (5.11)$$

The degrees/MU in this treatment is therefore

$$\frac{360°}{327} = 1.1°/\text{MU}$$

It is always a good precaution to do a trial rotation without the patient present, before the actual treatment begins, to verify that the number of degrees and the MU or the treatment time is correct. It is also good practice to manually rotate the machine 360° around the patient before leaving the treatment room to make sure that accidental collisions will not occur during the treatment.

Table 5.6   Tissue-Air Ratio Calculation for the 360° Rotation in Fig. 5.12 (4-MV Photons, 8 × 8 cm Field)

Radius No.	Length, cm	Fractional TAR
1	8.0	0.0338
2	8.0	0.0338
3	9.0	0.0323
4	11.0	0.0295
5	13.5	0.0260
6	16.0	0.0230
7	17.5	0.0214
8	18.5	0.0203
9	18.5	0.0203
10	17.0	0.0220
11	14.0	0.0254
12	12.5	0.0269
13	12.0	0.0280
14	12.5	0.0269
15	14.0	0.0254
16	17.0	0.0220
17	18.5	0.0203
18	18.5	0.0203
19	17.5	0.0214
20	16.0	0.0230
21	13.5	0.0260
22	11.0	0.0295
23	9.0	0.0323
24	8.0	0.0338
		TAR = **0.6236**

PROBLEMS

5.1   The %DD at a given depth
  (a) Increases with higher beam energies
  (b) Increases with lower beam energies
  (c) Beam energy does not matter

5.2   The amount of backscatter
  (a) Increases with lower beam energies
  (b) Increases with higher beam energies
  (c) Beam energy does not matter

5.3   Find the equivalent square for a 8 × 24 cm field using the area/perimeter method.

5.4   Subtracting the SMR from the TMR for a 10 × 10 cm field will give the
  (a) TAR
  (b) Scatter dose
  (c) TPR
  (d) Primary dose

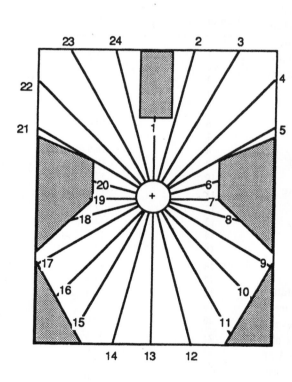

Radius #	Length	SAR
1		
2		
3		
4		
5		
6		
7		
8		
9		
10		
11		
12		
13		
14		
15		
16		
17		
18		
19		
20		
21		
22		
23		
24		

Figure 5.13   Calculate SAR at center of field.

5.5   Subtracting the TAR for a 0 × 0 cm field from the TAR for a 10 × 10 cm field will give the

(a) TAR for a 0 × 0 cm field

(b) Scatter dose for 10 × 10 a cm field

(c) Primary dose for 10 × 10 a cm field

(d) TMR for a 10 × 10 cm field

5.6   The OAR is the

(a) Ratio of the dose at a given depth along the central axis and the dose at a point off the central axis at the same depth

(b) Ratio of the dose at a given depth at a point away from the central axis and the dose at a point along the central axis at the same depth

(c) Ratio of the dose at a point at a given depth off the central axis and the dose on an isodose curve at the same depth

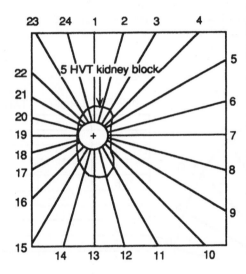

Radius#	Length	Frac. SAR	Blocked length	Subtr. Frac.SAR	SAR
1					
2					
3					
4					
5					
6					
7					
8					
9					
10					
11					
12					

Radius#	Length	Frac. SAR	Blocked length	Subtr. Frac.SAR	SAR
13					
14					
15					
16					
17					
18					
19					
20					
21					
22					
23					
24					

Figure 5.14 Calculate dose in the kidney. Use table to record length of each radius and fractional SAR. (Dimensions are only one-half of full size.)

5.7 A patient is receiving treatment to a lung tumor via parallel opposed 4-MV photon beams. The patient's diameter at the central axis of the beam is 20 cm. The treatment is isocentric and the field size is 12×18 cm at 80-cm SAD. 123 MU is delivered via each field. The cGy/MU for this field is 1.09. The dose in the spinal cord must be calculated at a point 7 cm cephalad from the central axis. The patient's diameter at this point is only 15 cm because of the slope of the anterior chest surface. The spinal cord is at 5 cm from the posterior surface and 10 cm from the anterior surface. The OAR for the posterior beam is 1.07; for the anterior beam, it is 1.035. What is the dose in the spinal cord? Use Table A.4 for TAR. There are no blocks and no wedges in this treatment.

5.8 Find the SAR at D_{max} at "+" in the field in Fig. 5.13. (Diagram is only one-half of full size.) Use Table A.8 for SAR.

5.9 Calculate the dose to the kidney at "+" under a 5-HVT block in Fig. 5.14. A 4-MV photon beam was used. The OAR at point "+" is 1.025 and the cGy/MU is 1.07. The 100 MU were delivered to one field only. The SSD was 80 cm and the depth was 12 cm. The tray factor is 0.96. (Dimensions are only one-half of full size.)

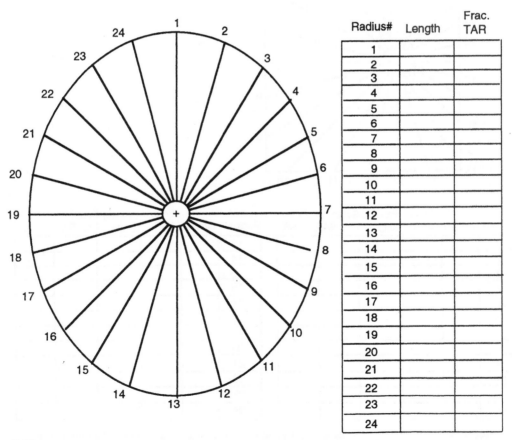

Figure 5.15 Find the TAR for the contour and use table to record fractional TAR.

5.10 A patient with the contour in Fig. 5.15 (diagram is only one-half of full size) is to be treated via a 360° rotation using an 8 × 8 cm cobalt-60 beam. The dose rate$_{ref}$ is 112.3 cGy/min for a 10 × 10 cm field and the area factor is 0.98. The 200 cGy is prescribed at the isocenter. What is the required treatment time? (Give the answer in minutes and seconds.)

5.11 In the above problem, how many degrees/minute must be set on the machine to deliver the prescribed dose while the machine rotates once through 360°?

REFERENCES

1. Batho HF, Theimer O, Theimer R: A consideration of equivalent circle method of calculating depth doses for rectangular x-ray fields. *J Can Assoc Radiol* 7:1951, 1956.
2. Day MJ: A note on the calculation of dose in x-ray fields. *Br J Radiol* 23:368, 1950.
3. Day MJ: The equivalent field method for axial dose determination in rectangular fields. *Br J Radiol Suppl* 10:77, 1961.
4. Jones DEA: A note on back-scatter and depth doses for elongated rectangular x-ray fields. *Br J Radiol* 22:342, 1949.
5. Sterling TD, Perry H, Katz L: Derivation of a mathematical expression for the percentage depth dose surface of cobalt-60 beams and visualization of multiple field dose distributions. *Br J Radiol* 37:544, 1964.
6. Clarkson JR: A note on depth dose in fields of irregular shape. *Br J Radiol* 14:265, 1941.
7. Chui CS, Mohan R: Off-center ratios for three-dimensional dose calculations. *Med Phys* 13:409, 1986.

Isodose Charts and Typical Field Arrangements

ISODOSE CHARTS

Isodose charts depicting the dose distribution from a single beam were explained in Chap. 3. Although such charts provide much more information about the radiation beam than central-axis percentage depth doses alone, it is important to recognize that they represent the dose distribution in only one plane and are usually available only for square or rectangular fields.

Isodose charts are almost exclusively obtained with the beam directed perpendicular to a water phantom that has a flat surface and uniform density. When the dose distribution is calculated for a patient —whose surface is rarely flat and whose internal density is never uniform—the isodose chart should be adjusted for the effects of irregular surface topography, oblique incidence, and inhomogeneities encountered in the path of the beam. In clinical practice, corrections for surface irregularities and beam obliquity are routinely made, but the effect of inhomogeneities is often disregarded because the size, location, and density of the inhomogeneities are frequently unknown. It should be borne in mind that as a result, most clinical data on which treatment decisions are based necessarily depend on dose calculations in which inhomogeneity corrections were not made.

CORRECTING ISODOSE CHARTS FOR IRREGULAR SURFACE CONTOUR

Photon Beams. Correcting photon isodose curves for irregular surface topography is quite simple in principle, but hand calculations are laborious and corrections are nowadays almost exclusively carried out with the help of computers. The manual method is considered first.

Figure 6.1 shows a single isodose chart superimposed on a sagittal chest contour. At A, the beam travels through 1.5 cm of air over and above the nominal SSD before it is intercepted by the patient. The absorbed dose along the line a to b is therefore higher than would be indicated by isodose curves *(solid lines)* measured in a flat water phantom. The increase in dose, compared to what would be ob-

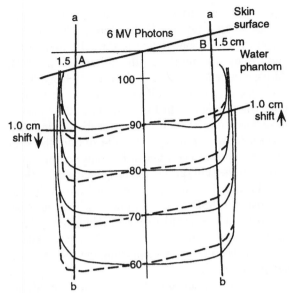

Figure 6.1   An isodose chart superimposed on a sloping patient contour. The isodose curves are corrected for the changes that occur as a result of the sloping surface contour. Since the contour slopes at a constant angle, the difference between the flat surface of the isodose chart and the patient's contour can be measured along only two ray lines (a to b).

tained at a given depth below a flat surface, is primarily caused by the reduced thickness of attenuating material above the point considered. Another factor altering the dose along this line is the smaller volume of scattering material due to the "missing tissue" near A. The increase in dose depends on the beam energy, field size, and shape of the block of "missing tissue," but it is, as an example, approximately 3 percent per centimeter of missing tissue thickness for 6-MV photons. Since the percent depth dose falls at a rate of approximately 5 percent per centimeter in tissue, a 3 percent increase in dose represents approximately two-thirds centimeter in tissue. Therefore, the distance by which the isodose curves must be shifted deeper along a given ray line is approximately two-thirds of the air gap. For lower energies, the shift is larger, and for higher energies, it is smaller. This is, of course, only an approximation. At B in Fig. 6.1, the opposite occurs. Here, the beam is intercepted by the patient at an SSD that is 1.5 cm shorter than the one used in measuring the isodose curves for flat surfaces. The effect on the isodose curves along a ray line is therefore in the opposite direction; each isodose line is shifted closer to the surface by two-thirds of the difference in SSD. Along the central axis, the dose is unchanged because the skin surface and the flat surface of the isodose chart coincide. In Fig. 6.1, the isodose curves have been corrected in this way for the sloping skin surface *(hashed lines)*. In this illustration, the skin surface sloped at a constant angle; however, in many situations the skin surface can be quite irregular (Fig. 6.2). In such situations, it is necessary to measure the difference in SSD at several points within the field and then to make a mark on each isodose curve along each ray line, as shown in Fig. 6.2. The new isodose lines are then drawn by connecting the marks made along each ray line.

This tedious manual method lends itself easily to computerization, and most commercial treatment-planning software corrects automatically for irregular skin contours and nonperpendicular incidence.

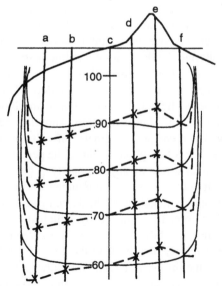

Figure 6.2   An isodose chart superimposed on an irregular patient contour. The isodose curves are corrected for the changes that occur as a result of the irregular surface contour. Here the difference between the flat surface of the isodose chart and the patient's contour must be measured along several ray lines.

Electron Beams.   When electron beams are used, the problems with irregular skin surfaces are the same as for photon beams. Correction of electron isodose curves for air gaps and oblique incidence is frequently needed because here the electron cone often cannot be placed directly on or perpendicular to the skin surface. When air gaps are encountered, it is a common practice to apply an inverse square law calculation.[1,2] It is first necessary to establish that the dose fall-off in fact follows the inverse square law.[3] The relative dose remains practically unchanged when the SSD is increased, but the actual dose is decreased. The penumbra is also wider when the cone-to-skin surface distance is increased, particularly when low energies and small fields are used.[4]

Oblique incidence presents a more complex situation, because here the side scatter at D_{max} depth is increased and the D_{max} itself is closer to the surface. The penetration of the beam is also reduced.[5] Khan *et al.* have determined obliquity factors as a function of energy and depth for various angles and have presented them in tabular form.[6,7] The changes in the dose distribution caused by air gaps and oblique incidence are quite tedious to carry out by hand; however, several methods of computer calculation are available.[8-10]

CORRECTING FOR INHOMOGENEITIES

Photon Beams.   Correcting isodose curves for inhomogeneities traversed by the beam is much more complex and often requires information that is unavailable. It is necessary to know, first, the electron density (electrons/cm^3) of the inhomogeneity and, second, the size, shape, and location of the inhomogeneous region. This information can best be obtained from a computed tomography (CT) scan of the area to be treated, but in most radiation therapy departments it is not routine to perform a CT scan for this purpose: the effect on the dose is instead estimated by one of several methods[7]:

1. A tissue-air ratio method takes into account the field size and the depth of the calculation point but does not take into account the position of the calculation point with respect to the inhomogeneity. It also assumes that the inhomogeneity has a constant thickness and that the width is infinite.

2. Another approach is the power law tissue-air ratio (TAR) method,[11-13] which takes into account the position of the calculation point with respect to the inhomogeneity but does not consider its width or the shape. Another form of the power law method allows for correction of dose within the inhomogeneity.[14] An equivalent TAR method also takes into account the effect of the geometric arrangement of the scattering structures with respect to the calculation point.[15] These methods are most practical when a point calculation only is required.

Though full adjustment of isodose curves for the effect of an inhomogeneity is very complex, it is similar to the shift method used to adjust for irregular surface topography. The amount of shift to be employed in this case depends on the beam energy, the electron density, and the thickness of the inhomogeneity that the beam traverses. For beam energies of 6 MV or lower, a shift of about 0.6 for air and 0.4 for lung can be used—i.e., when the beam traverses 10 cm of lung tissue (relative electron density less than 1.0), the isodose curves should be shifted 4 cm *deeper* (Fig. 6.3); whereas in bone, where the electron density is more than 1.0, the isodoses shift to shallower depths.

Another effect of inhomogeneities to consider is the dose buildup in the distal interfaces between muscle and less dense lung tissue (or air cavities) and the corresponding "builddown," where underdo-

sage can occur. The amount of underdosage at the proximal interfaces, which has been reported to be as high as 30 percent under extreme circumstances, depends to a large extent on the beam energy but also on the field size and on the geometry and density of the inhomogeneity.[16] It is difficult to ascertain the effects on the dose of low-density lung volume and of air cavities, either by measurements or calculations. The problem has been studied by several authors.[15,17-24]

Electron Beams. The effect of inhomogeneities on electron beam isodose distributions has also been studied by several authors.[25-30] Changes in the dose due to inhomogeneities can be significant, particularly when air cavities, lung, and bone are encountered. Compact bone attenuates the beam more than muscle and therefore reduces the dose beyond it. Spongy bone, such as the sternum, may have little effect; however, it is probably wise to assume that the surface of every bone is relatively compact. Therefore, when an electron beam is used to treat internal mammary lymph nodes, the lateral aspect of the sternum, where the beam direction can be parallel with the lateral surface of the bone, may attenuate the beam more than the central section, where the beam passes through only a thin wall of compact bone (Fig. 6.4). In lung tissue, the range of the electrons is increased by a factor of 3; thus the dose to the

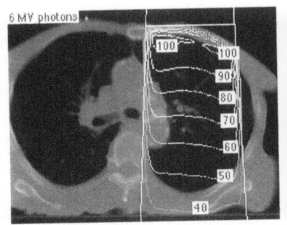
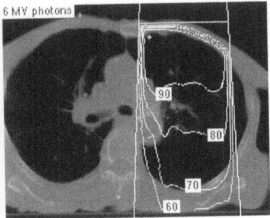

Figure 6.3 Isodose distribution calculated for a single 6-MV photon beam without (*left*) and with (*right*) correction for lung inhomogeneity. The dose is increased significantly when the lower density of the lung tissue is considered in the calculation.

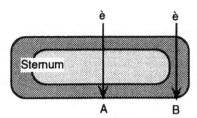

Figure 6.4 The thickness of dense bone *(darker shade)* that an electron beam encounters may vary across the beam. At A the beam passes through only two thin segments of denser bone, while at B the thickness of dense bone is greater.

lung and tissues beyond it is significantly higher than it would be at the same point if the inhomogeneity were absent. The change in dose can be corrected by using the coefficient of equivalent thickness (CET), where it is assumed that the attenuation by a given thickness of an inhomogeneity is equivalent to the attenuation by a certain thickness of water. The typical CET used for compact bone is 1.5 g/cm^3; for spongy bone, it is 1.1 g/cm^3. The electron density of lung tissue varies depending on depth and also on the patient's condition; however, an average value of 0.5 g/cm^3 is often used.[29] Due to changes in the scattering properties when electron beams traverse inhomogeneities, it is important to realize that the dose is dramatically altered. For example, backscatter can cause the dose to be about 5 percent higher in front of a compact bone and can cause the dose within the bone to be 10 to 15 percent higher than in soft tissues. In a similar fashion, the dose *in front of* a less dense area, such as an air cavity or a volume of lung tissue, is decreased because scattering is less, while *within* the less dense tissue, where the electron range is much longer than in muscle, a large volume of lung receives a higher dose.

The corrections just described represent changes in the isodose curves caused by the patient's skin-surface topography or the presence of an inhomogeneity in only one plane. The dose distribution on a plane in front of or behind this plane may be quite different, depending on the shape of the patient's surface and any inhomogeneous tissues in the path of the beam.

As with photon beams, manual isodose corrections for inhomogeneities are time-consuming and at

best provide no more than an estimate of the effect; however, computer algorithms to execute these calculations are emerging.[28,31–37] The calculations and measurements of dose in the presence of an inhomogeneity are complex, and significant errors in computer-aided dose estimation have been shown.[38]

BUILDUP REGION

Photon Beams. When cobalt-60 or higher-energy beams are used, the dose in the superficial layers of tissue is relatively low compared to the ionization maximum. This is due to the range of secondary electrons. The dose in this region gradually increases, or builds up, until it reaches a certain depth, and then it falls off due to the increasing thickness of attenuating tissue and the longer distance from the source (Fig. 6.5). The major factor determining the depth (D_{max}) at which dose maximum occurs is the beam energy.[39–41] For a given beam energy, the depth at which the maximum dose or equilibrium occurs is reduced as the field size is increased. As D_{max} is shifted closer to the surface, the dose on the surface is also increased. Another important condition under which the skin sparing is reduced is in obliquely incident beams.[42,43] In many treatments—for example, in the treatment of the chest wall or in most other situations where the beam "flashes" over the patient's skin surface (as in an extremity, the neck, or the perineum)—the beam intercepts the surface at a very steep angle and at some point is parallel with the surface immediately before it flashes over the skin surface (Fig. 6.6). When this occurs, the skin-sparing effect (Chap. 3), which is a great advantage of high-energy radiation beams, is reduced and may in some cases be completely lost.[42] In addition, the dose can be significantly higher in this region due to the smaller thickness of attenuating material that the beam often traverses in this shallow region.

A shift of D_{max} toward the surface is also caused by secondary electrons arising in the collimator and in various devices placed in the beam, such as wedges, compensators, field-shaping devices, and trays holding these devices.[44,45] It is also important to realize that the depth of D_{max} is shifted closer to the

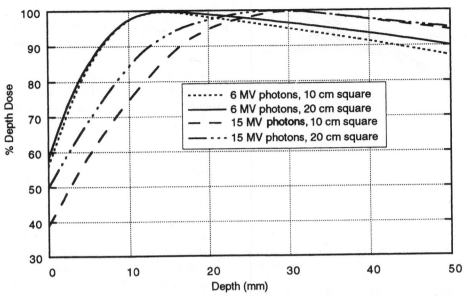

Figure 6.5 Percentage depth dose curves in the buildup region for 6- and 15-MV photon beams with two different field sizes. The depth of maximum dose (D_{max}) decreases with increased field size.

surface and the surface dose is increased when the beam is intercepted by sections of the treatment couch; immobilization devices; clothing, pads, or sheets placed on the treatment couch; or by casts or bandages on the patient. The effect on the surface dose of field size, beam energy, and photon beams traversing various materials has been studied by several authors.[40,44,46–53]

In some situations, it is necessary to shift D_{max} intentionally toward the skin surface while simultaneously treating a deep-seated lesion using a high-energy beam. An example of this situation would be when an incision on the skin surface must be treated at the same dose as the deeper primary tumor. In this situation, a piece of tissue-equivalent material (bolus) can be placed directly on the incision. There are other situations in which it is desirable to use a high-energy beam because of its superior dose uniformity but in which one wants at the same time to reduce the depth of the maximum dose while maintaining some degree of skin sparing. As an example, when a patient with Hodgkin's disease is treated with a mantle field, it is advantageous to use a high-energy beam to achieve an acceptable dose uniformity throughout the chest, but this may cause some of the superficial lymph nodes to fall in the buildup region of the beam, where they experience a lower and perhaps insufficient dose. To reduce the depth of the maximum dose, thus moving the lymph nodes into a higher-dose region while maintaining some skin sparing, a sheet of Lucite can be placed in the beam at a short distance from the skin surface.[54] The thickness of this ''beam spoiler'' and the distance at which it should be placed depends on the beam energy and the distance by which the maximum dose must be shifted.[55,56]

A note of caution is added here, because in some rare treatment situations the isocenter may be in the buildup region. When the dose distribution is calculated and is normalized to 100 percent at the isocenter, the dose elsewhere will be very high. For example, let us assume that the isocenter in a plan with a pair of wedges is at a depth in the buildup region that is equal to the depth of the 50 percent isodose line (Fig. 6.7). When the dose here is normalized to 100 percent, an increase by a factor of 2, all the other isodose values will also be multiplied by a factor of 2. In these situations, the isocenter must

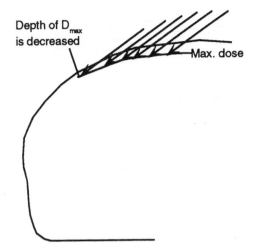

Figure 6.6 When a photon beam encounters a surface obliquely, D_{max} moves closer to the surface. Each arrow *(ray line)* passes through a thickness of tissue equal to D_{max}, but when the beam intersects the tissue at a steep angle, this distance can be very close to the surface; thus D_{max} is decreased.

be shifted and the fields adjusted, or a small thickness of bolus material must be added just over the isocenter to "force" the isocenter to be at a depth that is equal to or greater than D_{max}.

Electron Beams. Just as with photon beams, D_{max} for electrons increases at higher beam energies. However, unlike the photon case, the actual dose on the skin surface increases with higher energies. Figure 6.8 shows the percentage depth dose (%DD) in the buildup region for different electron-beam energies. The values shown in the figure should be used only as rough guides because they may vary from machine to machine, even when the beam energies are the same; therefore the data should always be measured for each particular machine prior to clinical use.[57] With lower-energy beams, the dose falls very rapidly with depth after it has reached 100 percent, while with higher-energy beams, the peak is less sharp and the dose remains close to 100 percent over several millimeters.

The therapeutic range of electrons (90 percent isodose line) is found by dividing the electron energy by 4, and the depth of the 80 percent line is usually

found by dividing the electron energy by 3. When using a 12-MeV electron beam, the 80 percent isodose line is therefore at about 4 cm depth (12/3) and the 90 percent isodose line is at about 3 cm (12/4). This is only an approximation, and to be certain of the depths, isodose curves measured for each electron beam must be consulted prior to writing the prescription.

COMBINING OF ISODOSE CHARTS

When a treatment consists of applying a single field of either photons or electrons, it is not usually necessary to display an isodose distribution on the patient's cross-sectional contour. Exceptions would be in situations where the patient's surface contour is very irregular or the beam traverses heterogeneous tissues; in such cases, the isodose chart requires correction, as described earlier, and the corrected version should be displayed on the contour. In practically all of radiation therapy, however, more than one field is used in the treatments.

The treatment can consist of a combination of either multiple fields using the same photon beam energy, several photon beams of different energy, a combination of photon and electron beams, or multi-

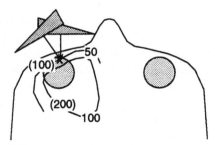

Figure 6.7 When the isocenter, where the dose usually is normalized to 100 percent, is in the buildup region, where the dose is low, all isodose lines will be affected by the dose normalization. In this plan, the isocenter is set in the buildup region, where the 50 percent isodose line falls. When the dose here is normalized to 100 percent *(parentheses)*, an increase by a factor of 2, the 100 percent isodose line in the plan will also increase by a factor of 2—i.e., it will become 200 percent *(parentheses)*.

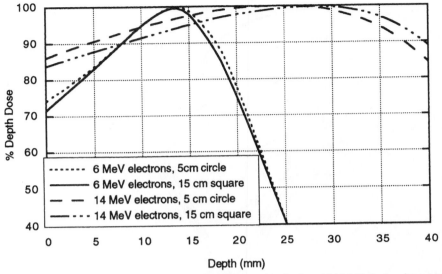

Figure 6.8 Percentage depth dose curves in the buildup region for 6- and 14-MeV electron beams with two different field sizes. The surface dose increases with higher beam energy and also with smaller fields.

ple electron beams. In many situations, it is also necessary to deliver a different amount of radiation from each field. In either of these situations, it is essential that the doses contributed by each field be added together and a composite isodose distribution be displayed on the contour. When this is done, one can easily see whether the dose uniformity within the target volume is acceptable and can make certain that the dose in the adjacent normal tissues is below tolerance. Such presentation also makes it easier to assess the effects of varying beam energy, weighting, beam angles, wedge dimension, and so on in achieving an acceptable dose distribution. The composite dose distribution is also very important in documenting the patient's treatment, and it should be clearly and completely labeled before it is inserted into the patient's treatment chart.

COMBINING TWO ISODOSE CHARTS

The sequence of steps leading up to the combination of isodose charts frequently is, in the absence of three-dimensional treatment-planning capabilities, that the target volume and radiosensitive structures in the vicinity are localized with respect to external reference marks. Next, the patient's external cross-sectional contour is obtained, indicating the reference marks used for target localization. The target volume and critical normal tissues are then indicated on the cross-sectional contour. The field arrangement, beam energy, and need for beam-modifying devices are determined. These steps are outlined in greater detail in Chap. 7.

The combining of isodose charts in this era of computers is almost never done manually. However, to understand the principle of the process, a brief review of manual isodose combination is presented. Isodose charts are, as already stated, produced by measuring the dose distribution in a water phantom; they therefore assume uniform density and a flat surface. We already know how to correct for the presence of an irregular surface, but to keep matters simple, we will assume that the patient's surface is flat in this case. In Fig. 6.9, two beams are directed so that the angle between them is 60°. Doses are added together at points where isodose lines from each chart intersect. Many points will have the same dose, and these points are connected in such a way that the doses along the line, interpolating between isodose values, are always the same. For example, we see

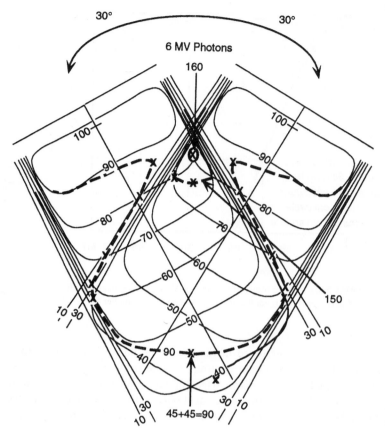

Figure 6.9 Isodose charts of two beams, angled 30° to each side, where the dose from the two is combined. The hatched lines indicate the combined dose (only 150 and 90 percent lines are shown).

that the 80 percent line of the left field in Fig. 6.9 intersects the 70 percent line of the right field. At this point the combined dose is 150 percent of the dose at D_{max} of one field only; i.e., when 100 cGy is delivered at D_{max} of each field, the dose at this point is 150 cGy. The same dose is found where the 80 percent line of the right field intersects the 70 percent line of the left field, also giving a combined dose of 150 percent at this point. The two points are connected, but not by a straight line. We must find some point between these two points where the dose is also 150 percent. In this case we must interpolate between the 70 percent and the 80 percent lines to find the 75 percent isodose line (not shown) of each field. The dose where the two 75 percent lines (which we have just interpolated) cross is also 150 percent; therefore, the 150 percent line connecting the two previously found 150 percent points must pass

through this new point. Closer to the surface, we see that the 80 percent lines of each field come together but do not cross one another. The dose here is therefore 160 percent. The 90 percent isodose line of each field remains unchanged until it is affected by the penumbra of the other beam. Although the lowest isodose line indicated is 10 percent, the dose continues to fall off gradually outside that line. As the 90 and 10 percent isodose lines approach one another, the combined dose increases; but since these lines do not intersect, the dose is less than 100 percent. At the point where the 5 percent isodose line is estimated to intersect the 85 percent line, the total dose is 90 percent; therefore, the 90 percent line must be modified so that it will go through this point. Interpolating between the lines, many points are found where the combined dose is 90 percent, and these points are connected as just described for the 150 percent line. In a similar manner, other isodose-curves representing the combined dose from the two fields are found. It is customary to trace out isodose curves only in 10 percent increments, particularly if an additional field must be added. Figure 6.10 demonstrates the combined isodose distribution in the example discussed above. This plan obviously does not result in desired dose uniformity but instead requires that wedges (Chap. 3) be used in the beams, as we shall show later in this chapter.

COMBINING MULTIPLE ISODOSE CHARTS

It is confusing and indeed almost impossible, using this simple technique, to add isodose charts from three or more fields simultaneously. Instead, it is easier to add the third field after the first two have been combined; when four fields are needed, it is best to first add together two pairs of fields sepa-

rately and then combine these. It must also be emphasized that when the isodose lines are being added, it is helpful if each chart is traced in a different color. The composite should also be traced in a different color to make it easier to distinguish the different lines.

COMBINING ISODOSE CHARTS WITH DIFFERENT WEIGHT

In many treatment plans, the dose delivered from one field may be different from that of the second field. In that case, the values along each isodose line are adjusted in the addition process to indicate the ratio of the dose delivered from each field before the isodose charts are combined. For example, if the dose through one field is half of that delivered through the other, the value of each isodose line of the less intense field is decreased by half. Alternatively, the

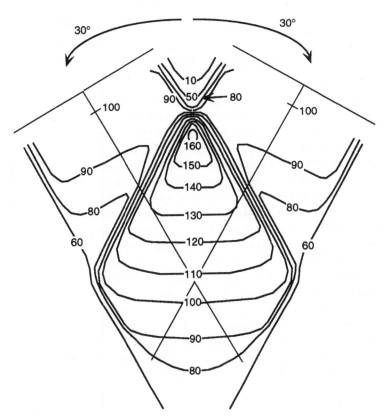

Figure 6.10 The isodose distribution resulting from combining the isodose charts in Fig. 6.9.

line values assigned to the field delivering the two-fold dose can be doubled. It is, however, critical to remember which method was used when the treatment time or MU is calculated. In the first method, the combined isodose values are the result of a total D_{max} dose of 150 percent (100 percent from one field and 50 percent from the field with the lower weight), while in the second method the total D_{max} dose is 300 percent (100 + 200). Using an isocentric treatment technique, all values should be reduced, so that the combined dose is 100% at the isocenter. In this example, a 2- to 1-weighting was used; hence the values are reduced by a factor of 1.5 and 3.0, respectively. The field delivering the higher dose will therefore deliver 66.66 percent, or two-thirds of the dose at the isocenter, and the field with the lower weight will deliver 33.33 percent, or one-third. Of course, other methods of normalizing the dose can be used, but it is critical that whatever method is used in combining the isodose lines be taken into consideration when the treatment time or MU is calculated.

COMBINING ISODOSE CHARTS OF DIFFERENT BEAM ENERGIES TREATING THE SAME FIELD

So far, we have combined isodose charts from beams aimed at a target from different directions. Here we shall combine isodose charts from two beams of the same size but with different beam energy, or with and without wedges, and aimed at the target through the same tissues. Sometimes the combination of an electron and a photon beam may be employed in the treatment of a single field—for example, in the treatment of a parotid tumor, where it is important to reduce the dose in the oral mucosa and the contralateral salivary glands, or in the treatment of the internal mammary lymph nodes, where it is important to spare the underlying mediastinal structures, such as lungs, heart, and esophagus. The isodose charts of the appropriate photon and electron beams are superimposed and the value of each isodose line is adjusted in the addition process to indicate the proportion of the dose delivered from each beam. Likewise, when two different photon-beam energies are mixed, the isodose charts are combined.

In some treatments requiring wedges, it may be necessary to produce isodose curves with an angle different from that produced by standard wedges. Most manufacturers make available wedges that are 15°, 30°, 45°, and 60°. If, for example, an isodose tilt of only 7.5° is needed, the isodose chart from an open beam and a 15° wedge with the same field size are combined (Fig. 6.11). In this case, the values along each isodose line in both charts are reduced to half. The two isodose charts are then superimposed, and the doses from the two charts are summed. The resulting isodose curves will have a 7.5° tilt. Similarly, isodose charts for two different wedge angles, for two different beam energies, or for a photon and an electron beam can be combined.

When the treatment time or MU is calculated for a mixed unwedged and wedged beam, it is necessary to use the wedge transmission factor only for the portion of the treatment delivered using the wedge —50 percent in the case described above. In the situation described here, where the same field is treated partially with an unwedged beam and partially with a wedge, it is a good practice to calculate the monitor

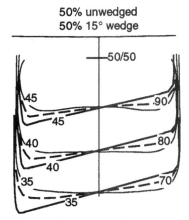

Figure 6.11 Combining two different isodose charts for treatment of the same field requires that the isodose charts be superimposed and the values of each isodose line adjusted with the fraction of the dose delivered from each beam. Here the two beams (unwedged and 15° wedge) are equally weighted (i.e., half of the dose is given with an unwedged beam and half with a 15° wedge to produce a 7.5° wedge effect). The combined dose is indicated by the hatched line.

units and carry the fields in the daily treatment chart as if they were different fields. The number of MU for the two fields will obviously be different, and it is important to indicate *clearly* which portions of the treatment were delivered with and without the wedge. In the rare event that a treatment machine breaks down during the treatment or the treatments are otherwise interrupted, it can be confusing to try to decipher what fraction of the dose was delivered with and without the wedge. Likewise, when two different wedge angles, two different photon energies, or photon and electron beams are combined, the fields should be carried as two different fields in the daily treatment record.

DOSE NORMALIZATION

A term often used in radiation therapy is *normalization*. It means that the dose at some point has been

"forced" to 100 percent and the dose everywhere else is changed by the same ratio. For example, in Fig. 6.12, the sum of the %DD at the middepth point for two opposed cobalt-60 beams is 130 percent and the maximum dose is 138 percent. When we "force" the middepth dose to be 100 percent, we decrease the middepth dose by a factor of 1.3 (or 130/100). All other dose values are also reduced by the same factor, and the maximum dose, as an example, is therefore 138/1.3 or 106.2 percent (numbers are rounded off).

In an SSD treatment technique, the dose is usually normalized to 100 percent at D_{max} of each field, and in an SAD technique, the normalization is routinely 100 percent at the isocenter. Other methods of dose normalization are possible. However, for the purpose of calculating MU or treatment time, it must be clear which method was used or serious errors in dose can occur. It is therefore a good practice, within a radia-

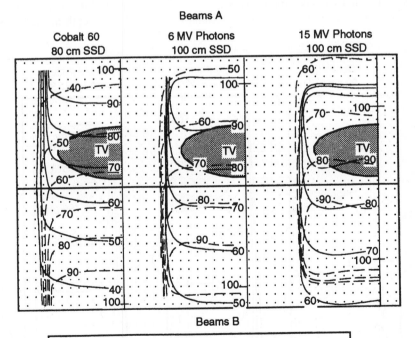

Figure 6.12 Parallel opposed beams comparing three different beam energies. The ratio of dose between D_{max} and middepth is decreased with the higher beam energy; in fact, the dose is almost the same (169 to 170 percent) when 15-MV photon beams are used, whereas with the cobalt-60 beams, the D_{max} dose is 138 percent, as opposed to 130 percent at middepth.

Fields	Cobalt 60 A+B	6 MV A+B	15 MV A+B
Mid-depth	65+65 =130	75+75 =150	85+85 =170
D_{max}	100+38 =138	100+52 =152	100+69 =169

tion therapy department, to establish a system with which everyone is familiar; thus the possibility of errors is reduced. Treatment-planning computers can frequently be the source of confusion concerning dose normalization; users must therefore become familiar with the convention used for dose normalization in their particular computer.

SINGLE-FIELD TREATMENT

PHOTON BEAMS

Treatment through a single photon field is rarely acceptable except for superficial targets such as the internal mammary and supraclavicular nodes or shallow tumors in an extremity. Before making a decision to use only one single-photon field, it is important to consider

1. The range of dose within the tumor
2. The maximum dose in the tissues
3. The exit dose (providing no skin sparing)

In general, the dose range within the target should be within ±5 percent, while the maximum dose should be < 110 percent of the prescribed dose. The maximum dose in a three-dimensional treatment plan, where the dose within the entire irradiated volume is known, is sometimes referred to as the "global" maximum dose. This dose gradient cannot always be achieved, but in patients where the required target dose is high, every attempt should be made to stay within these guidelines.

Figure 6.13 demonstrates that the use of a single 15-MV beam result in a smaller dose range within the tumor, D_{max} is at a greater depth in the patient, but the exit dose is higher than when a cobalt-60 or 6-MV photon beam is used to treat the same tumor. In this case, the low-energy beam is best in terms of exit dose, while the high-energy beam is best in terms of dose range within the tumor.

Tumors in and near the spinal cord are often treated through a single posterior field; however, the lumbar segment of the spine can be close to the mid-depth in many patients; in a large patient, the entire

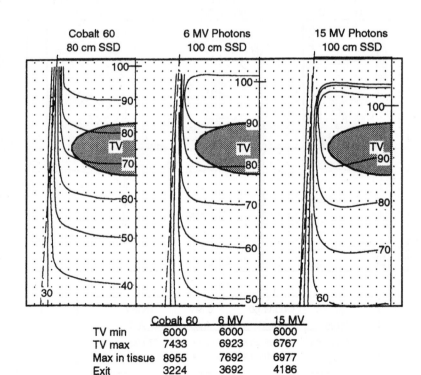

	Cobalt 60	6 MV	15 MV
TV min	6000	6000	6000
TV max	7433	6923	6767
Max in tissue	8955	7692	6977
Exit	3224	3692	4186

Figure 6.13 A single beam delivering a minimum tumor dose of 6000 cGy, comparing three different beam energies, shows that the dose range within the tumor is smaller with the 15-MV photon beam (6000 to 6767 cGy) versus 6000 to 7433 cGy with a cobalt-60 beam. The exit dose using the 15-MV photon beam is 4186 cGy, which is higher than that with the cobalt-60 beam (3224 cGy). The maximum dose within the field is 8955 cGy with a cobalt-60 beam versus 6977 cGy with the 15-MV beam.

spine can be at a significant depth. In the following example, we examine the virtues of a single field. In Fig. 6.14*A*, a single 6-MV photon beam using 100-cm SSD is employed to treat a tumor near the spinal canal. The tumor is encompassed by the 80 percent isodose curve (minimum tumor dose), while the maximum dose in the tumor is 92 percent. Thus, the dose range within the tumor is from 80 to 92 percent and the maximum dose in the patient is 100 percent. If a minimum tumor dose of 4500 cGy is delivered, the maximum tumor dose is 5175 cGy and the maximum dose in the patient is 5625 cGy. (It is important to recognize that the minimum and maximum doses specified here represent the dose on one plane only, while the doses in other planes are unknown.) This dose gradient exceeds the guidelines given for items

1 and 2 of the above list. However, it is often considered an acceptable treatment, since the prescribed dose is relatively low. If a lower-energy beam had been used, the range of dose within the tumor and in the patient would have been larger and probably unacceptable. On the other hand, using this lower energy results in a lower dose in the exit region in front of the spine than if two opposing fields were used. However, it is important to recognize that no skin sparing is provided in the exit region. The addition of an opposing field would result in a more uniform dose throughout the treatment area and would also provide some skin sparing in both entrance/exit regions.

Another situation where use of a single field may be useful is in treating a shallow soft tissue sarcoma

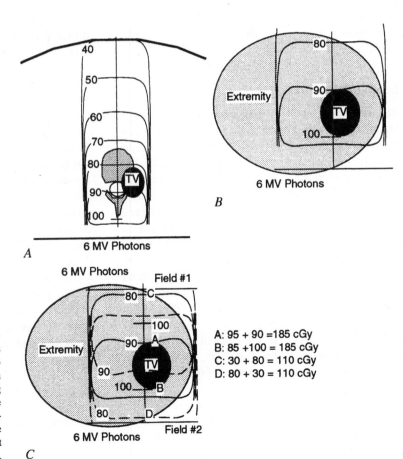

Figure 6.14 *A.* A single posterior 6-MV photon field to treat a paraspineous tumor. *B.* A single 6-MV photon field to treat a tumor in the arm results in a high exit dose, where there is no skin-sparing effect. *C.* When the beam is opposed, the dose uniformity is improved and skin sparing is achieved in both beams. The surface dose is estimated to be about 30 percent entrance and 80 percent exit in each beam.

A: 95 + 90 = 185 cGy
B: 85 + 100 = 185 cGy
C: 30 + 80 = 110 cGy
D: 80 + 30 = 110 cGy

of an extremity. In Fig. 6.14*B*, for example, the dose distribution from a single 6-MV photon beam (uncorrected for surface contour) is shown superimposed on a cross-sectional contour of an arm. The dose within the tumor ranges from 90 to 100 percent and the maximum dose in the arm is also 100 percent; thus the criteria for acceptability set forth earlier are met. Consideration should, however, be given to the dose on the skin surface in the exit region of the arm, where there is no skin sparing. In this treatment, the exit dose is 80 percent of the maximum dose in the arm, but it is almost the same as the minimum tumor dose. Let us assume that the minimum tumor dose is 6000 cGy (90 percent isodose line); then the exit dose, without any skin sparing, will be about 5330 cGy (80 percent isodose line) and the maximum tumor dose will be 6665 cGy (100 percent). An opposing field would improve the dose uniformity through the tumor and would result in the same skin sparing on each side of the arm (Fig. 6.14*C*).

ELECTRON BEAMS

Electron beams are most frequently used as a single beam or with two or more adjacent beams. Opposed electron beams are often used to treat posterior cervical lymph nodes when spinal cord tolerance has been reached in the treatment of head and neck malignancies. The beam energy must be selected so that no significant dose is delivered in the spinal cord and also so that the deep isodose lines from the two fields do not overlap at a depth (particularly in the spinal cord). When the dose in the spinal cord is calculated, it is important to consider also the contribution of the x-ray contamination, or *bremsstrahlung,* which always accompanies electron beams. This dose, caused by electron interaction with the collimator and other components in the head of the treatment machine, can be from 2 to 5 percent, depending on the electron energy and the design of the collimation system.

When electron fields are used, it is critical to be aware of the extent and maximum depth of the target volume and to choose an electron-beam energy and field margins so that the prescribed isodose line encompasses this volume. Since the dose falls off very rapidly beyond the 80 percent line, where the dose is often prescribed, knowledge of the depth is particularly important in electron-beam therapy. It is also important to recognize that when the dose is prescribed to the 80 percent line, the maximum dose (100 percent) is 25 percent higher (100/80). Depending on what tissues lie in the 100 percent area, the 25 percent higher dose may be acceptable. In the absence of radiosensitive tissues at a depth beyond the 80 percent line, the beam energy may be increased and the dose calculated to the 90 percent isodose line, effectively reducing the maximum dose. It is sometimes necessary to increase the surface dose (Fig. 6.15*A*) or to shift the isodose lines closer to the surface within a portion of the field so as to limit the dose to underlying tissues (Fig. 6.15*B*). In this case, a piece of tissue-equivalent material (bolus) of appropriate thickness can be placed directly on the skin surface.[58] The bolus must conform closely to the skin surface, leaving no air gaps between the bolus and the surface. A piece of bolus placed inside an electron field must have tapered edges to avoid very high dose in the tissue near the edges of the bolus.[6]

As in photon beams, the 50 percent isodose line is usually taken to be the geometric margin of the field. In electron beams, the isodose lines representing less than 50 percent tend to bulge out, thus unnecessarily including a large volume. The 80 and 90 percent isodose curves, on the other hand, tend to constrict, particularly in smaller fields and when higher-energy electron beams are used. At the depth of the 80 percent isodose line, the width of the region within which dose uniformity is acceptable may be reduced by 0.75 to 1.0 cm on each side (Fig. 6.15*C*). This unusual shape of the isodose curves must be considered when tumor margins are decided. In general, tumor margins must be more generous when electron beams are used than for photons.

PARALLEL OPPOSED FIELD TREATMENT

The term *parallel opposed* refers to two identical beams aimed toward each other from exactly opposite directions (i.e., the central axes are separated by

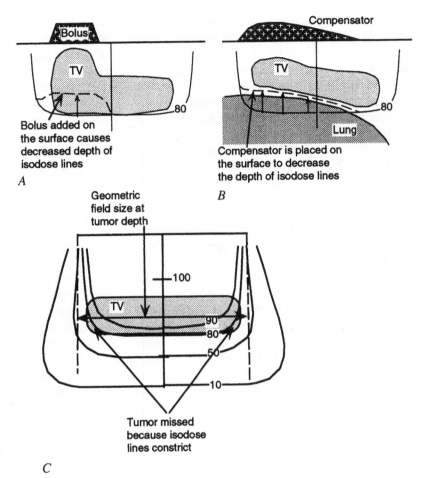

Figure 6.15 *A*. When a tumor extends near the surface at some point within an electron beam, bolus can be used to increase the surface dose and reduce the depth of dose maximum. However, at the same time, all isodose curves are moved to a shallower depth, possibly causing a tumor miss at a depth (for clarity, only the 80 percent isodose line is shown). *B*. The effect is the same as using a compensator on the skin surface to decrease the depth, now intentionally. *C*. When an electron beam is used, the tumor margins need to be considered, bearing in mind the characteristics of the electron isodose curves. The 80 and 90 percent isodose curves, where the dose usually is prescribed, tend to constrict at depth, causing the effective field size to be decreased by 0.75 to 1.0 cm on each side of the geometric field margins.

180°). Parallel opposed fields are probably the most commonly used field arrangement. They are often used to treat metastatic disease in various sites and are also frequently employed in treating large fields, such as the whole abdomen, or in half-body irradiation. They are also often used during a portion of the treatment of disease in the brain, pelvis, head and neck, lung, breast, pancreas, and extremities. In general, this field arrangement results in a uniform dose throughout the treated volume (Fig. 6.12). In this illustration, we notice that although the dose increases with higher beam energy, the ratio between the doses at a middepth and at D_{max} is decreased. If we were to normalize the dose to 100 percent at the middepth in all three plans, the dose at D_{max} would

be 106 percent for cobalt 60, 101 percent for 6 MV, and 100 percent for 15 MV. We also notice that the dose uniformity through the tumor is excellent except in the entrance/exit region of the cobalt-60 plan. This is caused by the gradual decrease in dose away from the central axis characteristic of cobalt-60 beams (Chap. 3).

Parallel opposed fields are often used when the depth of the target is uncertain, the target volume extends throughout the particular area treated, and multiple angled fields are impossible to set up. The arrangement is simple to set up, is more reproducible, and the risks of a tumor miss are reduced, particularly in uncooperative patients. The disadvantage of this beam arrangement is the incidental irradiation of large volumes of normal tissues situated within the fields, between the target and the skin surface. As we shall see in the following paragraphs, the dose in these areas can be very high, particularly if low energies are used or the thickness of the patient is large. To reduce the dose in these normal tissue regions, multiple field or rotational treatment techniques, described below, are needed.

When the thickness of the irradiated tissues is relatively small, the ratio between the dose at middepth and D_{max} remains within acceptable limits; however, as the thickness becomes larger or the beam energy decreases, this ratio increases.[59] Figure 6.16, where the dose is normalized to 100 percent at middepth, demonstrates, on a 20-cm-thick patient, the increase in dose closer to the beam entrance/exit points for three different beam energies. The increase is most severe when a cobalt-60 beam is used. In that case, the maximum dose is 13 percent (100/115) higher than at middepth, while for a 6-MV photon beam, it is less than 6 percent (100/106). Figure 6.17 shows the ratio between the middepth and D_{max} in a 30-cm-thick patient. Here we see that the maximum dose for a 6-MV photon beam is 18 percent (100/122) higher than the middepth dose—significantly higher than

when the separation is only 20 cm. For a 15-MV photon beam, the maximum dose is only 9 percent (100/110) higher than the middepth dose—a considerable improvement over the 6-MV photon beam.

When the %DD curve is closely examined, we find that within the first several centimeters from the surface, the dose falls off in a more or less linear pattern, while at greater depth, the fall-off is less rapid (Fig. 6.18). If the patient's thickness does not exceed the depth within which the dose fall-off is linear, we find, when opposing the curves, that the rate at which the %DD in one field falls off is the same as the rate at which it increases in the opposing field (Fig. 6.19). Therefore, when the doses from both fields are added together, we find that the dose is the same throughout the patient. When the patient's thickness is larger and extends beyond the linear portion of the %DD curve, we find that the dose near the entrance/exit region of the fields is higher than at middepth. This occurs because the %DD of one field does not fall off at the same rate as the opposing one increases—i.e., the fall-off is not linear throughout the patient (Fig. 6.20). The linear portion of the %DD curve continues to a greater depth in high-energy beams than in lower-energy

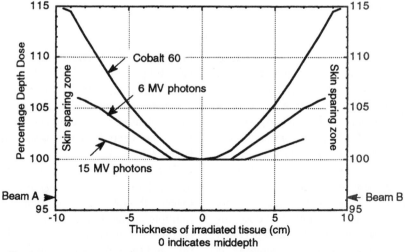

Figure 6.16 Percentage depth dose ratios normalized to 100 percent at middepth for parallel opposed fields. Shown here are dose profiles of opposed beams comparing three different beam energies on a 20-cm-thick patient. The dose in the entrance/exit region increases with decreased beam energy.

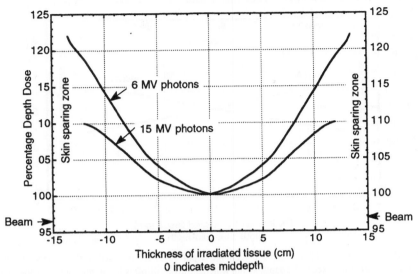

Figure 6.17 Percentage depth dose ratios normalized to 100 percent at middepth for parallel opposed fields. Shown here are dose profiles of opposed beams comparing two different beam energies on a 30-cm-thick patient. The dose in the entrance/exit region for both beam energies is increased when compared with that of Fig. 6.16, where the patient was smaller.

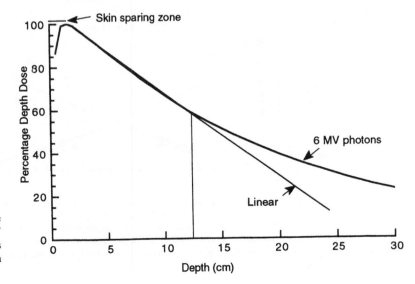

Figure 6.18 Percentage depth dose plotted as a function of depth for a 6-MV 100-cm SSD photon beam. The dose falls in a linear fashion within the first 13 cm and then falls less rapidly.

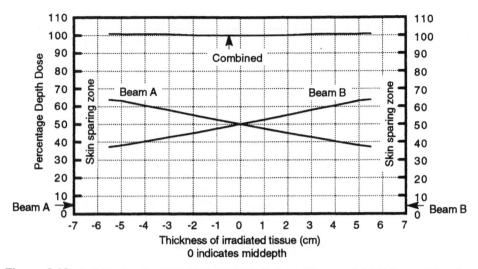

Figure 6.19 Individual and combined percentage depth doses for opposed 6-MV beams. When the patient's thickness does not exceed the depth within which the dose fall-off is linear, the combined dose of two opposed beams is uniform throughout the patient. This is because the dose fall-off in one field is equal to the dose increase in the opposing field.

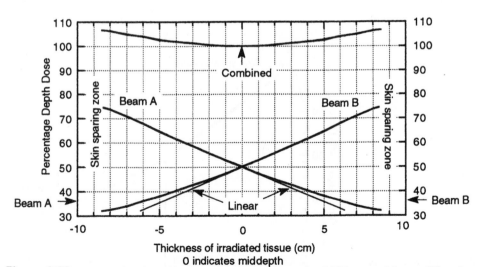

Figure 6.20 Individual and combined percentage depth doses for 6-MV opposed beams. When the patient's thickness exceeds the depth within which the dose fall-off is linear, the dose in the entrance/exit region increases because the dose in one field does not fall off at the same rate as the dose increases in the opposing field.

beams. It is therefore advantageous to use a higher-energy beam when a large patient is treated using parallel opposed fields.

DOSE WEIGHTING

In patients where the tumor is not situated at mid-depth, it is sometimes beneficial to deliver a higher fraction of the dose from the field where the tumor is shallower. Giving unequal doses from different beams is referred to as *weighting the beams*. This causes the dose to increase towards the entrance point of the field, delivering the higher dose away from the middepth location (Fig. 6.21). In many situations, this unequal weighting of beams is advantageous; however, the increased dose in the normal tissues situated between the tumor and the D_{max} region must be considered. Unequal weighting of the beams is also a useful tool to produce desired dose distributions in treatment plans where multiple fields are used. In an isocentric treatment technique, the depth of the isocenter can be very different for each

field. When the dose delivered at the isocenter is the same for all fields (equal weight), the D_{max} dose of fields with larger depth can be excessive. Delivering a smaller fraction of the isocenter dose from this field will reduce the dose in the region between the isocenter and the D_{max} point. In the past, changing the weight of an isodose chart manually was impossibly laborious and was therefore hardly ever done, but nowadays, treatment-planning computers permit the weighting to be changed quickly.

The practical application of unequal weighting is demonstrated in the chapters discussing treatment techniques in various anatomic regions (Chaps. 9–14).

DEPTH OF THE ISOCENTER

As already mentioned, the dose at D_{max} in a field depends on the depth of the prescription point, the dose to be delivered at this point, and on the beam energy. When the depth is large, the maximum dose is higher for a given beam energy than when the

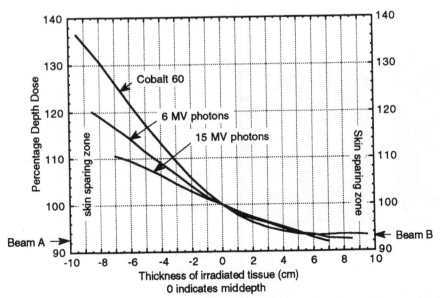

Figure 6.21   Percentage dose ratios normalized to 100 percent at middepth for parallel opposed fields, weighted 2 : 1. When the dose delivered from one field is higher than that from the opposing field, the dose in the entrance/exit region of the favored field increases.

prescription point is shallow. Simply speaking, one can say that to deliver the same dose at a greater depth as at a shallower depth, a higher dose is required at D_{max}. This is evident in Fig. 6.22 *(top)*, where two isodose charts are compared. The dose at the isocenter is normalized to 100 percent at the isocenter in both charts. In the left isodose chart, where the depth of the isocenter is 8 cm, the D_{max} dose is approximately 135 percent, while in the chart on the right, where the depth is 16 cm, it is 220 percent.

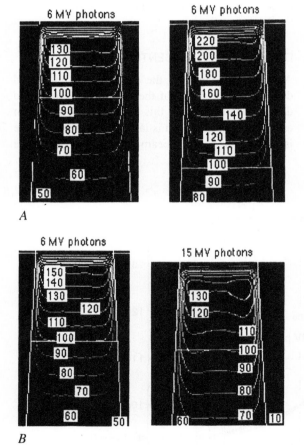

A

B

Figure 6.22 Comparison of two beams *(A)* where, on the left, the isocenter is at a depth of 8 cm and on the right at 16 cm. To deliver the same dose at the isocenter, the maximum dose is considerably higher when the isocenter is at a greater depth. Comparison of two beam energies *(B)* where the isocenter is at the same depth. To deliver the same dose at the isocenter, the maximum dose is higher with the lower beam energy.

Therefore, to deliver 100 cGy in the isocenter of the left field, a dose of approximately 135 cGy is required at D_{max}, while 220 cGy is required in the right field. The depth of the isocenter becomes an important consideration when isocentric treatment fields are used in multiple-field plans where the depth of the isocenter may be different for each field. To maintain the maximum dose of each field within an acceptable range, the amount of dose contributed at the isocenter by each field can be adjusted (weighted). The difference in D_{max} dose becomes less when the beam energy is increased (Fig. 6.22, *bottom*). In this illustration, the isodose charts from 6- and 15-MV photon beams with the dose normalized at the same depth (isocenter) are compared. As an example, we shall examine how the depth of the isocenter affects the dose in a practical example.

The advantage of using isocentric treatment techniques is that once the isocenter has been placed in the center of the target, the machine and the couch can be turned to practically any position while the target remains within the field. This is very convenient when, as an example, a boost treatment (a smaller field within a previously treated volume) is used in the management of pulmonary lesions, where it is customary to use parallel opposed oblique fields excluding the spinal cord. In setting up this arrangement, the isocenter is placed in the center of the target and the gantry is then turned until the spinal cord is out of the field (Fig. 6.23). However, it is not then unusual to find that the isocenter is not midway between the two entrance points. In Fig. 6.23A, the center of the tumor is determined from orthogonal radiographs and the isocenter is placed where the two central axes intersect. The gantry is then turned until the spinal cord is outside the beam. In Fig. 6.23B, we notice that the depth of the isocenter is quite different in the right anterior oblique (RAO) and the left posterior oblique (LPO) fields. If the same dose is delivered at the isocenter from both beams, the D_{max} dose of the RAO field will be much higher than in the LPO field (Fig. 6.23C). Unfortunately, isodose distributions resulting from parallel opposed fields are often not calculated, and this nonuniformity of the dose may go undetected. It is therefore recommended that the dose distribution for

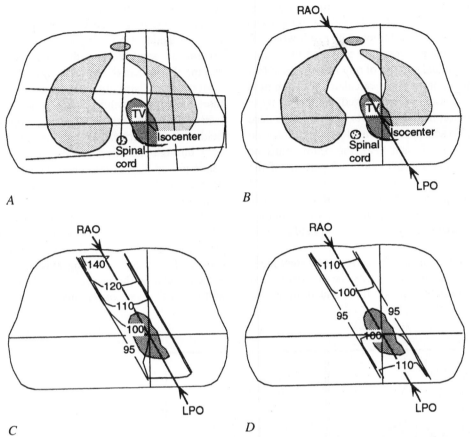

Figure 6.23   *A.* The isocenter is placed in the center of the tumor. *B.* The gantry is then turned until the spinal cord is excluded. *C.* Parallel, opposed, equally weighted beams (i.e., each field delivers 50 cGy in the isocenter) result in a high dose (148 cGy) in the entrance/exit region of the field with the larger isocenter depth. *D.* Improved dose uniformity can be achieved by weighting the beams delivering 38 cGy from the RAO field and 62 cGy from the LPO (weights: 0.38 to 0.62). The maximum dose is now 112 cGy.

parallel opposed fields be calculated when the isocenter is not in the midplane. "Hot spots" observed in such plans can be eliminated by changing the weighting until the D_{max} dose is the same for both fields (Fig. 6.23*D*). Alternatively, the isocenter can be moved along the central axes of the fields until it is at the midplane. Such isocenter shift made during the treatment simulation must obviously also be made in the treatment room.

We shall use the situation described above to examine how different methods of calculating the dose affect the D_{max} dose when the isocenter is not at middepth. In the first situation, the same dose is delivered at the isocenter from the two fields. Using a 6-MV photon beam and delivering 100 cGy at the isocenter from each field, the maximum dose (entrance and exit dose combined) on the central axis of the RAO field (18-cm depth) is 290 cGy, while in the LPO field (9-cm depth) it is 208 cGy. The dose is obviously not uniform in this situation. In the second situation, the difference in depths of the isocenter is not recognized and, inadvertently, the isocenter is *assumed* to be in the midplane. In this situation, although the MU calculated for each field is the same, the maximum dose on the central axis of the RAO field is 260 cGy; for the LPO field, it is 230 cGy;

while the dose in the isocenter is increased form the planned 200 cGy to 207 cGy. This also represents an unsatisfactory dose distribution. The result would be the same if it were incorrectly assumed that equal weight means equal number of monitor units and that as a result the monitor units calculated for each field in the first situation were averaged. Neither of these dose calculation methods results in acceptable dose uniformity. To achieve the same dose in the entrance and exit regions of each field, the beams must be weighted, so that approximately 63 percent of the dose in the isocenter is delivered through the LPO field and 37 percent through the RAO field—a weighting of 0.63 to 0.37. In this case, the combined entrance and exit doses at D_{max} of each field is about the same.

Other situations in which the isocenter may inadvertently be placed away from the middepth can occur. For example, a pelvic treatment is simulated for a four-field plan, and it is later decided not to treat the lateral fields. The isocenter, which could be anterior for bladder tumors or posterior for rectal tumors, remains as simulated, and the dose is calculated assuming that it is in the midplane, resulting in a nonuniform dose distribution. In yet another situation, a three-field plan designed to deliver a boost to the lateral pelvis is simulated, using opposed lateral fields and an anterior field. Later it is decided to treat only through the lateral fields, now with the isocenter placed well over to one side of the pelvis. The dose distribution is obviously nonuniform if the beams are equally weighted.

The same effect as described above can occur when the depth at which the dose is calculated (isocenter) varies within a field, as demonstrated in Fig. 6.24. In Fig. 6.24A, the long axis of the leg is not perpendicular to the central axis of the beam. This will cause the dose in the anterior part of the knee

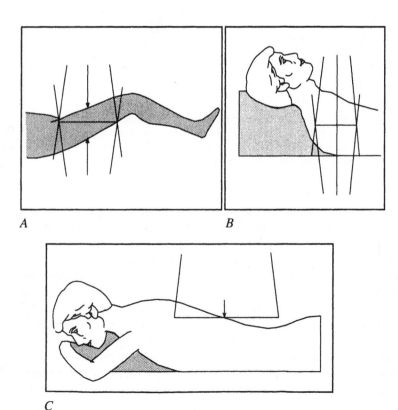

A   *B*

C

Figure 6.24 When the patient is not perpendicular to the beam, causing SSD and depth to vary within a field, high doses can occur where the SSD is shorter and the depth smaller. *A.* An extremity must be placed perpendicular to the beam; in this case, by lowering the knee. *B.* In a kyphotic patient, the dose can be high in the cephalad segment of an anterior field. The dose uniformity can be improved by changing the beam orientation (by rotation of the couch and the gantry). *C.* A posterior field to treat a spine tumor can cause a high dose in the thoracic spinal cord, where the SSD is shorter and the depth of the spinal cord is shallow. Lowering the chest to make the dorsal contour horizontal will improve the dose uniformity.

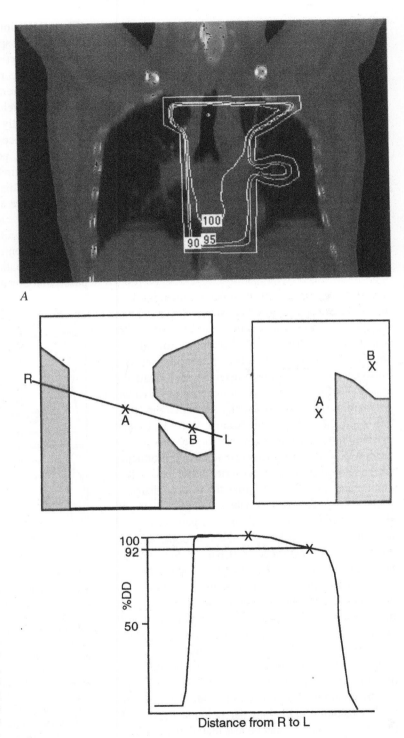

A

B

Figure 6.25   *A*. In segments that are small and remote from a larger field, the dose is lower due to less scatter. Such field shapes are sometimes seen in the treatment of lung tumors and when the paraaortic lymph nodes and the spleen are treated. A coronal dose distribution in a lung shows a very small area receiving 95 percent of the prescribed dose. *B*. A dose profile along the line from R to L in the lung field also shows a lower dose in the small peripheral segment.

and in the posterior aspect of the thigh near the buttocks to be higher because the SSD here is shorter. Contrarily, the dose in the anterior segment of the thigh near the inguinal area and in the posterior aspect of the knee will be lower because the SSD is longer. In Fig. 6.24*B*, a similar situation occurs. The dose will be higher in the cephalad portion of the anterior chest and in the caudal portion of the posterior chest because in these areas the distance is shorter. In Fig. 6.24*C*, where a single posterior field is used in the treatment of the spine, the dose is similarly higher where the SSD is shorter. Techniques to reduce these hot spots are demonstrated in the appropriate chapters describing treatment techniques in various anatomic sites (Chaps. 9–14).

FIELD SIZE AND BEAM DIVERGENCE

A very important aspect of treatment planning is to determine the appropriate field size and shape. Since the shapes of the isodose curves and the penumbra (Chap. 3) are different in different treatment machines, it is essential to first become familiar with the idiosyncrasies of these parameters in each treatment machine before making decisions about required target margins. Margins are usually set so that the target lies within the 95 percent isodose line. Additional margins are added to allow for organ and patient motion as well as for inconsistencies in reproducing the patient positioning, as described in Chap. 7. It is good practice to try to visualize the isodose distribution in three dimensions when the field size and shape are under consideration. The geometric field margin, in most machines, is taken to coincide with the 50 percent isodose level (Chap. 3, Fig. 3.16*A*); however, this may not always be true if the field is shaped so that the effect of the scatter is reduced. As an example, near the geometric corners of a square field, the dose is lower due to less scatter and the 50 percent isodose curve does not coincide with the geometric field margin (Chap. 3, Fig. 3.19). In an irregularly shaped field, the dose across the field may also vary due to the shape of the field. For example, in a treatment field designed to include the mediastinum and a tumor in the lung parenchyma, the dose to the peripheral tumor may be less than that calculated at the central axis of the beam near the hilar area

(Fig. 6.25). Similarly, when the paraaortic nodes and the spleen (or splenic pedicle) are treated, the dose in the spleen section of the field may be lower than in the paraaortic region because the spleen region is smaller and remote from the larger paraaortic segment of the field.

In practically all treatments with parallel opposed fields, the isocenter is placed at the midplane of the patient (lung, pelvis, abdomen, and so on) and the field size defined at the isocenter, is the same for both fields. This practice is usually acceptable; however, there are a few situations when the tumor also extends very close to the skin surface, where the beams enter and exit, and the tumor could be missed by the field entering from this direction. For example, when treating a rectal tumor using parallel opposed anterior and posterior fields using an isocen-

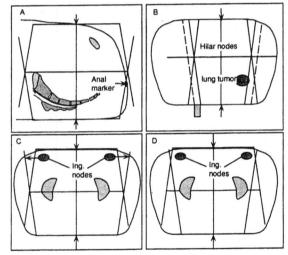

Figure 6.26 *A.* A marker on the anus may be included in the anterior field but not in the opposing posterior, because the fields are set to be identical anterior of the marker. *B.* A posteriorly located lung tumor may be missed in a posterior field even when it is well within the margins of an anterior field (*solid lines*). When the isocenter is set at middepth, the posterior field must be larger than the anterior field (*hatched lines*). This may cause the posterior field to include too much normal tissue on the other side; however, a block can be used to reduce this margin. *C.* When the inguinal lymph nodes are included in parallel-opposed anterior and posterior fields, the posterior field should be smaller (*solid lines*) or the margins around the lymph nodes will be excessive (*hatched lines*). *D.* Alternatively, the field size can be set at the depth of the lymph nodes.

tric technique, a marker indicating the anus may be included in the anterior field but not in the posterior (Fig. 6.26A). In a posteriorly located lung tumor, the posterior field must be larger than the anterior field, or the isocenter, where the field size is defined, should be at the depth of the tumor and the dose should be weighted appropriately (Fig. 6.26B). A posterior field, which is parallel opposed to an anterior field, shaped to include the inguinal nodes, may have too generous margins (Fig. 6.26C). The posterior field must be smaller than the anterior, but without compromising the margins around a deeper target (Fig. 6.26D).

MULTIPLE-FIELD TREATMENT

In the discussion of parallel opposed field arrangements, it was clear that the dose in the tissues near the entrance/exit point of the two beams can be quite high. These high-dose areas can be avoided by using a multiple-field arrangement in which all beams encompass the target but include different areas of surrounding normal tissues. In Fig. 6.27, for exam-

ple, we can see that while the target is treated via all fields, the normal tissues in the region are irradiated by some fields but not by others. As the number of fields increases, the dose in any given area of normal tissue decreases.

Multiple-field treatment plans can be designed to produce uniform dose distributions, particularly by using dose-modifying devices (wedges and compensators) and differential weighting and by selecting appropriate beam orientations, beam energies, and field sizes. There are, however, many restrictions in terms of selecting beam directions caused by the need for dose limitations of radiosensitive organs. Possible beam orientations may also be restricted by the presence of attenuating sections of a treatment couch, or because the head of the treatment machine, as it is moved, may not clear the patient or the couch.[60,61]

FOUR-FIELD TECHNIQUES

One commonly used four-field technique is two sets of opposed fields at right angles. Pelvic tumors, for example, are often treated using one set of opposed

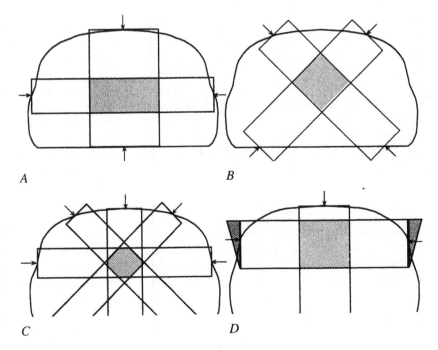

Figure 6.27 *A.* In a four-field technique, all fields encompass the target *(shaded)*, while the normal tissue between the skin surface and the target is only included within two of the four fields. *B.* The shape of the high-dose area can be altered by changing the beam angles. *C.* Combining the field arrangement in *(A)* and *(B)* causes the high-dose area to be octagonal, and the tissues between the skin surface and the target are receiving a lower dose because it is now included within only two of eight beams. *D.* A tree-field technique requires wedges to produce a uniform dose distribution.

A

B

C

D

fields in the anterior-posterior direction and a second set of opposed fields from the left-right direction (Fig. 6.27A). This is often referred to as a *box technique*—the name pertaining to the shape of the resulting high-dose area. In this technique, only the shaded area is irradiated through all four fields, while the tissues between the shaded area and the skin surface are irradiated through only two of the four fields, thus the dose here is lower. In large patients or when beam energies in the range of cobalt-60 and 4-MV photons are used, the dose in the entrance/exit region of the lateral fields may be excessive and the anterior/posterior fields may have to be more heavily weighted. Figure 6.28 illustrates two isodose distributions using an isocentric four-field technique with equal weighting; one using 4-MV and one using 15-MV photon beams. It is evident, in this illustration, that the higher beam energy delivers a better dose distribution. In general, higher-beam energies deliver a more uniform dose distribution because of the greater penetration, and, as a result, the dose falloff over a given distance is less than at lower beam energies. The dose uniformity in the 4-MV plan can be improved by increasing the weighting of the anterior-posterior fields (Fig. 6.28C).

As an alternative to the four-field box technique, two sets of opposing fields can be angled (Fig. 6.27B) and the high-dose area becomes diamond-shaped. This field arrangement is not very useful when centrally located prostate or gynecologic tumors are treated, because a larger volume of bladder and rectum is also within the high-dose area. A combination of these two techniques, consisting of four pairs of opposed fields, will yield a high-dose area that is octagonal, providing better sparing of the bladder and the rectum (Fig. 6.27C).

THREE-FIELD TECHNIQUES

A three-field arrangement is sometimes used when tumors in the pancreas, bladder, or rectum are treated. Figure 6.27D demonstrates such a plan using an anterior and two opposed lateral fields. The object is to achieve a uniform dose in the bladder while minimizing the dose in the rectum; therefore no posterior field used. The dose in the rectum is delivered

via the anterior field, which exits through the posterior pelvis. The dose distribution from the two opposing fields is relatively uniform, while the dose in the anterior field gradually decreases with depth as in any single field treatment; the uniform contribution of the opposing fields, when combined with the varying contribution of the anterior field, leads to some overall nonuniformity. Of course, the effect of the patient's external contour also contributes to the dose heterogeneity. Uniformity throughout the area may be improved by using wedges in the lateral fields. The purpose of the wedges is to cause the combined dose from the opposed fields to increase in a posterior direction at the same rate as the anterior field dose decreases in the same direction. The disadvantage of this plan is the high dose delivered in the lateral aspect of the pelvis, where the opposed fields contribute both entrance and exit doses. The dose here is also high because the separation between the entrance points is large, with the general consequences described above for parallel opposed fields. A larger fraction of the dose must therefore be given through the anterior field. That, on the other hand, increases the gradient of the dose through the high-dose volume (shaded) and a steeper wedge angle is needed in the lateral fields. When the weighting of a wedged field is low, the required wedge angle is increased because the effect of the wedge on the overall dose becomes less pronounced when the intensity is lower. The precise weighting of these fields and the needed wedge angle depend on the beam energy and the patient's size and shape. One very important point to observe in this type of plan is the possibility of a hot spot in the lateral aspect of the patient near the thin part of the wedge. In severe situations, it may be necessary to add a posterior field using a small weighting factor while at the same time reducing the weight from the lateral fields.

It is essential to select beam orientations so that the dose in normal tissues is minimized. Although each case must be considered individually, it is often an advantage to arrange the beams so that each one enters through tissues, not in the exit of another beam, and exits in tissues not otherwise irradiated (i.e., no beams are opposed). For example, in retreat-

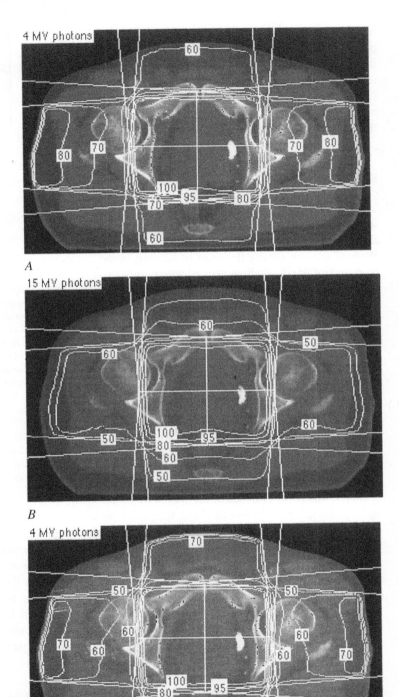

Figure 6.28 *A.* A four-field technique with equal weighting using 4-MV photons results in higher doses near the entrance/exit region of the lateral fields. This is due to the increased isocenter depth and the poorer penetration of the lower-energy beam. *B.* The same plan using 15-MV photon beams yields a more uniform dose distribution. *C.* The dose distribution in *(A)* can be improved by increasing the weight of the anterior and posterior fields, where the isocenter depth is smaller.

ment of previously irradiated brain tumors, noncoplanar beams can be arranged to enter and exit in different regions of the brain. Noncoplanar beams are beams where the central axes of all beams do not lie on a common plane. However, this type of field arrangement is difficult to produce in the absence of three-dimensional treatment-planning capabilities.

WEDGED FIELDS

Wedges used to alter the dose distribution in a beam were described in Chap. 3. In this section, some situations in which wedges are helpful are explained. Wedges were originally designed to be used in the treatment of small, shallow tumors where only two fields, separated by less than 180°, are used (Fig. 6.29). Examples of such treatment are unilateral brain and head-and-neck tumors. In these areas, the use of a wedged pair of fields spares the normal tissues on the opposite side, such as the opposite hemisphere of the brain, salivary glands, or areas of the oral mucosa. Since these fields are not opposed, the beams exit in unirradiated tissues. More recently, wedge techniques have been found useful in a wide variety of field arrangements in an effort to achieve dose uniformity in treating deep-seated tumors.

In Fig. 6.29A, two wedge fields at right angles (separated by 90°) are shown and the high-dose area is almost square. In Fig. 6.29B, the wedge fields are again separated by 90°, but this time they are both tilted at 45° to the vertical, so that the high-dose area, which is also tilted 45°, now appears as diamond-shaped, though in fact it is still square. The diagonal of the square has been rotated in space by altering the orientation of the arrangement with respect to the patient. In selecting beam orientations for different treatment situations, it is important to realize how the final dose distribution will appear. In Fig. 6.29C, the fields are separated by 120°, causing the diamond-shaped high-dose area to be elongated horizontally; in Fig. 6.29D, the beams are separated by 60°, causing the diamond-shaped high-dose area to be elongated in the vertical direction.

The wedge angle needed, or the degree by which the isodose curves should be tilted, depends on the

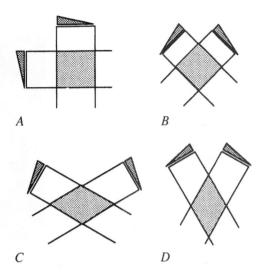

A   *B*

C   *D*

Figure 6.29   When two beams are separated by less than 180°, wedges may be necessary to improve the dose distribution. *A.* Two beams separated by 90° and with 45° wedges both include the target *(shaded),* while the tissue between the skin surface and the target is included within only one field. The dose under the thin portion of the wedges can be high, and when the isocenter is large, the dose in the normal tissue may in fact be higher than in the area included within both beams. *B.* When the same fields are used but the beam angles are changed, the high-dose area will have the same shape but the orientation with respect to the patient is different. *C.* To produce a high-dose area that is elongated in the horizontal direction, the angle between the fields (hinge angle) is increased and the wedge angle is decreased. *D.* When the elongation is needed in the vertical direction, the hinge angle is decreased and the wedge angle is increased.

hinge angle. The hinge angle is the angle separating the two central axes. If we assume that the isodose curves are not changed by the patient's surface topography, the wedge angle needed to produce uniform dose can be found by subtracting the hinge angle from 180° and dividing by two. For example, in a plan where the hinge angle is 90°, the needed wedge angle is $(180 - 90)/2 = 45°$; when the hinge is 120°, the wedge angle should be $(180 - 120)/2 = 30°$.

When only two unwedged fields are used and the central axes are separated by less than 180°, a hot spot will appear, as we have seen in Fig. 6.10. This can be eliminated by the addition of wedges in the beams, as shown in Fig. 6.30. There, in the plan la-

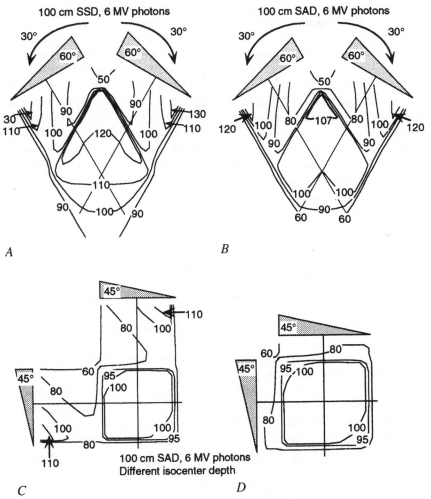

Figure 6.30 *A*. Two wedged fields (same as in Fig. 6.10) using an SSD technique, where the D_{max} dose of each field is 100 percent. There are three hot spots; one in each field under the thin portion of the wedge near the skin surface and another in the proximal side of the beam intersection. *B*. The same field arrangement, but now using an SAD technique where the dose is normalized to 100 percent at the isocenter. The dose uniformity within the region included within both fields is improved slightly. *C*. Two wedged fields separated by 90° and with 45° wedges in an SAD technique. There is still a hot spot under the thin portion of each wedge near the skin surface. *D*. The same plan as in *(C)*, but now with a smaller isocenter depth and the hot spots under the thin portion of the wedges is removed.

beled A, 60° wedges are inserted in an SSD treatment plan. The dose at the hot spot is now reduced from 160 to 120 percent; to reduce it further, the hinge angle must be increased or another field must be added that enters from the opposite side of the patient. There is also a hot spot under the thin portion

of each wedge near the skin surface. In Fig. 6.30*B*, the dose distribution is shown using the same field arrangement but with an SAD technique. The hot spot is now reduced to 107 percent, or about 7 percent higher than the dose in the isocenter while the hot spots under the thin portion of each wedge is basically unchanged. In Fig. 6.30C and D, an SAD technique is used, but the depth of the isocenter is different. In Fig. 6.30C, the depth is greater, leading to a hot spot (110 percent) near the surface under the thin part of the wedge. In Fig. 6.30D, the depth of the isocenter is smaller and the hot spot is eliminated.

In many situations, the available wedge angles may not be adequate, but one can then mix an unwedged beam to produce the needed isodose tilt, as described earlier. When wedges are used, it is essential that the plan is scrutinized carefully, as hot spots can occur near the skin surface, where the beam passes through the thin part of the wedge. The propensity for such hot spots to occur increases with increased field width, increased wedge angle, and increased weighting factor (i.e., in beams where the isocenter is at a greater depth or where a larger fraction of the dose is delivered). The width of the beam is important, because as the field becomes wider, an increasingly thinner part of the wedge, where the transmitted dose relative to the central axis dose is higher, lies within the field.

In a more sophisticated method, isodose curves with desired tilt can be produced by an independent jaw, and then, as the beam is turned on, the jaw is gradually moved across the field at a constant speed until it reaches the position where the entire field is irradiated. The segment where the collimator jaw was first set is irradiated during the entire treatment, while each segment across the field is irradiated a shorter and shorter time. Higher dose is therefore delivered where the jaw was first set; as the collimator jaw moves across the field, the dose is gradually decreasing. The tilt of the isodone curves can be varied by changing the speed with which the jaw moves or the rate at which the dose is delivered. In another, even more sophisticated technique, different isodose tilt can be produced within a given field.[62] Dynamic wedge treatment techniques, in which the collimator jaw is moved under computer control, are described in Chap. 3 (Fig. 3.24).

The practical implementation of wedges is further discussed in the various chapters describing treatment techniques in different anatomic regions (Chaps. 9–14).

MOVING-BEAM TREATMENT

In the treatment discussed so far in this chapter, it has been assumed that the beams and the patient are stationary. There are many techniques in which either the beam moves around the stationary patient or the patient moves with respect to the stationary beam, and in some very exotic techniques, both the patient and the beam move simultaneously in a predetermined pattern. In this section, only techniques in which the beam moves with respect to the patient will be discussed.

ROTATION THERAPY

A rotation therapy technique, in which the treatment is delivered while the radiation source continuously moves around the patient, can be thought of as an extension of the multiple-field technique already described. This technique is most useful when small symmetrically shaped, deep-seated tumors are treated. As in most other situations, rotation therapy using a high-energy beam results in a superior dose distribution.

In rotation techniques, the isocenter (the axis of rotation of the particular machine) is placed in the target, so that regardless of beam direction, the beam is always directed at the target while the normal tissues, farther out toward the periphery, remain in the beam for only a fraction of the treatment. As a result, the dose is highest in the target and gradually decreases toward the periphery (Fig. 6.31A). To illustrate, point A in Fig. 6.31A, lies outside the beam for orientations between 0° and about 30°. As the beam rotates beyond that, point A comes into the beam and receives radiation until the trailing edge of the field passes over it; at an orientation of 60°, for example, the beam has moved well past point A. On the other hand, point B, which is located closer to the target, is within the field when the beam is at 0° and is still being irradiated when the beam is at 60°. Of course, for each degree of rotation that the two points remain within the beam, the dose at point B is lower than at point A because the distance is longer and the thickness of attenuating tissue is greater. This relationship

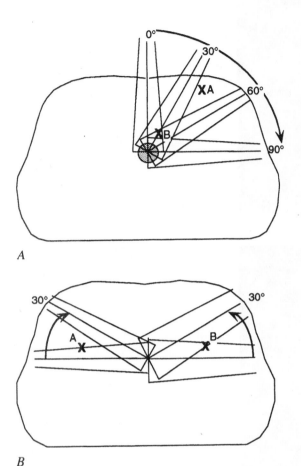

Figure 6.31 *A.* In a rotation technique, point A, located at some distance from the isocenter, remains within the moving beam during only a small fraction of the rotation while point B, located much closer to the isocenter, remains within the beam considerably longer. *B.* When a small field is used in a rotation treatment *(on the left),* point A remains within the beam during a smaller fraction of the rotation than point B *(on the right),* where a larger field is used.

is reversed when the radiation field has moved to the opposite position.

The rate at which the dose decreases as the point of interest moves toward the periphery depends on the field width and on the beam energy. When a wide field is used, the fall-off of dose in the periphery is less dramatic than when a smaller field is used. This occurs because when the field width increases, a

given point in the periphery remains inside the beam during a larger fraction of the treatment. Figure 6.31*B* shows the effect of the field width where point A remains within the radiation beam during a small fraction of the treatment when a small field is used *(left).* On the other hand, point B (identically located with respect to the isocenter) remains within the field during a larger fraction of the treatment because the field is larger. Figure 6.32*A* and *B* shows a 360° rotation with a 6-MV photon beam using two different field sizes. From this illustration, it is clear that rotational treatment techniques are less advantageous when large fields are used. To illustrate the effect of beam energy, a dose distribution for the same (360°) rotation as in Fig. 6.32*A*, using a 15-MV photon beam, is shown in Fig. 6.32*C*. As we would expect, the dose in the periphery is slightly lower when a 15-MV beam is used.

When a 360° rotation is performed in a cylindric phantom with the isocenter in the center of the phantom, the isodose curves in the cross-sectional plane will be circular. In a patient, where the external contour usually is more or less oval, the isodose curves showing the lower doses will also be oval (Fig. 6.32), but the longer dimension of the oval will be perpendicular to the long axis of the patient. This is caused by the varying thickness of attenuating tissue, causing the dose rate in the isocenter to vary. When the beam passes through the anterior and posterior region of the pelvis, for example, higher dose is delivered, causing the isodose curves to be elongated in the direction of the patient's smaller dimension.

The advantages of rotational techniques, originally introduced more than a half-century ago to overcome penetration difficulties at the low x-ray energies then available, over multiple (four to six) stationary fields are no longer clear cut when high-energy beams of adequate penetration are available. Unlike stationary treatment techniques, where each field can be shaped to conform to the target in the beam's eye view, the shape of rotational fields remains unchanged as the beam moves around the patient unless multileaf collimators capable of dynamic beam shaping are used. Furthermore, beam directions and field shapes in stationary techniques,

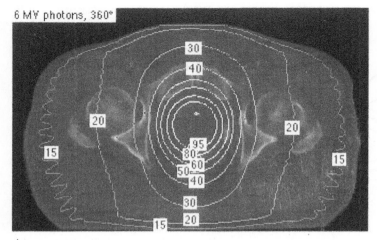

A

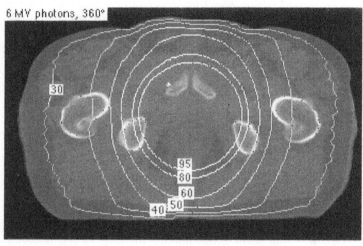

B

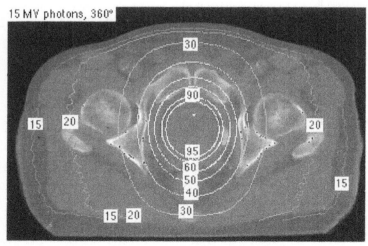

C

Figure 6.32 *A.* A dose distribution resulting from a 360° rotation using a 6-MV photon beam compared with *B*, where the same treatment is given but using a larger field. When the larger field is used, the dose fall-off in the periphery is less rapid. *C.* The same treatment as in *A*, but now using a 15-MV photon beam. There is not much gain using a higher-energy beam because, although the penetration is better, the exit dose is also higher.

though much less convenient than in rotation, have the advantage of being adjustable to minimize the dose in radiosensitive normal tissues.

ARC TREATMENT

In arc techniques, one or several sectors are skipped to reduce the dose in radiosensitive normal tissues —for example, the bladder and rectum. When a sector is skipped, the high-dose area is shifted away from the skipped sector (Fig. 6.33A). It is therefore necessary to move the isocenter toward the skipped sector (past-pointing) in order to bring the high-dose region back to the target (Fig. 6.33B). Similarly, when two asymmetrically arranged sectors are skipped, the isocenter must be shifted toward the direction where the larger section is skipped. When the target is off-centered on the cross-section contour, it is advantageous to treat only through the region where the depth of the isocenter is smaller and to skip a sector where the depth is larger.

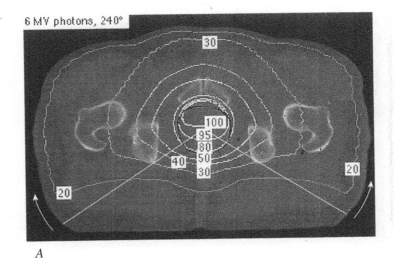

A

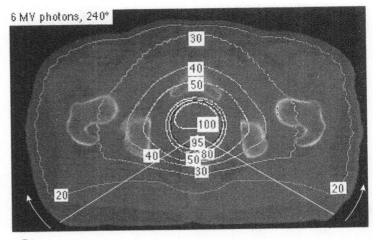

Figure 6.33 *A.* When a sector of the rotation is skipped (arc technique), the high-dose area is shifted away from the skipped sector. *B.* To move the high-dose area back to the target volume, the isocenter is moved toward the skipped sector.

B

COMBINING ARC AND WEDGE TECHNIQUES

In situations where a large sector is skipped, the resulting dose distribution will not only be displaced due to the asymmetric placement of the arc but it may also be non-uniform (Fig. 6.34). In an 140° arc, for example (Fig. 6.34A), the dose will gradually increase toward the irradiated sector. When this dose heterogeneity is undesirable, wedges can be added in the beam so that the thick side of the wedge always lies over the high-dose section; to achieve this, the wedge must be reversed midway through the arc (Fig. 6.34B).[63] The need for wedges is reduced with higher beam energies and increased with smaller arcs.

COMBINING FIXED- AND MOVING-BEAM TECHNIQUES

Moving-beam techniques are often used to treat a small area (boost) within a larger treatment field. For example, the entire pelvis may be treated using a stationary four-field technique followed by a boost to a smaller volume (prostate gland or the uterine cervix) delivered via a moving-beam technique.

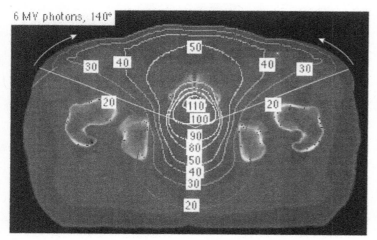

A

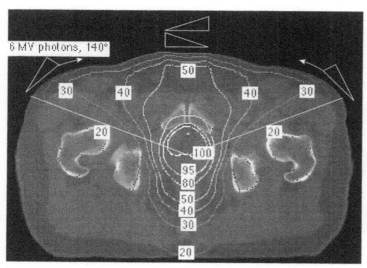

B

Figure 6.34 *A.* When a large sector is skipped (220° in this plan), a hot spot occurs toward the arc. *B.* Wedges can be used in the arc to reduce this hot spot. The wedge orientation must be such that the thick portion of the wedge is always over the hot spot (i.e., the wedge orientation must be reversed midway through the arc). In this 140° arc, 60° wedges were used.

DOSE PRESCRIPTION

Uniformity among radiation therapy centers is essential when doses are reported and information about the treatment is exchanged. It is also important if meaningful comparisons of results are to be made between therapy centers or even within a department. In an effort to improve uniformity, the International Commission on Radiation Units and Measurements (ICRU) has given some guidelines for reporting of doses.[63] The ICRU recommends that the dose be reported at a point, referred to as the ICRU reference point, within the planning target volume (PTV) (Chap. 7). This point should be selected according to the following criteria:

1. The point should be located at or near the center of the PTV.
2. The absorbed dose at the point should be clinically relevant and be representative of the dose throughout the PTV.
3. The point should be easy to define in a clear and unambiguous way.
4. The dose should be accurately determinable at the point.
5. The point should not be in a region of very steep dose gradient.

In some situations, the conditions do not allow for the ICRU reference point to be localized at or near the center of the PTV and at the same time also on the beam central axis in an area where the dose distribution is homogeneous. In such cases, the first criterion (i.e., the localization at or close to the center of the PTV) should be given preference. The ICRU reference dose is the dose at the ICRU reference point, and this should always be reported. A certain degree of dose inhomogeneity in the PTV cannot be avoided. As a minimum requirement, the maximum and minimum dose to the PTV should always be reported along with the dose at the ICRU reference point.

In many centers, the staff are so used to the prescription and treatment conventions in their own departments that they would be surprised to learn that their treatment reports are ambiguous, uncertain, or even incomprehensible to others. The ICRU therefore hopes that its recommendations in Report #50, which was in part developed because of the rapid changes and introduction of three-dimensional treatment-planning capabilities, will be adopted in day-to-day practice.

Methods of prescribing radiation dose vary among radiation therapy centers and sometimes also between physicians within the same center. For example, in multiple-beam or wedged-pair techniques, where the dose distribution is calculated on a cross-sectional contour of the patient, the dose is often prescribed to the "minimum target dose." Alternatively, the dose may be prescribed at the isocenter, or perhaps at the point of maximum dose shown on a plan that represents only one plane. In treatments where an isodose distribution is not usually calculated—for example, when parallel opposed fields are used—the dose is often prescribed at a point on the central axis, usually the isocenter in an SAD technique and at the midpoint between the entrance points of the two opposed fields in an SSD technique. The dose prescriptions in these examples are inconsistent and the treatments cannot therefore be compared.

DOSE PRESCRIPTION IN PRACTICE

In the following paragraphs, some more practical dose prescription and dose evaluation concepts are presented.

When a single anterior field is used to treat bilateral supraclavicular nodes, as is often the case in the treatment of head and neck malignancies, some physicians may prescribe the dose at D_{max} (0.5 cm for cobalt 60 and 1.5 cm for 6 MV) or at an estimated depth of the lymph nodes (3 to 4 cm) on the central axis. In a single field of this kind (Fig. 6.35A), the central axis is in the patient's midline and often under a block; therefore the dose at the prescription point is not representative of the dose in the supraclavicular lymph nodes. In Fig. 6.35B, it is evident that the dose on a single transverse plane through the patient can also vary significantly when parallel opposed fields are used in head and neck treatments. In spite of this, the dose is frequently prescribed at the midpoint on the central axis, though the dose there may not represent the dose in the tumor. At a certain

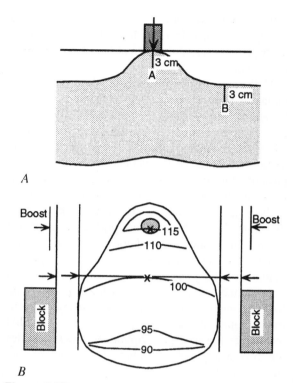

A

B

Figure 6.35 *A.* When a single anterior field is used to treat supraclavicular lymph nodes, the dose prescription point is sometimes made at 3-cm depth on the central axis. The dose at this point may not be representative of the dose in the intended target and may in some situations be under a midline spinal cord block. *B.* A transverse contour of the neck in a patient being treated with parallel opposed lateral fields. The dose prescription point is usually in the midline on the central axis. In the anterior portion of the neck, where the primary tumor site in this patient is located, the dose can be considerably higher due to the smaller diameter of the neck at this point.

dose level, while leaving the central axis (prescription point) fixed, the fields are reduced to exclude the spinal cord. Another field reduction (including the primary tumor site with a small margin) is later made, and this time the central axis is sometimes moved. When these small fields are treated, the original prescription point is frequently outside the fields and a new prescription point is therefore designated, usually on the central axis of the small fields. At times, the doses calculated at these two prescription points are inappropriately added together (see Chap. 9, Fig. 9.21). Due to variation in the thickness of the

neck, the dose delivered in the primary tumor site from the first sets of fields could be much higher than at the first prescription point. To prevent the risk of overdosage, the dose in the primary tumor should be calculated and recorded in the daily treatment record from the beginning of the treatment course. Alternatively, the dose should be prescribed at this point from the outset of the treatment.

As previously mentioned, the dose is often prescribed at a point on the central axis when parallel opposed fields are used. In some treatments, the field may be shaped so that the central axis is outside the treated area—for example, when a half-beam block is used. In this type of treatment setup, the dose obviously cannot be prescribed on the central axis. When opposed half-beam blocked fields are used in the treatment of head and neck malignancies, it is reasonable to measure the field separation in the center of the open area of the fields and calculate the prescribed dose at middepth. In other situations, the central axis may be blocked—for example, when a larynx or spinal cord block is used in an anterior bilateral supraclavicular field. In this setup, the dose must be calculated in the open area of the field.

Dose prescription for electron beam treatments varies depending on the underlying tissues. When the chest wall is treated, the beam energy is often chosen so that the 80 percent isodone line is at the chest wall–lung interface, bearing in mind that the maximum dose is about 25 percent (100/80) higher. When the underlying tissues are not particularly radiosensitive, the energy can be chosen so that the 90 percent isodose line includes the maximum depth of the target, thereby effectively reducing the maximum dose.

The dose uniformity recommended by the ICRU is that the actual dose fall within limits 7 percent greater and 5 percent less than the prescribed.[64-67] If the expected discrepancy is greater than this, it is up to the physician to decide whether it is acceptable or not. It is crucial to evaluate the location of the high-dose area with respect to normal tissues and to record the maximum dose in the daily treatment record. Unpleasant consequences can be avoided by reducing the fields to exclude the hot spot or by changing the field arrangement. Dose incidentally delivered in radiosensitive organs such as the spinal cord or lens of the eye should also be calculated and recorded in the daily treatment record to avoid unpleasant surprises. In some cases, a higher dose may be found in a part of the PTV where the highest tumor cell concentration is expected; in such a situation, this high dose may be advantageous.

For three-dimensional treatment plans, a high dose volume is considered clinically meaningful if the diameter of the total volume exceeds 15 mm. A smaller volume is, in most cases, not crucial to normal tissue tolerance for large organs such as the liver, lungs, kidney, and skin. However, for smaller organs— such as the eye, optic nerve, and the larynx—a high dose volume even smaller than 15 mm must be considered.

The dose uniformity recommended for a two-dimensional dose distribution, where only limited dose information is displayed, may be difficult to achieve when the same dose distribution is viewed in three dimensions. This is because isodose distributions calculated in three-dimensions yield much more information about the dose within the entire irradiated volume than the traditional two-dimensional dose calculations. In three-dimensional dose calculations, consideration is also given to the shape of the field and the external surface contour within the entire volume. Hot spots that were not detected in traditional two-dimensional dose distributions, because they were out of the single plane of the calculation, show up clearly in three-dimensional dose displays. If high-dose areas cannot be avoided, the prescription may need to be modified either by reducing the fraction size or the total dose.

Three-dimensional treatment-planning systems also permits one to evaluate the dose by calculating dose-volume histograms (DVH). A DVH shows the volume of a given organ receiving various dose levels. For example, the DVH shown in Fig. 6.36 is calculated for the cervical spinal cord and indicates that a very small volume (about 2 percent) receives 90 percent of the dose and that all of the cervical spinal cord receives 40 percent or less. One shortcoming of a DVH is that it does not, for example, reveal whether the small volume of spinal cord receiving 90 percent of the dose is a long narrow strip

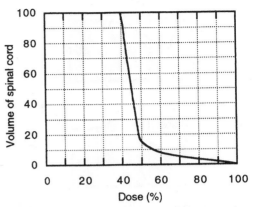

Figure 6.36 A dose-volume histogram demonstrating the volume of the cervical spinal cord receiving various dose levels. For example, a very small volume receives 95 percent of the prescribed dose, and all of the spinal cord receive 40 percent or less.

on one side or a small segment across the entire circumference—obviously a difference of serious consequence. Therefore, information given by a DVH should never by used *alone* to make decisions regarding the patient's treatment but should be used *in conjunction* with a dose distribution calculated within the entire irradiated volume.

DOSE DISTRIBUTION AT MULTIPLE PLANES

IRREGULAR CONTOUR

In general, treatment plans are generated in only one transverse plane within an often large treatment volume. This plane is usually chosen to contain the central axes of the treatment fields. It is often sufficient to view the dose distribution in this single plane, because from previous experience we know that in very many situations the dose distribution is nearly the same in other transverse planes parallel to the first. There are, however, situations when further planning, including examination of dose in other planes, should be carried out. Typical examples would be in the treatment of the chest, either through anterior and posterior or oblique fields; treatment of breast carcinoma through tangential fields; and in treatment of the pelvis in an obese patient through

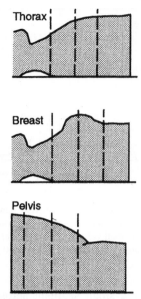

Thorax

Breast

Pelvis

Figure 6.37 Regions where isodose distributions in more than one level may be warranted include the thorax, breast, and pelvis of an obese patient.

anterior and posterior fields (Fig. 6.37). In such areas, the dose can vary significantly within the treatment volume, particularly when lower-energy beams are used.

Yet another example is in the head and neck region; even though relatively small fields are usually used in this site, there may be a severe dose variation within the treated volume because of the irregular

patient contour and also because multiple wedged fields are often used. For example, the lateral diameter of the patient's neck varies a great deal, both in the transverse and the coronal planes, causing the dose to vary even when opposed lateral fields are used (Fig. 6.38). Calculation of isodose distributions in multiple planes should therefore be considered in such cases.

In areas where the SSD is shorter than on the central axis, due to an irregular surface, the D_{max} dose will be higher, on the other hand, the depth dose will be lower than in the central axis because of the greater thickness of attenuating tissues that the beam has to traverse (Fig. 6.39). For example, when an anterior field is used in the treatment of maxillary antrum tumors, the dose will be higher in the nose than in the surrounding area. Similar changes in the SSD within a field may occur as a result of the patient's position with respect to the beam. As an example, when the chin is extended in treatment of maxillary antrum tumors, the SSD in the lower segment of the field will be shorter than at the central axis (Fig. 6.40). Similarly, when the neck and upper thorax of a kyphotic patient is treated through anterior and posterior fields and the patient's chest is not perpendicular to the beam, dose inhomogeneities will occur as a result of variations in the SSD. In Fig. 6.41, the anterior SSD in the cephalad segment of the field is shorter than at the central axis, causing a hot spot in the anterior neck; similarly, the posterior SSD is shorter in the caudal segment of the field, also causing a hot spot.

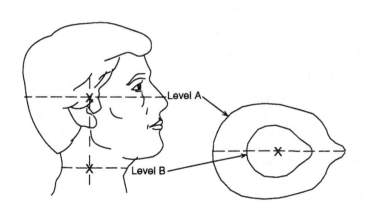

Figure 6.38 In the head and neck area, the patient's contour may vary considerably, and isodose distributions in one or more planes may be of benefit even when only opposed lateral fields are used.

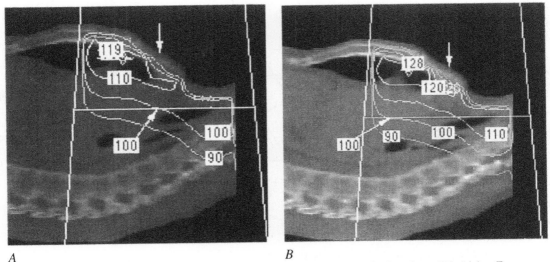

A   *B*

Figure 6.39   In areas where the SSD is shorter than at the central axis, the D_{max} dose will be higher. To deliver the same dose at the same SAD, the D_{max} dose will be higher where the SSD is decreased and the depth is larger. In *A*, 100 cGy is delivered at 100-cm SAD and the D_{max} dose along the central axis is approximately 110 cGy (119 cGy where the SSD is shorter). In *B*, the same dose (100 cGy) is delivered at the same SAD (100 cm), but at the point where the SSD is decreased and the depth is increased. The maximum dose is now approximately 128 cGy.

The "irregular" surfaces caused by the patient's position can, to a large extent, be eliminated by altering either the patient's position with respect to the beam or by altering the beam's orientation with respect to the patient.

WEDGES

Dose variations at other levels within a treatment area, as previously described, should also be examined when wedges are used in the treatment plan. It is particularly important to calculate the dose distribu-

Figure 6.40   The patient's position may cause the SSD to be decreased, and thus the dose is increased near the surface. *A*. When the patient's head is in neutral position, the SSD is fairly uniform within an anterior field. *B*. When the chin is extended as in the treatment of a maxillary antrum tumor, the dose in the caudal area of an anterior field (nose and mouth), where the SSD is decreased, will be increased.

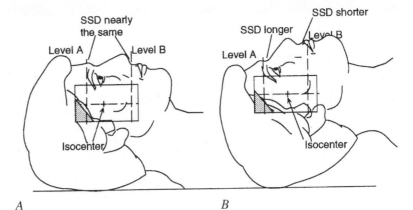

A   *B*

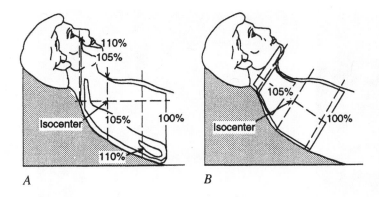

A   *B*

Figure 6.41 *A.* In a kyphotic patient, treated with opposed anterior and posterior fields, the dose can be very high in the cephalad region of the anterior field and in the caudal region of the posterior field. *B.* The beam can be arranged perpendicular to the patient by rotating the couch 90° and then turning the gantry to the appropriate angle.

tions in other planes when the treatment fields are shaped, so that the radiation goes through a thinner section of the wedge in a plane other than the primary plane. A hot spot, which often occurs under the thinner portion of a wedge, would be hidden to the casual observer unless a dose distribution were also displayed at such a level (Fig. 6.42).

THREE-DIMENSIONAL DOSE CALCULATION

Traditional treatment-planning systems are only capable of calculating and displaying dose in two dimensions on one plane, usually the central axis plane, because information about the patient's shape

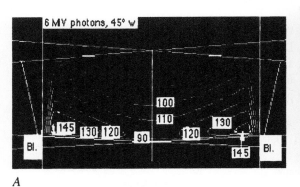

A

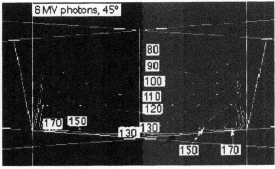

B

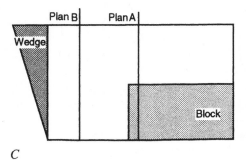

C

Figure 6.42 When wedges are used in a treatment, unexpected hot spots can occur under the thin portion of a wedge at levels other than where the isodose distribution is displayed. In the isodose distribution *(A)* calculated at the central axis *(see diagram, C)* in a plan using just opposed wedged fields, the hot spot is about 145 percent. At this level, the thinnest portion of the wedge is blocked. In an isodose distribution calculated for the same field arrangement *(B)* but at another level *(diagram, C),* where the thin portion of the wedge is not blocked, the hot spot is about 170 percent—a significant increase in dose.

and the beam outline in the third dimension is often not available. The field arrangement is also limited to coplanar beams only (i.e., the central axes of all fields must be on a common plane). Historically, very little consideration has therefore been given to the dose in structures not visible on the central plane. Three-dimensional treatment-planning systems, on the other hand, use information about both the patient and the beams in three dimensions and are capable of calculating dose within the entire irradiated volume. The information used, such as the location of tissues of different densities and the shape of the patient's external surface, is usually obtained from the CT data. The choice of beam orientation is unrestricted and the central axes do not have to be on a common plane (i.e., they can be noncoplanar). In utilizing all of the information, three-dimensional dose calculations are usually more accurate than conventional dose calculations and yield much more information about the dose within the treated volume.

Complex beam arrangements, with compound angles, sometimes designed with the help of three-dimensional treatment planning tools may not yield the optimal dose distribution. There are, however, many methods by which the dose distribution can be improved. The most commonly used beam modifier is a wedge. In such complex beam arrangements, it may be necessary also to angle the collimator in which the wedge is usually fixed, so that the wedge direction is unconventional, in order to produce a uniform dose distribution (Chap. 10, Fig. 10.24). Computer programs to calculate the needed wedge angle and wedge direction have been described.[68,69]

ADJACENT FIELDS

A frequently occurring problem that causes much concerns on the part of radiation oncologists is the treatment of adjacent fields, particularly when the gap between fields occurs over the spinal cord. The difficulties arise because the beam edges diverge, leading to nonuniformity in the overlap region. However, the divergence is perfectly predictable and can be determined from graphs as shown in Fig. 6.43 or from

$$\text{Tan } \theta = \frac{\text{half-field length}}{\text{distance}} \qquad (6.1)$$

If the fields are abutting on the skin surface, there will be an overlap with high dose at depth; when there is a small gap between the fields, there will be a cold area in the shallow region. These dose heterogeneities and techniques to minimize them has been the subject of study by many investigators.[70–95]

Lance and Morgan have described a technique in which the beam's central rays are angled slightly away from one another, so that the diverging beam edges are parallel (Fig. 6.44A). This technique is only applicable when the fields are treated concurrently or if the addition of an adjacent field is anticipated when the first field is treated. Williamson, Hopfan, and Chiang described a technique using half-beam blocks to eliminate beam divergence (Fig. 6.44B), while Armstrong, Fraass, Griffin, and Hale have described a technique in which small penumbra generators (small wedges) are inserted at the field margins to increase the width of the penumbra (Fig. 6.44C). Wider penumbra makes the dose less sensitive to small errors in the field separation because the dose fall-off is more gradual (Fig. 6.44D1 and D2). Lutz recommends using a small spinal-cord block with a thickness of 1 HVT at the junction (Fig. 6.44E) in situations where the patient's position is changed from supine for anterior field treatment to prone for posterior field irradiation.[91] Several authors have described moving the calculated gap during the course of treatment (Fig. 6.44F).[74,86,96] Caution must be used here because, even when the gap location is shifted, high-dose areas can be inadvertently produced if the dose is not the same in the adjoining areas.[72] Starchman described a technique in which large areas with multiple fields are treated without gaps by rotating the head of the therapy unit around the source. Field-shaping blocks are placed on a table over the patient and the beam then sweeps over the table and patient. A similar technique was

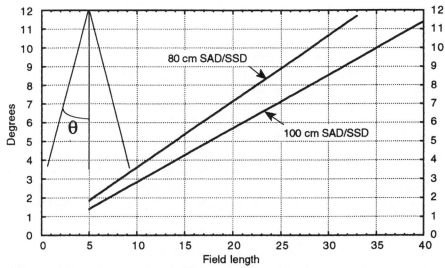

Figure 6.43   The angle of a diverging field margin as a function of field length and distance.

described by Kosnik, where the head of the machine is fixed but the couch with the patient is moved in the beam.[88]

The most commonly employed field-matching method is that of allowing a gap between the fields on the skin surface so that the beam edges converge at a certain depth (Fig. 6.45). This method considers only the geometry; however, it is necessary also to consider the dosimetry in the gap region.

DOSE CONSIDERATIONS

The dose in the triangular gap region above the beam convergence (labeled a in Fig. 6.45) will be lower than at the point where the beams converge because the triangle lies outside the geometric margins of either field. The dose in the region beyond the beam convergence (labeled b in Fig. 6.45), on the other hand, will be higher because it lies within the geometric boundaries of both fields. When adjacent posterior fields are used to treat the spinal axis, this higher dose will occur in the abdomen, chest, or throat, depending on where the field junction is located. To prevent this overlap from occurring in the same tissues throughout the course of treatment, causing the dose to be very high in one area, the gap

is moved to a new location a few times during the course of the treatment—for example, every 1000 cGy. This will not eliminate the overlap, but the area of dose inhomogeneity is shifted to other locations, thus reducing the magnitude of the inhomogeneity and therefore also the risks of adverse consequences in normal tissues such as the spinal cord, bowel, heart, esophagus, and larynx. It is preferable to make the necessary field separation in a location where there is no tumor. In cases where this is not possible, the field separation should be calculated so that the beams converge at a depth that is shallower than the tumor.

In most radiation beams, the dose at the geometric field margin is 50 percent of the dose at the central axis at the same depth—i.e., at a depth where the dose is 60 percent on the central axis, the dose at the geometric field edge is 30 percent, and so on (Chap. 3, Figs. 3.16 and 3.19). Thus, the dose contributed at the point where the geometric boundaries of two fields converge will be 50 percent of the dose on the central axis of each field. For example, when 200 cGy is delivered on the central axis of each of two adjacent fields, 100 cGy (50 percent) from each field (100 + 100 cGy) is delivered at the point where the field margins converge; thus the dose on a

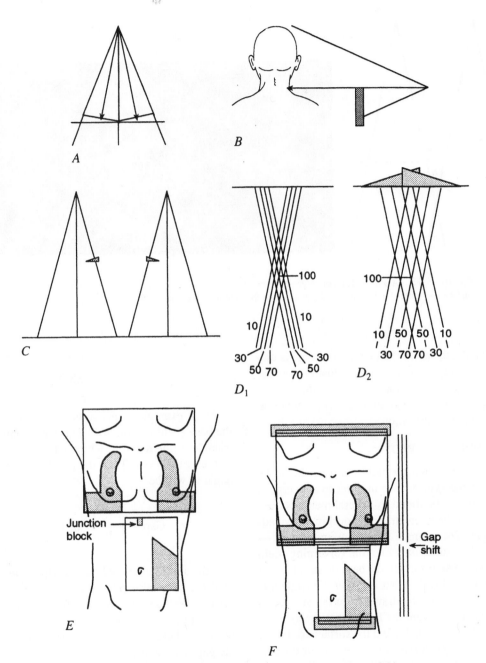

Figure 6.44   *A – E*. Different techniques for matching adjacent fields.

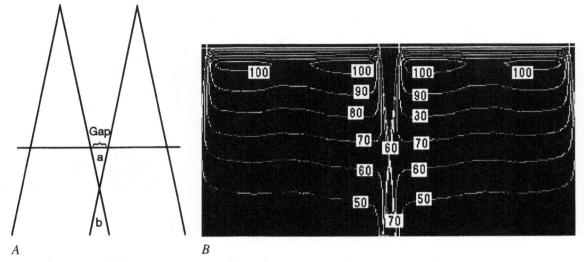

A   B

Figure 6.45 *A* and *B*. The convergence of two adjacent beams at a depth causes a cold spot near the surface and a hot spot beyond the depth at which the field margins converge.

plane at the depth where the beams converge is uniform. This is only a theoretical conclusion, because there are many other factors that affect the dose— for example, the beam penumbra, surface topography, and scatter contribution.

DETERMINING GAP WIDTH

The distance by which the field margins should be separated on the skin surface in order to converge at a given depth can be found by several methods. Figure 6.46 shows the geometric relationship of two adjacent fields. The triangle labeled A in field #1— formed by the central axis line, the (diverging) field margin, and the skin surface (or base of the triangle) —is similar to triangle a but is larger. Triangle a is formed by a vertical line drawn from the surface to the point where we want the beams to converge, the diverging edge of the field, and the surface (or base). The base of triangle a represents the gap, or the distance between the field side to the vertical line drawn from the surface to the point where the beams converge (d) in Fig. 6.46. This distance can be found from the following consideration. The SSD (in A) is to d (in a) as the base of triangle A is to the base of triangle a. Therefore,

$$Gap = \frac{d \times b}{SSD} \qquad (6.2)$$

As an example, suppose that the SSD is 100 cm, the base (field length, or FL) in A is 15 cm, and d in triangle a (the depth at which we want the fields to converge) is 7 cm. Then the gap (or the base of triangle a) will be

$$Gap = \frac{7 \times 15}{100} \text{ or } 1.05 \text{ cm}$$

If the adjacent field #2 has the same dimensions as field #1, the total gap between the two fields will be 2.1 cm. We can see from Fig. 6.46 and this calculation that when the SSD becomes shorter or the depth where the beam sides converge increases, the size of the gap will be larger.

In the next example, we calculate the gap needed between two fields with different geometry. In field #1, the SSD is 100 cm, the base (or half-field length) is 12 cm, and the depth (d) is 5 cm. In field #2, the SSD is 80 cm, half-field length is 16 cm, and d is also 5 cm. The total gap is found from

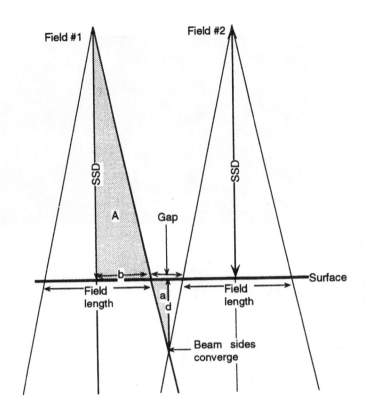

Figure 6.46   The gap needed on the surface between two adjacent beams depends on the distance (SSD or SAD), the field length (FL) in the direction of the gap, and the depth (d) at which the field margins should converge.

$$\text{Gap} = \left(\frac{5 \times 12}{100}\right) + \left(\frac{5 \times 16}{80}\right) \text{ or } 1.6 \text{ cm}$$
$$(0.6 + 1.0)$$

When the necessary gap has been found, it is advisable to make the separation slightly larger to compensate for uncertainties associated with the setup, including the possibility of small discrepancies in the beam-light coincidence, vague lines on the skin surface indicating the field margins, and involuntary patient motion. When the gap is over the spinal cord, a small block can be added in the fields over the spinal cord, thus reducing the risks of injury.[91] Overdosage, even to a narrow strip across the spinal cord, can lead to transverse myelitis—a devastating disability.

GAP BETWEEN OPPOSED ADJACENT FIELDS

In treatments where adjacent fields are opposed, the problem is similar, but here the most uniform dose in the gap region is achieved if the beam edges are calculated to converge at the patient's middepth (Fig. 6.47A). The shallow areas, described in the previous section as being outside both field margins, are now included in both of the opposing fields as they exit the patient. The region which earlier was in the overlap area is now excluded from the opposite fields, eliminating the high-dose area. The entire treatment area is included in two fields; however, the two triangles created above and below the point where the beams converge lie in the exit of two fields, resulting in a slightly lower dose than at middepth.

Figure 6.47B illustrates two opposed adjacent fields labeled #1 through #4. We will assume that each field delivers 100 cGy at middepth on the central axis. The darkest shaded areas, labeled 1 + 2 and 3 + 4, then receive approximately 200 cGy. The triangles labeled 2 + 4 and 1 + 3 lie within the exit areas of these beams thus receiving a somewhat lower dose. Each of the areas labeled 1, 2, 3, and 4 is

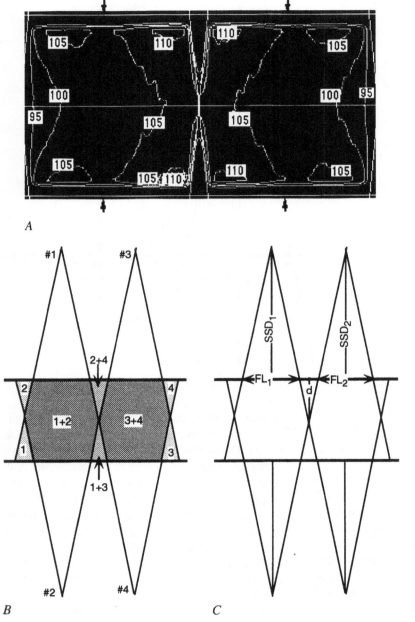

A

B

C

Figure 6.47 *A.* When adjacent fields are opposed, the best dose distribution is achieved if the fields converge at middepth. *B.* The dose in the region anterior and posterior to the point where the beams converge will be lower because each region is included only in the exit of two beams. *C.* The geometry of the gap calculation.

included in the exit of only one beam and therefore receives a low dose.

In Fig. 6.47*B*, the fields have been drawn so that they are identical; therefore, the diverging field margins in the diagonally opposing fields are perfectly matched. For example, the diverging line of field #1 matches the diverging line of field #4. Likewise, the diverging lines of fields #2 and #3 match. As we shall see later, this match is lost when the two sets of opposing fields are geometrically different (Fig. 6.48).

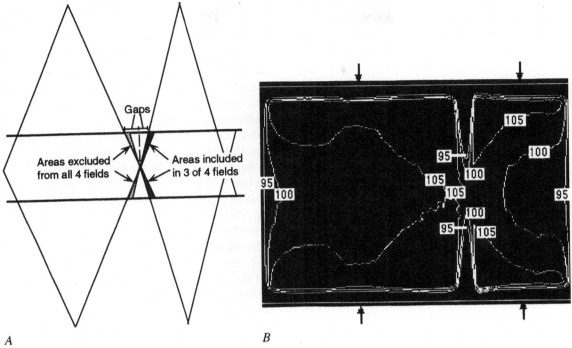

A   *B*

Figure 6.48 *A* and *B*. When two sets of opposed fields are not of the same size or the distance is different, the "perfect match" is lost.

In the next example, we shall calculate the gap between two fields (Fig. 6.47*C*) using a simpler approach. In most gap calculations, it is not necessary to calculate the needed gap for each field separately, so we can find the total gap in a simpler way.

$$\text{Gap} = \frac{d}{2}\left(\frac{FL_1}{SSD_1} + \frac{FL_2}{SSD_2}\right) \qquad (6.3)$$

In this example, we will assume that the SSD in both fields is 100 cm, the FL is 22 cm, and d is 10 cm. The gap between the two sets of fields is therefore

$$\frac{10}{2}\left(\frac{22}{100} + \frac{22}{100}\right) = 2.2 \text{ cm}$$

In yet another example, we shall assume that all fields are treated using an SAD technique. It is important to remember that the distance to be used in the calculation must be the distance at which the field length is defined, whether an SSD or SAD technique is used. When an SAD treatment technique is used, it is simpler to use the field length at the source-axis distance rather than the distance and field on the surface where the gap will ultimately be measured. The result is the same as we shall find in the following calculations.

In the first calculation, we will use the source-axis distance and the field length at this distance. The SAD_1 is 100 cm and FL_1 is 12 cm in one field, the SAD_2 is 80 cm and FL_2 is 28 cm in the second field, and d is 12.5 cm. The needed gap then is

$$\frac{12.5}{2}\left(\frac{12}{100} + \frac{28}{80}\right) = 2.9 \text{ cm}$$

We next shall show that the answer is the same if we use the distance to the surface and the field length at that distance. Here SSD_1 is 87.5 cm $(100 - 12.5)$, FL_1 is 10.5 cm $(12 \times 87.5/100)$, SSD_2 is 67.5 $(80 - 12.5)$, and FL_2 is 23.6 cm $(28 \times 67.5/80)$, while the depth is unchanged at 12.5 cm. The needed gap is then

$$\frac{12.5}{2} \left(\frac{10.5}{87.5} + \frac{23.6}{67.5} \right) = 2.9 \text{ cm}$$

The answer is, as we predicted, identical and was found with less difficulty in the first example.

The distances and field lengths are not the same in the two sets of opposing fields where the gap was just calculated; therefore, the field margins do not match precisely as shown in Fig. 6.48. Of course, in clinical practice we know that these field margins do not match perfectly due to small discrepancies, including rounding out of numbers, small variations in setting up the treatment daily, and patient motion. These uncertainties can lead to under- or overdosage at the field junction.

In the examples above, it was assumed that the surface on which the gap was determined was flat and that the patient's thickness was the same over the whole treated area. In many situations, the gap is in a region where the patient's surface is uneven and the patient's thickness may also be different in the two adjacent fields. The depth at which the field margins need to converge should be based on the patient's thickness measured at the location where the gap will occur. The problem of matching field margins on sloping surfaces has been studied.[85,87,91]

FIELD SEPARATION IN IRREGULARLY SHAPED FIELDS

In the examples shown so far, the geometry was simple and the gap calculation straightforward. It is almost always assumed that the field edges of the two adjacent fields are defined by the collimator and thus are perfectly straight. In such a situation, we can calculate the necessary gap by using simple geometry as shown in the previous sections. However, with increasing frequency, these field edges are created by customized blocks. For example, in a mantle treatment, the field margin is usually defined by the collimator, whereas in the adjacent paraaortic field, the margin is often defined by a block (Fig. 6.49). This often occurs when the paraaortic field must extend cephalad to include the spleen and thus also inadvertently extends into the previously irradiated mantle field. The spleen usually lies within the region shielded by the left lung block during the mantle field irradiation. In the patient's midline, where the mantle field was unshielded, the paraaortic field must be shaped by a block to create the necessary gap. This block must be made so that a straight line is formed across the spinal cord.

In the situation where the margins of the previously treated fields were defined by the collimator and the gap must be created by inserting a block in the new fields, it is difficult to define precisely where the block should be drawn on the simulation film. Calculation of the necessary gap should be made using the distance from the central axis of the new field to where the field gap is anticipated. Placing a lead marker at this point on the anterior surface would indicate where the block must be placed. If both the previous and the new fields are treated while the patient is supine, the anterior and posterior fields will be identical at the gap and both beam-shaping blocks can be produced from the same radiograph. Caution should be used here, since the splenic portion of the field may need to be different on the anterior and the posterior film because the spleen usually lies in the posterior portion of the abdomen (Chap. 14, Fig. 14.9).

In the following example, we calculate the necessary gap between the previous mantle field and the new paraaortic field shown in Fig. 6.49. The mantle field is treated at 100 cm SAD and the field length is 38 cm. The paraaortic field is also treated at 100 cm SAD and the length is 20 cm. The depth where the fields converge is 10 cm. The gap between the mantle and the paraaortic field is achieved by blocking three cm of the paraaortic field. Therefore, the distance from the central axis to the field edge is half the field length (10 cm) minus the blocked area (3 cm), leaving the half-field length at 7 cm. Using Eq. (6.2),

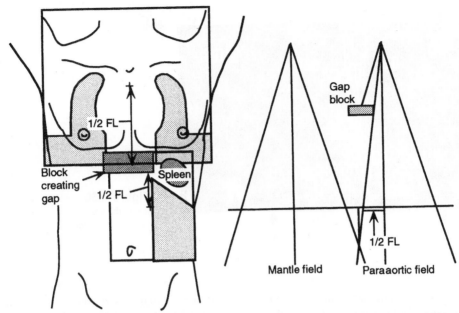

Figure 6.49 Anterior mantle and paraaortic fields where the separation between them is defined with a customized block. The spleen, in this case, lies under the lung block previously used in the mantle field. For calculating the gap between the mantle and the paraaortic field, only the distance from the central axis to the block edge is used as half the beam length.

the necessary gap between the two fields is therefore

$$\left(\frac{10 \times 19}{100}\right) + \left(\frac{10 \times 7}{100}\right) = 2.6 \text{ cm}$$

SHIFTING THE LOCATION OF THE GAP

When adjacent fields are treated concurrently or in planned sequence, the field margins are often shifted to blur out the dose inhomogeneities between the adjacent areas (Fig. 6.50). Such instances would be, for example, in the treatment of the entire central nervous system, where all fields are usually treated concurrently, and the treatment of Hodgkin's disease, where the planned fields are treated sequentially but with a planned break between treatment courses. The doses in the region affected by the gap shift must be very carefully calculated and documented, because high-dose regions can unintentionally occur.[72] The proper gap shift can be achieved by increasing the size of one field and at the same time reducing the size of the adjacent field, as illustrated in Fig. 6.44F. A shield is placed in the cephalad and caudal margin of the treated area to prevent the radiation beams from extending beyond the intended target area when the field sizes are changed.

PATIENT POSITIONING

The ideal situation for matching adjacent fields is to maintain just one patient position (i.e., either supine or prone) when all fields are treated. This is, of course, impractical in many situations. For example, mantle fields are often too large for posterior treatment in the supine position through the tabletop window, and the patient is therefore positioned prone for treatment of the posterior field. This presents a very difficult field-matching problem when the patient returns for treatment of the paraaortic/spleen fields. In this situation, it is safest to treat the adjacent fields

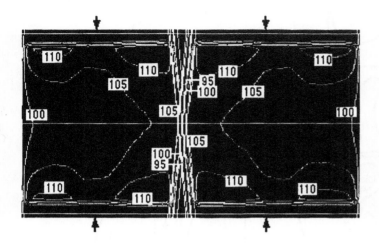

Figure 6.50 When the gap is shifted three times, the areas of dose inhomogeneity are moved to a new location.

with the patient in the same two positions, even if the new posterior field could be treated through the window with the patient in the supine position. The radiographs of these fields must be carefully examined so that a possible overlap in the spinal cord can be prevented. The use of a small spinal cord block with a thickness of 1 HVT (50 percent dose transmission) has been proposed at the junction between such adjacent fields.[91]

MATCHING NEW FIELDS WITH PREVIOUSLY TREATED FIELDS

Where adjacent fields in a patient are treated concurrently or with a short rest period between treatment courses—for example, the mantle and paraaortic fields—the appropriate gap can be determined with confidence. This is because tattoos indicating previously treated fields are reliable, since the patient's weight likely would not have changed much and the immobilization device is usually saved so the position can be reproduced. In a patient who returns possibly years later for further treatment of an adjacent area, tattoos may have shifted due to weight change, the position is uncertain, and treatment documentation, including radiographs of previous treatment area, may be unavailable. The need for careful documentation of treatments can not be overemphasized.

When radiographs of previously treated fields are available, these fields should, with the use of a simulator, be reproduced with respect to bony anatomy and be marked on the patient's skin. If at all possible, port (rather than simulation) films of previous treatment fields should be consulted, since the field may have been changed following the simulation. The treatment fields may also have been changed during the treatment course, and it is therefore important to examine the chart carefully for changes in collimator setting, block configurations, and so on as the original treatment progressed.

When a patient returns for additional treatment and new anterior and posterior fields must be matched with previously treated anterior and posterior fields over the spinal cord, it is prudent to consult port films of both of the previously treated fields to determine which segment of the spinal cord has been irradiated. If tolerance doses have already been delivered, the new fields should be designed so that the previously treated segment of the spinal cord is excluded.

Patients previously treated through parallel opposed anterior and posterior fields are usually patients with lung carcinoma treated in the supine position. They often return with metastatic disease in the spine or with a spinal-cord compression requiring immediate intervention. Often, the new fields must be adjacent to the previously treated area and the needed gap on the skin surface is calculated in the usual fashion. Even if a posterior field only is contemplated to treat the spine and the previous treatment was delivered with the patient in the supine position, the supine position should be strongly considered in the new treatments in order to maintain optimal geometry in the gap region. Modern equipment allows many treatments to be delivered uninterrupted through a window in the treatment couch. Furthermore, the supine position is often more reproducible and most patients, especially those with painful metastatic disease, are more comfortable.

USING A HALF-BEAM BLOCK

A technique in which the gap between the previously treated field and the new field can be minimized is to use a half-beam block. In this technique, the central axis of the "new" field is set near the margin of the "old" field and then a half-beam block is inserted over the previously treated field. The same effect can be achieved by closing the independent collimator jaw (when available) to the central axis. This eliminates any beam divergence of the new field into the previously treated area and thus minimizes the size of the unirradiated area. The gap required between the margin of the old field and the central axis of the new one must be calculated to account for the divergence of the old field only (Fig. 6.51). This technique may be advantageous in situations where the disease is very close to a previously treated area and it is important to minimize the size of the gap—for example, when a spinal cord compression is very close to the previously treated area.

Some patients present with a spinal cord compression in more than one site. When two sites are close

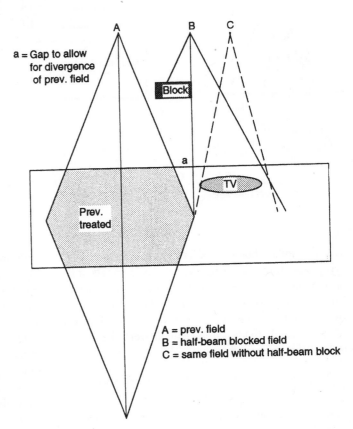

Figure 6.51 When retreatment near a previously treated area is necessary, the size of the gap can be reduced by using a half-beam block or closing an independent collimator jaw to the central axis.

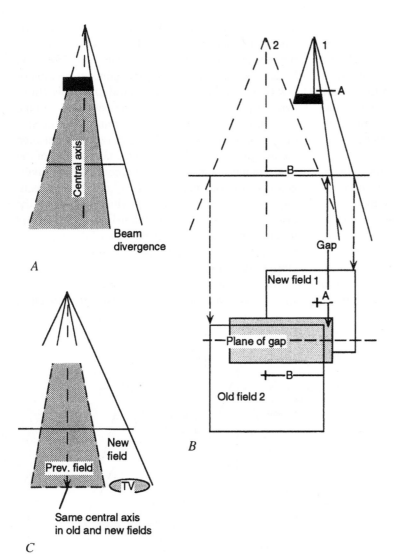

A

B

C

Figure 6.52 *A.* When a block or an independent jaw is extended across the central axis of the beam, both field margins diverge in the same direction. *B.* When the beam is blocked across the central axis (field 1), the divergence of the field margin is in the same direction as in the previously treated field (field 2). Thus, the divergence is negative. *C.* The central axis of the new field can be set at the same point as in the previous treatment. The field size is then set to include the adjacent target, and the previously treated area is blocked.

to one another but the patient does not have any symptoms from disease between these segments, it is best, in most instances, to include this region as well. Microscopic disease may already be present, and from a field-matching viewpoint, it is almost impossible to match fields safely and to treat the small in-between segment later on.

EXTENDING THE BLOCK OR INDEPENDENT JAW ACROSS THE CENTRAL AXIS

In some situations, an independent collimator jaw or a block may extend across the central axis, blocking

more than half of the beam. In this case, both field edges diverge in the same direction but at different angles (Fig. 6.52*A*). This is an important consideration when a gap must be calculated between the fields.

The gap needed between a field in which the block or independent jaw extends across the central axis and a new adjacent field must be calculated keeping in mind that the previous beam divergence was in the same direction as the new (Fig. 6.52). The gap needed as a result of divergence of the new field is subtracted from the divergence of the proximal side of the previous field. For example, in field 1 in Fig. 6.52B (new field), the distance from the central axis to the block edge (A) is 5 cm, and in field 2 (old field), the distance from the central axis to the beam edge (B) is 11 cm. The SSD is 100 cm in both fields and the gap is calculated so that the beam edges converge at 10-cm depth. The needed gap is found from

$$Gap = \left(\frac{10 \times 11}{100} \right) - \left(\frac{10 \times 5}{100} \right)$$

or

$$1.1 - 0.5 = 0.6\text{-cm gap}$$

Another method to match an adjacent field with a field that is blocked across the central axis is to set the central axis of the new field at the same point as in the previous field and then block the previously treated area (Fig. 6.52C). This will achieve the same geometry as in the previous field; however, a small gap should be used as a precaution, since tissues tend to move and marks are not totally reliable.

ADJACENT ORTHOGONAL FIELDS

In the previous sections, the discussion has been with regard to adjacent fields where the central axes were either parallel or opposed. In many situations, adjacent fields are angled from different directions, most commonly in an orthogonal right-angled fashion. For example, in craniospinal irradiation, lateral fields are used to treat the brain and cervical spine and a posterior field is used to treat the spinal axis. An orthogonal field arrangement is also used to treat head and neck malignancies, where lateral fields are used to treat the tumor above the shoulders and an anterior field is used to treat the lower neck and supraclavicular lymph nodes. An even more complex field-matching technique is used to match tangential breast or chest wall fields and anterior supraclavicular fields. In this field match the beams are not orthogonal, since the supraclavicular field is angled about 15° away from the midline and the tangential fields across the chest are angled about 30 to 60°. Orthogonal field-matching techniques have been described by many authors.[74,79,81,95,97–99] Details of these techniques as they apply to different anatomic regions and can be found in the appropriate chapters in this text.

GENERAL CONSIDERATIONS

When customized field-shaping blocks are used, the field margin can be drawn so that it crosses the spinal canal at an angle, making field matching very difficult. Superior field-matching geometry can be achieved when the patient returns for additional

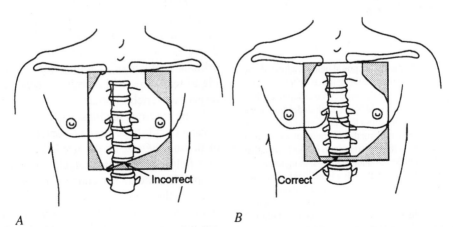

A   *B*

Figure 6.53 *A* and *B*. When customized block shaping is used, fields should be shaped so that the margins cross the spine in a straight line perpendicular to the spine to accommodate proper field matching across the spinal cord.

treatment if field edges cross the spinal cord in a line perpendicular to the spine (Fig. 6.53). Examples of areas where a field edge may be defined by a custom-shaped block across the spinal cord is in the treatment of malignancies in the thorax and the head and neck area.

It is sometimes thought that the cephalad and caudal margins of fields that include the spinal cord should be set so that the field margins are between two vertebral bodies. These margins are often determined while viewing an anterior radiograph, while the appearance of the spinal column in the posterior view is disregarded. It is only possible to have these field margins pass between two vertebral bodies in both the anterior and the posterior radiograph when the fields are defined at the depth of the spinal cord. In Fig. 6.54, field a includes the T9 vertebra, while field b does not. On the other hand, field c includes T9, while field d does not. As shown earlier, the optimal dose distribution is achieved when two pairs of adjacent opposing fields converge at the patient's middepth as in Fig. 6.54. When the fields are defined

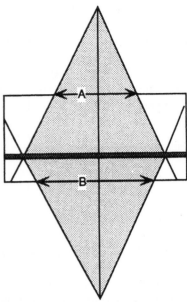

Figure 6.55 A and B. Two opposed fields can be set to include the same length of the spine; however, the field size must be specified at the depth of the spine.

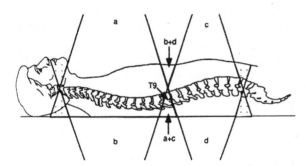

Figure 6.54 When two parallel opposed fields are treated, the field margins of each field will cross the spine at different levels because the spine lies posterior to the patient's middepth. In field a, T9 vertebra is included; but in field b, it is excluded. Making the field size such that both margins cross the spinal cord at the same intervertebral space while maintaining the geometry of a matching set of fields is not possible. In this illustration, it is also shown that fields a and d cross the spine at the same level—one includes T9, while in the other it is excluded. On the other hand, field c includes T9 while in field b it is excluded. To verify a gap calculation, an anterior mantle field (a) should cross the spine at the same point as a posterior paraaortic field (d), and a posterior mantle field (b) should cross the spine at the same point as the anterior paraaortic field (c).

at the more posteriorly situated spine (Fig. 6.55), the dose uniformity is compromised. In most instances, the diverging beam margins will cross the vertebral bodies at an angle, and when the beams are opposed, the divergence is in opposite directions, making it impossible to have the beam edges go through the intervertebral space (Fig. 6.55). Again, it is necessary to study the dose distribution in the field-junction area as well as calculating the geometric gap. There is no need to further complicate an already difficult problem of matching adjacent fields by trying to make the field margins appear the same with respect to vertebral bodies.

In the previous sections, gap calculations to match adjacent fields have been presented. Another method of finding the size of the needed gap between adjacent fields without any calculation is to first set up the previous field. The couch with the patient is then lowered the same distance as the desired depth of beam convergence. The field will now appear larger because the distance is increased. The field margin, in the direction of the second field, is marked on the

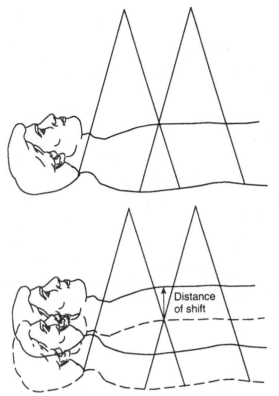

Figure 6.56 A simple method of matching fields can be made without a calculation. The previous field is first set such that the field size on the skin surface now equals the field size previously used at the depth where the fields are to converge. This field is then marked on the skin surface. The new field is then set so that it abuts the old field. The couch is then elevated a distance that is equal to the depth where the fields are to converge.

patient. The second field is then set adjacent to the first field and the couch is then raised to the treatment distance (Fig. 6.56).

Although this section has primarily dealt with the problems of matching adjacent fields in the sagittal plane and in the spinal cord, gaps between fields are dealt with in the same way in all parts of the body even when it is necessary to match adjacent fields in more than one direction.

MATCHING TWO ADJACENT ELECTRON BEAMS

In many treatment situations, the area to be treated may be larger than can be encompassed in one electron field, or the shape of the patient's contour may require that multiple electron fields be used. Clinical judgment must be used in deciding about field matching. If two electron fields abut on the skin surface, a hot spot will occur at a depth (Fig. 6.57), just as with photon beams. If the beam edges are separated, on the other hand, a low-dose area occurs in the superficial tissues. The magnitude of this dose nonuniformity can be reduced by moving the location of the field junction at approximately every 1000 cGy to reduce the risks of normal tissue injury or tumor recurrence. It is preferable to arrange the fields so that the location of field junctions does not occur in known tumor or in a critical organ—for example, the heart when a chest wall is irradiated.

In patients with breast carcinoma, electron beams

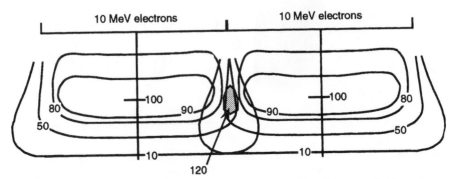

Figure 6.57 Two electron fields without a gap result in a hot spot at depth.

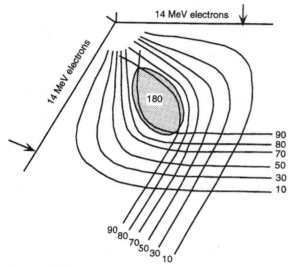

Figure 6.58   When two electron beams are angled in toward one another, a very hot spot occurs at depth.

are sometimes used to treat the chest wall or to boost the dose to an incision or to the area of the primary tumor. Because of the curvature of the chest wall and the breast, it is difficult to deliver a uniform dose to the entire area through a single field. An anterior field is often supplemented by a lateral or oblique field to treat the lateral aspect of the chest wall. Very high doses can occur at a depth where these beams intersect (Fig. 6.58). Rib fractures and even death from ventricular perforation have been reported as a result of poor matching of adjacent electron beams on the chest wall.[100] In cases where multiple fields must be used, polystyrene absorbers can be inserted in the junction between the fields (Fig. 6.59). Matching of angled electron beams must be preceded by a very careful determination of the dose distribution across the junction. It is also necessary to shift the location of the field junction in these situations to reduce the risks of injuring normal tissue.

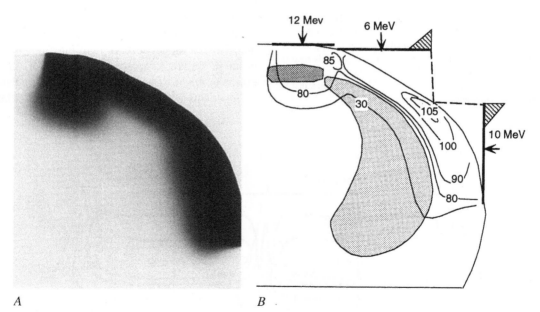

A   *B*

Figure 6.59   *A*. A radiograph, shaped to the patient's contour and exposed to the proposed electron beam arrangement, before its implementation. *B*. The dose distribution from the angled electron fields in *A*, using a wedge absorber at the junction.

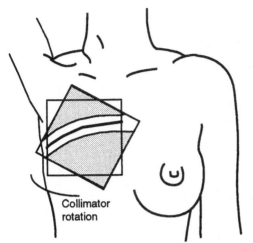

Figure 6.60   When an area, which is longer than the largest electron cone, must be treated, the cone can be turned to take advantage of the larger diagonal dimension.

When a long narrow area such as an incision is treated, the target may be too long to be encompassed by the largest available cone. Increasing the distance to achieve a larger field will cause the width of the penumbra to increase. Alternatively, the collimator can be turned with respect to the target, taking advantage of the larger diagonal dimension of the cone (Fig. 6.60).

MATCHING PHOTON AND ELECTRON BEAMS

It is often necessary to use an electron beam to treat an area adjacent to a photon field. In the head and neck area, for example, it is common practice to treat the lymph nodes in the posterior neck using an electron beam so as to spare the spinal cord, while the primary tumor site and the lymph nodes in the anterior neck are treated using a photon beam. If these beam edges are set up without a gap between them, a hot spot occurs at a depth (Fig. 6.61). If a gap is left between the two beam edges on the skin surface, considerable underdosage could occur in the superficial tissues. Because it is difficult to place the end of the electron cone directly on the skin surface in this area, an air gap is almost always present. This causes the electron-beam penumbra to increase in width,[41] lowering the risks of a hot spot. Judgment about whether to leave a gap or to abut the fields must be based on the clinical situation, taking into consideration the combined dose distribution across the junction, the depth of the tumor, the location of radiosensitive tissues with respect to hot spots, the size and location of high- or low-dose areas, the magnitude of the dose variation, and the total dose to be delivered. If the tumor volume lies at a shallow depth, it may be advantageous to make the field edges abut so that the tumor receives a full dose. If the fields abut on the surface, it is advisable to move the location of the junction a few times during the course of the treatment to decrease the magnitude of potential hot spots.

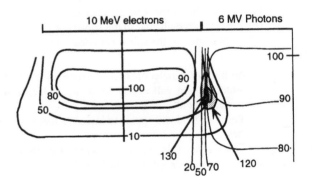

Figure 6.61   Dose distribution when an electron beam and a photon beam abut on the skin surface. The dose at a depth can be very high.

PROBLEMS

6.1   Photon isodose curves used in dose calculation on a patient usually require the following corrections:
   (*a*) Surface irregularities only
   (*b*) Oblique incidence and inhomogeneities only
   (*c*) Oblique incidence and surface irregularities
   (*d*) Inhomogeneities only

6.2   Electron isodose curves used in dose calculation on a patient usually require
   (*a*) No corrections
   (*b*) Corrections for beam obliquity only
   (*c*) Inhomogeneity corrections only
   (*d*) Corrections for beam obliquity and surface irregularities

6.3   The maximum dose from a single 6-MV photon beam occurs at approximately
   (*a*) 1.5-cm depth
   (*b*) 2.0-cm depth
   (*c*) 0.5-cm depth
   (*d*) 3.0-cm depth

6.4   The depth of maximum dose (D_{max}) for any photon-beam energy is reduced by
   (*a*) Smaller field size and oblique incidence
   (*b*) Larger field size and oblique incidence
   (*c*) Smaller field size and longer SSD
   (*d*) Smaller field size and shorter SSD

6.5   A beam spoiler is
   (*a*) A sheet of Lucite placed in large fields to reduce the dose rate
   (*b*) A sheet of Lucite placed in large fields to improve the beam penetration
   (*c*) A sheet of Lucite placed in the beam to deliver the treatment faster
   (*d*) A sheet of Lucite placed in the beam to reduce the depth of D_{max}

6.6   Treatment fields should always be shaped so that the beam edge
   (*a*) Crosses the spinal cord at an angle
   (*b*) Crosses perpendicular to the spinal cord
   (*c*) With respect to the spinal cord does not matter

6.7   In port films of parallel opposed isocentric fields of a lung tumor, the
   (*a*) Anterior field will appear to include a longer segment of the spinal cord than the posterior field
   (*b*) Posterior field will appear to include a longer segment of spinal cord than the anterior field
   (*c*) The anterior field appears to include a shorter segment of the spinal cord
   (*d*) Two fields will appear to include the same segment of spinal cord

6.8   To minimize the gap between two adjacent fields,
   (*a*) A posterior field alone can be used
   (*b*) An anterior field alone can be used
   (*c*) A half-beam block can be used
   (*d*) The two fields can be treated simultaneously

6.9   When adjacent areas must be treated, it is best to
   (*a*) Calculate the gap necessary between the fields to prevent an overlap
   (*b*) Set a 2-cm gap between all fields
   (*c*) Rely on tattoos to prevent an overlap
   (*d*) Always use a 3-cm separation on the skin

6.10 When an isodose tilt of about 22° is needed,
   (a) Isodose charts for a 30 and a 45° wedge can be combined
   (b) Isodose charts for an open and a 45° wedge can be combined
   (c) Isodose charts for an open and a 30° wedge can be combined
   (d) Isodose charts for a 45 and a 60° wedge can be combined

6.11 To estimate the needed wedge angle in oblique fields,
   (a) Subtract the hinge angle from 180 and divide by 2
   (b) Subtract the hinge angle from 90 and divide by 2
   (c) Add the hinge angle to 180 and divide by 2
   (d) Add the hinge angle to 90 and divide by 2

6.12 In an isocentric treatment technique, it is routine to normalize the dose
   (a) At D_{max} of each beam
   (b) At isocenter
   (c) At D_{max} of each beam and then find the average
   (d) At D_{max} of the beam with the largest depth

6.13 In an electron beam,
   (a) The 80 percent isodose curve bulges out and the 20 percent curve constricts
   (b) All of the isodose curves bulge out
   (c) The 20 percent isodose curve bulges out and the 90 percent curve constricts
   (d) The 80 percent isodose curve bulges out and the 20 percent curve constricts

6.14 When parallel opposed 6-MV photon beams are used in a 20-cm-thick patient, the maximum dose will occur at
   (a) The entrance/exit of each field
   (b) The dose will be uniform throughout the patient
   (c) The tumor
   (d) The midplane in the patient

6.15 When 4- and a 15-MV photon beams are used to treat parallel opposed fields in a 20-cm-thick patient, the dose in the entrance/exit region
   (a) Is highest when the 15-MV photon beams are used
   (b) Is the same for both energies
   (c) Is the same throughout the patient with both energies
   (d) Is highest when the 4-MV photon beams are used

6.16 When a sector is skipped in an arc technique,
   (a) The high-dose area is shifted toward the skipped sector
   (b) The high-dose area remain centered on the isocenter
   (c) The high-dose area becomes twice as large
   (d) The high-dose area is shifted away from the skipped sector

6.17 When parallel opposed fields are used with the isocenter at middepth and one field is weighted twice as much as the other, the maximum dose is in the
   (a) Entrance/exit region of the field with lower weight
   (b) Entrance/exit region of the field with higher weight
   (c) Isocenter
   (d) The dose is the same throughout the patient

6.18 To minimize the risks of hot or cold spots in the junction between two photon fields, the gap should
  (*a*) Be moved several times during the treatment course
  (*b*) Be increased by 0.5 cm each week
  (*c*) Be increased and shifted once during the treatment course
  (*d*) Be moved and decreased several times during the treatment course

6.19 To obtain optimal geometry in the gap region, the patient should
  (*a*) Remain in the prone position for posterior and supine for anterior treatments
  (*b*) Be supine during the treatment of one and prone for the other sets of fields
  (*c*) Remain in the supine position for all treatments
  (*d*) The patient's position is irrelevant

6.20 Matching of electron beams on a chest wall is
  (*a*) Unusually easy because the electron beams do not diverge
  (*b*) More difficult because some isodose curves bulge out and others constrict
  (*c*) Never done because it is not needed
  (*d*) Unusually easy because the fields can be abutting

REFERENCES

1. Khan FM, Lee JMF: Computer algorithm for electron beam treatment planning. *Med Phys* 6:142, 1979.
2. Okumura Y: Correction of dose distribution for air space in high energy electron therapy. *Radiology* 103:183, 1972.
3. Khan FM, Sewchand W, Levitt SH: Effects of air space on depth dose in electron beam therapy. *Radiology* 126:249, 1978.
4. Johnson JM, Khan FM: Dosimetric effects of abutting extended source to surface distance electron fields with photon fields in the treatment of head and neck cancers. *Int J Radiat Oncol Biol Phys* 28:741, 1994.
5. Ekstrand KE, Dixon RL: The problem of obliquely incident beams and electron-beam treatment planning. *Med Phys* 9:276, 1982.
6. Khan FM, Deibel FC, Soleimani-Meigooni A: Obliquity correction for electron beams. *Med Phys* 12:749, 1985.
7. Khan FM: *The Physics of Radiation Therapy,* 2d ed. Baltimore-London: Williams & Wilkins, 1994.
8. Deibel FC, Khan FM, Werner BL: Electron beam treatment planning with strip beams (abstr). *Med Phys* 10:527, 1983.
9. McKenzie AL: Air-gap correction in electron treatment planning. *Phys Med Biol* 24:628, 1979.
10. Werner BL, Khan FM, Deibel FC: Model for calculating electron beam scattering in treatment planning. *Med Phys* 9:180, 1982.
11. Batho HF: Lung corrections in cobalt 60 beam therapy. *J Can Assoc Radiol* 15:79, 1964.
12. Young MEJ, Gaylord JD: Experimental tests of corrections for tissue inhomogeneities in radiotherapy. *Br J Radiol* 43:349, 1970.
13. Young MEJ, Kornelson RD: Dose corrections for low-density tissue inhomogeneities and air channels for 10-MV x-rays. *Med Phys* 10:450, 1983.
14. Sontag MR, Cunningham JR: Corrections to absorbed dose calculations for tissue inhomogeneities. *Med Phys* 4:431, 1977.
15. Sontag MR, Cunningham JR: The equivalent tissue-air ratio method for making absorbed dose calculations in a heterogeneous medium. *Radiology* 129:787, 1978.
16. Klein EE, Chin LM, Rice RK, Mijnheer BJ: The influence of air cavities on interface doses for photon beams. *Int J Radiat Oncol Biol Phys* 27:419, 1993.
17. Beach JL, Mendiondo MS, Mendiondo OA: A comparison of air-cavity inhomogeneity effects for cobalt-60, 6- and 10-MV X-ray beams. *Med Phys* 14:140, 1987.
18. Epp ER, Lougheed MN, McKay JW: Ionization build-up in upper respiratory air passages during teletherapy units with cobalt-60 radiation. *Brit J Radiol* 31:361, 1958.
19. Epp ER, Boyer AL, Doppke KP: Underdosing of lesions resulting from lack of electronic equilibrium in upper respiratory air cavities irradiated by 10 MV x-ray beams. *Int J Radiat Oncol Biol Phys* 2:613, 1977.
20. Koskinen MO, Spring E: Build-up and build-down measurements with thin LiF-Teflon dosimeters with special reference to radiotherapy of carcinoma of the larynx. *Strahlenth* 145:565, 1973.
21. Nilsson B, Schnell PO: Build-up studies at air cavities measured with thin thermoluminiscent dosimeters. *Acta Radiol (Ther)* 15:427, 1976.

22. Scrimger JW: Effect of air gap on absorbed dose in tissue. *Radiology* 102:171, 1972.

23. Sontag MR, Battista JJ, Bronskill MJ, Cunningham JR: Implications of computed tomography for inhomogeneity corrections in photon beam dose calculations. *Radiology* 124:143, 1977.

24. van de Geijn J: The extended net fractional depth dose: Correction for inhomogeneities including effects of electron transport in photon beam dose calculation. *Med Phys* 14:84, 1987.

25. Almond PR, Wright AE, Boone ML: High energy electron dose perturbations in regions of tissue heterogeneity. *Radiology* 88:1146, 1967.

26. Dahler A, Baker AS, Laughlin JS: Comprehensive electron-beam treatment planning. *Ann NY Acad Sci* 161:189, 1969.

27. Hogstrom KR, Mills MD, Almond PR: Electron beam dose calculations. *Phys Med Biol* 26:445, 1981.

28. Jette D, Walker S: Electron dose calculation using multiple-scattering theory: Evaluation of a new model for inhomogeneities. *Med Phys* 19:1241, 1992.

29. Laughlin JS: High energy electron treatment planning for inhomogeneities. *Br J Radiol* 38:143, 1965.

30. Laughlin JS, Lundy A, Phillips R, et al: Electron-beam treatment planning in inhomogeneous tissue. *Radiology* 85:524, 1965.

31. Brahme A: Current algorithms for computed electron beam dose planning. *Radiother Oncol* 3:347, 1985.

32. Cygler J, Battista JJ, Scrimger JW, et al: Electron dose distributions in experimental phantoms: A comparison with 2-D pencil beam calculations. *Phys Med Biol* 32:1073, 1987.

33. Hogstrom KR, Mills MD, Meyer JA, et al: Dosimetric evaluation of a pencil beam algorithm for electrons employing a two dimensional heterogeneity correction. *Int J Radiat Oncol Biol Phys* 10:561, 1984.

34. Kooy HM, Rashid H: A three dimensional electron pencil-beam algorithm. *Phys Med Biol* 34:229, 1989.

35. Lax I: Accuracy in clinical electron beam dose planning using pencil beam algorithms. *Radiother Oncol* 10:307, 1987.

36. Mah E, Antolak J, Scrimger JW, Battista JJ: Experimental evaluation of a 2-D and 3-D pencil beam algorithm. *Phys Med Biol* 34:1179, 1989.

37. Starkshall G, Shui AS, Bujnowski SW, et al: Effect of dimensionality of heterogeneity corrections on the implementation of a three dimensional electron pencil beam algorithm. *Phys Med Biol* 36:207, 1991.

38. Ostwald PM, Metcalfe PE, Denham JW, Hamilton CS: A comparison of three electron planning algorithms for 16 MEV electron beam. *Int J Radiat Oncol Biol Phys* 28:731, 1994.

39. Biggs PJ, Ling CC: Electrons as the cause of the observed d_{max} shift with field size in high energy photon beams. *Med Phys* 6:291, 1979.

40. Petti PL, Goodman MS, Gabriel TA, Mohan R: Investigation of buildup dose from electron contamination of clinical photon beams. *Med Phys* 10:18, 1983.

41. Sixel KE, Podgorsak EB: Buildup region and depth of dose maximum of megavoltage x-ray beams. *Med Phys* 21:411, 1994.

42. Gerbi BJ, Meigooni AS, Khan FM: Dose buildup for oblique incident photon beams. *Med Phys* 14:393, 1987.

43. Jackson W: Surface effects of high energy x-rays at oblique incidence. *Br J Radiol* 44:109, 1971.

44. Fontenla DP, Napoli JJ, Hunt M, et al: Effects of beam modifiers and immobilization devices on the dose in the build-up region. *Int J Radiat Oncol Biol Phys* 30:211, 1994.

45. McParland BJ: The effect of a universal wedge and beam obliquity upon the central axis dose buildup for 6MV x-rays. *Med Phys* 18:740, 1991.

46. Gagnon WF, Grant WG: Surface dose from megavoltage therapy machines. *Radiology* 117:705, 1973.

47. Gagnon WF, Horton JL: Physical factors affecting absorbed dose to the skin from cobalt-60 gamma rays and 25 MV x-rays. *Med Phys* 6:285, 1979.

48. Gerbi BJ, Khan FM: Measurement of dose in the buildup region using fixed-separation plane-parallel ionization chambers. *Med Phys* 17:1, 1990.

49. Klein EE, Purdy JA: Entrance and exit dose regions for Clinac-2100C. *Int J Radiat Oncol Biol Phys* 27:429, 1993.

50. Purdy JA: Buildup/surface and exit dose measurements for a 6-MV linear accelerator. *Med Phys* 13:259, 1986.

51. Rao PS, Pillac K, Gregg EC: Effects of shadow trays on surface dose and build-up for megavoltage radiation. *Am J Roentgenol* 117:168, 1973.

52. Tannous NBJ, Gagnon WF, Almond PR: Buildup region and skin dose measurements for the Therac 6 linear accelerator for radiation therapy. *Med Phys* 8:378, 1981.

53. Velkley DE, Manson DJ, Purdy JA, Oliver GD: Build-up region of megavoltage photon radiation sources. *Med Phys* 2:14, 1975.

54. Doppke KP, Novack D, Wang CC: Physical considerations in the treatment of advanced carcinomas of the larynx and pyriform sinuses using 10 MV x-rays. *Int J Radiat Oncol Biol Phys* 6:1251, 1980.

55. Kubo H, Russel M, Wang CC: Use of 10 MV spoiled x-ray beam for the treatment of head and neck tumors. *Int J Radiat Oncol Biol Phys* 8:1795, 1982.

56. Lee PC, Thomason C, Glasgow GP: Characteristics of a spoiled 6-MV beam from a dual-energy linear accelerator. *Med Phys* 20:717, 1993.

57. Shiu AS, Tung SS, Nyerick CE, et al: Comprehensive analysis of electron beam central axis dose for a radiotherapy linear accelerator. *Med Phys* 21:559, 1994.

58. Sharma SC, Derbel FC, Khan RM: Tissue-equivalence of bolus materials for electron beam. *Radiology* 146:854, 1983.

59. Carleson-Bentel G: A rapid method to determine the maximum dose from parallel opposed fields. *Int J Radiat Oncol Biol Phys* 2:367, 1977.

60. Bentel GC: Collimator and treatment couch design in radiation therapy equipment. *Rad Ther J Rad Oncol Sci* 1:250, 1992.

61. Humm JL: Collision avoidance in computer optimized treatment planning. *Med Phys* 21:1053, 1994.

62. Leavitt DD, Martin M, Moeller JH, Lee WL: Dynamic wedge field technique through computer-controlled collimator motion and dose delivery. *Med Phys* 17:87, 1990.

63. Larsen RD, Svensson GK, Bjärngard BE: The use of wedge filters to improve dose distribution with the partial rotation. *Radiology* 117:441, 1975.

64. ICRU: *Prescribing, Recording, and Reporting Photon Beam Therapy.* Washington, DC: International Commission on Radiation Units and Measurements, 1993.

65. Brahme A, Chavaudra J, McCullough E, et al: Accuracy requirements and quality assurance of external beam therapy with photons and electrons. *Acta Oncol Stockholm* (suppl 1, special issue), 1988.

66. Mijnheer BJ, Batterman JJ, Wambersie A: What degree of accuracy is required and can be achieved in photon and neutron therapy. *Radiother Oncol* 8:237, 1987.

67. Wittkämper FW, Mijnheer BJ, Van Kleffens HJ: Dose intercomparison at the radiotherapy centers in The Netherlands: 1. Photon beams under reference conditions and for prostatic cancer treatment. *Radiother Oncol* 9:30, 1987.

68. Sherouse GW: A mathematical basis for selection of wedge angle and orientation. *Med Phys* 20:1211, 1993.

69. Sherouse GW: A simple method for achieving uniform dose from arbitrary arrangement of possibly noncoplanar fixed fields. (Abstract.) *Int J Rad Onc Biol Phys* 30(suppl 1):241, 1994.

70. Agarwal SK, Marks RD, Constable WC: Adjacent field separation for homogeneous dosage at a given depth for the 8 MV (Mevatron 8) linear accelerator. *Am J Roentgenol* 114:623, 1972.

71. Armstrong DI, Tait J: The matching of adjacent fields in radiotherapy. *Radiology* 108:419, 1973.

72. Bentel GC, Halperin EC: High dose areas are unintentionally created as a result of gap shifts when the prescribed doses in the two adjacent areas are different. *Med Dosim* 15:179, 1990.

73. Bianciardi L, Breschi R, Chiaradia P, et al: Field separation in radiation therapy with opposing fields. *Radiology* 122:493, 1977.

74. Bukovitz AG, Deutsch M, Slayton R: Orthogonal fields: Variations in dose vs. gap size for treatment of the central nervous system. *Radiology* 126:795, 1978.

75. Chiang TC, Culbert H, Wyman B, et al: The half field technique of radiation therapy for the cancers of head and neck. *Int J Radiat Oncol Biol Phys* 5:1899, 1979.

76. Faw FL, Glenn DW: Further investigations of physical aspects of multiple field radiation therapy. *Am J Roentgenol* 108:184, 1970.

77. Fraass BA, Tepper JE, Glatstein E, van de Geijn J: Clinical use of a match-line wedge for adjacent megavoltage radiation field matching. *Int J Radiat Oncol Biol Phys* 9:209, 1983.

78. Garavaglia G: Field separation of adjoining therapy fields. *Med Phys* 8:882, 1981.

79. Gillin MT, Kline RW: Field separation between lateral and anterior fields on a 6 MV linear accelerator. *Int J Radiat Oncol Biol Phys* 6:233, 1980.

80. Glenn DW, Faw FL, Kagan RA, Johnson RE: Field separation in multiple portal radiation therapy. *Am J Roentgenol* 102:199, 1968.

81. Griffin TW, Schumacher D, Berry HC: A technique for cranial-spinal irradiation. *Br J Radiol* 49:887, 1976.

82. Hale J, Davis LW, Block P: Portal separation for pairs of parallel opposed portals at 2 MV and 6 MV. *Am J Roentgenol* 114:172, 1972.

83. Hopfan S, Reid A, Simpson L, Ager P: Clinical complications arising from overlapping of adjacent radiation fields —Physical and technical considerations. *Int J Radiat Oncol Biol Phys* 2:801, 1977.

84. Holupka EJ, Humm JL, Tarbell NJ, Svensson GK: Effect of set-up error on the dose across the junction of matching cranial-spinal fields in the treatment of medulloblastoma. *Int J Radiat Oncol Biol Phys* 27:345, 1993.

85. Jani SK, Pennington EC, Wacha JE, Hussey DH: Megavoltage radiation field matching on uneven surface. *Int J Radiat Oncol Biol Phys* 15:1247, 1988.

86. Johnson PM, Kepka AG: A double-junction technique for total central nervous system irradiation with a 4-MV accelerator. *Radiology* 145:467, 1982.

87. Keys R, Grigsby PW: Gapping fields on sloping surfaces. *Int J Radiat Oncol Biol Phys* 18:1183, 1990.

88. Kosnik LT, Mantel J, Sheer AC: Large-field telecobalt therapy with a moving table: Physical considerations. *Radiology* 104:653, 1972.

89. Kurup RG, Glasgow GP, Leybovich LB: Design of electron beam wedges for increasing the penumbra of abutting fields. *Phys Med Biol* 38:667, 1993.

90. Lance JS, Morgan JE: Dose distribution between adjoining therapy fields. *Radiology* 79:24, 1962.

91. Lutz WR, Larsen RD: Technique to match mantle and para-aortic fields. *Int J Radiat Oncol Biol Phys* 9:1753, 1983.

92. Starchman DE, Loeffler RK, Sommer RD: Achievement of uniform dose without overlap in multi-port treatment fields, including interport shaped blocks. *Radiology* 108:695, 1973.

93. Van Dyk J, Jenkin RDT, Leung PMK, Cunningham JR: Medulloblastoma: Treatment technique and radiation dosimetry. *Int J Radiat Oncol Biol Phys* 2:993, 1977.

94. Werner BL, Khan FM, Sharma SC, et al: Border separa-

tion for adjacent orthogonal fields. *Med Dosim* 16:79, 1991.

95. Williamson TJ: A technique for matching orthogonal megavoltage fields. *Int J Radiat Oncol Biol Phys* 5:111, 1979.

96. Hale C, Schlienger M, Constans JP, et al: Results of radiation treatment of medulloblastoma in adults. *Int J Radiat Oncol Biol Phys* 11:2051, 1985.

97. Datta R, Mira JG, Pomeroy TC, Datta S: Dosimetry study of split beam technique using megavoltage beams and its clinical implications—I. *Int J Radiat Oncol Biol Phys* 5:565, 1979.

98. Gillin MT, Kline RW, Kun LE: Cranial dose distribution. *Int J Radiat Oncol Biol Phys* 5:1903, 1979.

99. Werner BL, Khan FM, Sharma SC, et al: A method for calculating field border separation when treating with adjacent orthogonal fields (abstr). *Annual Meeting of the American Society of Therapeutic Radiologists,* Dallas, 1980.

100. Chu FCH: Electron beam therapy of breast cancer, in Chu FCH, Laughlin JS (eds): *Proceedings of the Symposium on Electron Beam Therapy.* New York: Memorial Sloan-Kettering Cancer Center, 1981.

CHAPTER

7

The Treatment Preparation Process—I: Target Localization, Treatment Uncertainties, and Patient Immobilization

Although the term *treatment planning* properly refers to all aspects of planning of the patient's course of therapy (surgery, chemotherapy, radiation therapy, and so on), in radiation therapy it is usually associated with the tasks of determining the volume to be treated, the dose to give and the fractionation schema, deciding what field arrangement to use, designing beam modifying devices, and producing an appropriate isodose distribution.

Following the decision to utilize radiation therapy

in the management of the patient's disease, a technically very complex set of procedures must be carried out with utmost precision and usually within a short period of time. It is the period of time during which the team of physicians, physicists, dosimetrists, and technologists share in the preparations of the treatment. Figure 7.1 shows a typical flowchart for the process of radiation therapy, with emphasis on the treatment preparations. In some situations, not all procedures are needed; in others, the order may be

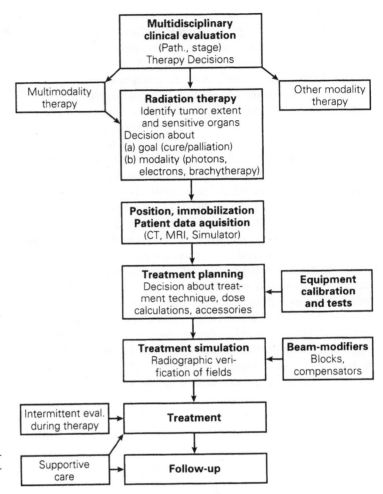

Figure 7.1   Flowchart for the processes in radiation therapy, emphasizing the treatment planning process.

changed. The physician—based on information gained through inspection, palpation, and various imaging studies—determines the target volume. With the assistance of other staff, the treatment approach is decided. This includes, for example, decisions about patient positioning and immobilization, beam energy, beam orientations, and the use of beam-modifying devices that may be required. In many radiation therapy departments, standard procedures are in place for preparation and administration of radiation therapy for patients with commonly seen diseases. Examples of these include uncomplicated cases of gynecologic tumors, breast cancer, prostate cancer, head and neck malignancies, and some

tumors of the central nervous system. In less routine situations, however, the preparations require intense planning and the collaboration of many staff members. Before embarking on a description of the procedures involved in the treatment preparation, it is appropriate to present some background of the issues at hand.

TARGET LOCALIZATION AND TREATMENT SIMULATION

Many of the technical difficulties encountered in radiation therapy are related to determination of the relative positions of the target and certain radiosensitive anatomic organs to the external surface of the patient. Many diagnostic imaging studies help to define the target volume and positions of internal organs. In radiation therapy, however, it is necessary to know these positions in relation to recognizable external marks. Traditionally, radiation oncologists have been limited to the use of a simulation unit (Chap. 2) capable of producing radiographs of diagnostic imaging quality and using contrast media to demonstrate the positions of relevant internal organs otherwise not visualized. More recently, however, the use of computed tomography (CT) and magnetic resonance imaging (MRI) in radiation therapy localization procedures has improved the accuracy of target localization and made the procedure easier. The ability to determine target volumes better has led to other very important considerations. For example, smaller volumes of normal tissue may be irradiated because the margins around the target can be made tighter. Consequently, the patient's position must be reproduced with greater accuracy in the daily setup to reduce the risk of missing the target. Finally, because there is less room for variation in the patients'

positioning, the use of beam-alignment laser systems and immobilization devices has become a very important element in radiation therapy.

NOMENCLATURE

The many terms used in radiation therapy must be clearly understood by everyone caring for the patient. The term *tumor volume* is sometimes confused with *target volume*. The two are different, and a misinterpretation can lead to serious errors in treatment choice. The International Commission on Radiation Units and Measurements (ICRU) has recommended definitions of these and other important concepts in radiation therapy.[1] The term *gross tumor volume* (GTV) is the gross palpable or visible/demonstrable extent and location of malignant growth. The GTV usually correspond to those parts of a tumor where the tumor cell density is greatest. This may consist of primary tumor, metastatic lymphadenopathy, or other metastasis. The extent of the GTV can be determined through clinical examination and various imaging studies. If the gross tumor has been removed, no GTV can be defined. The *clinical target*

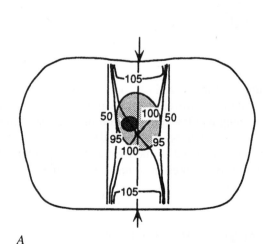

A

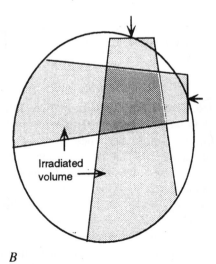

B

Figure 7.2 *A*. The gross tumor volume (■) is always smaller than the planning target volume (▣). The treated volume is the volume of normal tissues receiving essentially the same dose or more than the prescribed dose (95 percent). *B*. The irradiated volume is the volume of tissues that receives a significant dose relative to the tissue tolerance—for example, in the exit region of two nonopposed beams.

volume (CTV) is a tissue volume that contains a de-monstrable GTV and/or subclinical microscopic ma-lignant disease that must be eliminated. This volume thus has to be treated adequately in order to achieve the aim of therapy.[1] The *planning target volume* (PTV) contains the tissues that are to be irradiated to a specified dose according to a specified time-dose pattern.[1] This volume consists of the tumor and adja-cent tissues where tumor is presumed to be present, and, in some instances, also the regional lymph nodes (Fig. 7.2A). In some instances the tumor may have been removed but radiation treatments are needed to eradicate microscopic disease that may be present in the tumor bed. Thorough knowledge of the behavior and the pattern of spread of different tumors is needed in order to determine the PTV. Because the PTV includes the GTV in addition to other tissues, the PTV is always larger than the GTV.

The *treated volume* is the volume enclosed by an isodose surface, selected and specified by the radia-tion oncologist as being appropriate to achieve the purpose of the treatment (i.e., tumor eradication or palliation).[1] Because of limitations in treatment de-livery, it is often impossible to design a treatment plan that limits the prescribed dose to the PTV only. Unintentionally, some tissues near the target are also irradiated to the same dose as the target. The treated volume is therefore always larger than the PTV and has a simpler shape. For example, in the treatment of the pelvis or chest wall through opposed fields, a large volume of normal tissue is incidentally irra-diated to the same dose as the target volume (Fig. 7.2A).

The *irradiated volume* is the volume of tissue that receives a dose considered significant in relation to tissue tolerance.[1] This dose level can be expressed as a percentage of the prescribed target dose. For ex-ample, when two nonopposed fields are used in a treatment plan, the tissues beyond the target where the beam exits can receive a significant dose (Fig. 7.2B). The tissue that is irradiated in the penumbra region also receives a significant dose.

BEAM GEOMETRY

Treatment Fields.   Before discussing localiza-tion procedures and treatment simulation, it is im-portant to understand the geometry particular to ra-diation therapy. The size of the radiation field is defined by two pairs of secondary collimator jaws. The field can be square if both sets of jaws are opened the same distance or rectangular if one set is opened more than the other. The central axis (CA) of the radiation field is, under these conditions, at the geometric center of the field, as the name implies (Fig. 7.3A and B). In more modern machines, one or all four secondary collimator jaws can be moved in-dependently. If one jaw is moved more than the op-posite jaw, the CA of the beam is not at the geometric center of the field (Fig. 7.3C). In modern radiation therapy, most treatment fields are irregular in shape and are often defined by custom-made blocks with beveled inner walls that correspond to the diverging

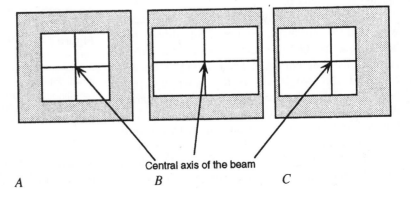

Figure 7.3   The central axis is in the center of a beam defined by fixed leaves that only move in pairs, forming a square *(A)* or a rectangular field *(B)*. In machines where the leaves of the collimator move independently, the central axis may not be in the geometric center of the field *(C)*.

Central axis of the beam

A   B   C beam. In such fields, the CA of the beam can be anywhere in the treated field and can even be outside the actually irradiated area. It is important to consider this situation in prescribing and calculating the dose. Dose prescriptions usually refer to the dose on the CA of the beam; however, when the CA is outside the radiation field or near the edge, the dose prescription should be made at a more relevant point inside the field. This matter is also discussed in Chap. 6.

The field size (FS) is usually defined at the rotational axis of the machine, usually 100 cm in linear accelerators. The maximum FS at this distance is often 40 × 40 cm, but in some machines the circular radiation field, defined by the primary collimator, is only slightly more than 40 cm in diameter. Therefore, the corners of the projected square field are outside the radiation beam (Fig. 7.4A and B).[2]

Beam Divergence. As the radiation beam exits from the head of the machine, it is spreading or diverging in a predictable pattern. Figure 7.5A illustrates that the angle of the divergence is more acute farther from the CA while the beam CA is pointing straight down, indicating no divergence. The following equation gives the angle of the divergence:

$$\text{Tan } \theta = \frac{\text{half-field length}}{\text{distance}} \qquad (7.1)$$

Figure 7.5B also shows that the divergence occurs in all directions away from the beam CA. It becomes very important to understanding the beam divergence when one is trying to match adjacent fields, as discussed in Chap. 6.

The angle of beam divergence is also more acute with shorter distances. Figure 7.6A shows two beams, one at 100-cm source-axis distance (SAD) and another at 80 cm SAD. The field size at the isocenter of the two beams is the same; however, beyond the isocenter, the 80-cm SAD beam is larger than the 100-cm beam due to the divergence. Caution should be used in the event that the treatment is simulated at one distance and treated at another. Figure 7.6B shows that the target is inside field b (shorter source-surface distance, or SSD); however,

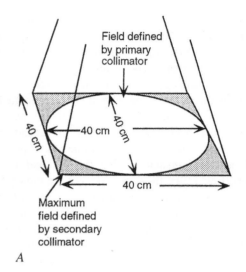

A

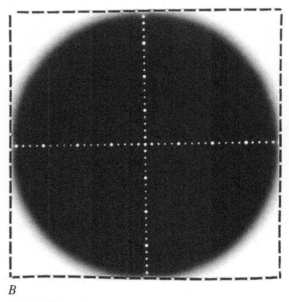

B

Figure 7.4   *A.* When the collimator is opened to the maximum field size, the radiation beam is often circular because it is now defined by the primary circular collimator.   *B.* A radiograph exposed with maximum collimator opening (40 × 40 cm field) showing no radiation dose in the corners. This problem can become severe when large fields are treated.

in beam a (longer SSD), the target is partially outside the radiation beam. The field size on the surface is the same in the two beams.

Figure 7.5 *A.* As the radiation beam exits from the collimator, it is diverging in a predictable pattern. The angle depends on the distance from the target (origin) and the distance from the central axis.   *B.* Often in radiation therapy, the beam is thought of as if it diverged only in the planes along and across the field, but it is really diverging in all directions.

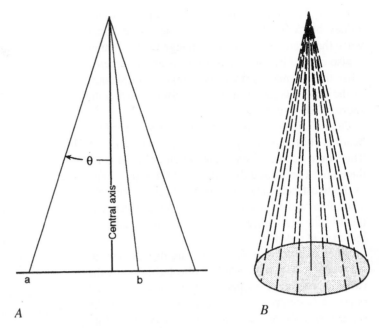

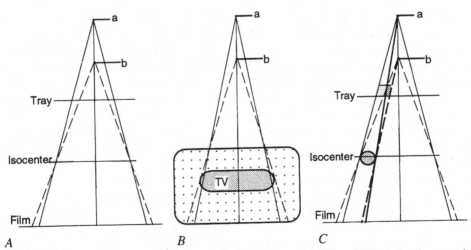

Figure 7.6 *A.* When the same field size is set at the isocenter using 100-cm SAD (a), the divergence is different from setting 80-cm SAD (b).   *B.* The beam spreads more beyond the isocenter when the SAD is shorter; therefore, a target that was simulated using 80-cm SAD may be missed if it is treated at 100-cm SSD.   *C.* When the SSD is changed, a block positioned on a tray in the beam to shield an organ inside the patient must be shifted and the size changed.

Figure 7.6*C* shows how the size and position of a kidney block must be changed at the tray distance when the treatment distance is changed. This change is also caused by the difference in beam divergence when the treatment distance is changed. The shadow of the kidney is larger at the film distance when the shorter SSD is used.

Figure 7.7 shows that when the central axis of the beam is shifted, the target may be partially missed. This could occur, for example, when the field is reduced for a boost and the CA is shifted to the center of the boost field. The treatment field is entering the same area on the surface, but, due to the difference in the way the beam edges diverge, the same area is not included at a depth.

When parallel opposed fields* are used, beam divergence becomes further complicated because the two beams diverge in opposite directions. In parallel opposed isocentric fields, the two beams treat the same area only at the depth of the isocenter (Fig. 7.8). Therefore, a posterior port film cannot be compared with an anterior simulation film unless anatomic structures at the depth of the isocenter are used for comparison. Figure 7.8 demonstrates that the length of the spine included in the anterior field is longer than that in the posterior field. This is because the spine lies farther posterior than the isocenter. In the chest, the carina, which usually lies at the middepth in the chest, is a reliable reference structure when comparing anterior and posterior radiographs. It would be impossible to make both the anterior and posterior field margins transect the spinal cord at an interspace between two vertebral bodies without making the two fields of different lengths. That would, of course, make subsequent field matching more complicated.

Another area where caution should be used is in treating narrow strips of tissue away from the CA—for example, in treating the paraaortic lymph nodes and the spleen (Fig. 7.9). When the two parallel opposed fields are shaped as in Fig. 7.9, only a small diamond-shaped volume at middepth is included in both fields, as shown on the axial contour caudad of

---

* Parallel opposed fields are fields identical in size and shape and with central axes separated by 180°.

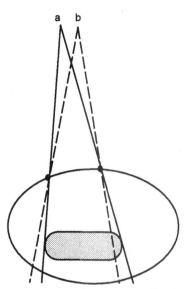

Figure 7.7 When the location of the central axis is shifted—for example, to deliver a boost—the target can be missed.

the beam central axis. The posteriorly located spleen can be missed in the posterior field.

A similar situation can occur in a lung field that includes the supraclavicular lymph nodes (Fig. 7.10). The anteriorly located supraclavicular lymph nodes may be missed by the posterior field. Another example of this problem occurs when a brain field shaped as in Fig. 7.11 is treated. The blocks, added to shield the pituitary gland and the optic chiasm, could as well have been enlarged to also shield the narrow strip of tissue now being irradiated caudally. Due to the divergence, only a small diamond-shaped volume of tissue in the midbrain is being irradiated by both fields. Figure 7.12 demonstrates a similar situation in the pelvis, where a boost field is treated without shifting the isocenter.

Magnification Devices. As we have seen in the previous sections, the radiation beam "spreads" or diverges in all directions and becomes larger as the distance increases. This divergence is directly proportional to the distance and is therefore predictable. Since, in many procedures, a radiograph—which represents an enlarged image of the patient—is used to determine various dimensions of the patient, it is

Figure 7.8   *A.* The fields include only the same tissues at the depth of the isocenter or where the field sizes are identical. When the isocenter is at middepth in the patient, the length of spinal cord included within the two fields is different because the spinal cord is located farther posterior than the isocenter, where the fields are identical.   *B.* When two pairs of opposed fields are adjacent, the beam edge A and B₁ follows the same divergence (line A and line B₁ should demarcate the same anatomical reference, since A includes what B₁ excludes); therefore, tissues inside beam 1 is outside beam 4. Likewise, tissue inside beam 3 is outside beam 2.   *C.* Parallel opposed beams always diverge in opposite directions.

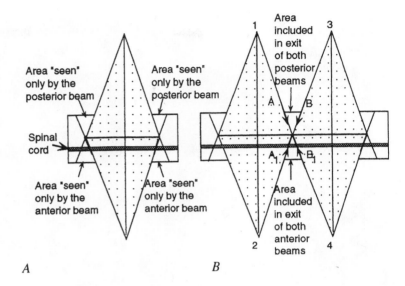

necessary to know just how much the radiographic image is enlarged. For this purpose, the magnification factor for each radiograph must be found. In this section, we discuss the virtues of various devices placed in the beam and used to determine the magnification factor.

Radiation therapy simulators usually display the field size via thin radiopaque wires, which can be moved in pairs much like the secondary collimator jaws of the treatment machines. A cross hair, or in some machines a small circle, indicates the CA of the beam, and some simulators also display a scale in the beam (Fig. 7.13). This scale, projected as a large crosshair in the center of the field, indicates each centimeter along and across the field. The distance between each centimeter mark is 1 cm at the isocenter; as the distance increases, the marks are projected farther apart. Thus this scale is an excellent magnification device. Such scale helps to quickly reduce any measurements made on the radiograph to real size in the patient. For example, in transferring anatomic information from the radiograph to a cross-section contour of the patient, one can quickly determine the distance from the CA to any relevant anatomic landmark and then indicate this distance on the contour. Such a magnification device is safe and reliable; however, in many instances this feature may

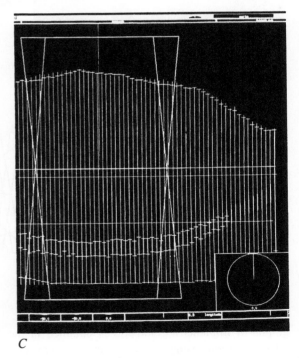

C

be absent, and other magnification devices are needed.

Sometimes radiographs are obtained without the benefit of a treatment simulator or with a simulator that does not have the features just described. Radio-

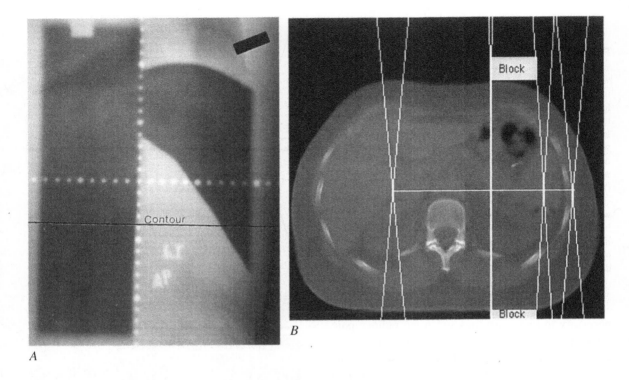

A

B

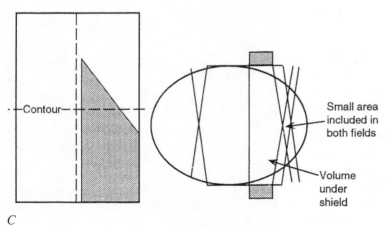

C

Figure 7.9 When a narrow strip of tissue located at some distance from the central axis *(A)* is treated using parallel opposed fields, only a very small volume of tissue is included within both fields *(B)*. This is demonstrated in a typical paraaortic and spleen fields *(C)*. The spleen, located posterior of the isocenter, could be missed in the posterior field. The dose within this narrow strip of tissue consists mostly of penumbra.

graphs of implants are sometimes obtained in the operating room using a diagnostic-type x-ray machine and the target-to-film distance (TFD) may not be known. In these situations, some type of magnification device placed in the path of the beam is necessary in order to determine needed dimensions in the patient. As discussed above, both the size and the position of such devices in the beam are very important. It is also important that the device be chosen so that its dimensions measured on the radiograph are correct. For example, use of the long dimension of a Fletcher-Suit ovoid to determine the magnification factor on a radiograph may result in an error, as shown in Fig. 7.14A. A magnification device placed

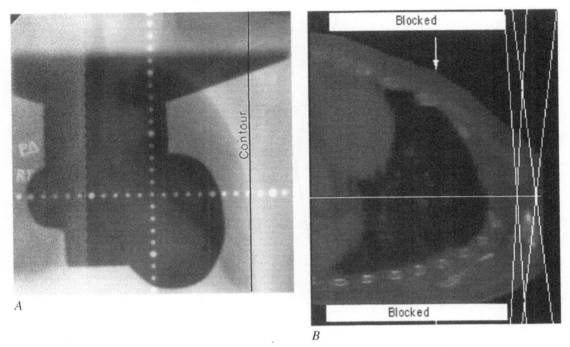

Figure 7.10   When the supraclavicular lymph nodes are treated in a lung field, they may be missed in a parallel opposed posterior field *(A)*. The posterior field exits cephalad of the anterior and a very small area, consisting mostly of penumbra, is included in both fields *(B)*.

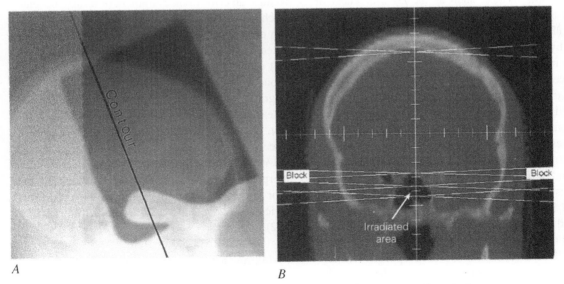

Figure 7.11   *A* and *B*. Efforts to block the optic chiasm in a brain field result in a very small area in the center being included within the geometric margins of the two opposing fields.

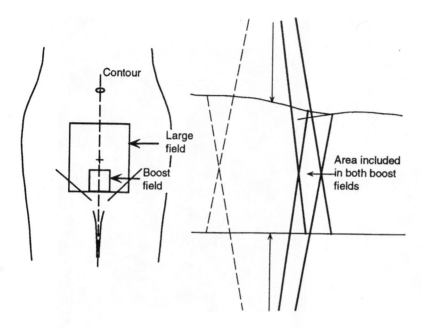

Figure 7.12 When large parallel opposed pelvic fields are reduced for a boost without shifting the isocenter, the opposing fields diverge in opposite directions.

on the patient's anterior surface when radiographs of a tandem and ovoid are obtained (Chap. 16), will be enlarged more than the tandem and ovoid, which usually are close to the midplane of the patient. A ruler with radiopaque centimeter marks placed on a sloping skin surface, such as the anterior chest or pelvic area, will appear foreshortened on a radiograph (Fig. 7.14*B*). If the slope is severe, 1 cm indicated by the marks could even appear smaller than 1 cm on the radiograph.

Since it is always the outermost dimensions of an object that will determine the size on the radiograph, a round object is most accurate and the precise orientation is then irrelevant (Fig. 7.14*C*). There is, however, a problem with a round object, because as the beam passes through a diminishing thickness of attenuating material in the periphery, the precise margins may not be appreciated on the radiograph (Fig. 7.15). The transverse diameter of an ovoid can be used as a magnification device as long as its outermost dimensions can be clearly seen on the radiograph. Two metal markers placed opposite one another near the surface of a vaginal cylinder cannot be used as a magnification gauge because the way they

are projected on the radiograph depends on how the cylinder is positioned with respect to the beam. In the most extreme case, the two markers could be superimposed (Fig. 7.16).

The size of a magnification device is important, because an error in measurement of its size becomes much more critical when the device is small. A 1-mm error in measuring a magnification device projected as 20 mm on a radiograph represents a 5 percent error (21/20 = 1.05). As a result of using this erroneous magnification factor in interpreting a radiograph, the error in the width of the bony pelvis, for example, could be almost 1 cm, which is significant. A 1-mm error made in measuring a larger magnification device results in a smaller percent error and would therefore represent a smaller error when interpreting the radiograph. For example, a 1-mm error in the measurement of a 50-mm magnification device results in only a 2 percent error (51/50 = 1.02).

Magnification Factors. An understanding of the phenomenon of magnification is crucial to practically all technical aspects of radiation therapy. The

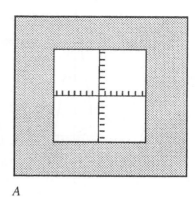

Figure 7.13   *A.* A crosshair or a circle, inserted in the path of the beam, indicates the central axis of the beam. Some crosshairs have a centimeter scale that can be used as a magnification gauge when measurements are taken on the radiograph. In these radiographs (*B* and *C*), a vaginal cylinder with centimeter markers is also used.

A

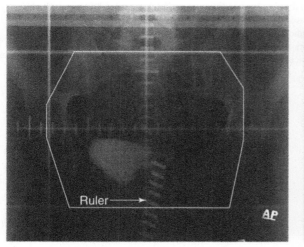

B

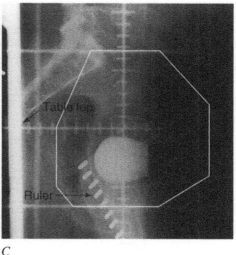

C

radiation field spreads and becomes larger, or magnified, with increased distance from the source or target.* The divergence, or spread of the beam, is directly proportional to the distance from the target. A field that is 5 cm at an 80-cm distance will have spread to 10 cm at a 160-cm distance (i.e., the field

---

* The origin of the radiation is often referred to as the *source or target.* Source is often thought of as a cobalt-60 source and target as the target in a linear accelerator which, when bombarded by electrons, produces photons. In this text, the words are used interchangeably. However, this target should not be confused with the target at which the radiation beam is aimed.

size is doubled when the distance doubles). Since the beam is diverging in a predictable pattern, it is possible to calculate the field size or the size of a marker at any point along the path of the beam as long as some dimension is known at a given distance in the beam.

The field size and distance affect the dose that is delivered. It also affects how devices inserted in the beam are imaged, and it affect the appearance of the patient on a radiograph. The size and shape of beam-defining blocks, for example, depend on the distance along the beam at which they are inserted and also at what distance the patient is positioned. Beam-defin-

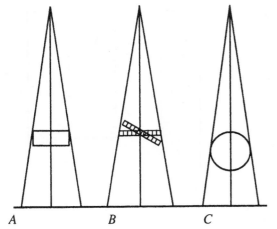

Figure 7.14 *A.* A rectangular object may appear larger on the radiograph because it is the part of the device that is closest to the target to be shadowed on the film. *B.* A centimeter ruler placed at an angle in the beam will appear foreshortened on the radiograph, as was also seen with the vaginal cylinder, which appears at an angle in the radiograph in Fig. 7.13. *C.* Magnification devices should ideally be circular, with known dimensions.

ing blocks are always placed in the beam at a distance that is shorter than the distance to the patient: therefore, the field size at this distance is always smaller than that on the patient. Radiographs always represent an enlarged image of the patient, because the film captures the image as the beam exits the patient. The degree to which something is enlarged or decreased in size depend on where in the path of the beam it is positioned.

The most frequently required calculation is that of reducing or magnifying dimensions on a radiograph to the actual dimension in the patient. When the source-to-film distance (SFD) or target-to-film distance (TFD) is known, it is straightforward to find the actual size of anything at a given distance in the beam. For example, when the TFD is 140 cm and the SAD is 100 cm, the magnification factor is 140/100 or 1.4 on the film. That is, anything at a distance of 100 cm in the beam is enlarged by a factor of 1.4 on the radiograph. Anything at a distance of 90 cm in

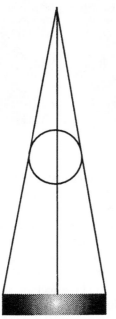

Figure 7.15 The precise margins of a coin or other circular object may not be appreciated on a radiograph due to the diminishing thickness of attenuating material in the periphery.

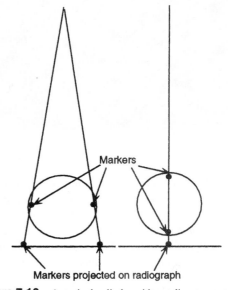

Figure 7.16 A vaginal cylinder with a radiopaque marker in the periphery can be used as a magnification device only if it happens to be turned so that the two markers are maximally separated with respect to the beam. Depending on how the cylinder is turned, the two markers could be superimposed. This is, therefore, an unreliable magnification device.

the beam is enlarged by 140/90 or 1.55; at 110 cm in the beam the magnification factor is 140/110 or 1.27.

Sometimes the TFD of a port film is unknown, but if the field size is known at a known distance, the TFD can be found by a simple calculation. For example, the field size is 15 × 15 cm at 80-cm SAD and measures 20 × 20 cm on the port film. The TFD is found as follows:

$$\text{TFD} = \frac{\text{SAD} \times \text{FS}_{\text{TFD}}}{\text{FS}_{\text{SAD}}} \qquad (7.2)$$

or

$$\frac{80 \text{ cm} \times 20 \text{ cm}}{15 \text{ cm}} = 106.5 \text{ cm TFD}$$

The treatment field in Fig. 7.17, which appears to be 17 × 17 cm on the radiograph at 130 cm TFD, is smaller at the SAD (100 cm). The following equation must be solved to find the field size (FS) at 100 cm:

$$\text{FS}_{100} = \frac{\text{SAD} \times \text{FS}_{130}}{\text{TFD}} \qquad (7.3)$$

or

$$\frac{100 \times 17 \text{ cm}}{130} = 13 \text{ cm}$$

In other situations it may be necessary to calculate, from known dimensions on the patient, where to place a block or a compensator on a tray that is closer to the radiation source. For example, in Fig. 7.17, the SAD is 100 cm at the midplane of the patient and the target-to-tray distance (TTD) where beam-defining blocks are placed is 65 cm. To find the size of a treatment field at 65 cm that will project a 20 × 20 cm field at 100 cm, the following calculation is required:

$$\text{FS}_{65} = \frac{\text{FS}_{100} \times \text{TTD}}{\text{SAD}} \qquad (7.4)$$

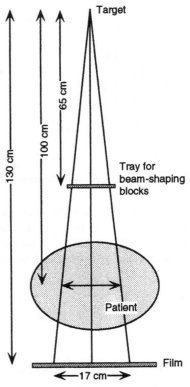

Figure 7.17 Geometric arrangement of the patient, film, and tray.

or

$$\frac{20 \text{ cm} \times 65}{100} = 13 \text{ cm}$$

In Fig. 7.18A, a contrast-filled lymph node (a) appears on the simulation film (125-cm TFD) at 7 cm from the central axis of the beam (b). The lymph node is at the midplane of the patient, which is at 100-cm SAD in the beam. To find the distance from the CA of the beam to the lymph node at 100-cm SAD the following calculation is required:

$$\frac{100 \times 7 \text{ cm}}{125} = 5.6 \text{ cm}$$

In Fig. 7.18B, a marker has been placed on an

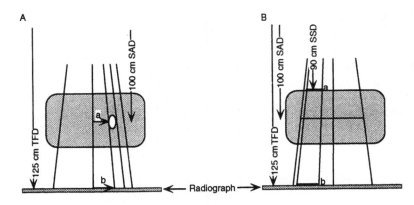

Figure 7.18 To reduce dimensions from a radiograph to real size in the patient, knowledge of the geometry of the setup is necessary.

incision (a) on the patient's skin surface (90-cm SSD). This marker is 5 cm long on a simulation film (b), which is at 125-cm TFD. To find the actual length at 90 cm, the following calculation is required:

$$\frac{90 \times 5 \text{ cm}}{125} = 3.6 \text{ cm}$$

COORDINATE SYSTEM AND PLANES

Localization of the target volume and adjacent normal organs in preparation for radiation therapy requires a thorough knowledge of the geometric relationship between the patient and the therapy machine. An understanding of how the spatial coordinate system is applied in the patient is also necessary. The goal of localization procedures is to identify the precise position of relevant internal structures with respect to external landmarks. Prior to any treatments, one must be certain that the treatment fields, as marked on the patient's skin or on an immobilization device, truly include only the intended volume.

The geometric relationship between the patient and the radiation beam is best described using a coordinate system that can be applied in three dimensions. This system allows one to describe the location of any point with respect to a known point (the origin). It also requires a description of the motions of the machine and the orientations of three planes in the patient. Figure 7.19 demonstrates the three planes

in the patient: sagittal, coronal, and transverse or axial, as well as the x-, y-, and z-axes. The orientation of these axes with respect to the patient is optional but must be consistent so that no confusion will occur (i.e., the convention used during the localization procedure, treatment planning, and treat

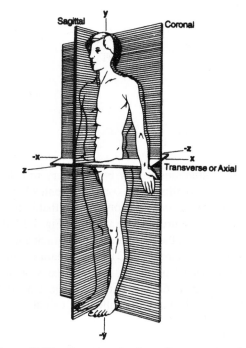

Figure 7.19 The conventional coordinate system and planes with respect to the patient.

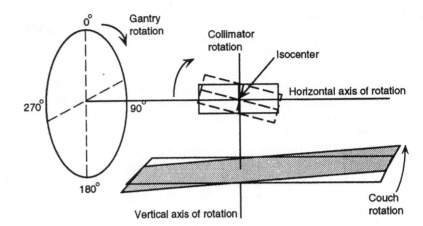

Figure 7.20 Motions of the gantry, couch, and collimator in a typical treatment machine.

ment setup must be the same). It is also highly recommended that the convention within one department be consistent. The location of a point with respect to the origin is described by the distance measured along each axis and also by indicating on which side of the axis the point is located. The latter is indicated by a positive or negative sign in front of the measured distance. Throughout this text, the following convention is used. The x-axis represents the patient's right-to-left direction, with a negative number indicating a location to the left of the origin when facing the patient (the patient's right). The y-axis represents the cephalad-to-caudal direction, with a negative number being caudal to the origin. The z-axis represents the anterior-to-posterior direction, with a negative number indicating a position posterior to the origin. The origin is usually chosen to represent the isocenter but can be any known point that can easily be identified.

The moving parts of the treatment machine are the gantry, collimator, and couch (Fig. 7.20). The gantry rotates around a horizontal axis that is parallel to the normal treatment couch position, usually 0°. The angles are expressed from 0 to 360° in the clockwise direction, with the 0° position being when the beam is vertical and pointing down toward the floor. The horizontal axis around which the gantry rotates also represents the y axis in the patient—an important point to remember when realigning the patient for

treatment. When the gantry is in the 0° position, the collimator and couch rotate around a vertical axis and the angles are expressed from 0 to 360° in the clockwise direction in the beam's eye view* (Fig. 7.21). The vertical axis of rotation also represents the z-axis in the patient. The intersection of the horizontal and vertical axes of rotation is referred to as the *isocenter*.

* International Electrotechnical Commission standards.

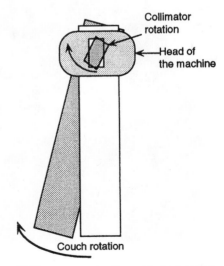

Figure 7.21   Couch and collimator angles in the "beam's-eye view."

LASER ALIGNMENT SYSTEMS

Repositioning of the patient with respect to the radiation beam, either from the simulation room to the treatment room or from day to day in the same treatment room, is very difficult without an alignment system.[3] Alignment systems, mounted so that lines representing the three planes described above intersect at the isocenter of a particular machine, are essential (Fig. 7.22). The projection of these lines is set so that they intersect at the isocenter, but they should also be set so that they are parallel with the sagittal, coronal, and axial planes. It is insufficient to align the patient with the isocenter only. To assure patient-repositioning with respect to the beam, the entire patient must be aligned correctly in the coordinate system described above. Figure 7.23 illustrates what can happen if the patient is misaligned with the sagittal axis by 10°, even when the alignment marks match correctly at the isocenter.

A small misalignment in the transverse plane can cause the beam, although set up to marks on the skin surface, to miss a deep-seated tumor in the pelvis (Fig. 7.24) or inadvertently include the spinal cord in the chest.

CONTOURS

The most common field arrangement in radiation therapy is parallel opposed fields, where the dose is

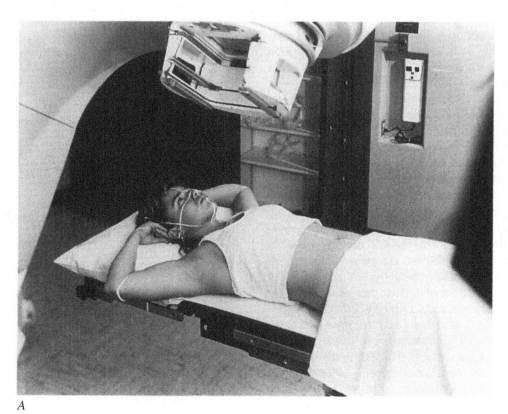

A

Figure 7.22   Laser alignment systems used to re-position the patient with the radiation beam. (Courtesy of Gammex RMI.)

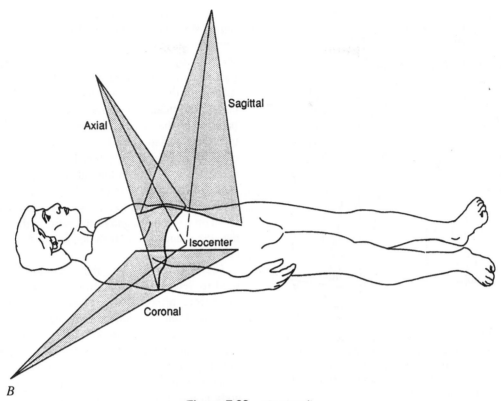

Sagittal

Axial

Isocenter

Coronal

B

Figure 7.22   *(Continued).*

prescribed at the middepth on the central axis. In these instances, it is sufficient to know the separation between the two entrance points. However, in situations where multiple fields are anticipated, a contour, or cross-section outline, of the patient's external surface is also necessary. A contour for treatment-planning purpose also calls for outlines of the planning target volume (PTV) and adjacent dose-limiting normal organs. Most frequently, a contour in the transverse, or axial, plane at the CA of the beam is obtained. In areas where the external surface is irregular, it may be necessary to obtain contours in multiple planes. Examples of such irregular surfaces are the head and neck area, breast, chest, pelvis of an obese patient, and an extremity, especially when long fields are treated. In many of these areas, a sagittal contour may also be helpful in developing a treatment plan.

PLASTER-OF-PARIS CONTOURS

There are many different ways of obtaining a true outline of the patient's external surface. Obviously, any contour must be taken with the patient in treatment position and with some reference marks that are traceable to the patient indicated on the contour. A strip of plaster of Paris—long enough to reach from the couch top on one side, over the patient, and down to the couch top on the opposite side—provides a fairly good representation of the patient's contour. If the patient's body rests on the couch, the posterior contour can be assumed to be horizontal. Extra-fast-setting 4-in-wide plaster-of-Paris strips can be used for plaster contours. The strips are folded lengthwise two times, making each strip four layers thick and 1 in wide. The strips are dipped in hot water and, after most of the water has been squeezed

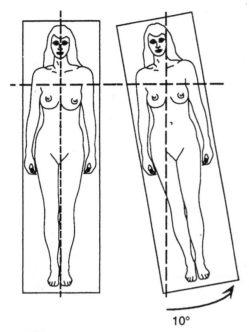

10°

Figure 7.23 It is insufficient to align the patient only at the isocenter. A small angle of the patient's position on the couch will have the same effect as a couch angle. In this situation, the extremes of a treatment field can be misaligned even when the isocenter is in the planned location.

out, placed along the transverse plane of the patient. If alignment lasers are available, the direction of the strip should follow the transverse laser lines. This type of plaster, when dipped in hot water, becomes hard within a couple of minutes.

It is necessary to make some marks on the patient's skin surface that are also marked on the contour. This is essential in order to transpose and mark the position of the planned treatment fields on the patient correctly. These marks must, of course, remain until the patient returns for the simulation procedure and treatment. If the contour is taken with the patient on the simulator couch and an isocentric technique is used, the alignment lasers at 0°, or vertical, and at 90° and 270°, or right and left, are marked on the contour and on the patient's skin surface for future reference. The intersection of these three lines represents the isocenter. These lines should be indicated on the contour and be traceable to the patient so that the planned treatment fields can be positioned correctly.

The distance scale on the simulator can also be used to determine the depth of the isocenter at the same three reference points and at the posterior or 180° position. By subtracting the SSD from the SAD, the depth from the skin surface to the isocenter is given for each location (Fig. 7.25A). In determining the posterior isocenter depth, the thickness of the couch top must be considered, and, if the patient's body is not resting directly on the couch, the additional space must be added to the SSD observed at the couch top. The areas where the patient's body is frequently not resting directly on the couch top is in the lumbar spine and the head and neck (Fig. 7.26). During the hardening of the plaster strip, the markings can be made and the SSDs obtained, as described above.

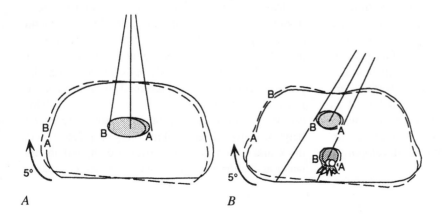

A *B*

Figure 7.24 A small rotation of the patient's body can cause the tumor to be moved out of the beam (*A*) or the spinal cord to be moved in (*B*).

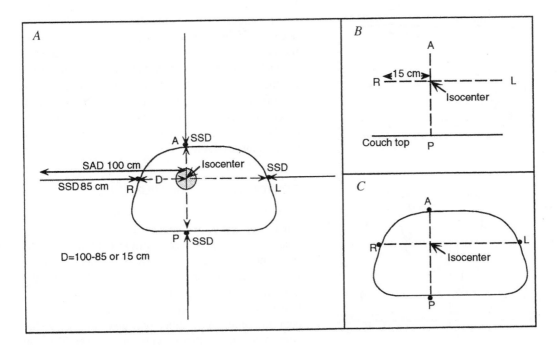

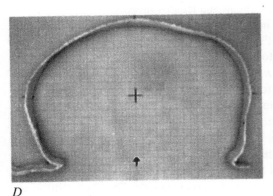

Figure 7.25 *A.* Subtracting the SSD from the SAD gives the depth of the isocenter at each location. *B.* The isocenter is marked on a piece of graph paper. The distance from this point to the skin surface is indicated at the four alignment-laser positions. *C.* The marks on the plaster contour, indicating the alignment lasers, are then aligned with the marks on the paper. *D.* The plaster contour is very carefully transferred to the paper, and it is the inside of the plaster that represents the patient's contour.

Before the plaster strip is removed from the patient, a point indicating the isocenter should be marked on the paper where the contour will be traced. Horizontal and vertical lines should be drawn through this point. Each reference point is marked on these lines in the appropriate direction (anterior, posterior, right, and left) and at the correct isocenter-surface distance as determined during the contouring procedure (Fig. 7.25B). The reference marks on the plaster strip are then aligned with the marks on the paper. The plaster strip may become slightly bent while it is transferred from the patient to the paper

where the contour is traced. Once the isocenter and the distances from the isocenter to the three laser reference points have been marked, the shape of the plaster strip can be restored by lining up the three marks on the contour with the three marks on the paper (Fig. 7.25C). In the contouring method just described, the inside of the plaster strip represents the patient's external contour—an important point to consider when the contour is traced on the paper (Fig. 7.25D).

In the situation where the patient's posterior surface does not rest on the couch surface, a posterior

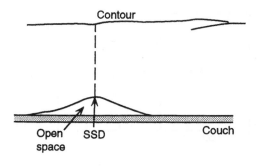

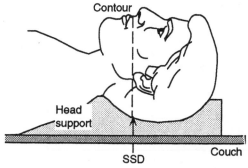

Figure 7.26   In some areas, the patient's body may not be resting on the couch—for example, in the cervical and lumbar spine.

contour may also have to be obtained with a separate plaster strip. In this case, it is necessary to pull the strip on each side until it follows the posterior skin surface. This strip must be sufficiently long that the two lateral laser alignment lines can be indicated. By superimposing the lateral laser marks on the anterior and posterior contours, the two contours can be correctly positioned with respect to one another.

Many patients are treated while positioned in a mold. It may then be difficult to contour the entire cross section of the patient. However, the portion of the patient's body that lies within the mold can be contoured by marking the transverse laser line on the mold on each side of the patient. With the patient removed, the mold is aligned with the alignment mark and the inside of the mold can be contoured. One must remember that the *outer* surface of the plaster strip now represent the patient's skin surface. Again, marks must be made on both the anterior and the posterior contour representing the same height above the couch top, so that the anterior and the pos-

terior contours can be connected correctly. It is often necessary, when contouring a patient, to also indicate the position of devices that potentially would be in the path of the beam or could prevent the head of the treatment machine from clearing as it is rotated from one orientation to another. Devices that may prevent a certain beam orientation from being used include head rests, immobilization devices, and metal bars in the treatment couch.

CONTOURING IN MULTIPLE LEVELS

As previously mentioned, there are some situations where one transverse contour is not sufficient. One example of areas where multiple contours may be necessary is in the breast. Here, it is often necessary to obtain a contour near the cephalad and caudal margins of the treatment fields in addition to a contour representing the central axis plane. These three contours should be outlined on a piece of paper in the correct position with respect to one another. This can be a difficult and tedious process.

The three plaster strips are placed around the patient's chest as previously described when taking one contour (Fig. 7.27). The three laser alignment lines are marked on all three plaster strips and the SSDs are found as described earlier, but now on all three contours. Because breast patients are usually treated with the arm on the uninvolved side down by the side, it can be difficult to contour and read the SSDs on this side. In that situation, it is often sufficient to read SSDs on the anterior surface and in the lateral position on the involved side. The plaster strips are placed over the involved side and as far to the opposite side as possible. The treatment couch must be moved, but only in and out from the gantry, until the central axis of the beam is at the particular plaster strip where the SSDs are determined.

The procedure for transferring the contours to a piece of paper is the same as previously described. A separate piece of paper should be used for each contour because it can be confusing to have all three contours on one paper (Fig. 7.27). It is a good practice to superimpose the origin or "isocenter" of all three contours and evaluate the relationship between the contours.

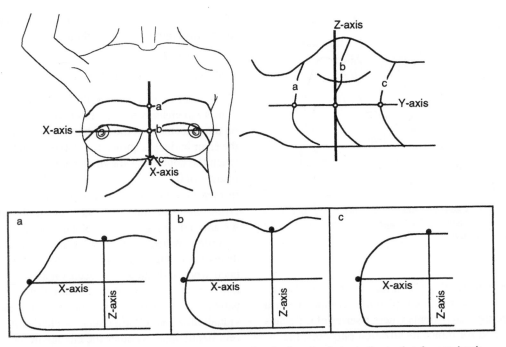

Figure 7.27   The procedure for contouring a patient in three levels is similar to that for one level; however, the three levels must be placed correctly with respect to one another in the coordinate system.

CONTOURS FROM COMPUTED TOMOGRAPHY

Computed tomography (CT) is rapidly becoming an essential tool in treatment planning. Many radiation therapy departments now have access to a CT scanner in the imaging department or have a dedicated unit of their own for data acquisition. Information with respect to the patient's anatomy provided by a CT scan includes an outline of the external contour and also very accurate information with respect to the position of internal anatomy. Computed tomography scans used for treatment planning are different from diagnostic images because they are obtained with the patient in treatment position on a flat-table insert on the CT table and with some external reference marks that are visible on the CT images.

If diagnostic CT images are used for outlining internal anatomy, caution should be used, because the patient's position may have been different and the shape of the couch top tends to change the relative positions of the internal organs. Furthermore, it is very difficult to determine precisely in the cephalad-caudad direction which CT image in fact represents the actual level of the contour. Diagnostic CT scans in the head and neck area are particularly unreliable because the head position during CT imaging is often different than during treatment and the plane of the CT image may therefore be quite different from that of the contour plane (Fig. 7.28).

Measurements on a small CT image can lead to a significant error in the scaling factor, as we saw earlier. The measurements (magnification factor) should instead be obtained from an enlarged image. The images can be enlarged to real size using a photographic enlarger. Caution must be used with such an enlarger because the periphery of the image can be distorted due to the convexity of the lens.

If a treatment-planning CT is available, both the external contour and internal anatomy can be outlined from the enlarged image and then transferred to the treatment-planning computer via a digitizer. In

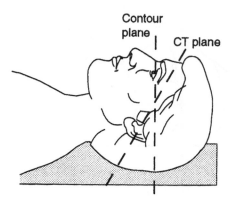

Figure 7.28   Caution should be used when transposing information from a diagnostic CT image to a contour because the planes may be different.

many instances, the CT information can also be transferred to a treatment-planning computer via a magnetic tape. In patients where a series of CT scans are obtained for tumor localization purposes, the information can be reconstructed and displayed in three dimensions. When only a single CT image obtained at the beam's CA is available, consideration

of the position of the target and normal organs within the entire region is quite difficult.

ACCURACY OF CONTOURS

The accuracy of the external contour and of the patient's dimensions has an effect on both the dose and on the placement of the treatment fields. In Fig. 7.29, the error in dose is shown for different beam energies when the contour or the dimensions of the patient is in error of 0.5 and 1.0 cm. It is not only discrepancies in measurements or contouring that can cause such errors in dose but also changes in the patient's weight and changes in size of superficial tumors. Intermittent verification of SSDs and the patient's dimensions is suggested. The dose should be recalculated when indicated. The decision as to whether or not to recalculate the dose based on changes in the patient's dimensions should be made for each individual situation. Criteria such as change in the percent depth dose, whether the change in the patient's dimensions is sustained over a long period of time, and so on may be used.

Changes in the field location also affect the dose

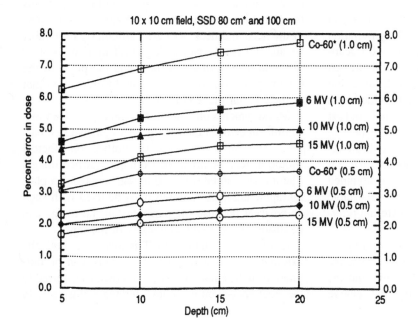

Figure 7.29   The magnitude of error in dose caused by 0.5- and 1.0-cm errors in depth for various beam energies.

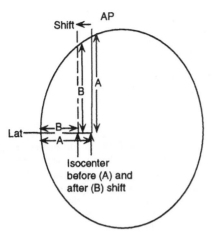

Figure 7.30 A field shift can cause a change in depth and consequently also a change in dose. When the isocenter is shifted 1 cm laterally, both the anterior and lateral depths were reduced, causing the dose to increase.

in the same way. When a treatment field is misaligned or when the location of the isocenter is intentionally shifted, the depth of the calculation point also often changes, affecting the dose. When parallel opposed fields are treated, the dose is often not

changed when the isocenter is shifted; however, if a pair of wedged fields are used and the isocenter is shifted, the effect on the dose can be considerable and a change in the dose calculation may be necessary (Fig. 7.30).

The effect on the field placement is evident in Fig. 7.31, where the depth of the isocenter is measured from the contour on the left (Fig. 7.31B). However, the slope of the chest, combined with a small discrepancy in where (in the cephalad/caudal direction) the depth of the isocenter is measured when the gantry is turned to the treatment angle can cause the isocenter to be set too far posterior, as shown on the right (Fig. 7.31C). In this situation, the target volume is partially missed and the deep margin of the treatment field is too close to the spinal canal. Similar misplacements of the isocenter occur if the chest contour is obtained with the patient's arms down by the sides but the treatment is set up with the arms raised above the head. Marks on the skin surface made when the arms are down along the torso will move cephalad when the arms are raised, causing a change in the relative position of the skin marks and underlying tissues (Fig. 7.32).

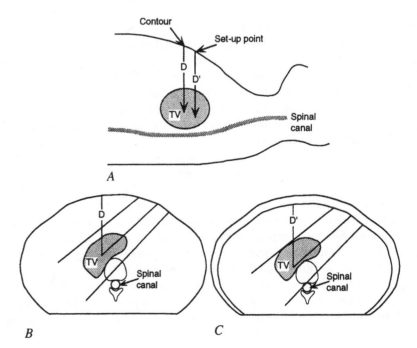

Figure 7.31 The isocenter of a field can inadvertently be placed at the wrong depth when it is measured on a very steep-sloping surface. When the beam is then angled "off the spinal cord," it may in fact be too close to the spinal cord.

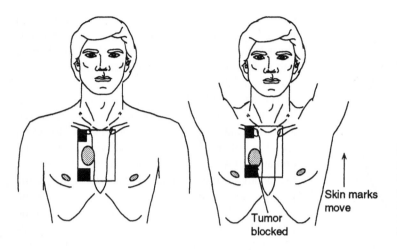

Figure 7.32 Marks that are made on the chest when the patient's arms are down by the sides will shift with respect to the deeper tissues when the arms are raised. This can cause the depth of the isocenter to shift as well, and a field angled off the spinal cord may, in fact, include it.

LOCALIZATION AND SIMULATION PROCEDURES

The terms *localization* and *simulation* are sometimes used interchangeably. A localization procedure in radiation therapy is the procedure in which the target volume and dose-limiting normal tissues in the region to be treated are delineated with respect to the patient's external surface This is one of the most important initial phases of treatment planning. An error in this process can lead to a tumor miss or inadvertent irradiation of radiosensitive organs. The field arrangement, beam energies, and beam-modifying devices are then selected so that the desired dose distribution is produced. The desired dose distribution is one that results in a uniform high dose including the target, while minimal doses are delivered in the adjacent normal tissues.

A treatment simulation procedure is one in which the planned field arrangement is verified using a simulator unit that mimics the geometry of the therapy machine and produces diagnostic-quality radiographs. Ideally, all treatment aids—such as beam-shaping blocks, compensating filters, and so on (Chap. 8)—should be verified prior to the treatment.

In some situations, the field arrangement and target volume are so standardized that the treatment fields are simulated without a prior localization procedure. For example, malignancies in the head and neck area are usually treated through parallel opposed lateral fields covering the primary lesion and the cervical lymph nodes above the shoulders. The separation between the two entrance points is recorded for subsequent CA dose calculation. An anterior field is used to treat the lymph nodes in the lower neck and the supraclavicular fossae. The extremes of the field margins are determined under fluoroscopic guidance. The fields are then designed on a simulation radiograph and beam-defining shields are fabricated prior to treatment.

Most malignancies in the pelvis are treated through a four-field technique consisting of opposed anterior/posterior and opposed lateral fields and often do not require a localization procedure, only treatment simulation. Radiation fields used in the treatment of pelvic malignancies are often designed with contrast material in the bladder and the rectum, and, in female patients, a radiopaque marker in the vagina. The cervix, uterus, prostate, and relevant lymph nodes are not visualized on the radiograph, but with knowledge of normal anatomy and visualization of contrast-filled organs, radiation fields can be designed to include the target with optimal sparing of adjacent normal organs. A contour is obtained and the dose distribution is calculated following the simulation procedure.

In outlining a contrast-filled cavity, it is important to remember that the contrast occupies the cavity.

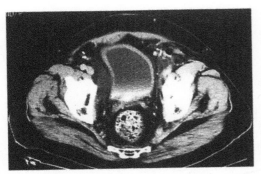

Figure 7.33   It is important to realize that the contrast observed on a radiograph represents only the cavity and that the walls of the contrast-filled organ actually is larger.

Therefore, a margin around the contrast may have to be added to also include the mucosa of the organ under consideration (Fig. 7.33).

There are other situations where neither a localization or simulation procedure is necessary. For example, skin lesions that are easily visualized or palpated can be treated with a single field setup clinically. Whole-brain treatment for metastatic disease is often set up clinically using external anatomic landmarks as reference points.

TRADITIONAL LOCALIZATION PROCEDURES

Over the past couple of decades, procedures in which the target volume and relevant internal anatomic structures can be localized with respect to external marks have been markedly improved. Many years ago, diagnostic-type x-ray machines were used to take orthogonal films from which recognizable internal structures were demagnified and transposed to a transverse contour of the patient. Orthogonal radiographs consists of two films taken from two angles separated by 90° (Fig. 7.34). These x-ray machines had no mark identifying the CA of the beam, nor did they have any beam-defining wires indicating the field size. Distances to the patient and to the cassette were not easily determined. These shortcomings often caused the beam divergence to be different from that of the therapy machine, with consequences as previously described in the discussion of beam divergence. In Fig. 7.35A, the central axis of the localization beam (a) is not known, but the marks on the skin surface indicate where the beam must enter in order to include the target *(shaded area)*. When the treatment field (b) is set up to the skin marks and with the central axis of the beam in the center of the field, the change in beam divergence causes some of the target to be missed. Figure 7.35B shows a situation where the localization (b) was made at a shorter SSD than the treatment SSD (a), also resulting in some of the target being missed. Similar difficulties still exist with localization of implants when the radiographs are taken in the operating room using a diagnostic-type x-ray machine.

Localization procedures using a diagnostic-type x-ray machine was usually limited to exposing an anterior and a lateral radiograph with a magnification device on the patient's skin surface and with a radiopaque marker (lead wire) indicating ink marks on the patient's skin. Recognizable bony landmarks or contrast-filled cavities seen on the radiograph were then demagnified and outlined on the contour with respect to the skin marks indicated on the contour.

The method of using the patient's external contour or an external skin mark as a reference point when indicating the position of internal organs is associated with uncertainty and should be avoided. The patient's skin surface, for example, cannot be ob-

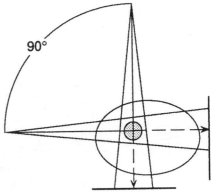

Figure 7.34   Orthogonal radiographs consist of two films taken from two angles separated by 90°.

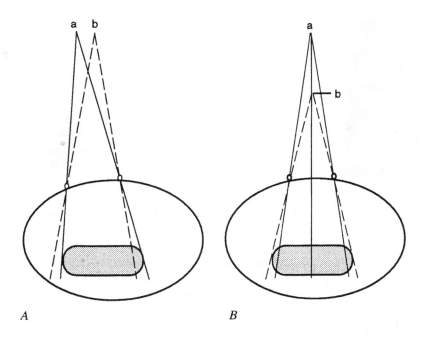

A   *B*

Figure 7.35 *A.* A target that is localized using a diagnostic x-ray machine and the field borders marked on the skin surface can be missed when it is treated, because the geometry is different. *B.* A target simulated at one SSD and treated at another can also be missed or an unnecessarily large volume of normal tissue can be irradiated.

served on most lateral radiographs. In the event that it can be seen, it is not clear which part of the skin surface is being observed. Although a supine patient is resting on the couch top, one cannot assume that the posterior skin surface is represented by the couch top as it is observed on a lateral radiograph (Fig. 7.36; also see Fig. 7.13). Radiopaque markers placed on the anterior and the posterior skin surface along the patient's midline reveal information with regard to the location of the midline skin surface on a lateral radiograph. With knowledge of the magnification factor on the radiograph, one can find the separation between the two radiopaque wires. The anterior/posterior dimension of the contour should match the separation between the two wires measured on the radiograph. Additional information is necessary with regard to where in the cephalad/caudal direction a contour was obtained before internal anatomy can be transposed.

The uncertainties associated with these procedures, now rarely necessary, required generous margins around the intended target. In modern radiation

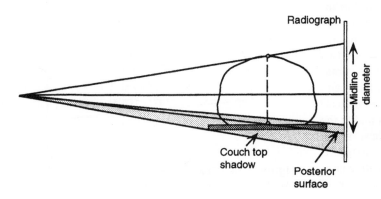

Figure 7.36 One cannot assume that the couch top, observed on a cross-table lateral radiograph, represent the patient's posterior skin surface. Due to the beam's divergence, the posterior surface appears somewhere inside the shadow of the couch on the radiograph.

therapy, however, increased accuracy of contouring, delineation of the target, use of positioning and immobilization devices, and use of linear accelerators with small penumbras have led to smaller tumor margins and subsequently to inclusion of smaller volumes of normal tissue.

LOCALIZATION PROCEDURES
USING A SIMULATOR

Treatment simulators, described in Chap. 2, have greatly improved the accuracy of localization and treatment simulation. The ability to simulate the geometry of the treatment and to identify the central axis and the extremes of the desired treatment field under fluoroscopic visualization improves the accuracy and reduces the time required for the procedure. A graticule in the beam displays a scale that can be used as a magnification device for quick transposition of internal information onto a transverse contour of the patient (Fig. 7.13).

In many situations, particularly when multiple angled fields are anticipated, the best field arrangement must be determined following careful localization of the target and of normal dose-limiting organs. In that situation, it might be necessary to bring the patient to the simulation room twice; first for a localization procedure and then, after the field arrangement has been designed, for a simulation procedure to verify the treatment plan.

From a set of orthogonal radiographs, the position of internal anatomy can be outlined in three dimensions (Fig. 7.37). The anterior radiograph reveals information in the right/left and cephalad/caudal directions while the lateral radiograph reveals information in the anterior/posterior and cephalad/caudal directions. The information from the localization radiographs is then transposed onto a cross-section outline of the patient's external contour.

It is extremely important that the laser alignment lines and the central axis marks indicated on each localization radiograph be marked on the patient's skin surface during the localization procedure. These marks, representing reference lines only, are used to reposition the patient for the simulation procedure and to determine the position of the planned treatment fields.

The position of internal anatomic structures, often visible on radiographs as bone and contrast-filled cavities, is outlined on the contour through measurements on the localization or simulation radiographs. The position of the isocenter is a known point on both the localization and simulation radiographs and on the contour as described previously. This point is therefore ideal to use as a reference point in transposing information from the radiographs to the contour. For example, the distance measured on the radiograph from the isocenter, indicated by the cross hair, to the anterior aspect of the rectal contrast (measured slightly caudal to the isocenter) in Fig. 7.37B is 2.0 cm. Reduced by the magnification factor on the film (SAD, 100 cm, and TFD, 135 cm = 135/100 or 1.35), this distance is 1.48 cm (2.2/1.35) on the contour. From the isocenter to the posterior aspect of the rectal contrast, the distance is 7.0 cm on the lateral radiograph. Reduced by 1.35 it is 5.2 cm on the contour. The right-to-left direction, which is determined on an anterior radiograph, cannot with certainty be determined here, since there is no rectal contrast. However, since the precise position from right to left is not important in this patient because the anterior field includes the entire pelvis, we can assume that the rectum is centered on the rectal tube. Rectal contrast is usually not introduced until after radiographs of the anterior or posterior fields have been obtained, since it would obscure other important landmarks (i.e., metal markers or the isocenter mark, as in this patient). Each point that must be transposed from the radiograph to the contour is measured in a similar fashion from the isocenter on the radiograph. The distance is reduced by the magnification factor and then marked on the contour (Fig. 7.38). In most situations, the position of pertinent anatomic structures should be outlined only as it appears at the level of the contour. In some situations, however, it may be of some importance to know the maximal dimensions in each direction—for example, the target or the rectum and so on.

The type of target localization just described provides limited information about the target volume and normal anatomy. It does not give information with respect to the shape of the organs involved but

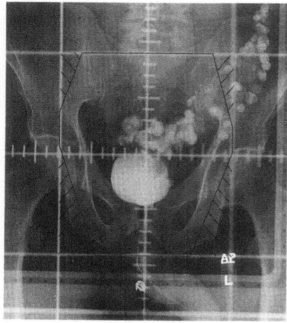

A

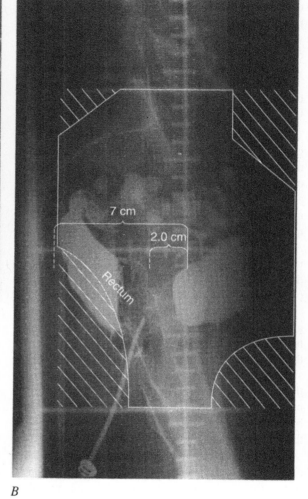

B

Figure 7.37 *A* and *B*. Anterior and lateral (orthogonal) radiographs of the pelvis. When the contrast-filled organs are outlined on the contour, the measurements are with respect to the isocenter —a known point on the contour and in the patient.

indicates the extremes of each organ in three directions.

Localization procedures as they pertain to each particular anatomic area are explained in the appropriate chapter later in this text.

LOCALIZATION PROCEDURES USING COMPUTED TOMOGRAPHY

The use of CT and MRI has made the determination of tumor extent more precise and the position of the target with respect to adjacent anatomy easier to ap-

preciate. Although CT and MRI images obtained for diagnostic purposes cannot be used directly in radiation therapy, as previously mentioned, the technology has had a tremendous impact on the accuracy with which treatment planning can be achieved.

In the section describing contouring methods, some discussion about the use of CT in radiation therapy planning was presented; however, a more thorough discussion is needed in order to clarify their proper use. The widespread use of CT and MRI in treatment planning, along with an explosion of developments in computerized treatment planning and

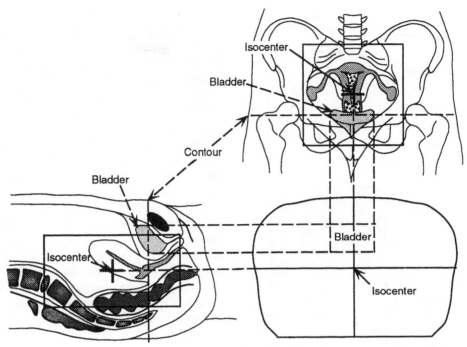

Figure 7.38 Outlining anatomic structures from orthogonal radiographs to a contour of the patient.

the application of sophisticated computer graphics, has led to three-dimensional (3-D) display of the anatomy and dose distributions.[4-12] Three-dimensional treatment-planning software programs, to which many radiation therapy departments now have access, require CT- or MRI-based patient information. Three-dimensional treatment-planning methods are discussed elsewhere in this text; however, data accession for traditional use of CT information is similar to that of 3-D systems and is therefore explained simultaneously.

Acquisition of Data. Tomographic images of the patient, primarily CT, provide an excellent 3-D representation of the patient on the basis of which treatment plans can be designed with greater accuracy than ever before. Although MRI yields very detailed images, many immobilization devices are too large to fit inside the small tunnel in most MRI units, often precluding this modality from being used for treatment-planning purposes. A laser alignment sys-

tem is needed in the CT room to define a coordinate system in the data set. This laser system can be mounted outside the scanning tunnel so that the laser lines intersect at the center of the CT reconstruction circle or at some other known point (Fig. 7.39). With the patient in treatment position, the laser alignment lines are marked on the patient and/or on the immobilization device. Radiopaque plastic tubes are taped onto these marks so that they can be visualized on the CT image; they are then used when the planned field orientations are transferred to the patient. The alignment marks, which are used in repositioning the patient, must be maintained throughout the course of the treatment. The patient's y-axis (cephalad/caudal) should be aligned with the sagittal laser (Fig. 7.40). The horizontal (or coronal) laser lines on each side of the patient are marked after the table height (z-axis) for the scan has been set. The CT couch is fixed in the x-axis (right to left); therefore, the patient can only be moved along the y-axis during the scan. For 3-D treatment planning, a series of scans throughout the treatment region is needed. Before the scan is

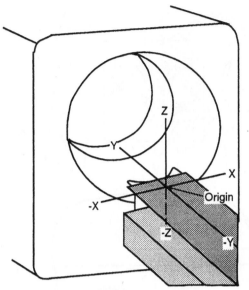

Figure 7.39   A laser alignment system in a CT unit mounted so that the lines coincide at the center of the reconstruction circle. The coordinate system is also shown.

begun, it is necessary to set an 0-level scan, which usually indicates the scan on which the point of origin in the coordinate system is set. This level must also be marked on the patient, so that the planned treatment fields can be set up at the correct y-level.

The data set is transferred to a treatment-planning computer via modem or a magnetic tape. The images are then displayed and anatomic structures relevant to the treatment are contoured. Beam orientations are determined, and dose distributions are calculated on one or multiple images. Treatment-planning computers capable of displaying a 3-D image of the patient builds an image of the patient around the coordinate system used during the scanning process. The external surface, relevant internal anatomic structures, and the target volume are contoured on all images (Fig. 7.41). The contour surface from each axial image of each structure is then displayed, giving a 3-D appearance of the patient and the internal structures that were contoured (Fig. 7.41).

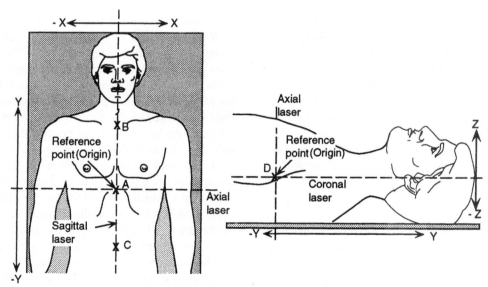

Figure 7.40   *(A, B, C).* The patient should be aligned with the alignment system in the CT unit system. To carry out the treatment as planned, the same position with respect to the coordinate system must be maintained throughout the patient's treatment.

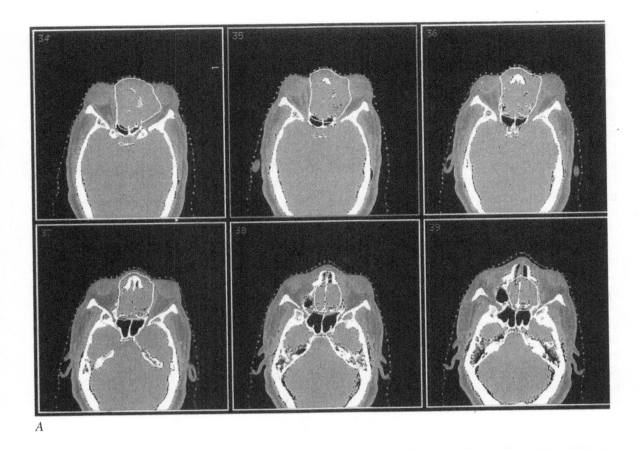

A

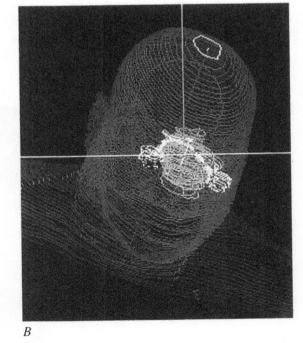

B

Figure 7.41 *A.* The target volume and pertinent anatomy are outlined on each CT image. *B.* A three-dimensional image of the patient is built exactly as the patient was positioned during the data acquisition.

Using CT Images in Treatment Planning. It is insufficient to determine the needed field size from the target-volume outline on a single CT image even if it is the image where the target appears to be largest. For example, the shape of the target volume may be such that on images obtained in other parallel planes (cephalad or caudal), part of the target lies outside the boundaries of the field or the curved spinal cord lies inside the field at another level (Fig. 7.42). It is therefore necessary to outline, on the CA contour, the position of the target and pertinent anatomy on all images as it appears with respect to the origin.

A simple method of how to use the CT information to determine beam directions and field sizes is described here. The plastic tubes, taped to the patient's skin surface during the CT scan, should be marked on each external contour (Fig. 7.43A). A horizontal line drawn between the right and the left plastic tubes represents the horizontal or coronal laser alignment line and indicates a common height for all CT contours. A vertical line drawn perpendicular to the CT couch through the anterior marker represents the sagittal laser alignment line and indicates the right-left or x-axis position on each contour. The intersection of these lines on the 0-level scan image represents the origin in the coordinate system. From this point, all other points can be described using the designations of the x-, y-, and z-axes. The vertical and horizontal lines on each image are superimposed onto the contour outline representing the CA of the anticipated beams. The target and other internal structures of interest are then traced onto this single contour (Fig. 7.43A, *lower diagram*).

In the lower contour (level 0) in Fig. 7.43A, the target volume, and bony anatomy from each of the seven CT images have been transposed to the CA contour in the correct position with respect to the intersection of the laser alignment lines. To treat this target, large anterior and lateral fields will include the target in all levels but will also include a substantial volume of normal tissue. This method of transposing the target does not yield information about the shape of the target but merely gives information about the location of the target in the x- and z-directions. Beam angles and field sizes, but not field shape, can be determined from this information.

Figure 7.44 shows a chest wall tumor outlined by the method just described. Should the beam size, location, and angle be determined on the CA image only (0 level), portions of the target would obviously be missed, as shown on the composite drawing (Fig. 7.44, *lower left*). In looking at the composite outline of the target, it appears as if the tumor were outside

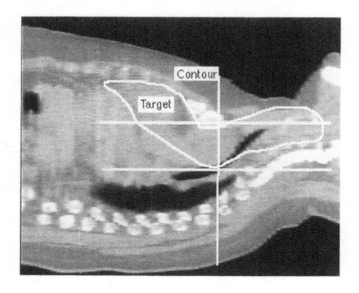

Figure 7.42 The target volume and pertinent anatomic structures are outlined in only one CT image. Often, if field sizes are determined in the plane where the target appears to be largest, portions of the target volume can be missed or the spinal cord can fall within the treatment field. In all CT images, it is necessary to know the position of both the target and normal anatomy with respect to one another in the coordinate system.

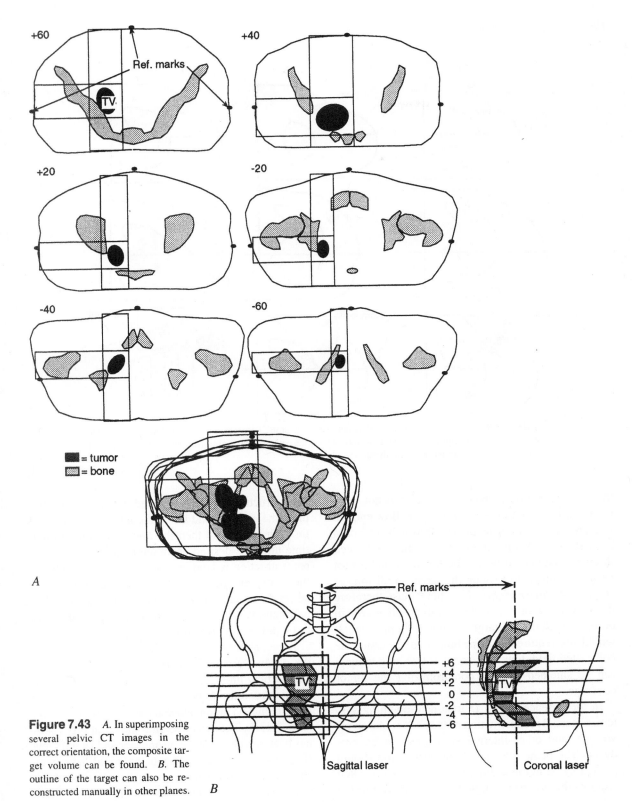

Figure 7.43 *A.* In superimposing several pelvic CT images in the correct orientation, the composite target volume can be found. *B.* The outline of the target can also be reconstructed manually in other planes.

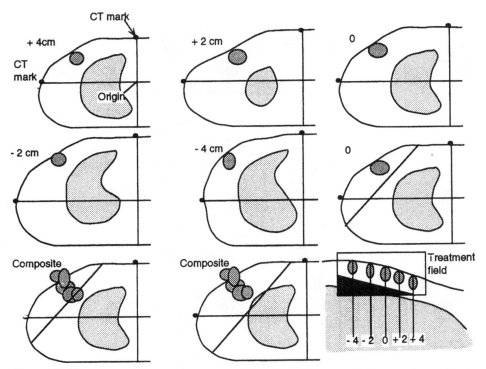

Figure 7.44   A tumor on the chest wall is outlined in several CT images, which are superimposed on the central axis image. It appears as if the tumor were outside the patient's external contour due to the curvature of the chest wall in the cephalad/caudad direction.

the external contour, which it obviously is not. As a matter of fact, the tumor is probably shallow enough in each individual image that an electron beam could be used to treat this tumor. If the tumor is treated through a tangential beam, the treatment field must be large enough to include the target in all images (Fig. 7.44, *lower right*). This field must therefore flash over the patient's chest wall in all levels in order to include the target in the − 4 cm level. It would also require that some lung tissue be inside the collimated field; however, some of this lung volume can be shielded without compromising the tumor coverage.

In the absence of a 3-D treatment-planning system, a manual reconstruction of the patient, the target volume, and other internal structures can be produced. The plane selected for reconstruction should preferably be in the beam's-eye view; however, that requires that the beam angle be selected prior to the

reconstruction. In the calculated 3-D computer display, the external and internal contours are outlined on each image and then the image is turned in real time until the desired beam angle is found. Manual reconstruction is laborious and is not as accurate as the computer-calculated image. Only 2-D views can be produced manually. External contours and internal anatomy must be outlined on several axial planes through the treatment region.

A reconstructed view is produced by measuring the distance from the intersection of the horizontal and vertical lines (origin) to the extremes of the internal structure to be reconstructed and marking these points on graph paper at the appropriate y-level (Fig. 7.43*B*). The target volume shown in Fig. 7.43*A* has been reconstructed in an anterior and lateral view (Fig. 7.43*B*), but any other plane could have been chosen. The information about the position of the target with respect to the surrounding anatomy provided by CT imaging, enables the radiation oncologist to conform the beam to the shape of the target and thus spare more normal tissue.

In Fig. 7.45, a lung tumor and the spinal canal have been reconstructed in anterior and lateral views. Obviously, this tumor cannot be treated through lateral or anterior-posterior fields without also including the spinal canal. A suitable beam angle would have to be selected first; then the target and the spinal canal can be reconstructed in the beam's-eye view. In deciding on the best beam direction, it is important also to consider the ability to spare normal tissues at a given beam angle. It is sometimes difficult to determine the best beam angles in the treatment of malignancies of the chest because of the extent of tumor and the presence of large volumes of normal tissues, including normal lung, heart, and spinal cord. To minimize radiation to these tissues, the shape of the target volume in the beam's-eye view must be known.

TREATMENT SIMULATION

Following the localization and treatment-planning process, the designed treatment must be tested for accuracy. This is what a simulator is designed to do, although—to a very large extent—it is also used for taking orthogonal radiographs for the purpose of localizing various internal organs, as described above. It is during the simulation procedure that the marks, first made on the patient during the data-acquisition procedure, must be realigned with the alignment system. This is not always achievable to the desired precision due to some minor discrepancies between the alignment systems in the different rooms and also because there may be some difference in the sagging of the couches in the different rooms, and so on.[13]

During the treatment-simulation procedure, the position of the isocenter of the planned fields is determined by measuring the distance from the origin of the coordinate system, indicated by reference marks. The right/left direction is determined from the anterior mark and the anterior-to-posterior direction is determined from the horizontal or lateral marks. The cephalad-to-caudal direction can be determined from either of the marks made on the pa-

tient. Under fluoroscopic guidance, the position of the beam's central axis with respect to recognizable bony landmarks is verified.

When the position of the isocenter is set, the planned field size is set and the machine is turned to the planned gantry, collimator, and couch angles. The position of each field with respect to the patient's anatomy is verified in fluoroscopy and a radiograph of each field is obtained for later comparison with port films. The TFD must be recorded for each field so that beam-shaping blocks can be formed from the outlines on the radiographs. The treatment fields are also marked on the patient, along with the alignment laser lines indicating the isocenter.

Many treatment machines have some limitations in terms of beam angles. A couch angle of more than 20° often will not allow a lateral tangential chest wall field to be treated without the head of the machine colliding with the couch. A posterior oblique head and neck field may not clear the couch posteriorly, particularly if the isocenter is high above the treatment couch. Often these difficulties cannot be determined with the simulator unit, since each therapy unit may have different limitations. Ideally, the simulator should be capable of indicating limitations on any treatment machine, but this is probably not possible in the foreseeable future. Before the treatment is planned, it is a good idea to test, on the treatment machine, whether a certain beam angle can be used in a particular setup.

THREE-DIMENSIONAL TREATMENT PLANNING AND SIMULATION

Three-dimensional treatment-planning systems have the capability of building a 3-D image of the patient and pertinent anatomic structures from sequential CT or MRI scans in precisely the same geometric relationship as it was during the data-acquisition procedure. The patient's external surface and any internal structure of interest is contoured on each CT image. The contours (external and internal) appearing as wire frames and arranged in precisely the right spatial position can then be displayed on a computer monitor. Each anatomic structure, distinguished by a unique color, can be turned on or off as the need arises during the treatment-planning session. The ability to visualize the contoured internal structures, as if the patient had transparent skin, allows the user to select beam angles that will minimize inclusion of radiosensitive structures within the beam.

The Virtual Simulator. A 3-D system referred to as the Virtual Simulator™* and developed at the University of North Carolina[11,12] is described here,

* Sherouse Systems, Inc.™, Charleston, S.C.

but many other 3-D systems are being used.[7-9] The Virtual Simulator is unique in that the entire process between acquisition of the data set to treatment is carried out on the computer system. No conventional treatment simulation is necessary. The relevant anatomic structures and the tumor or target volumes are outlined on each CT image (Fig. 7.46*A*). A 3-D image of the patient is then displayed on the computer monitor. The computer monitor displays simultaneous windows with pertinent treatment-planning options (Fig. 7.46*B*). Three windows display

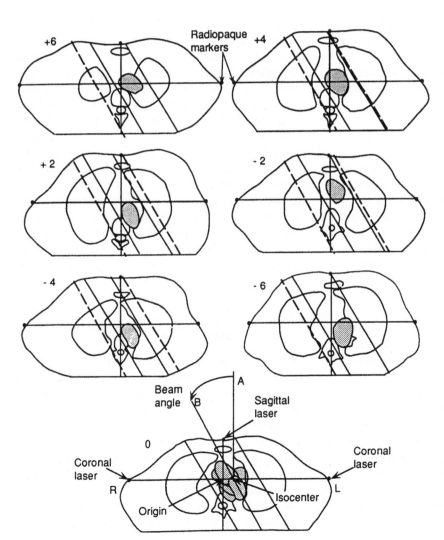

A

Figure 7.45 *A.* To include the entire lung tumor at a 30° beam angle *(lower image),* the field appears to also include the spinal cord. Spinal cord sparing is, however, possible because of the curvature of the spinal cord and the ability to shape the beam to the tumor (solid lines in images +6 to −6). *B.* The same tumor reconstructed in anterior and lateral views.

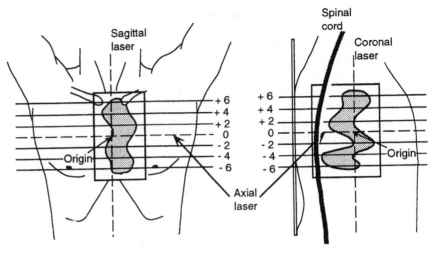

Figure 7.45 *(Continued)*. *B*

outlines in different colors of the patient's anatomy as they were drawn on each sequential CT image. One image displays the patient as seen from the radiation source (beam's-eye view), with an overlay of the field and the beam cross hair. This beam's-eye view (BEV) is supplemented by two other views perpendicular to the BEV. One window displays icons of the gantry, the collimator, and the treatment couch, allowing the user to observe the motion of these icons as the patient is moved into desired orientation in the beam. Various control panels and knobs—used for setting the isocenter, field size, gantry, collimator, and couch angles—are displayed. One window displays the vertical, lateral, and longitudinal settings of the isocenter with respect to the point of origin of the coordinate system used when the scan was made on the CT unit, as explained above. Another control panel allows the user to select the treatment machine and beam-modifying devices and to design the shape of treatment field.

The ability to turn the patient in space around either of the three axes simultaneously is very useful when one is trying to find a suitable beam orientation. The optimal beam direction is one in which the separation between the target and critical organs allows the beam edge to pass between the two entities with maximal margins. When the desired beam

direction is attained, the user can design the size and shape of the treatment field via a mouse control. The beam can then be copied and opposed, if desired, or copied and moved in another direction and then redrawn to fit the shape around the target in the new BEV.

When all beams are designed, the dose is calculated, and—unlike in 2-D dose calculations—the beam and patient geometry are considered in 3-D (Fig. 7.46C). In most routine clinical practice, the density and 3-D shape of inhomogeneities cannot be considered, and the dose given to structures away from the central plane is often not considered. Evaluation of 3-D dose distributions is tedious and often requires the physician's presence to view the dose distributions superimposed on reconstructed CT images in many pertinent planes directly on the computer monitor. Another useful tool to evaluate dose distributions is the dose-volume histogram (Chap. 6, Fig. 6.36), where the vertical axis represent the volume of an organ that receives the dose on the horizontal axis. Dose-volume histograms, although helpful in the evaluation process, do not yield information about the spatial distribution of the dose (Chap. 6).

When exiting the simulation program, setup instructions for each beam are printed. The setup instructions give the particulars about SSD, SAD, field size, and field position with respect to the origin previously marked on the patient. They also give the gantry, collimator, and couch angle readout for the particular therapy unit selected for the treatment. A template of the designed field shape, used for producing a customized beam-shaping block, is plotted for each beam. Digitally reconstructed radiographs (DRRs) are finally generated from the CT data in a plane perpendicular to the central axis of each beam (Fig. 7.46D).[14] Superimposed on the radiograph are the wire contours of selected internal structures that were previously contoured. The beam-defining wires, cross hairs with centimeter markers, and beam outline are also superimposed on the DRR. These DRRs serve as reference images for verification of the computer-designed treatment and are used for comparison when port films are reviewed during the course of treatment. When treatment plans are designed on the Virtual Simulator, the traditional localization and simulation procedures becomes obsolete. Conventional treatment simulation procedures should still be considered when the treatment is to be delivered to the chest. Involuntary motions—such as respiration, coughing, swallowing, and so on—not appreciated on CT images may require that field

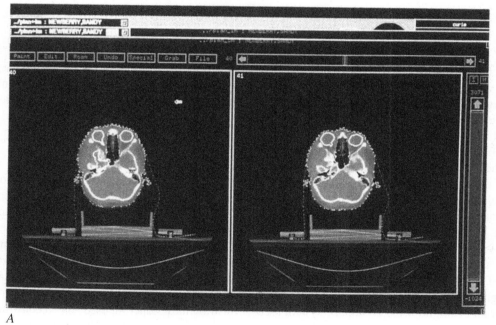

A

Figure 7.46 *A.* The target and pertinent anatomy is outlined in all CT images. *B.* The three-dimensional image of the patient is built. In the left lower corner are the icons showing the motions of the couch, gantry, and collimator as the beam directions are determined. In the lower right corner are dials for setting the field size and isocenter. Above is a three-dimensional rendering of the structures drawn on the CT images and the two perpendicular views of the patient. In the lower left of the screen is a CT image of the patient with outlined anatomy; while the planning takes place, the beams can be visualized on the image. Any CT image can be viewed in this window. At the top of the screen are the dials for choosing beam energy, wedges, trays, and other accessories along with options for outlining the treatment field in the beam's-eye view. An autocontour option allows the user to set the desired margin around the target; the program will then automatically draw the field around the target. *C.* Dose calculations in three dimensions are viewed on the screen or plotted on paper. *D.* Digitally reconstructed radiographs are calculated from the CT data for each field. (See color illustration 1, which appears between pages 532 and 533.)

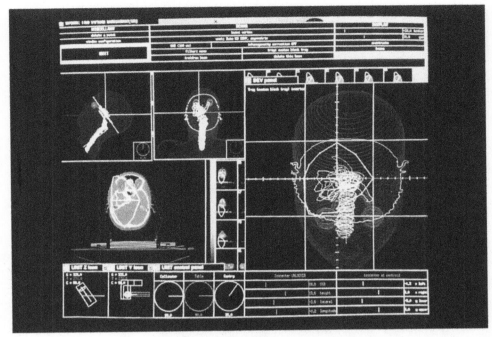

B

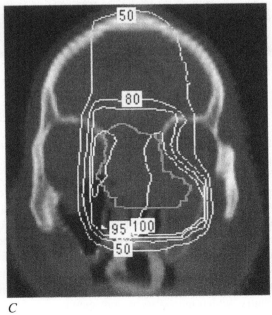

C

Figure 7.46   (*Continued*).

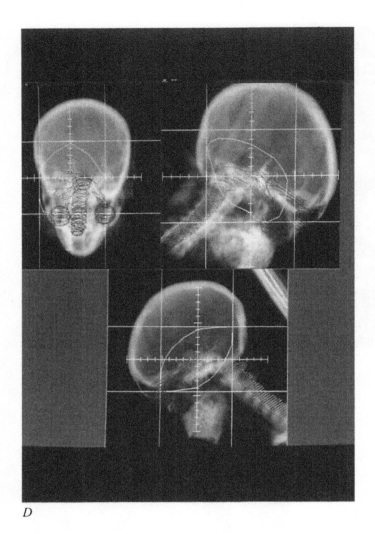

D

Figure 7.46 *(Continued).*

margins be made more generous than those planned on the computer.

The geometric relationship between the CT images and the therapy machine must be maintained to get the desired result. The patient's position during the acquisition of the data set must therefore be reproduced during each therapy session. The geometry on the CT unit is quite simple; however, in the simulation or treatment room, there are many other motions, such as those of the couch, collimator, and gantry, which must also be considered.

Three-dimensional treatment design often calls for unusual beam angles. Unlike the traditional treatment planning methods, this approach offers the capability of visualizing the target with respect to dose-limiting organs in the vicinity of the target from any direction. The radiation oncologist can, with much more confidence than earlier, outline the radiation beam to the shape of the target with minimal margins. Such conformal beams assume that the patient can be repositioned precisely for each treatment.

UNCERTAINTIES IN RADIATION THERAPY

To plan and deliver external beam radiation therapy is a complicated process, and it is always associated with a large number of uncertainties. Yet the precision required is probably the most critical of all disciplines in oncology. The uncertainties can be divided into two major groups; uncertainties of dose (i.e., inhomogeneities, dose calculations, variables in machine output; Chap. 3) and uncertainties in patient-beam geometry (spatial uncertainties). Although different in character, these two types of uncertainties are closely tied together. For example, if a portion of the tumor is missed once or twice during a course of treatment, the dose to that portion of the tumor is also in error. Geometric uncertainties can be broadly divided into those inherent in mechanical inaccuracies in the treatment machine (beam-angle indicators, beam-light coincidence, isocenter accuracy, and so on)[15,16] and those related to target determination and localization and patient positioning. It is important to recognize and to understand the cause and the magnitude of the uncertainties when the treatment plan is designed in order to minimize their effect. Although the emphasis here is on uncertainties in patient-beam geometry, uncertainties with respect to dose cannot be excluded.

TREATMENT UNCERTAINTIES

Even under the most favorable circumstances, there are many uncertainties associated with the delivery of radiation therapy.[17] First, defining the target volume is associated with many uncertainties mainly because the precise spread of the disease is unknown. Other uncertainties lie in the reproducibility of the patient's position during CT, simulation, and treatment and from treatment to treatment. Other changes that affect both the dose and patient-beam geometry are weight loss or gain and tumor regression, which can occur during the course of treatment. These spatial uncertainties are considered by the radiation oncologist, who is likely to draw field margins around the target with these uncertainties in mind.

Another source of uncertainty is the dose delivery.

Regardless of how carefully the treatment machine has been calibrated, there are some uncertainties in measurement and there may be small variations in output from day to day. The dose may also vary slightly with small inconsistencies in the setup of the patient each day. Interpreting between and rounding of numbers during the calibration of the machine and during the calculation of the dose accounts for small uncertainties in dose. No matter how precisely the dose is calculated, there are still small discrepancies. These uncertainties must be kept to a minimum by being precise in determining patient topography and calculating the dose.

It is important to recognize that there are uncertainties in the treatment so that remedial action can be taken. Acceptable levels of uncertainty must be established and one must take steps to keep these uncertainties within those levels. One must also understand the magnitude and the implications of the uncertainties.

Spatial Uncertainties. Geometric discrepancies caused by mechanical limitations/problems in the machine can, in theory, be eliminated by very rigorous testing and adjustment. In everyday practice, however, we accept the fact that not all discrepancies can be corrected. It has been suggested that displacements caused by mechanical machine inaccuracies, even when they are within the specified minimum requirements, can range up to 5 mm. Uncertainties in the extent of the target volume, patient and organ motion, and in the treatment setup can cause errors of up to 8 mm. The combined uncertainty can therefore be up to 10 mm.[18] Variations in the day-to-day setup are difficult to contend with because patients tend to move, and there are inaccuracies in aligning the treatment beam to the setup marks. Several studies[19–21] show that present practice does not meet the < 5 mm uncertainty recommended by the American Association of Physicists in Medicine.[22] Methods to deal with these uncertainties are presented here.

It is important to distinguish between localization errors and positioning errors, although both can lead to failure to control the disease. Localization errors result from failure to determine the extent of the disease or from the design of inadequate treatment fields. Positioning errors, on the other hand, are the displacement of the treatment field with respect to the intended position. The latter can be caused either by patient motion or failure to reposition the patient.

Determination of the PTV—which includes the tumor, adjacent tissues, and sometimes the regional lymph nodes—is a difficult task, often associated with uncertainties. The physician must integrate information gained from various imaging studies, surgical reports, and physical examinations before deciding what area must be treated and what dose should be delivered. To compensate for uncertainties in outlining the target volume and in patient-beam alignment, margins are routinely added around the target. It is, however, important to recognize that when margins are added, more normal tissues are inevitably irradiated. The use of 3-D treatment-planning systems, taking advantage of the CT and MRI information, may reduce some of the uncertainties leading to the use of smaller tumor margins. The ability to limit the volume of normal tissue in some instances may allow higher doses to be delivered to the target, possibly also increasing the probability of local tumor control.[23,24] However, precision and effective immobilization techniques are essential when the tumor margins are reduced. It is important to recognize that the diagnostic (CT or MRI) information used in 3-D treatment-planning systems may not be ideal. If the extent of tumor involvement is underestimated, marginal misses may occur. Considerations with respect to tumor margins are important and are discussed in the following section.

Tumor Margins. In general, most treatment fields are designed to treat the target volume plus "a margin." This margin is added to account for three factors: dose fall-off at the beam edge (penumbra), inaccuracies in defining the target volume, and inaccuracies in patient-beam alignment, including organ and patient motion. The edge of the beam-defining field light usually coincides with the 50 percent isodose level (Chap. 3, Fig. 3.16). The distance from this geometric field margin to the 95 percent line (often used for dose prescription) varies from machine to machine but is often ~ 5 mm on a linear

accelerator. A 5-mm margin for inaccuracies in target identification is a minimum value, given the difficulties in interpreting conventional diagnostic images and transferring this information to the simulator films as previously described. The third area of uncertainty lies in the reproducibility of the patient-beam alignment and the probability of organ and patient motion. Many radiation oncologists add a modest 5-mm margin to compensate for these uncertainties. A combined margin of 15 mm is thus commonly added around the target volume. Under optimal circumstances, including the use of a linear accelerator, rigid patient immobilization, a 3-D treatment planning system, and conformal beam shaping, this margin may be sufficient. In the absence of these technologies, however, larger margins may be necessary.

When margins are added around the target to compensate for uncertainties, a larger volume of normal tissue is inevitably irradiated. Even a small increase of the margin can have a significant effect on the volume of normal tissues that is exposed (Fig. 7.47). For example, adding a 5-mm margin to a 5 × 5 cm field increases the *area* by 5 cm² (> 40 percent), while the addition of a 5-mm margin to a 20 × 20 cm field increases the irradiated *area* by about 40 cm² (10 percent). If we then consider the third dimension of these fields, the *volume* is much larger. Consideration must be given to the fact that the largest volumes of normal tissue being irradiated lie in the path of the beam before it reaches the target and in the exit region beyond the target. Treatment techniques consisting of several fields directed from different angles and shaped to conform to the target in the beam's-eye view can reduce the dose in the normal tissues surrounding the target in all directions (Chap. 1, Fig. 1.3).

The change from cobalt-60 machines to linear accelerators, where the penumbra is much sharper and the dose is more uniform within the geometric edges of the field, has made it possible to reduce the tumor margins. The rapid fall-off of dose near the edges, however, makes even small beam displacements more critical. The introduction of customized beam-shaping blocks with divergent edges (Chap. 8) has further reduced the penumbra. It has also made it

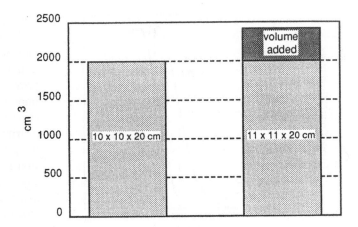

Figure 7.47 When 0.5-cm margins are added around a 10 × 10 cm field in a 20-cm-thick patient, a large volume of normal tissue is added within the irradiated field.

possible to shape the beam so that it more closely conforms to the shape of the tumor. Prior to custom shielding capabilities, tumor margins were sometimes excessive because blocks were generally limited to square or rectangular shapes. Areas that previously could not have been shielded can now be blocked, thus reducing the volume of irradiated nor-

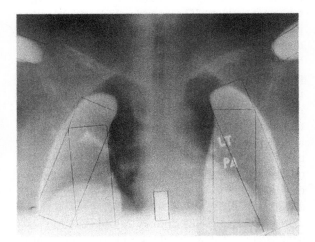

Figure 7.48 Using treatment fields that are shaped to conform to the target minimizes the volume of normal tissue within the irradiated field. With only square or rectangular blocks, which were used in the past, the tumor margins were often more generous; thus normal tissues were unnecessarily irradiated. In some situations part of the tumor may also have been unintentionally blocked because it was more difficult to shape the fields.

mal tissue (Fig. 7.48). There were also risks that tumors were inadvertently blocked due to the limited block shapes.

When the margins are reduced, the need for precision in the execution of the treatment plan is increased. Aggressive patient immobilization and highly trained, meticulous technologists who take the time to carefully set up the treatment and pay close attention to details are crucial.

The Effect of Uncertainties and the Need for Precision. Although uncertainties are being reduced with the use of improved imaging techniques and 3-D treatment-planning computers, problems related to patient motion and uncertainties in repositioning still remain and must be addressed. Field placement errors involve displacement of the treatment field relative to the intended treatment volume, resulting in reduction of the dose delivered in the missed part of the target. At the same time, a segment of normal tissue on the opposite side is moved into the beam and inadvertently irradiated. Such errors result from movement during treatment and from failure to reproduce the treatment fields or to reposition the patient accurately from treatment to treatment. The dose-response curve for many tumors is quite steep, and a small error in dose can have a profound effect on tumor control and normal tissue injury (Fig. 7.49). Missing the tumor once or twice could lead to failure to control the tumor and, if the segment of normal tissue moved into the beam was

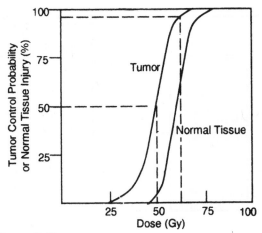

Figure 7.49 Typical dose-response curve showing a hypothetical situation where, by giving the tumor 5000 cGy, there is a 50 percent probability of tumor control with almost no risk of injury to normal tissue. If the dose is increased to about 6200 cGy, the probability of tumor control increases to about 95 percent, but the risk of injury to normal tissue has also increased to almost 60 percent.

the spinal cord, a kidney, or the lens of the eye, the result could be devastating for the patient. It must be recognized that complications from the radiation do not occur in unirradiated tissue; it is therefore important to limit the irradiated volume of normal tissue as much as possible.[25] It is also important to realize that structures located outside the geometric field margins receive some dose that could give rise to complications.[26]

The need for precision in therapy and the effect on the outcome has been studied by several authors.[17,27-34] Generally, a high degree of precision is required in all phases of radiation treatment if frequent tumor control without excessive complications is the desired endpoint. The International Commission on Radiation Units and Measurements (ICRU) recommends an accuracy of ± 5 percent in the delivery of an absorbed dose to the target if tumor eradication is desired.[35] More recently, other authors have suggested a more precise accuracy requirement.[36-38] Cunningham has pointed out that the standards recommended by the ICRU are difficult to achieve.[39]

Failure to deliver the prescribed dose can, of course, be caused not only by geometric tumor-beam

misalignments but also by uncertainties in dose calculation, machine calibration, measurement of the patient's size, and determination of tissue composition (inhomogeneities and so on). Although improvements have been made in these areas, further improvements are necessary, particularly with respect to determination of the patient's size and the distribution and density of inhomogeneities within the patient. Another important area requiring precision is the geometric alignment of the patient on a day-to-day basis and the accuracy with which each machine parameter is set by the technologists. Although impossible to eliminate, uncertainties caused by patient motion can be reduced by using an aggressive immobilization system. In the following pages, some considerations with respect to patient positioning and immobilization are presented.

POSITIONING AND IMMOBILIZATION

One element of radiation therapy that requires serious consideration is patient positioning and immobilization. This is just one of the many preparations aimed at reducing uncertainties associated with treatment delivery. The goal should be to place the patient in a position that is comfortable, easily reproduced, and yet practical (i.e., not interfering with the beam orientation or the head of the machine). To precisely reproduce the patient's position approximately 30 times during a course of treatment is a monumental task requiring highly competent technologists with great patience. Extensive literature on the subject during the past 20 years indicates that the difficulty of repositioning of patients for treatments is of great concern within the radiation therapy community and that the issue is being addressed.[19-21,40-55]

In addition to giving primary consideration to patient safety and comfort, the geometry of the setup must be reproduced from simulation to treatment and from day to day in later treatments. Small discrepancies in patient-beam alignment between the simulator room and the treatment room are sometimes observed on the first set of port films.[13,20,21,47,56,57] This may be due to small differences in the two alignment systems as well as to varying amounts of sag of the two couches. For example, the surfaces of some simulation couches are rigid while the couch in the treatment room may have ''windows'' to allow a posterior or oblique field to be treated without interception of the beam by the treatment couch. Many treatment couches have openings arranged differently in each end and, by reversing the tabletop, the most appropriate arrangement for a given situation can be selected. For example, at one end, there may be a thick bar in the center of the couch, while each side of the couch is open to allow oblique or tangential fields to enter uninterrupted. At the opposite end, the central section may be open, allowing posterior fields to be treated, while a bar on each side of the couch offers stability (Chap. 2, Figs. 2.11 and 2.12). A thin Mylar sheet stretched across the window or an insert consisting of a tennis-racket-type net will sag under the patient's weight, disturbing the relationship between skin marks and internal anatomy that existed during the simulation procedure. The integrity of these special couch supports must therefore be maintained, and they may have to be replaced frequently. These differences may appear trivial, but they can cause serious errors and should therefore be minimized. It is crucial that port films be obtained on the first treatment and corrections made for subsequent treatments. There are also some reasons for small changes in the patient-beam relationship that cannot be eliminated—for example, respiration.

The practice of pulling the patient's clothing away from the treatment area, rather than having the patient undress, creates rolls of clothing under the patient on either side of the treatment area. These rolls of clothing may not be in precisely the same place for each treatment and may be of various sizes, depending on what kind of clothing the patient wears on a given day. Variation in the rolled-up clothing under the patient will change the curvature of the spine, and the patient's position is then not precisely reproduced. Having the patient undress for each treatment eliminates these inconsistencies.

Changes in the patient's weight during a course of treatment and changes in swelling or tumor size may cause changes in the position of skin marks with respect to underlying anatomy. New positioning and restraining devices, in addition to resimulation of the treatment fields, may be required to ensure continuous correct patient-beam alignment when weight changes occur. Such changes may also require that the dose calculation to be repeated, as previously described.

The elevation of the patient's arms above the head—routinely practiced for treatment of breast carcinoma. Hodgkin's disease, and lateral or oblique fields in the thorax—must be very carefully reproduced for each treatment session. Positioning devices, such as Alpha Cradles®,* described below, are essential for comfortable and reproducible patient positioning.[58–61]

Elderly patients who are confused and patients with compromised coordination must be strapped to the treatment couch during the treatment and require close supervision via closed-circuit television to prevent serious accidents during the treatment.

As shown in the previous sections, the position of the patient during the radiation treatments is not a trivial matter but requires serious consideration.

PATIENT POSITIONING

The design of older therapy machines often limited the choice of beam orientations (Chap. 2, Fig. 2.13), and it was not unusual, instead, to change the patient's position between treatment fields. For example, an anterior field was treated with the patient in the supine position while the posterior field was treated with the patient in the prone position. Opposed lateral head and neck fields were often treated while the patient was positioned on alternate sides. In both of these situations, the beam was directed vertically toward the floor of the room (i.e., the angle at which the beam was directed at the tumor was changed by altering the patient's position). Conversely, in modern radiation therapy, the patient remains motionless while the radiation source is moved to the desired position. A major development in radiation therapy is the design and manufacture of treatment equipment that make it feasible to direct the beam at the tumor from practically any angle

---

* Smithers Medical Products, Inc., Akron, Ohio.

while the patient remains in the same position on the treatment couch.

It is also recognized that once the position of the target volume with respect to skin marks has been established, the patient's position must remain unchanged to prevent internal structures and skin marks from moving with respect to one another. Even a slight change in the patient's position can cause skin marks to move with respect to the deeper target; thus, the target can be missed when the treatment is set up to the skin marks (Fig. 7.32). Other concerns are the risks of over- or underdosage that can arise as a result of the movement of internal tissues as the patient's position is changed from supine to prone. For example, a given segment of small bowel may be located at middepth in the pelvis when an anterior field is treated with the patient in the supine position, and the same segment of small bowel may be displaced anteriorly when the patient is prone for the treatment of a posterior field. Thus, when the anterior field is treated, the dose is as calculated in the middepth; however, when the posterior field is treated, the dose is lower than calculated because of the increased depth. Thus the bowel receives a dose that is lower than prescribed.

The practice of using a source-surface distance (SSD) technique when multiple fields are treated also gives rise to concern with respect to both the beam position and dose accuracy, even when the patient's position is unchanged. In this technique, the fields are marked on the patient's skin surface and the treatment fields are set up to coincide with the marks. The SSD is adjusted so that it is the same for each field, which requires that the couch be moved in order to navigate the patient to the appropriate beam entry point and SSD.

Using an isocentric technique (source-axis distance, or SAD), where the position of the isocenter is set once during each treatment session (usually in the center of the target), after which the gantry is turned to the appropriate angle, is a much more reliable technique. The dose is also more precise in this technique, because if the distance is slightly longer from one side, causing the dose to be lower, it is compensated for in an opposing field, where the effect is in the opposite direction. In the SSD technique, the dis-

tance can possibly be off in the same direction in all fields, and there would be no countereffect; instead, there would be a cumulative effect.

Comfort.   The first consideration in patient positioning should be patient comfort and safety during the treatments.

A triangular pillow under the patient's knees will relax the back and make the patient feel more comfortable (Fig. 7.50). This position changes the curvature of the lumbar spine and must be reproduced during each treatment.

Most treatment couches are narrow and do not provide a comfortable resting place for the patient's arms. Removable arm supports of thin Plexiglas can be added to the width of the couch (Fig. 7.50). The Plexiglas can be anchored by placing part of it under the patient's body. Such arm supports should be used with caution if the chest is treated, as they may cause patient-beam misalignment. An alternative arrangement is to place a large sheet of Plexiglas, wide enough to extend about 6 in beyond the couch on each side, across the treatment couch under the chest to eliminate patient rotation. The use of arm supports effectively increases the width of the couch and may therefore prevent the head of the machine from clearing when lateral or rotational fields are used.

Allowing the patient to cross the legs will cause marks on the lateral aspect of the pelvis to change

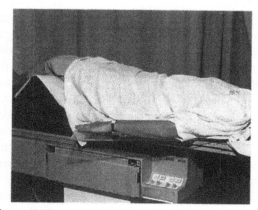

Figure 7.50   Providing patients with some supports—for example, under the knees or under the arms—make them feel more comfortable.

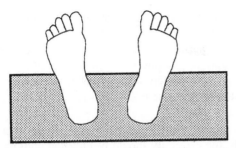

Figure 7.51   A simple device made of Styrofoam can be used to maintain leg separation during the treatment.

with respect to internal anatomy and should therefore be avoided. A rigid support, which fixes the separation of the patient's legs, can be made of Styrofoam. When used for patients being treated to the abdomen, pelvis, and lower extremities, this will help to reproduce the leg position (Fig. 7.51).

General Considerations.   The angle at which the beam impinges on the patient can be set either by changing the orientation of the beam or changing the patient's position with respect to the beam, as previ-

ously explained. In a kyphotic patient, for example, it would be difficult to place the patient in a position such that the axis of the torso is perpendicular to the vertical beam. Instead, the desired patient-beam relationship can be achieved by turning the couch 90° and then turning the gantry until the incident beam is perpendicular to the axis of the patient's torso (Fig. 7.52).

A patient with superior vena cava obstruction may not be able to breathe while lying down and may have to be treated in an upright position. Such patients are often unable to get out of bed and can be treated while in bed, with the head of the bed elevated. Until the patient's condition allows conventional positioning, treatment through a single anterior high-energy photon field may be necessary. A patient sitting in bed may be supported by providing a foot board. This will reduce the risk of the patient slipping down and causing target-beam misalignment. Some patients may also benefit from having a firm support behind the back to maintain their position during the treatment.

Most treatment equipment is designed to facilitate

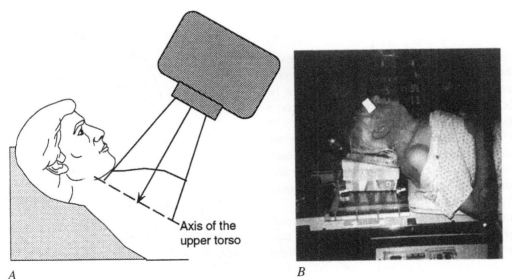

Axis of the upper torso

A   *B*

Figure 7.52   *A* and *B*. The axis of the torso should be perpendicular to the beam. A kyphotic patient may therefore have to be treated with the couch turned 90° and the gantry rotated until the beam is perpendicular to the torso.

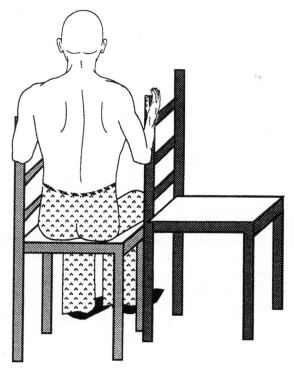

Figure 7.53 A patient who must be treated in a sitting position is better supported if given a second chair to hold onto during the treatment.

to cause the anterior surface of the abdomen to be flattened against the couch top. In most patients, the posterior surface is fairly flat and less mobile than the anterior. This position is therefore preferable for the marking of setup lines, and it improves treatment-field reproducibility. This is discussed in more detail in Chap. 13.

In treating an extremity through parallel opposed fields, the extremity should be elevated until its axis is parallel with the axis of gantry rotation; that is, the extremity should be at right angles to the direction of the beam (Fig. 7.54). With the patient in the supine position and using parallel opposed anterior and posterior fields, the extremity should be horizontal. When oblique opposed beams are used, the center of the extremity should still be parallel with the axis of the gantry rotation, so that the treatment distance to the center of the extremity is the same everywhere within the treated segment.

PATIENT IMMOBILIZATION

Effective immobilization is fundamental to successful radiation therapy when radiosensitive structures

the treatment of patients lying on the treatment couch; therefore treating a sitting patient is not easy. Also, the patient's position is often difficult to reproduce, and normal treatment distances may not be possible. If the patient is able to sit sideways on a chair, both an anterior and a posterior field may be treated without allowing the beam to traverse the chair back. The patient can rest one arm on the back of one chair and the other arm on the back of a second chair placed beside him or her on the opposite side (Fig. 7.53).

In situations where the patient's weight exceeds the tolerance of the treatment couch, the patient may have to be treated either standing or sitting. Under these circumstances, the patient-beam reproducibility is very poor and alternatives should be considered. Other difficulties are the treatment of obese patients. An obese patient may be positioned prone

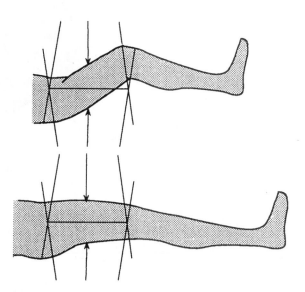

Figure 7.54 An extremity must also be positioned so that the axis is perpendicular to the beam.

are adjacent to the target and when the tumor margins are small. The advantages gained by the ability to conform the fields to the target, as discussed earlier, may be lost by poor immobilization techniques. The need for effective patient immobilization is well recognized, as evidenced by the large number of articles in the literature.[58-74]

The term *immobilized* (meaning incapable of motion) is used loosely in radiation therapy, where it usually refers to a patient placed in some type of positioning device. In this text, as in most other literature, the expression *patient immobilization* is used to describe positioning or stabilization devices used in radiation therapy to aid in patient repositioning.

Certain characteristics are desirable in immobilization devices. One is that they be built from materials that only minimally attenuate the radiation beam. Metal parts may obscure important anatomic reference structures otherwise visualized on radiographs, or they may cause artifacts on CT images, preventing visualization of important information needed in the treatment-planning process. When only a small segment of a radiation beam passes through such attenuating material, including part of an immobilization device, the dose is reduced in only that portion of the radiation field giving rise to dose inhomogeneities across the field. Furthermore, the dose on the skin surface may be increased due to secondary scatter from the metal. Immobilization devices made of plastic materials are therefore preferable, but, depending on the thickness, these may also perturb the radiation beam. Another but less important characteristic is that the device be transparent, to allow visibility of the beam light and the distance indicator. It is also important to have an immobilization device that is light in weight, strong, and durable. The ability to make setup marks on the immobilization device is also desirable, since these marks generally are more reliable than skin marks.

As in all immobilization, it is crucial to secure the part of the body that is being treated and to include at least one joint on each side of this area within the device. For example, when the upper extremity is immobilized, the entire arm and chest should be included; and when immobilizing a breast patient, the chest, arms, head, and hips should be included within

the device. This requires fairly large immobilization devices and consideration may be necessary for storage in the treatment room.

Alpha Cradles. An immobilization system called Alpha Cradles is widely used to aid in the repositioning of patients for radiation therapy. This system consists of Styrofoam forms that roughly match the shape of the part of the patient's body for which they are intended (Fig. 7.55). A foam mixture is used, which—when prepared and used as directed by the supplier—fills the space between the form and the patient's body and becomes a mold. The success of these Alpha Cradles depends to a large extent on the care with which they are made. A description and some helpful hints are therefore given in the following paragraphs.

The patient's position in the Styrofoam form should be tested prior to fabrication of the device. This provides an opportunity to test the anticipated position and to give the patient a chance to feel what it is like to hold the position while lying down in the device. It also helps in making decisions about possible modifications to the form before the foam is prepared. Once the foam is mixed and prepared, there is very little time to make changes to the form or to explain the position to the patient. The amount of foam needed for a given Alpha Cradle can be reduced by filling empty spaces around the patient with pieces of Styrofoam left over from the block-cutting room or from trimming off the Styrofoam form. When the form is ready, it is enclosed in a polyvinyl bag, which is approximately 1 ft wider and 1 ft longer than the Styrofoam form. The contents of the two bottles of foaming agents are mixed and prepared as directed by the supplier. They are then evenly distributed in the form inside the bag. Air is allowed to circulate inside the bag for about 1 min. The air is then forced out and the bag is sealed before the patient returns to the form.

The foam will feel warm to the patient as it expands and sets. It is important to make sure that the foam is forced up against the patient's body while it is expanding. This requires that there be enough space in the bag to allow the foam to expand in the desired direction. The foam, which is very light in

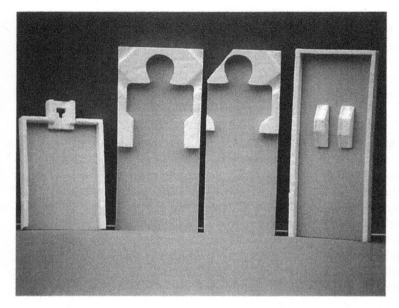

Figure 7.55   Various Styrofoam forms are available for foam molds used in immobilization of patients undergoing radiation therapy. The space between the form and the patient's body is filled with foam, which expands around the patient. From left to right are molds for treatment of craniospinal axes, Hodgkin's disease, breast, and pelvis. (Courtesy of Smithers Medical Products, Inc.)

weight, will expand in the direction of least resistance. It therefore has a tendency to move away from the patient and must be guided toward the patient. This can be achieved in different ways. For example, a tape can be attached to one side of the Alpha Cradle and then be stretched tightly across to the opposite side, forcing the two sides together toward the patient. When the bag is too small or there is too much foam, resulting in insufficient space for the foam to expand, the foam will displace the patient instead of forming a mold around the patient's body. The foam can be redistributed while it is still soft by guiding it from places with too much to places with less foam. It will then harden and begin to cool within 5 to 10 min.

Patients should always be asked to think about how it feels to lie in the finished Alpha Cradle, so that when they return for future simulation and treatment, they can twist and turn until the position feels the same. Setup marks are made on the Alpha Cradle and on the patient's skin. However, marks made on the immobilization device are considered more reliable than skin marks, since skin marks tends to move over deeper tissues. In the majority of patients immobilized in an Alpha Cradle at Duke University Medical Center, the device is made long enough to allow alignment marks to be made both above the head and between the knees, or a long line is made from between the feet to between the thighs as well as on each side of the patient's torso. Realigning the patient with these marks for each treatment assures that the patient is positioned correctly on the couch before the isocenter is setup.

Styrofoam forms are available for different parts of the body or can be built to suit the need for each patient. Forms for breast patients are available with an opening for the elevated arm on the affected side. Some are designed so that they fit better through the opening of the CT aperture; however, when a large patient is scanned, the finished Alpha Cradle may need more trimming off of excess foam. Alpha Cradles consist primarily of lightweight foam; thus, treatment through the material, using linear accelerators, has little effect on the beam.[75]

The setups are more reproducible when these immobilization devices are used, thus the need for field shifts and repeat port films is reduced. Customized positioning devices, such as Alpha Cradles, also help patients to feel secure while laying alone on a narrow couch in the treatment room. Similar immobilization systems are available on the market. One system uses bags of different shapes and sizes that are filled with small polyurethane spheres. The patient is placed on the bag and the contents are forced toward the patient's body, the air is then evacuated, causing the device to assume the shape of the patient and to harden. These bags are reusable, thus requiring cleaning and removal of setup marks between patients.

A more detailed description of immobilization as it applies to each anatomic area can be found in the appropriate chapters.

PROBLEMS

7.1 The term *gross tumor volume,* as defined by ICRU, means
   (a) The tissues that are to be irradiated to a specified dose according to a specified time-dose pattern
   (b) The gross palpable or visible/demonstrable tumor extent to be irradiated to a specified dose
   (c) The gross palpable or visible/demonstrable tumor extent and location of malignant growth
   (d) The tissues that are to be irradiated

7.2 The term *clinical target volume,* as defined by the ICRU, means
   (a) A tissue volume that contains a demonstrable GTV and/or subclinical microscopic malignant disease, which has to be eliminated
   (b) The gross palpable or visible/demonstrable tumor extent and location of malignant growth
   (c) The primary tumor, metastatic lymphadenopathy, or other metastasis
   (d) The tissues that are to be irradiated to a specified dose according to a specified time-dose pattern

7.3 The field size when using an SSD technique and a photon beam is usually defined
   (a) On the skin surface
   (b) Where the beam exits the patient
   (c) At the block tray distance
   (d) At the rotational axis of the machine

7.4 The angle of beam divergence is
   (a) The same within the field
   (b) Larger farther from the central axis
   (c) Largest on the central axis
   (d) Smaller farther from the central axis

7.5 When parallel opposed fields are used and the isocenter is at middepth in the chest, the length of the spinal cord is
   (a) The same in both fields
   (b) Longer in the posterior field than in the anterior
   (c) Shorter in the anterior field than in the posterior
   (d) Longer in the anterior field than in the posterior

7.6 When parallel opposed fields are used and the isocenter is at middepth in the chest,
   (a) The anterior port film should appear exactly as the anterior simulation film with respect to the anatomy

(b) The anterior port film should appear exactly as the posterior simulation film with respect to the anatomy

(c) The posterior port film should appear exactly as the anterior simulation film with respect to the anatomy

(d) The anterior and the posterior port films should appear to be identical with respect to the anatomy

7.7   The size of a magnification device is

(a) Totally unimportant

(b) Important because a large device is more likely to lead to errors in the magnification factor

(c) Important because a small device is more likely to lead to errors in the magnification factor

(d) Important because a small device is much more accurate than a large device

7.8   A circular magnification device, which is 5 cm in diameter, is placed on the patient's anterior surface where the SSD is 100 cm. The simulation film is at 135 cm from the target (TFD). The magnification of the device is

(a) 1.35

(b) 1.00

(c) 1.40

(d) 1.25

7.9   A three-dimensional coordinate system is used in radiation therapy to describe a point in the patient with respect to a known point (the origin). A point described as $+2$ cm on the y-axis would be located

(a) 2 cm to the patients right side from the origin

(b) 2 cm cephalad of the origin

(c) 2 cm caudal of the origin

(d) 2 cm posterior of the origin

7.10   The gantry rotates around a horizontal axis which is

(a) Parallel with the collimator rotation

(b) Parallel with the x-axis of the patient when he is supine on the couch and the couch position is $0°$

(c) Parallel with the normal couch position

(d) Parallel with the couch motion in the $70°$ position

7.11   The three planes in a patient are across the body, along the body in a lateral view, and along the body in an anterior view. Respectively, they are referred to as

(a) Axial, coronal, and sagittal

(b) Coronal, axial, and sagittal

(c) Axial, sagittal, and coronal

(d) Sagittal, axial, and coronal

7.12   When a patient is realigned with a laser alignment system,

(a) It is necessary to align three points indicating the isocenter

(b) It is necessary to align the marks on the anterior skin surface

(c) It is necessary to align the lateral marks

(d) It is necessary to align two points separated by a long distance

7.13   A treatment-planning CT scan is different from a diagnostic CT scan because
  (a) In a treatment planning CT scan, the patient's position must always be with the arms above the head
  (b) In a treatment planning CT scan, the patient must be in treatment position on a flat surface
  (c) In a treatment planning CT scan, the patient is never given contrast
  (d) In a treatment planning CT scan, the patient must be supine on a flat surface

7.14   A contour of a patient taken for calculating an isodose distribution
  (a) Must be accurate because it has an effect on the dose
  (b) Must represent the patient's shape, but the size is not important
  (c) Must represent the size of the patient, but the shape is not important
  (d) Does not have to be accurate because it has no effect on the dose

7.15   The anterior and posterior skin surfaces seen on a lateral radiograph of a patient's pelvis
  (a) Truly represent the largest diameter of the pelvis in the anterior-posterior direction
  (b) Does not represent the patient's skin surface in the midline
  (c) Represent the patient's skin surface in the midline
  (d) The posterior skin surface cannot always be seen but the distance from the tabletop to the anterior skin surface represents the patient's midline diameter in the anterior-posterior direction

7.16   When the location of a contrast-filled bladder is transposed from a set of orthogonal radiographs (anterior and lateral) to a transverse contour of the pelvis,
  (a) The anterior film yields information in the anterior/posterior directions and the lateral film yields information in the cephalad/caudal directions
  (b) The anterior film yields information in the cephalad/caudal directions and the lateral film yields information in the right/left directions
  (c) The anterior film yields information in the right/left and cephalad/caudal directions and the lateral film yields information in the anterior/posterior and cephalad/caudal directions
  (d) The anterior film yields information in the anterior/posterior and cephalad/caudal directions and the lateral film yields information in the right/left and cephalad/caudal direction

7.17   Discrepancies in the patient/beam alignment between the first port film and the simulation film may be due to
  (a) Differences in laser alignment systems, difference in clothing under the patient, and weight gain
  (b) Differences in laser alignment systems, different couch tops, and difference in clothing under the patient
  (c) Differences in couch tops, difference in clothing under the patient, and different technologists treating the patient
  (d) Differences in laser alignment systems, different couch tops, respiration

7.18   Uncertainties associated with delivering radiation therapy can be totally avoided by
  (a) Having the same technologists treat each patient, daily machine calibration, and using vigorous patient immobilization
  (b) Having the same physicist calibrate the machine daily, using vigorous patient immobilization, and taking port films of each field daily

(c) Daily machine calibration, vigorous patient immobilization, and using CT for treatment planning of all patients

(d) No special means, since there is no method by which all uncertainties can be avoided

7.19 When the treatment fields are designed by the radiation oncologist, margins are always added around a tumor because of

(a) Uncertainties in determining the tumor extent, penumbra of the beam, and patient motion

(b) Uncertainties in the penumbra of the beam, patient motion, and changes due to weight gain during the course of treatment

(c) Uncertainties in determining the tumor extent, patient motion, and changes of the tumor during the course of treatment

(d) Uncertainties in the penumbra of the beam, respiration, and weight gain during the course of treatment

7.20 When an 0.5-cm margin is added to all sides of a 15×15 cm field, the added area is

(a) 15 cm^2

(b) 25 cm^2

(c) 31 cm^2

(d) 21.5 cm^2

REFERENCES

1. ICRU: Prescribing, recording, and reporting photon beam therapy. Washington, DC: International Commission on Radiation Units and Measurements, 1993.

2. Prasad SC, Bassano DA: Corner transmission in several linear accelerator photon beams. *Med Phys* 18:763, 1991.

3. Bentel GC: Laser repositioning in radiation oncology. *Appl Radiol* 13:24, 1984.

4. Fraass BA, McShan DL: 3-D treatment planning: Overview of a clinical planning system, in Bruinvis IAD, Van Der Giessen PH, Van Kleffens HJ, Wittkamper FW (eds): *The use of Computers in Radiation Therapy.* North Holland: Elsevier, 1987.

5. Goitein M, Abrams M, Rowell D, et al: Multi-dimensional treatment planning: II. Beam's-eye view back projection, and projection through CT sections. *Int J Radiat Oncol Biol Phys* 9:789, 1983.

6. Goitein M, Abrams M: Multi-dimensional treatment planning: I. Delineation of anatomy. *Int J Radiat Oncol Biol Phys* 9:777, 1983.

7. McShan DL, Fraass BA, Lichter AS: Full integration of the beam's-eye view concept into computerized treatment planning. *Int J Radiat Oncol Biol Phys* 18:1485, 1990.

8. Mohan R, Barest G, Brewster LJ, et al: A comprehensive three-dimensional radiation treatment planning system. *Int J Radiat Oncol Biol Phys* 15:481, 1988.

9. Reinstein LE, McShan D, Webber BM, Glicksman AS: A computer-assisted three-dimensional treatment planning system. *Radiology* 127:259, 1978.

10. Rosenman J, Sherouse GW, Fuchs H, et al: Three-dimensional display techniques in radiation therapy treatment planning. *Int J Radiat Oncol Biol Phys* 16:263, 1989.

11. Sherouse GW, Bourland JD, Reynolds K, et al: Virtual simulator in the clinical setting: Some practical considerations. *Int J Radiat Oncol Biol Phys* 19:1059, 1990.

12. Sherouse GW, Chaney EL: The portable virtual simulator. *Int J Radiat Oncol Biol Phys* 21:475, 1991.

13. McCullough EC, McCullough KP: Improving agreement between radiation-delineated field edges on simulation and portal films: The edge tolerance test tool. *Med Phys* 20:375, 1993.

14. Sherouse GW, Novins K, Chaney LE: Computation of digitally reconstructed radiographs for use in radiotherapy treatment design. *Int J Radiat Oncol Biol Phys* 18:651, 1990.

15. Hudson FR: A simple isocenter checking procedure for radiotherapy treatment machines using the optical pointer. *Med Phys* 15:72, 1988.

16. Lutz WR, Larsen RD, Bjärngard BE: Beam alignment tests for therapy accelerators. *Int J Radiat Oncol Biol Phys* 7:1727, 1981.

17. Goitein M: Calculation of the uncertainty in the dose delivery during radiation therapy. *Med Phys* 12:608, 1985.

18. Svensson GK: Quality assurance in radiation therapy: Physics efforts. *Int J Radiat Oncol Biol Phys* 10(suppl 1): 23, 1984.

19. Byhardt RW, Cox JD, Hornburg A, Liermann G: Weekly localization films and detection of field placement errors. *Int J Radiat Oncol Biol Phys* 4:881, 1978.

20. Rabinowitz I, Broomberg J, Goitein M, et al: Accuracy of radiation field alignment in clinical practice. *Int J Radiat Oncol Biol Phys* 11:1857, 1985.

21. Rosenthal SA, Galvin JM, Goldwein JW, et al: Improved methods for determination of variability in patient positioning for radiation therapy using simulation and serial portal film measurements. *Int J Radiat Oncol Biol Phys* 23:621, 1992.

22. AAPM: *AAPM Report No. 24: Radiotherapy Portal Imaging Quality.* New York: American Institute of Physics, 1987.

23. Suit HD: Potential for improving survival rates for the cancer patient by increasing the efficacy of treatment of the primary lesion. *Cancer* 50:1227, 1982.

24. Suit HD, Westgate SJ: Impact of improved local control on survival. *Int J Radiat Oncol Biol Phys* 12:453, 1986.

25. Suit HD, duBois W: The importance of optimal treatment planning in radiation therapy. *Int J Radiat Oncol Biol Phys* 21:1471, 1991.

26. Foo ML, McCullough EC, Foote RL, et al: Doses to radiation sensitive organs and structures located outside the radiotherapeutic target volume for four treatment situations. *Int J Radiat Oncol Biol Phys* 27:403, 1993.

27. Daftari I, Petti PL, Collier JM, et al: The effect of patient motion on dose uncertainty in charged particle irradiation for lesions encircling the brain stem and spinal cord. *Med Phys* 18:1105, 1991.

28. Hendrickson FR: Precision in radiation oncology. *Int J Radiat Oncol Biol Phys* 8:311, 1982.

29. Herring DF, Compton DMJ: The degree of precision required in radiation dose delivered in cancer radiotherapy, in Glicksman AJ, Cohen M, Cunningham JR (eds): *Computers in Radiotherapy.* Br J Radiol Special Report Series No. 5, 1971.

30. Herring DF: The consequences of dose response curves for tumor control and normal tissue injury on the precision necessary in patient management. *Laryngoscope* 85:1112, 1975.

31. Mijnheer BJ, Batterman JJ, Wambersie A: What degree of accuracy is required and can be achieved in photon and neutron therapy. *Radiother Oncol* 8:237, 1987.

32. Shukovsky LJ: Dose, time, volume relationships in squamous cell carcinoma of the supraglottic larynx. *Am J Roentgenol* 108:27, 1970.

33. Stewart JG, Jackson AW: The steepness of the dose response curve both for tumor cure and normal tissue injury. *Laryngoscope* 85:1107, 1975.

34. Wambersie A, Dutreix J, Dutreix A: Precision dosimetrique requise en radiotherapie: Consequences concernant le choix et les performances exigees des detecteurs. *J Belge Radiol* 52:94, 1969.

35. ICRU: *Determination of Absorbed Dose in a Patient Irradiated by Beams of X- or Gamma-Rays in Radiotherapy Procedures.* Washington DC: International Commission on Radiation Units and Measurements, 1976.

36. Brahme A: Dosimetric precision requirements in radiation therapy. *Acta Radiol Oncol* 23:379, 1984.

37. Goitein M: Nonstandard deviations. *Med Phys* 10:709, 1983.

38. Rassow J: Quality control of radiation therapy equipment. *Radiother Oncol* 12:45, 1988.

39. Cunningham JR: Development of computer algorithms for radiation treatment planning. *Int J Radiat Oncol Biol Phys* 16:1367, 1989.

40. Ding GX, Shalev S, Gluchey G: A ρ θ technique for treatment verification in radiotherapy and its clinical applications. *Med Phys* 20:1135, 1993.

41. Dutreix A: Keynote address: Prescription, precision and decision in treatment planning. *Int J Radiat Oncol Biol Phys* 13:1291, 1987.

42. El-Gayed AAH, Bel A, Vijbrief R, et al: Time trend of patient setup deviations during pelvic irradiation using electronic portal imaging. *Radiother Oncol* 26:162, 1993.

43. Gall KP, Verhey LJ: Computer-assisted positioning of radiotherapy patients using implanted radiopaque fiducials. *Med Phys* 20:1153, 1993.

44. Goitein M, Busse J: Immobilization error: Some theoretical considerations. *Radiology* 117:407, 1975.

45. Griffiths SE, Pearcey RG, Thorogood J: Quality control in radiotherapy: The reduction of field placement errors. *Int J Radiat Oncol Biol Phys* 13:1583, 1987.

46. Huizenga H, Levendag PC, DePorre PMZR: Accuracy in radiation field alignment in head and neck cancers: A prospective study. *Radiother Oncol* 11:181, 1988.

47. Kihlén B, Rudén B-I: Reproducibility of field alignment in radiation therapy. *Acta Oncol* 28:689, 1989.

48. Kligerman MM, Hogstrom KR, Lane RG, Somers JW: Prior immobilization and positioning for more efficient radiotherapy. *Int J Radiat Oncol Biol Phys* 2:1141, 1977.

49. Lam KL, TenHaken RK, McShan DL, Thornton AF: Automated determination of patient setup errors in radiation therapy using spherical radio-opaque markers. *Med Phys* 20:1145, 1993.

50. Leong J, Shimm D: A method for consistent precision radiation therapy. *Radiother Oncol* 3:89, 1985.

51. Marks JE, Haus AG, Sutton HG, Griem ML: Localization error in the radiotherapy of Hodgkin's disease and malignant lymphoma with extended mantle fields. *Cancer* 34:83, 1974.

52. Marks JE, Haus AG: The effect of immobilization on localization error in the radiotherapy of head and neck cancer. *Clin Radiol* 27:175, 1976.

53. Pearcey RG, Griffiths SE: An investigation into the daily reproducibility of patient positioning for "mantle" treatments. *Clin Radiol* 37:43, 1986.

54. Tatsuzaki H, Urie M: Importance of precise positioning for proton beam therapy in the base of skull and cervical spine. *Int J Radiat Oncol Biol Phys* 21:757, 1991.

55. Verhey LJ, Goitein M, McNulty P, Munzenrider JE, Suit HD: Precise positioning of patients for radiation therapy. *Int J Radiat Oncol Biol Phys* 2:289, 1982.

56. Creutzberg AL, Althog VG, Huizenga H, Visser AG: Quality assurance using portal imaging: The accuracy of patient positioning in irradiation of breast cancer. *Int J Radiat Oncol Biol Phys* 25:529, 1993.

57. Griffith SE, Khoury GG, Eddy A: Quality control of radiotherapy during pelvic irradiation. *Radiother Oncol* 20:103, 1991.

58. Bentel GC: Positioning and immobilization device for patients receiving radiation therapy for carcinoma of the breast. *Med Dosim* 15:3, 1990.

59. Bentel GC: Positioning and immobilization of patients undergoing radiation therapy for Hodgkin's disease. *Med Dosim* 16:111, 1991.

60. Bentel GC, Marks LB, Sherouse GW, et al: The effectiveness of immobilization during prostate irradiation. *Int J Radiat Oncol Biol Phys* 31:143, 1995.

61. Bentel GC, Marks LB, Sherouse GW, Spencer DP: Customized head immobilization system. *Int J Radiat Oncol Biol Phys* 32:245, 1995.

62. Barish RJ, Lerch IA: Patient immobilization with low-temperature splint/brace material. *Radiology* 127:548, 1978.

63. Devereux C, Grundy G, Littman P: Plastic molds for patient immobilization. *Int J Radiat Oncol Biol Phys* 1:553, 1976.

64. Gerber RL, Marks JE, Purdy JA: The use of thermal plastics for immobilization of patients during radiotherapy. *Int J Radiat Oncol Biol Phys* 8:1461, 1982.

65. Goldson AL, Young J, Espinoza MC, Henschke UK: Simple but sophisticated immobilization casts. *Int J Radiat Oncol Biol Phys* 4:1105, 1978.

66. Hauskins LA, Thompson RW: Patient positioning device for external-beam radiation therapy of the head and neck. *Radiology* 106:706, 1973.

67. Jones D, Hafermann MD: A radiolucent bite-block apparatus. *Int J Radiat Oncol Biol Phys* 13:129, 1987.

68. Kooy HM, Dunbar SF, Tarbell NJ, et al: Adaptation and verification of the relocatable Gill-Thomas-Cosman frame in stereotactic radiotherapy. *Int J Radiat Oncol Biol Phys* 30:685, 1994.

69. Landberg T, Swahn-Tapper G, Bengtsson CG: Whole body casts for patient immobilization in mantle treatment, treatment of the inverted Y and moving strip. *Int J Radiat Oncol Biol Phys* 2:809, 1977.

70. Schlegel W, Pastyr O, Bortfeld T, et al: Computer systems and mechanical tools for stereotactically guided conformation therapy with linear accelerators. *Int J Radiat Oncol Biol Phys* 24:781, 1992.

71. Sørenson NE, Sell A: Immobilization, compensation and field shaping in megavoltage therapy. *Acta Radiol Ther Biol Phys* 11:129, 1972.

72. Thornton AF, TenHaken RK, Weeks KJ, et al: A head immobilization system for radiation simulation, CT, MRI, and PET imaging. *Med Dosim* 16:51, 1991.

73. van de Geijn J, Harrington FS, Lichter AS, Glatstein E: Simplified bite-block immobilization of the head. *Radiology* 149:851, 1983.

74. Wang CC, Boyer A, Dosoretz D: A head holder for treatment of head and neck cancers. *Int J Radiat Oncol Biol Phys* 6:95, 1980.

75. Mondalek PM, Orton CG: Transmission and build-up characteristics of polyurethane-foam immobilization devices. *Medical Dosimetry* 7:5, 1982.

Treatment Preparation—II: Beam-Modifying Devices and Quality Assurance

BEAM-MODIFYING DEVICES

FIELD SHAPING: PHOTON BEAMS

As previously discussed, it is often necessary to modify the shape of the square or rectangular radiation field as it exits the collimator so that it conforms to the shape of the target. Prior to 1980, irregularly shaped photon therapy fields were commonly defined by multiple lead bricks arranged on a tray inserted in the collimator or on a coffee-table-type cart wheeled in across the patient in the path of the beam.

In the first arrangement, the blocks were at a fixed distance in the beam and the tray was fixed with respect to the beam. In the second arrangement, the height of the table above the patient could be changed, thus changing the target-to-tray distance and consequently also the size of the block shadow on the patient. The blocks were not fixed with respect to the beam or the patient (Fig. 8.1). In this context, it is important to realize that optimally, the beam, patient, and any devices between them should be fixed with respect to one another. In Fig. 8.1A, the

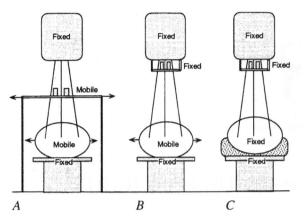

A   *B*   *C*

Figure 8.1 *A.* When beam-shaping blocks are placed on a coffee-table–like cart over the patient, the blocks are not fixed with respect to either the beam, the patient, or the couch. Misalignments could easily occur. *B.* When the blocks are fixed with respect to the beam, the risk of misalignment is reduced. Ideally, both the patient and the blocks should be fixed with respect to the beam *C*, but unfortunately, due to patient motion, that is not always possible.

vertently blocking tumor-bearing areas (Chap. 7, Fig. 7.48). Furthermore, reproducing the shape of the field from day to day was a tedious task even when templates, placed on the tray, were used. In some departments, blocks for mantle fields were milled out of lead to resemble the shape of the lungs, and the same blocks were used for all patients. To adjust for the difference in size of the lungs from one patient to the next, the blocks were placed at different distances in the beam by changing the height of the coffee-table-type cart. This cart was used to support the blocks for many types of fields requiring complex blocking.

Neither of the two arrangements discussed above allowed any gantry angle other than that for a vertical beam. A gantry rotation would cause the blocks, stacked on a tray fixed to the collimator, to fall off, with obvious consequences (Fig. 8.3A). In the case of blocks on the coffee table, a gantry angle would

beam is fixed only with respect to the treatment couch, while the patient and the blocking arrangement are mobile.

In Fig. 8.1*B*, the blocks are fixed with respect to the beam and the couch while the patient is mobile, and in Fig. 8.1*C*, the beam, blocks, and patient are fixed. This is, of course, an idealized situation, since there is always some patient motion that we cannot totally avoid. Figure 8.2 represents a common arrangement where a customized block is fixed on a tray that is secured in the collimator. The field outline on the port film placed in the exit beam is always the same; however, the position of the patient relative to the outline may vary depending on patient motion and accuracy of the setup.

The lead bricks were usually square or rectangular with vertical edges and with a 5-half-value thickness (HVT), transmitting about 3 percent of the dose. Even when these bricks were stacked in two tiers, the desired field shape was difficult to achieve and the weight was excessive. Shielding the lungs in a mantle field was very difficult because the blocks rarely projected the shape or size of the lungs. It was difficult to shield normal lung tissue without also inad-

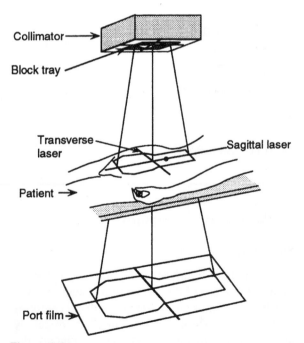

Figure 8.2 With the beam-shaping blocks fixed on a tray that is fixed in the beam, the shape of the treatment field is reproduced during every treatment. Misalignments between the beam and the patient can be observed on port films.

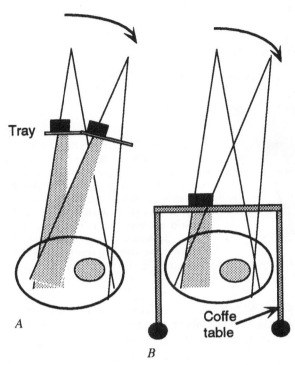

Tray

Coffe table

A

B

Figure 8.3 *A.* Beam-shaping blocks loosely placed on a tray that is fixed in the collimator would fall off the tray when the gantry was angled. *B.* Blocks placed on a coffee-table–like cart over the patient would not fall when the gantry was angled but the beam shape would change and the beam would not pass through full thickness of the blocks.

cause the beam to pass through the blocks obliquely rather than through the 5-HVT, and the field shape would be changed (Fig. 8.3*B*). In later years, lead bricks that could be fastened onto the tray were introduced, allowing gantry angles to be used while maintaining the field shape.

In Fig. 8.3*A*, the field-shaping blocks are loosely placed on a tray that is fixed with respect to the beam. A gantry angle will cause the blocks to move or fall off unless they are fixed to the tray. In Fig. 8.3*B*, field-shaping blocks on a coffee-table-type cart have been added in the beam. A gantry angle will cause the field to change shape because the beam-block relationship is disturbed.

Independent Collimator Leaves. In supervoltage therapy machines, the treatment field is de-

fined by two pairs of secondary collimator leaves arranged symmetrically with respect to the central axis of the beam (Chap. 2). Some linear accelerators are built to offer the option of moving one or all four leaves independently. In some treatment setups, beam divergence must be avoided—for example, when matching field margins of an anterior supraclavicular field with tangential breast fields. In these situations, the central axis of the field is placed at the cephalad edge of the tangential fields and the caudal half of the field is then blocked using a half-beam block (HBB). A universal HBB can be used in most situations; however, when the open half of the field requires additional shielding adjacent to the HBB, a custom-made shield is necessary, since placing two blocks adjacent to one another will result in "leakage" between them. It is therefore necessary to produce individualized shielding blocks for each patient. These blocks, which shield half of the beam and provide the additional shielding desired, can be quite heavy and cumbersome. The ability to close in the collimator leaf to the central axis on one side of the field would eliminate the HBB, and additional shielding can still be accomplished. In machines where only one leaf can be moved independently, a collimator rotation may be necessary in order to move that leaf to the side of the field where the field reduction is needed. This creates a problem when a wedge is used in the beam, since wedges usually fit into the beam in a fixed position. Machines where all four collimator leaves can be moved independently provide more flexibility both in terms of closing in more than one collimator leaf simultaneously and in combining wedges with independently moving leaves. Of course, recording of the field size becomes more complex because the setting of each separate leaf is necessary for each field. Even in two opposing fields, the setting will be different, because when the gantry angle is changed by 180°, the right and left leaves (with respect to the normal position of the patient on the couch) will be reversed.

In some situations, it may be desirable to enable the independent leaf to travel across the central axis of the field, thus causing more than half of the "regular" field to be untreated (Fig. 8.4). When this type of setup is used, one must consider the change in the

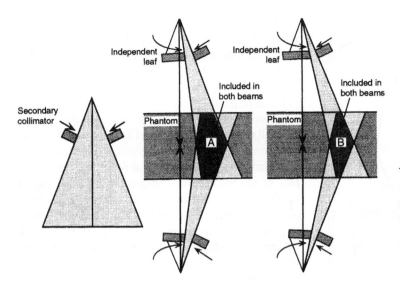

Figure 8.4 When independent collimator jaws are closed across the central axis of the beam, the beam divergence changes, so that both field edges diverge in the same direction but at different angles. When the fields are opposed, the area included within both fields is largest at middepth (A) but becomes smaller closer to the surface. When the collimator jaw is closed farther across the central axis (B), the area closer to the surface is further decreased.

''normal'' beam divergence, both in terms of opposing the fields and in matching of adjacent fields (Chap. 6). In Fig. 8.4, both field margins are diverging in the same, not the opposite direction, as in the ''normal'' beam divergence. When the independent jaw is set past the central axis of the beam, the divergence is similar to that shown in Chap. 7, Figs. 7.9 to 7.12. It is also important to consider the effect on the dose when independent collimator leaves are used to shape the field.[1-7]

Customized Beam-Shaping Blocks. Although several less cumbersome systems of field shaping were tried in the 1960s and early 1970s,[8-14] the most successful one was introduced by Powers *et al.* in 1973.[15] This technique, which eliminates many of the difficulties associated with the stacking of lead bricks above the patient, has been so successful that it is now routinely used in practically every radiation therapy department in the United States and in many other countries. In this system, a low-melting-point alloy—known in the United States as Lipowitz metal* (Cerrobend®, Ostalloy®, or Wood's metals®™)—is used. This alloy, which melts at about 70°C, consists of 50 percent bismuth, 26.7 percent lead, 13.3 percent tin, and 10 percent cadmium. The attenuation capability of this alloy is about 85 percent of lead density, meaning that these blocks must be about 15 percent thicker than lead blocks to produce the same attenuation. For megavoltage photon beams, the blocks must be about 7.5 cm thick to reduce the transmission to about 3 percent.

Block Fabrication.   The shape of the shields is formed by using a block-cutting machine in which the treatment geometry can be mimicked. The distance between the target, the blocking tray, and the radiograph from which the shield is formed can be adjusted to match that of practically any treatment situation. A typical block-cutting machine is shown in Fig. 8.5. The block-cutting device consists of a light box placed horizontally at comfortable working height. A rigid vertical arm, attached to a swivel joint, has a segment consisting of a nichrome wire, which becomes hot when an electric current is turned on. The stability of the arm along the nichrome wire is maintained by two C bars. The lower end of the vertical arm has a pointed Teflon®† stylus that is used to trace the shape of the shielding block. The swivel joint holding the vertical arm is connected via a horizontal bar to a strong vertical column at the back of the device. This column is marked with a centimeter scale, and the swivel joint—representing

---

* Brand name: Cerrobend, Cerro Metal Products, Bellefonte, PA.

† Dupont, Wilmington, DE.

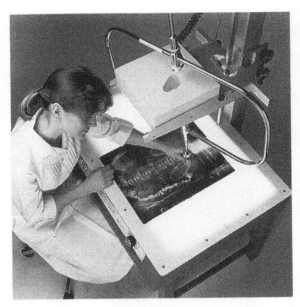

Figure 8.5. A typical block-cutting apparatus. (Courtesy of Huestis Machine Corporation.)

the target in the geometric arrangement—can be raised or lowered to mimic the target-to-film distance (TFD). Also attached to the back column are two horizontal bars which support a block of Styrofoam®*, from which the shape of the shielding block is formed. These bars can also be raised and lowered to mimic the target-to-tray distance (TTD) in the beam.

The shape of the shielding blocks is indicated on a radiograph, usually a simulation film, exposed with the same geometric arrangement as that which will be used in the treatment. The shield can also be produced from a template indicating the central axis of the beam. The radiograph or the template, with a known TFD, is fastened on the light box so that the beam central-axis mark coincides with the cross-hair marking the point at which the Teflon stylus of the vertical arm is in fact vertical. The orientation of the radiograph should be in the beam's-eye view (BEV), so that when the shield is mounted in the beam, the orientation is correct. A Styrofoam block of the same

* Registered trade name by Dow Chemical, Midland, MI.

thickness as the desired shield is then placed on the two horizontal bars. The Styrofoam block must be positioned so that its side is parallel with the collimator lines on the radiograph or template that indicates the collimated field margins. The swivel joint is raised until it corresponds to the TFD at which the radiograph was exposed, and the Styrofoam block is raised or lowered until its position corresponds to the TTD.

The electric current is turned on through the nichrome wire and, as the Teflon stylus is moved in to the point marking the central axis of the beam, the hot nichrome wire melts the Styrofoam and cuts it. The outline of the shield, as it is marked on the radiograph, is slowly traced with the stylus. The hot nichrome wire will cut through the Styrofoam block, cutting out pieces of Styrofoam that match the shape of the desired shields and with sides that follow the beam divergence. The pieces of Styrofoam that represent the shielding blocks are removed from the Styrofoam block and discarded, leaving openings that are later filled with the alloy (Fig. 8.6A). The size of the cavities in the Styrofoam block are obviously much smaller than the blocks marked on the radiograph, because the blocks will be mounted closer to the target. It is very important throughout this process that the central axis of the beam and the orientation of the Styrofoam block with respect to the patient be clearly marked and labeled.

The Styrofoam block is fastened to a plastic tray with a crosshair indicating the central axis. The crosshair indicated on the Styrofoam is aligned precisely with the central axis mark on the tray, and the orientation of the Styrofoam on the tray must match that of the field indicated on the radiograph. Normally, by mounting the Styrofoam block tightly on the two horizontal bars on the block-cutting equipment, the sides of the Styrofoam block are parallel with the beam crosshair. These alignments must be verified intermittently on the block-cutting equipment to assure continuous alignment. It is usually the practice to mount the shielding blocks so that the beam passes through the shields before passing through the tray (i.e., the shielding blocks are fastened on top of the tray). The Styrofoam block is secured to the tray and the assembly is placed on a

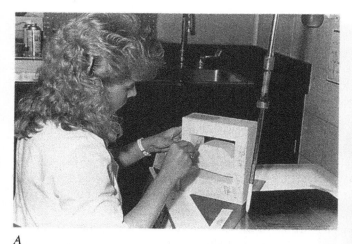

A

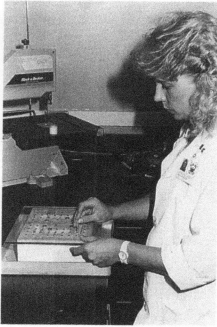

B

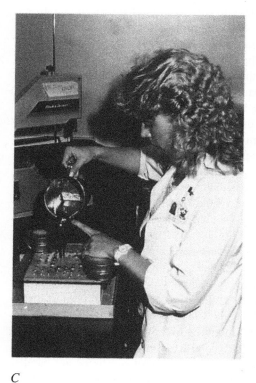

C

Figure 8.6 *A.* The opening where the hot wire entered the Styrofoam is sealed by tape to prevent leaks. *B.* A tray is attached to the Styrofoam by pushing nails through holes in the tray into the Styrofoam. *C.* The melted alloy is poured into the cavities left by the Styrofoam through small holes in the tray.

cooling plate (Fig. 8.6*B*). It is necessary to weigh down the Styrofoam to prevent it from floating, since it is much lighter than the alloy. The cavities can be sprayed with a silicone release formula prior to pouring the alloy. This makes separation of the fin- ished shield and the Styrofoam easier. The alloy is poured through small holes in the tray, filling the cavities in the Styrofoam block (Fig. 8.6*C*). It is nec- essary to pour the alloy slowly to prevent air bubbles from forming in the shield. Several screws are then inserted into the liquid alloy through small holes in the tray (Fig. 8.6*B*). These screws will secure the shields to the tray throughout the course of treatment. At least two screws must be inserted into each of the shields to prevent the block from turning around a single screw; also, one screw may not be strong enough to hold the heavy block.

After approximately 2 h, the alloy is hard and cool and can be removed from the Styrofoam (Fig. 8.7). With the block removed from the tray, sharp edges or corners that may have formed during the cooling process are filed off and the dust is wiped off the tray and the shields. It is also important to inspect the tray carefully to make sure that no alloy has inadvertently spilled onto the tray anywhere inside the radiation field, causing perturbation of the radiation. A light source on the block-cutting machine, mounted so that it can be moved into the position of the swivel point (representing the beam source), is turned on to verify the shape and mounting of the blocks on the tray.[16] The radiograph or template from which the blocks were produced is secured again on the light box and the tray holding the finished blocks is placed on the two arms where the Styrofoam was placed earlier. The target-to-film and target-to-tray dis-

tances are verified. When the light source is turned on, the shadow of the blocks should match that of the blocks traced on the radiograph. When the tray is inserted correctly into the collimator of the therapy machine, the radiation field is projected precisely as outlined on the radiograph. The size and shape of the cavities can also be verified prior to pouring the alloy by painting the inside walls of the cavities with barium and then inserting the tray with the Styrofoam block at the appropriate distance in the collimator of the simulator.[17] This can be done with or without the patient present. The ultimate confirmation of the accuracy of the blocks is a port film with the blocks in place. This will assure not only that the block is producing the correct field shape and size but also that it is aligned correctly with the patient.

More recently, a computer-driven block-cutting device has become available.[18] The shapes of the desired shields are either digitized or electronically transmitted from the treatment-planning system into a computer that operates a wire cutter which will cut out the desired cavities in a block of Styrofoam. This system can be used to produce shielding blocks for both photon and electron beams.

Safety. The potential hazards of working in a mold room where alloy shields are made consist primarily of inhalation of vapors and dust particles, ingestion of small fragments of the metal, skin penetration, and burns.

The risk of inhaling vapors from the melted alloy, primarily lead and cadmium, has been an area of concern. As a result, some hospitals have elected to install a special exhaust system in the block fabrication rooms. Many users have surveyed the work areas where block making takes place and have found that the measured air concentration generally is well below the permissible exposure limit (PEL) established by the Occupational Safety and Health Administration (OSHA).[19–21] The PEL established by OSHA is 5 μg/m^3 of air for cadmium[22] and 50 μg/m^3 of air for lead[23] averaged over an 8-h work period. Regular testing of air concentrations of these metals in the mold room along with monitoring of employees' blood levels is required.

The melting point (158°F or 70°C) of the alloy used in block making is considerably lower than the

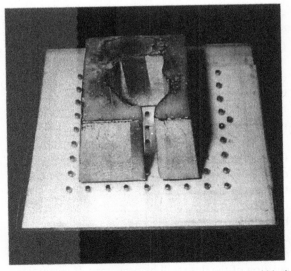

Figure 8.7   Sharp edges are removed from the finished block and it is dusted before it is brought to the treatment room.

temperature at which vaporization of lead and cadmium occurs (approximately 500 to 700°F or 260 to 370°C, respectively), practically eliminating the risks associated with inhalation during normal procedures. A higher risk of vaporization occur when a soldering iron is used to alter a block, since the temperature of the soldering iron can reach several hundred degrees Fahrenheit. Ingestion is also a potential route of entry if safety precautions are not followed. Smoking, eating, and drinking should not be permitted in the block-making area. Small fragments of alloy on the counters and on hands may inadvertently be ingested along with food. Good hygiene is essential, not only for the staff making the blocks but also for the technologists who handle the blocks daily in the treatment rooms. Hand washing before eating, drinking, and smoking is necessary to prevent ingestion of metal dust. Proper ventilation and the use of protective clothing, including gloves when handling the alloy, will reduce the risks of inhalation, ingestion, skin penetration, and burns associated with block making.

Dust and small metal fragments on the floors, countertops, and other areas in the block-making room should be removed by vacuuming. The vacuum cleaner should be equipped with a special filter and bag, which is sealed and disposed of without allowing the metal dust to become airborne. The waste should not be disposed of along with other hospital trash. Hospital waste is often incinerated at very high temperatures; thus these metallic fragments may pose a health hazard for employees involved in the incineration. The content should instead be disposed of in a special toxic metal landfill or by being returned to the supplier.

Cadmium-free alloys are available but contain a higher concentration of lead and melt at a higher temperature, thus the risks of vaporization and burns are increased.

Potentially, hazardous inhalation of vapors containing styrene, Freon, and methyl chloride can occur during the cutting of polystyrene with a hot wire. The release agent often sprayed into the cavities in the polystyrene foam blocks also poses a health hazard and should be used sparingly.

Effect on the Dose. Customized beam-shaping blocks, produced as described above, make it possible to produce radiation fields with very complex shapes. The tailoring of the radiation beam to the shape of the target also minimizes irradiation of adjacent normal tissues.[24] Furthermore, the focused edges of these shields reduce the penumbra of the radiation beam (Fig. 8.8)—an advantage in many situations where the target lies very close to critical radiosensitive organs. On the other hand, the dose under the shield is higher than outside the collimated field edge due to about 3 percent transmission of dose through the block (Fig. 8.8). In a situation where it is important to have small penumbra and the dose transmitted through the block is less important, the choice would be to define the field edge with a focused block. On the other hand, in a situation where the penumbra is less important but the dose outside the field is critical, it is preferable to define the field edge with the collimator. There are, of course, many situations in which one cannot choose a field-defining method because it could introduce problems with having to add an adjacent field, thus introducing field-matching problems.

Secondary electrons, produced when the photon beam interacts with different materials in its path, travel primarily in a forward direction. The tray on which the shields are secured is usually thick enough to absorb most of the secondary scatter produced by photon interaction in the lead shields. The secondary electrons produced by interaction in the tray, however, may cause an increased skin-surface dose. In photon beam therapy, there are two reasons for placing the shields at some distance from the patient: (1) to reduce the contamination of secondary electrons on the skin surface and (2) to maintain maximal clearance around the patient so as to prevent machine-patient collisions.

Moving the Treatment to a Machine with Different Geometry. Treatment machines sometimes break down or require preventive maintenance, but patient treatments must continue. If the treatment is moved to a treatment machine with different geometry and beam energy, the changeover may require that a change be made in the field size, and it may also require resimulation. In many instances, only recalculation of the dose will be necessary. If customized beam-defining blocks are used, these may have to be made for the geometry of the new treatment ma-

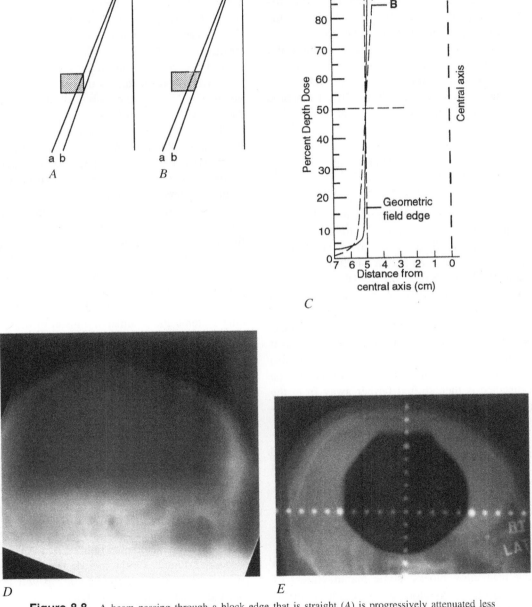

Figure 8.8 A beam passing through a block edge that is straight (*A*) is progressively attenuated less toward the open beam, causing the penumbra to be wide. When a beam passes through a block with focused edges, (*B*), the beam either passes through full block thickness or none at all, causing the penumbra to be sharp. The graph shows the dose gradient using a beam edge defined by a focused block (*curve* A) and the collimator (*curve* B). Port films obtained with a cobalt-60 beam (*D*) and a linear accelerator (*E*). Only the superior margin in *E* is defined by the collimator; and the remainder of the field, showing a sharper beam edge, is defined by blocks with focused edges.

chine. This is a simple procedure if the treatment distance remains the same and only the target-to-tray distance is different on the new machine. However, if the treatment distance is different, the film distance will have to be adjusted accordingly on the block-cutting equipment when the new blocks are constructed. For example, if the simulation film from which the blocks were originally cut was taken with 80-cm source-axis distance (SAD) and the patient's treatments are changed to a machine with 100-cm SAD, the following equation must be applied:

$$\text{Film distance} = \frac{\text{TFD} \times 100}{80} \qquad (8.1)$$

In some situations, due to limitations in the planning equipment, it is not possible to simulate the extended treatment distance needed for large fields. Beam-shaping blocks can still be produced by alternative methods.[25,26] Nair et al. describe a technique in which the radiograph is taken at a focus-to-skin distance less than the required source-to-skin distance, and a tray-distance shift is made on the block-cutting device. Douglas et al. describe a film-shift technique. Here the focus-to-skin distance is also less than the required source-to-skin distance, but the film distance is then shifted farther away from the pivot point on the block-cutting equipment. The required film shift (f) is found from

$$f = \frac{(\text{SSD} - \text{FSD})\,(s + a + d)}{(\text{FSD} + d)} \qquad (8.2)$$

where s is the patient thickness, a the exit surface-to-film distance, and d the depth of the outer limit of the volume to be shielded.

Multileaf Collimators. As an alternative to casting lead alloy blocks, some manufacturers of medical linear accelerators are offering multileaf collimators (MLC) (Chap. 2). Several authors have studied the dosimetry of MLCs, particularly with respect to the effect of the steplike field edge and "leakage" between the leaves.[27-31] Although, conceptually, MLCs could replace lead alloy shields,

some limitations still exist. Because of limitations in field size, "scalloped" isodose curves in the penumbra and sometimes inability to form the desired field shape with the leaves, their use is limited to certain fields. The weight of an MLC also makes it impractical to use, since it would have to be removed for the treatment of patients where it could not be used. In some large centers, one therapy machine equipped with MLC is dedicated to treatment of all patients where MLC fields are possible, eliminating the need for removal of the MLC between patients.

The use of computers in radiation therapy has been extended to drive MLCs in moving-beam treatments so that the shape of the beam matches the shape of the target in the beam's-eye view (BEV) from any direction. As the radiation beam moves around the patient, the shape of the beam is changed by moving independent leaves in or out of the radiation beam to maintain the shape of the target. Such computer-controlled conformal therapy (CCCT) techniques are becoming increasingly popular, but potential problems must be addressed to make their application practical.[32] Development of dose-planning systems and automated transfer of the resultant settings for each collimator leaf to the treatment-unit control computer must be available before widespread use of MLCs can become a reality.

FIELD SHAPING: ELECTRON BEAMS

Field shaping for electron beams is usually accomplished either through placing wax-coated lead shields directly on the patient's skin surface or by inserting lead shields at the distal end on the electron cone. One disadvantage of securing the shield to the collimator rather than to the patient is that small shifts of the patient's position can cause the target to move out of the irradiated field. When the shielding is secured directly on the patient, small shifts in the patient-collimator (cone) relationship will not disturb the target-beam relationship (Fig. 8.9). In treating uncooperative, very ill, or neurologically compromised patients, using a large cone and then shielding a large area around the target would prevent target misses even when large shifts occur. In photon beam therapy, there is no other option than to

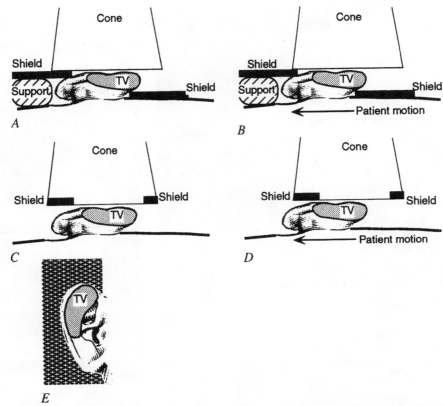

Figure 8.9 *A.* Shielding of small superficial lesions, when either electron beams or low-energy x-rays are used, should be placed directly on the patient and cover a large area surrounding the lesion. This allows a large field to be used. *B.* Should the patient inadvertently move during the treatment, the lesion remains within the irradiated field. When the same field is defined by a shield fixed to the end of the electron cone (*C*), the lesion would be outside the irradiated field when the patient moves (*D*). When a lesion on the ear is treated, for example, a shield should be placed behind the ear to prevent unnecessary irradiation of tissues behind it. *E.* The same consideration should be given to shielding in the nose, eyes, and other cavities, where a thin lead sheet can be inserted distal to the tumor.

place the blocks at some distance from the patient, as already described.

Shields inserted in an electron cone (Fig. 8.10*A*) can be manufactured from the alloy used in photon beam–shaping blocks; however, the procedure is quite different.[33] Electron beam–shaping blocks are inserted in the distal end of the electron cone, close to the patient's skin surface; therefore, the size of the opening in the block is practically the same as the desired field on the skin surface. These blocks are also much thinner than the photon blocks—about 1 to 2 cm for most electron energies,[34] eliminating the

need for focused edges. The shape and size of the treatment field is traced onto a template, made either by tracing the field drawn on the skin surface or from a radiograph, but reduced to the size on the skin surface. The field size on a radiograph can usually be reduced using a treatment-planning computer. When electron shields are made, it is the shape of the field rather than the shield that is cut from a piece of Styrofoam. This can be accomplished by using either the hot wire in the block-cutting machine or a band saw. The piece of Styrofoam representing the treatment field is placed inside a replica of the distal end

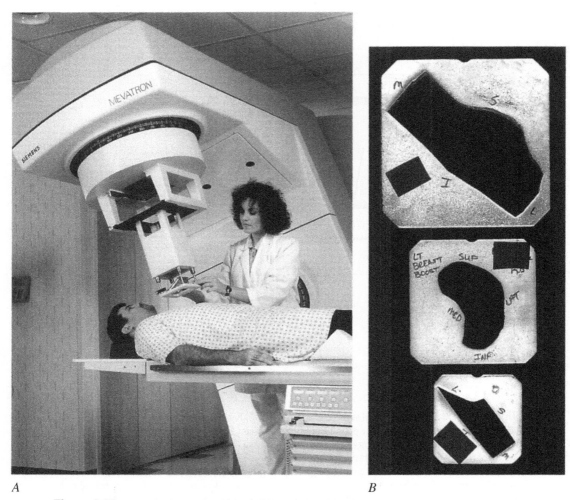

A   *B*

Figure 8.10   *A* and *B*. Custom shielding blocks for electron beams are placed directly in the cone and can be much thinner than the blocks used for photon beams. (*A* is courtesy of Siemens Medical Systems, Inc.)

of the particular electron cone to be used. This replica, which is usually supplied by the manufacturer of the linear accelerator, is made of a pliable material, facilitating easy removal of the finished shield. Liquid alloy is poured around the Styrofoam, which is weighted down on a cooling tray. These shields are usually quite small and will cool and harden in about 30 min (Fig. 8.10*B*). The effect on the dose rate of irregularly shaped electron beams must be considered when doses are calculated.[35]

FIELD SHAPING: ORTHOVOLTAGE AND SUPERFICIAL BEAMS

In orthovoltage and superficial therapy, the shielding, or beam-shaping material, is usually placed directly on the patient's skin surface. This is possible because only a very thin layer of lead, usually on the order of millimeters, depending on the beam energy or penetration, is needed. Secondary scatter arising from the interaction in the lead is absorbed within the lead or by a thin layer of wax placed between the lead sheet and the skin surface. The same principle as described for electron therapy applies here with respect to whether the shields are placed on the skin surface or in the cone (Fig. 8.9).

INTERNAL SHIELDS

When photon beams interact with fillings in the teeth, secondary electron scatter is caused, which significantly increases the dose in the buccal mucosa, the tongue, or other tissues immediately adjacent to the filling. To reduce the effect of the secondary electrons, a wax mold or other tissue-equivalent material, shaped to conform to the teeth, can be used during the treatment (Chap. 9). Separating the mucosa from the fillings by a couple of millimeters may be sufficient.[36,37]

When electron beams are used in the treatment of lesions in the lip, buccal mucosa, or gingival sulcus, it is sometimes possible to place an internal lead shield in the mouth to protect normal tissues beyond or around the target. Secondary electrons, backscattered when an electron beam interacts with the lead, can cause very high doses in the tissue-metal interface. This phenomenon has been studied by several authors.[38-41] To disperse the backscatter, a bolus material (wax) can be placed between the lead shield and the beam entrance side. Other materials, such as aluminum or dental acrylic, can also be used.[42] In a similar way, protective shielding is used when superficial tumors on or near the eyelids are treated using either superficial or electron beams. It is always a good idea to cover both the entrance and exit sides of a lead shield with a coat of wax, aluminum, or dental acrylic to reduce any secondary scatter that may be present on the surface of the shield. The coating is also better secured to the shield if it envelopes the entire shield.

TISSUE COMPENSATORS

PHOTON BEAMS

Missing-Tissue Compensators. In areas where the patient's surface topography perpendicular to the

incident beam is irregular, the shape of the isodose curves will be affected, as described in Chaps. 3 and 6. The lack of dose uniformity within the beam, illustrated in Fig. 8.11, can have adverse effects in the irradiated tissues. In some areas (B in Fig. 8.11) the dose is higher than at the same depth on the central axis of the beam (A in Fig. 8.11), because the beam traverses less attenuating tissue or lower because it traverses more attenuating tissue than at the central axis point (C in Fig. 8.11). To produce the same dose at A, B, and C, we need to "compensate" for the "missing tissue" at B. A bag of water or other tissue-equivalent material (bolus) could be used to produce a flat surface, and thus the thickness of attenuating material would be the same at A and B. This solution, however, would not address the problem of lower dose at C and would cause loss of the skin-sparing advantage of megavoltage radiation. The first problem could be solved by calculating the prescribed dose at C and then filling the entire space

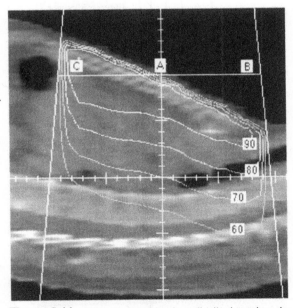

Figure 8.11   The effect on the dose distribution when the beam enters through a sloping surface. Here, the dose along a vertical line at B is higher and at C lower than at the same distance in the beam along the central axis (A). The dose can be made uniform by inserting a compensator in the beam.

within the field with tissue-equivalent material. The problem with loss of skin sparing can only be addressed by placing the compensating material at some distance (15 to 20 cm) from the patient's skin surface, similar to the placement of the beam-shaping blocks. In fact, compensators for megavoltage therapy are often placed on the same tray as the blocks but on the opposite side (downstream in the beam) to avoid having either one interfere with the placement of the other. Compensators can also be placed on a separate tray in the beam. When compensators are fabricated, it is important to bear in mind that, as with beam-shaping blocks placed closer to the radiation target, the size of the compensator in the BEV must be reduced, while the thickness remains unchanged. Compensators need not be made from tissue-equivalent material but can be constructed from any material with a known attenua-

tion coefficient. Commonly used materials are wax, paraffin, Lucite, brass, aluminum, or, more recently, a gypsum mixture.[43,44] Lead and Lipowitz metal have also been proposed as compensator materials. When these or other materials with high density (high Z) are used, a very small error in the thickness will cause a large error in dose. Materials with lower density are therefore safer, since they are less sensitive to small errors in thickness.

The design and fabrication of missing-tissue compensators for megavoltage therapy is difficult and tedious, since the dimensions must be reduced in size while the needed thickness along each ray line of the beam must be calculated for the particular material used (Fig. 8.12). The needed reduction can be found by SSD/target-to-compensator distance. For example, if the compensator is placed at 50 cm from the target in an 80-cm SSD treatment, the dimensions of

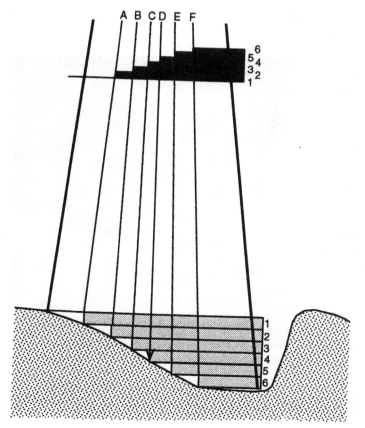

Figure 8.12   A missing-tissue compensator can be constructed by finding the thickness of missing tissue along ray lines drawn from the source. Appropriate number of sheets of a compensating material with known attenuation is then placed in the beam.

the compensator must be reduced by a factor of 1.6 (80/50). To precisely reproduce the shape of the missing-tissue segment, but on a smaller scale, several techniques have been suggested.[45–53]

Compensators are often needed when an anterior and posterior field arrangement is used in the chest, where the anterior chest surface almost always slopes toward the neck. The simplest compensating method consists of a wedge inserted in the beam so that the "heel" of the wedge (the thicker side) lies over the segment where the patient is thinner. Most wedges must be inserted to cover the entire field; however, in many situations only a small portion of the field requires a compensator. In this case, sheets of attenuating material (copper, brass, or Lucite) can be stacked in a steplike fashion over the area requiring compensation only (Fig. 8.12). In these two methods, the compensation is made in the cephalad-caudal direction only. The dose can also be reduced in the cephalad margin by inserting a block during a few treatments. The need for tissue compensators is particularly important in the treatment of anterior and posterior mantle fields, where the thickness of tissue usually varies considerably.[54,55] Sheets of brass, shaped to match the shape of the major segments of a typical mantle field but reduced to appropriate size, are stacked in a steplike fashion on a tray above the patient. In this technique, attempts are made to consider the variation of the irregular surface within the entire field.

In one method, compensating filters are constructed of brass or aluminum blocks with columns that correspond to the irregular surface. Each column follows the diverging beam and is reduced in size. In another method, the missing-tissue volume is determined by rods that slide down to the patient's skin surface along the diverging path of the beam.[48] The rods are locked in place when they touch the skin and the upper ends of the rods produce a cavity that corresponds to the shape of the missing tissue, but appropriately reduced in size. This cavity is then filled with a tissue-equivalent material such as wax. Other authors have described a method in which the shape and thickness of the compensator is determined from the exit dose measured on port films.[56,57]

Beck *et al.* and Boge *et al.* have described a technique in which a routing device is used to hollow out the shape and size of the missing-tissue segment in a Styrofoam block (Fig. 8.13).[45,46] The hollow, which is appropriately reduced in size, is then filled with a tissue-equivalent material. The routing device is attached to the machine usually used in the construction of beam-shaping blocks.

In recent years, computer-assisted compensator design has become very popular.[53,58–61] In these techniques, information about the patient's topography is obtained from CT images and, using a special computer, the needed compensator is calculated. The computer then drives a router, which hollows out a block of Styrofoam to form the size and shape of the required compensator, and the cavity is filled with tissue-equivalent material. Computer-driven milling machines that can produce the needed cavity into which to fill the tissue-equivalent compensating material are commercially available (Fig. 8.14).

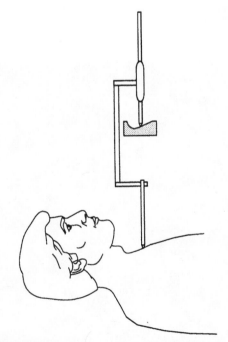

Figure 8.13 A technique can be used in which a Styrofoam block is hollowed out to the shape of the missing tissue. The hollow is then filled with tissue-equivalent material.

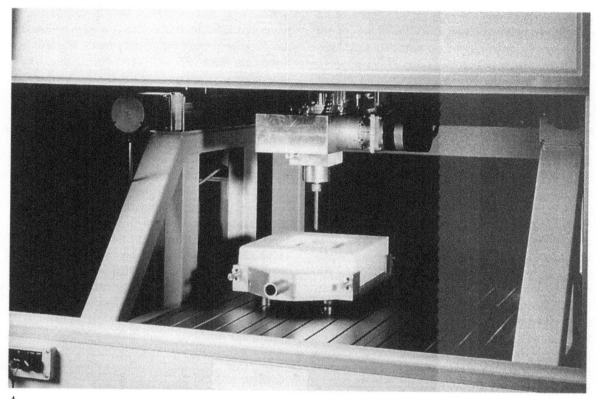

A

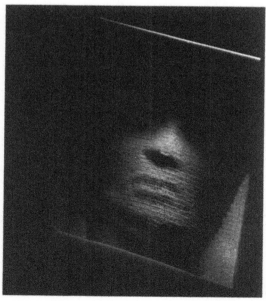

B

Figure 8.14 *A* and *B*. A computer-driven milling machine can hollow out very fine details of the missing-tissue volume. (Courtesy of Par Scientific AS.)

Renner et al.[51,52] have described a photogramme-tric technique in which a grid, inserted in the field light of the simulator or treatment machine, projects lines on the patient's skin. The grid lines appear curved on the patient's irregular surface and provide three-dimensional information about the topography of the patient's external surface. The grid pattern is photographed and entered into a computer for calcu-lation of the needed size and shape of the compensa-tor.

Compensators designed with the same thickness as the missing-tissue segment tend to overcompen-sate (i.e., reduce the dose too much). This is because the missing-tissue compensating material is placed on a tray away from the patient, in effect removing the scattered dose that otherwise would have been produced by the missing-tissue volume.[49,62–66] This can be overcome by making the compensators slightly thinner, so that more primary dose is trans-mitted. Missing-tissue compensators cannot be de-signed to produce uniform dose across an entire field and at all depths. Many variables—such as beam energy, field size, depth, missing-tissue thickness, and compensator-surface distance—affect the dose distribution. It is also important to bear in mind that the effect of missing tissue on the dose is decreased with higher beam energies; for example, the dose heterogeneity within a mantle field is more severe when a cobalt-60 beam is used than if a 6-MV pho-ton beam is used. The need for compensators is de-creasing, as higher beam energies are often used. Meanwhile, other applications for compensators have been found; these are described in the following sections.

Other Applications for Compensators. Beam compensators were originally designed to compen-sate for topographic irregularities of the patient's surface; however, they have subsequently also been used to compensate for dose variations caused by tissue inhomogeneities.[67–70] Attempts have also been made to compensate for the "horns" often observed in overflattened beams from linear accelerators.[71] Recently, compensators have also been used to achieve intentional dose heterogeneities within a field. For example, a technique in which the boost, or

a higher dose to a smaller area within the field, is delivered concurrently has been described.[72,73] In this technique, the boost area receives a higher dose while the dose in the rest of the field is reduced by a compensator. The thickness of this compensator de-pends on the dose prescription for the two areas (Fig. 8.15). In this treatment, a beam attenuator is cast so that it covers the entire large field with the exception of the boost area. Therefore, while the boost area receives, for example, 200 cGy, the remainder of the field, which is "compensated," simultaneously re-ceives a lower dose; maybe 180 cGy. The dose dif-ferential can be achieved by varying either the thick-ness or the density of the compensator.

In total-body irradiation (TBI), opposed lateral fields are often used. Here, the patient's thickness varies dramatically between the maximum width (usually across the arms and thorax) to the minimum (usually across the head and feet). In the thorax, the dose is often excessive due to the large thickness of the low-density lung tissue that the beam traverses. Placing the patient's arms along the sides of the chest reduces the dose in this area, but additional compen-

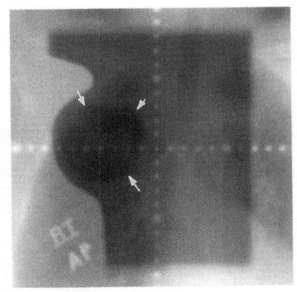

Figure 8.15 A compensator can also be used to deliver dif-ferent doses to a tumor simultaneously. The darker area in the right lung is receiving a higher dose than the surrounding area, where the compensator is inserted.

sation may be necessary. In the head and the lower legs, compensation can be accomplished by stacking sheets of brass or Lucite of appropriate thickness on a tray in the beam. When anterior and posterior TBI fields are used, lung compensators must be reduced in size until they match the size and shape of the lung volume at the distance in the beam where they will be placed.[70,74] The soft tissues anterior and posterior to the lungs are then treated using electron beams.

ELECTRON BEAMS

Selection of the beam energy for electron treatments is usually made so that the deepest part of the target is included. Meanwhile, radiosensitive tissues that may be located at a shallower depth within the same field must be avoided. It is then possible to place tissue-equivalent material directly on the skin surface overlying the areas of concern so as to reduce the depth of the electron beam in these areas (Fig. 8.16). For example, when the chest wall is treated with electrons, the beam energy is selected such that the deepest portion of the chest wall is included within the prescribed isodose line; then a compensator is used in areas where the chest wall is thinner. The appropriate thickness and position of such a compensator can be obtained from CT images throughout the chest wall. Sheets of wax, softened in

hot water, can be molded to the shape of the chest wall and to appropriate thickness. Verification of the placement and the thickness of the compensator can be made by repeating the CT scans through the area with the compensator in place.

PLACEMENT OF COMPENSATORS

Tissue compensators for megavoltage beams must be placed at some distance from the patient's skin surface to preserve the skin-sparing effect of high-energy beams. Compensators made from tissue-equivalent material that are used in orthovoltage treatments can be placed directly on the skin surface, since there is no skin-sparing effect to be concerned about. Compensators used in electron beams must of necessity be placed on the skin surface at the distal end of the cone; the skin-sparing effect is then lost. Compensators should not be used without first verifying that they are placed correctly in the beam and that the desired and the resulting isodose distributions agree.

OTHER BEAM- AND DOSE-MODIFYING TECHNIQUES

In the compensating techniques described so far, the goal has been to produce a device that is placed in the

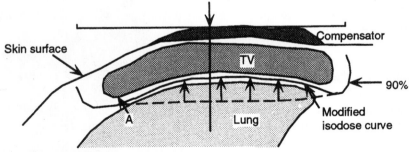

Figure 8.16   A compensator can also be used to modify the shape of an electron beam by placing an appropriate thickness of a tissue-equivalent material directly on the skin surface. Here an electron energy was selected so that the 90 percent isodose curve would include the target at the deepest point. A. The dose in the underlying lung tissue would have been irradiated to a high dose as well (*hatched lines*). (The change in the isodose curve caused by the lung inhomogeneity is not shown.) Tissue-equivalent material was added on the skin, so that the combined thickness of soft tissue and the compensator was the same within the field when measured in the beam direction.

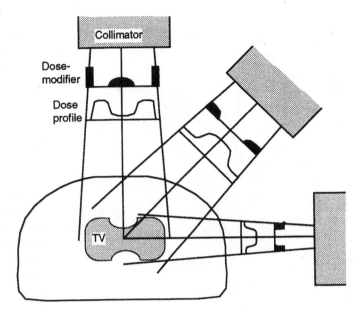

Figure 8.17 A beam modifier is built so that in the anterior field, a lower dose is delivered in radiosensitive tissues (bladder and rectum). In the lateral field, the highest dose is desired in the center of the beam where the prostate is located and a lower dose is desired in the anterior and posterior segment of the field where the bladder and rectum are located. Isodose distributions can be shaped by varying the intensity of the radiation depending on the beam angle.

beam so as to produce the desired dose in the patient. A unique approach to calculating the required shape of a beam modifier (not to be confused with missing-tissue compensators) is an inverse method by which the optimal dose distribution is derived first, and then the needed dose intensity within each field is calculated.[75–89] For example, within segments of a beam where radiosensitive organs or tissues are located, a lower dose or perhaps no dose is desired (Fig. 8.17). Variations of dose intensity across the beam can be produced by placing a compensator or attenuator in part of the field or by varying the position of dynamic jaws or multileaf collimator leaves.[90,91] The effect is similar to that of differential weighting of a particular beam, although here the differential weighting is *within* a beam. Combining this partial dose reduction with differential weighting *among* the beams can also be used to produce the desired dose distribution. These techniques can be used to produce dose distributions of practically any shape but, they require powerful computers to calculate the desired dose intensity. With the ability to obtain detailed information about the patient's anatomy, the availability of computer software, and the manufacture of treatment machines allowing a wide variety of options, inverse treatment planning may be commonly used in the future.

The principle of intensity-modulated beams just described is similar to that described by Proimos in the late 1950s and early 1960s.[92–97]

Proimos described a rotation technique in which gravity-oriented dose-modifying devices are inserted in the beam.[93,94,96] Figure 8.18 demonstrates the principle of this cyclotherapy technique. A tumor model, made of light material (Styrofoam) and reduced to appropriate size, is inserted into a cylinder-shaped can and the remaining space around the model is filled with lead shot (Fig. 8.19). The cylinder is suspended in the beam such that the axis of the cylinder coincides with the central axis of the beam and is parallel to the axis of rotation. A weight is attached to the cylinder to maintain the initial orientation of the model during the gantry's rotation. Due to the curvature of the cylinder, parts of the beam traverse a smaller thickness of lead shots, giving rise to a slightly higher dose. This effect is eliminated by the addition of a sleeve placed around the cylinder.

Proimos has also described a technique in which the dose to radiosensitive organs can be reduced while some or all of the surrounding tissues are

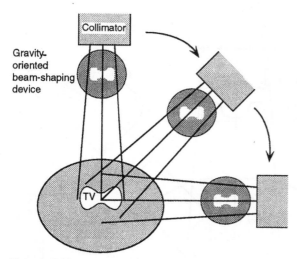

Figure 8.18   Another method to shape the dose distribution to the target is using a moving-beam technique in which a gravity-oriented shield accomplishes practically the same normal-tissue sparing as shown in Fig. 8.17.

treated.[92,94] For example, in a synchronous shielding technique, the dose in the spinal cord can be reduced by about 50 percent while the surrounding tissues are irradiated. The shape of the area that needs protection is formed by lead or other high-density material. In the case of the spinal cord, a lead or tungsten rod, appropriately reduced in size and shaped to match the curvature of the spinal cord, is inserted in the beam in a fashion similar to that of the tumor model described in the previous paragraph (Fig. 8.20). As the radiation source rotates around the patient, the shield remains in the same position with respect to the patient (i.e., the spinal cord always lies in the shadow of the shield). Because the shield is relatively thin (roughly the same diameter as the spinal cord), the attenuation of the beam may be only about 50 percent. Delivering 6000 cGy in the surrounding tissues, the spinal cord dose would be approximately 3000 cGy—a dose usually tolerated by the spinal cord. The dose uniformity within the unshielded part of the field is quite unsatisfactory with this technique; however, it can be improved by the insertion of a specially constructed wedge filter.[98]

Proimos has also described synchronous shielding devices for a variety of shapes,[97] including one that

shields both eyes while the surrounding tissues are irradiated.[94] The arrangement of the synchronous eye shields is more complex in that the long axes of the two shielding cylinders must always be oriented such that they are parallel with the beam direction (5 HVT) and that they are constantly shielding the eyes (Fig. 8.21). In this treatment technique, the dose near and between the eyes is also reduced. This can be improved by the insertion of a compensator in the remainder of the field not affected by the eye shields.[99]

Another technique to conform the dose distribution to the target has been described.[100] In this technique, the treatment is delivered through computer-controlled simultaneous motions of the collimator setting, couch, and gantry. A narrow slit in the collimator is moved along the patient's long axis by motion of the couch in and away from the gantry; simultaneously, the field width is changed by opening and closing of the collimator leaves while the gantry moves around the patient.

Mantel et al. described use of conformation therapy coupled with variations in the dose rate during rotation therapy to improve the dose distribution.[101] Takahashi et al. described use of dynamic multileaf collimators to define asymmetric irregular fields and coined the term *conformational therapy*.[102–104]

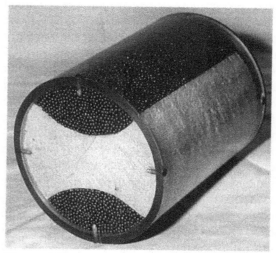

Figure 8.19   Photograph of the device used in Fig. 8.18.

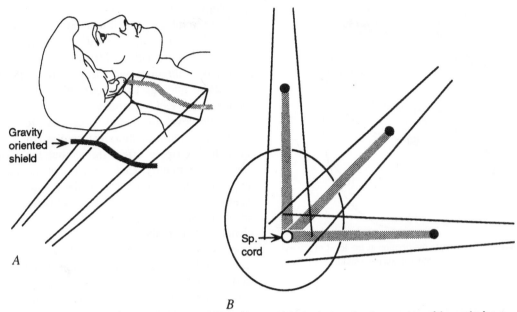

Figure 8.20   *A* and *B*. A gravity-oriented spinal cord shield that is shaped to the curvature of the particular segment of the spinal cord to be shielded. The shield is suspended in the beam in such a way that it always shields the spinal cord as the machine rotates around the patient.

The very complex treatment techniques described here, where the field shape and dose rate are changing dynamically, require interplay between the planning computer and the computer driving the treatment machine. This technology will probably become commercially available before the end of this century; however, potential problems must be addressed before they become practical.[32] Treatment documentation is just one of the problems envisioned.

Dose-modifying devices used in the techniques described above should not be confused with the missing-tissue compensators described earlier.

BOLUS

Tissue-equivalent materials used in megavoltage radiation therapy to reduce the depth of the maximum dose (D_{max}) are referred to as *bolus*. Bolus material must be pliable so that it conforms to the curvature of the patient's skin surface. A commonly used material called Superflab is available in different thicknesses and can be formed to the desired size and shape by cutting it with scissors.[105] It should be wrapped in a thin plastic protective sheet when used and be stored in an airtight bag. This material can be reused for many patients but needs thorough cleaning between patients.

A bolus material that can be made in most clinics consists of water (200 mL), glycerin (100 mL), and gelatin (100 g). The water and gelatin are mixed well and then heated in a water bath until liquified. The glycerin is added and the mixture is stirred until it is smooth. A small amount of propylparaben can be added to the mixture to prevent deterioration of the material if it is to be stored for a long time. The mixture is poured to desired thickness into a Teflon pan. When it is cool and solid, the sheet can be removed and stored in an airtight bag. Bolusused to bring the maximum dose closer to the surface should not be confused with a compensator consisting of the same material and placed on the skin surface.

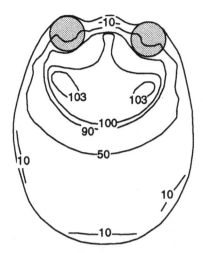

Figure 8.21 An isodose distribution at the level of the eyes resulting from the use of a synchronous eye-shielding technique.

QUALITY ASSURANCE

The increasing complexity of radiation therapy, coupled with the growing pressure by credentialing organizations in recent years, has led to mandatory requirements for quality assurance programs in radiation therapy. Standards set forth by the American College of Radiology can be found in a document published in April 1990.[106] A comprehensive QA protocol by the American Association of Physicists in Medicine (AAPM) was published in 1994.[107] The consistency of treatments demanded by multiinstitutional treatment protocols also requires that the participating centers maintain a high standard of quality assurance.[108] The Radiological Physics Center (RPC), established on the recommendation of the Committee on Radiation Oncology Studies, plays an important role in quality assurance in radiation oncology and has suggested parameters to be included in all radiation therapy treatment charts.[109] This organization, sponsored by the AAPM, aims to assure consistency and correctness of data in radiation therapy clinical trials, to provide feedback to participating institutions for correction of discrepancies, to assist and advise clinical study groups on quality-control procedures in radiation therapy, and to communicate instructive findings to the radiation

oncology community. The major activities of the RPC are to review patient treatment records, dosimetry calibration of equipment used in the treatment of patients enrolled in clinical trials, remote monitoring of beam calibrations via TLDs, and communicate instructive findings to the clinical study groups.[110] Although the RPC's primary function is to maintain a certain level of quality assurance for patients enrolled in multi-institutional studies, their efforts have had a ripple effect throughout the radiation therapy community. Chances are that the standards applied to the treatment of patients enrolled on a protocol are also being applied to all patients treated in participating institutions and perhaps also to patients treated at other centers.

A comprehensive quality-assurance program aimed at delivering the best possible care to patients and at establishing and documenting all operating procedures is necessary in every radiation therapy department. Such a quality-assurance program should include written treatment policies and procedures describing the management of each pathologic entity to ensure uniform care, to obtain consistent data for evaluating results, and to guide the physician in treatment decisions. Treatment-planning factors such as the treatment technique, use of treatment aids, description of the target volume, dose prescription, tumor doses, and fractionation schedules should be reviewed by both the physician and the physics/dosimetry staff. Radiographic images from which the target volume was established and simulation films of the treatment fields are required in order to document the appropriateness of the treatment ports. Weekly dosimetry review of all treatment charts in order to verify appropriate documentation of accumulated dose and make sure that intended changes in the treatment in fact occur is essential to ensure that the treatment is carried out as intended.

A radiation oncology record, separate from the hospital medical record, should be kept on file for easy access by radiation oncologists, technical staff, and the referring physician. The radiation oncology chart should contain consultation notes with a detailed but concise report of history and physical examination. It should also contain reports of laboratory and radiographic studies, histology or cytologic reports documenting cancer and, when appropriate, surgical reports detailing the findings at the time of surgery. Diagrams or photographs illustrating the extent, location, and appearance of the disease as well as the stage of the disease should be an integral part of the chart.

Intermittent quality assurance of equipment in terms of output and performance is essential. The extent and frequency of such quality assurance is usually specified by each state's regulatory body. Departmental written procedures should be designed jointly by a qualified radiation physicist and a radiation oncologist. Results of periodic quality assurance procedures should be accurately documented and readily available. Any malfunction or other problem with the machine discovered by the technologists during warmup or routine operation should be reported and recorded.

Details of the treatment planning—including the target volume, isodose distributions, dose prescription, dose calculation, simulation, and port films—should also be an integral part of the treatment documentation. Polaroid pictures showing the patient's position, immobilization devices, treatment fields, shields, and beam-modifying devices should be in every patient's treatment chart. Records of the daily monitor units or treatment time per field and the cumulative dose at various points should be maintained and verified at least weekly by physics/dosimetry staff as well as by the radiation oncologist.

Weekly chart reviews should include verification of the following:

1. Statement of diagnosis and histology as well as the stage of the disease
2. Presence of pathology report or acceptable reasons why no histologic proof is available
3. Presence of report describing history and physical examination
4. Presence of consent for treatment
5. Dose prescription dated and signed by the radiation oncologists prior to initiation of therapy
6. Statement of treatment technique, site of the treatments, and dose to various sites within the target volume (i.e., boost, etc.)
7. Weekly port films of each field, approved, signed, and dated by the radiation oncologist

8. Dose calculation and isodose distributions approved, signed, and dated by radiation physicist
9. Treatment records checked and signed weekly by the radiation physicist or dosimetrist
10. Evidence of weekly evaluation of the patient's progress by the physician

Appropriate forms for demographic information, staging, dose prescription, and recording of external beam and brachytherapy treatments should be present in every department. At the completion of therapy, the chart is checked for the presence of a completion note summarizing the treatment actually delivered and that a follow-up plan for the patient has been made. Copies of the appropriate sections of the chart should be provided to other physicians involved in the care of the patient to ensure proper continued care.

Every radiation therapy department should also maintain a tumor registry, statistics with respect to number of patients seen in consultation and treated, anatomic site of tumors treated, number of procedures (simulations, treatments, fields treated, treatment plans, brachytherapy procedures, follow-ups), and outcome of treatment.

In the early 1980s, an international conference on quality assurance in radiation therapy was held in the United States, during which various aspects of this important topic were presented. The reader is referred to the special issue of the *International Journal of Radiation Oncology Biology and Physics* for the details of this meeting.[111-122]

Specific quality-assurance procedures for radiation therapy equipment (linear accelerators, cobalt-60 machines, simulators, treatment-planning computers, brachytherapy sources, and remote afterloading equipment) are published elsewhere.[42,123,124]

The quality-assurance procedures particular to the technical staff are discussed in more detail in the following sections.

DOCUMENTATION OF TREATMENT PARAMETERS

Delivering high doses of radiation to a human being requires responsible documentation of where and how much radiation has been delivered. The radiation dose delivered in a tumor is often limited by the tolerance of the adjacent normal tissue; thus, further radiation to the same tissues would be harmful and could even be fatal. It is therefore imperative that a detailed description of the treatment, both in terms of dose and areas included in the radiation field, be given very clearly in the patient's records. Since the effect of the radiation remains throughout the patient's lifetime and cancer patients are surviving longer than in previous decades, it is critical to preserve such records for many years.

The population has become more mobile, and in many instances patients receive radiation treatments in more than one clinic. Thus, treatment records are frequently sent to other radiation therapy departments, where they will be studied in great detail to determine whether further treatments can safely be given. The complex legal issues that could arise should the patient later develop complications from the radiation therapy are best avoided by giving all treatments within the same radiation therapy practice. This is however, not always possible, due to relocation and also because patients are sometimes referred to larger centers for specialized care or complex treatments (brachytherapy, hyperthermia, and so on). Records of patients who are treated on multi-institutional protocols are sent to review centers, where the staff must interpret the treatment charts and make sure that treatment has, in fact, been delivered as outlined by the protocol. The staff at these other radiation therapy centers may not be familiar with the peculiarities of a given radiation therapy department. Therefore, consistent terminology particular to radiation therapy and a uniform treatment chart can make it easier for others, unfamiliar with the peculiarities of a given center, to understand the treatment. However, because each department has its own system, which works well within the department, changes cannot be expected in the foreseeable future. It is therefore incumbent on each department to clearly document every variable of the patient's treatment in great detail and in such a way that it can be understood by everyone. The International Commission on Radiation Units and Measurements has made specific recommendations for documenting and reporting of radiation treatments.[125,126]

Over the last decades, treatment techniques have become more complex and therefore require a more detailed description. For example, in the past, treatment fields were almost always square or rectangular, the central axis was in the center of the field, and sometimes a couple of corners were blocked. In more recent years, fields are often shaped to more closely resemble the shape of the target and can therefore have very irregular shapes. The central axis of the field may not be in the center and might even be outside the treated area. Collimators with independent jaws can be closed from either side, causing the central axis of the field to be anywhere inside or outside the field.

An anterior field used in the treatment of the maxillary antrum will exit through the patient's brain. Exactly what part of the brain was in the field can only be determined if the head position is also known. In order to determine where the previous treatment was delivered, a simulation film or port film is necessary. In addition, a diagram, photograph, or tattoo is needed. The patient's chart and the isodose distribution may also be helpful in determining what dose the different areas have already received.

TREATMENT CHARTS

A radiation therapy treatment chart represents an important document for communication between staff regarding the details of the patient's treatment.[127-129] It must therefore contain the information necessary to deliver the treatments accurately. This document should also represent the history of the patient's treatment in a form that is clear, concise, and understandable to anyone involved in the care of the patient.

There is no uniform agreement as to how and what should be documented about the patient's radiotherapy treatments. Minimally, a radiation therapy treatment record should contain all the particulars of the patient's treatment in such detail that it could be reproduced if necessary. The chart should therefore contain information with regard to the patient's position and dimensions in the irradiated area. It should also contain information with respect to the treatment beam, such as beam energy, beam angles, field sizes, the use of beam-modifying devices, treatment distances, and point(s) of the dose calculation. There must also be details about the dose in terms of dose calculations, monitor units or treatment time, and dose delivered per fraction in addition to the cumulative dose at prescribed points. Such points could be in the target, in a dose-limiting normal organ inside the field, or even be in a radiosensitive organ outside the field. Any changes made in the dose or treatment fields during the course of treatment should also be clearly indicated.

Treatment records are often designed by the staff of each clinic; thus contain treatment descriptions and jargon commonly used in that department. While this chart is easily understood by the department's staff, it might cause confusion when the patient's care is transferred to another clinic. The terminology used in the two different clinics may be different, leading to uncertainties about the treatment.[130] Some treatment charts contain every possible detail about the treatment in a very well organized way, while others have minimal amounts of information. One treatment chart recently received for a multi-institutional protocol quality assurance review contained no information regarding the daily treatment with the exception of the cumulative tumor dose and the date of each treatment. Some treatment charts have columns labeled for a certain treatment parameter but, without a change in the heading, the column is used for another piece of information. With increasing pressure by accrediting organizations to improve quality assurance, one may hope that these and similar problems will be eliminated.

The increasing complexity of treatments make detailed documentation very difficult. For example, treatments designed for a three-dimensional system often contain beams that are noncoplanar (i.e., the beams do not have a common plane on which to display the dose distribution). Dose distributions may therefore be displayed on a contour through an arbitrary plane that is difficult to describe. In some treatments, the beam direction is such that it prevents port films from being obtained—for example, a ver-

tex field. In dynamic field-shaping treatments, where multileaf collimators constantly change the field size and shape, documentation of the field dimensions is impossible.

Many treatment machines are now computer-operated and others also have a "record and verify" system that prevents treatment unless the various parameters of the treatment are followed exactly. At any time during the course of treatment, the patient's treatment record can be printed out. These computer printouts of the treatment are different from system to system and the validity of such records is questionable.

In the following paragraphs, the treatment chart currently used at Duke University is described (see Figs. 8.22 through 8.28).

The first page of the treatment chart, shown in Fig. 8.22, is the prescription page, which also contains demographic information about the patient as well as the diagnosis and other details that make it easier for nurses and technical staff to care for the patient. When the patient returns for further treatments, there is separate area for a second prescription. In the event that more space is needed, a new page is added.

The second page (Fig. 8.23) contains treatment setup information. This page, which is printed on the back of the prescription page, is filled out by the simulation technologist and the dosimetry staff following completion of the simulation and treatment-planning procedures. The circle is used to indicate wedge directions and beam angles as they pertain to the particular machine on which the patient is treated. If multiple areas are treated simultaneously, another circle is loosely taped over the current circle and each is labeled with the field numbers for which it is intended.

Figure 8.24 shows the details of the treatment simulation and is used as a "scratch pad" during the simulation procedure. It is not unusual for anticipated fields to be set up and radiographs obtained, later to be changed when the radiograph is examined in more detail. The technologist will therefore have to record the settings for each radiograph as they are obtained. This page also serves as a reminder, so that the correct numbers (field size, SSD, TFD, and so on) can later be recorded on the radiographs. In ad-

DUKE UNIVERSITY | **RADIATION**
MEDICAL CENTER | **ONCOLOGY**

Name				Duke No.	
Age	Race	Sex		R.O. No.	
Diagnosis					
M.D.	Resident			Protocol # or short description	
	Staff				

	Narrative plan:		Goal:	Cure/Palliation	
_____ Course Prescription					
Port Films:					
Blood Tests:					
Other:		Staff M.D. signature: _____			

Date	Technique and Anatomic Site	Beam Energy	Depth or isod.	Fr/ day	Fr/ wk	Tot. Fr.	cGy/ Frac.	Subtotal Dose	Total Dose	Init.

	Narrative plan:		Goal:	Cure/Palliation	
_____ Course Prescription					
Port Films:					
Blood Tests:					
Other:		Staff M.D. signature: _____			

Date	Technique and Anatomic Site	Beam Energy	Depth or isod.	Fr/ day	Fr/ wk	Tot. Fr.	cGy/ Frac.	Subtotal Dose	Total Dose	Init.

Figure 8.22   A prescription page from a treatment chart.

TREATMENT FIELDS

Field No	Description	SSD(s) or SAD (a)	Dir	Collimator WxL (cm)	Gantry Angle	Coll Angle	Tray	Comp- ensator	Bolus	Wedge	Init

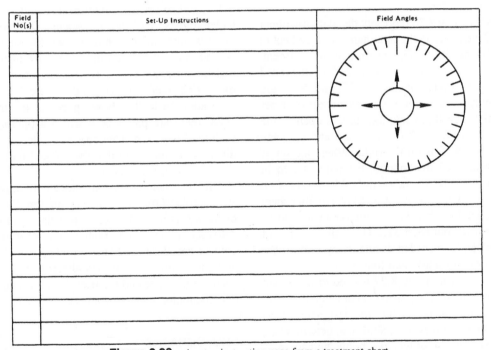

Figure 8.23 A setup instruction page from a treatment chart.

dition, this page helps the dosimetrist to record various off-axis measurements for subsequent dose calculation. It can also be used to draw a diagram of where each measurement was obtained. The simulation page is usually placed in the chart after the daily treatment record.

Figure 8.25 represents the reverse side of the simulation page. These diagrams and the text are self-explanatory. Suffice it to say that calculation and documentation of gaps between adjacent fields are considered important enough to warrant a special page.

Figure 8.26 shows a typical page for the calculation of monitor units or treatment time. In many departments including ours, dose calculations are performed on computers and a printout containing these same parameters is then inserted into the chart. This information is usually inserted after the daily treatment documentation.

Figures 8.27 and 8.28 represent the daily treatment log. All of the pages in the treatment chart are kept in a three-ring binder during the course of treatment. Therefore, new pages can be added as the need arises. Pages shown in Figs. 8.27 and 8.28 are printed on opposite sides of the same sheet of paper and inserted such that when the chart is opened, the page shown in Fig. 8.27 is on the left and the page shown in Fig. 8.28 is on the right. When one set of pages is filled (25 treatments), the page shown in Fig. 8.28 is turned over and on the back of it, now on the left, is the page shown in Fig. 8.27. Another sheet is then inserted so that the cumulative dose, and so on, can be filled out each day. Thus, any number of treatments can be recorded during many years if the patient returns for additional treatment.

The page shown in Fig. 8.27 is used to document the daily treatment. The particulars of each treatment field (the limit is six)—such as the designated treatment machine, beam energy, field size, field number, field description, use of wedges, bolus, and so on—are recorded here. One column is reserved for recording the rare occasion when the patient's treatment must be delivered on another machine or with another beam energy, or when there is a change in the collimator setting. In the left upper corner is an icon showing a manufacturer's designation of four independent collimator jaws.

The page shown in Fig. 8.28 has enough columns to accumulate dose at six different locations during a course of treatment. This is needed, for example, when a mantle field is treated and the dose is carried in many different sites. The site of the dose accumulation is described in the heading of the column in addition to the identifying number of the field(s) contributing dose to that site. There is also a place to record previous dose delivered to the same area and to record the depth of the dose calculation point or the isodose line at which the dose is calculated.

In the right upper corner is a space where the technologists can keep notes about the treatment that will help them quickly perform related jobs, such as sending the patient for laboratory tests. It also gives information with respect to frequency of port films, whether the patient has an immobilization device, bolus, and so on. Each treatment is initialed by two technologists and the physician. Dosimetry and physics staff initial each time a weekly chart review is made or any time during the course of treatment that the chart requires a review, as when the treatment is changed, requiring a dose calculation.

In addition to the shown pages of the treatment chart, there are pages onto which a photograph of each field is pasted. That space can also be used for diagrams in the event that they would more clearly show the treatment fields.

This treatment chart is included here only to give an example of treatment documentation. Clear documentation is needed to show that the treatment was delivered as intended, both in terms of treatment volume and dose fractionation schema. Federal regulations with respect to the delivery of radiation are becoming stricter and the need for clear and concise documentation cannot be stressed enough.

PHOTOGRAPHS

Many years ago, treatments were given using orthovoltage levels of radiation, which provided very little or no skin sparing. The dose on the skin surface was therefore often so high that permanent skin changes (telangiectasia), which often occurred, could be observed for many years. Such skin changes could sometimes be used to determine the location of

DUKE UNIVERSITY MEDICAL CENTER
Department of Radiation Oncology
Simulation Parameters

Patient's Name: _____   Rad. Onc. #: _____

Date	Tx Unit	Field Number	Field Description	Field Size	SAD	SSD	TFD	Gantry Angle	Collim. Angle	Couch Angle	Thickness

Remarks:

Off-axis calculation points:

Anatomic site	SSD	IFD	Depth	Off-axis dist.	Other

_____
Simulation Technologist

Figure 8.24   A treatment-simulation page.

GAP CALCULATION

Gap calculation between fields no. ____ & ____

Two sets of opposed pairs of fields must be calculated to converge at the patient's mid-depth.

Two posterior fields treating the spinal cord must be calculated to converge at the depth of the spinal cord.

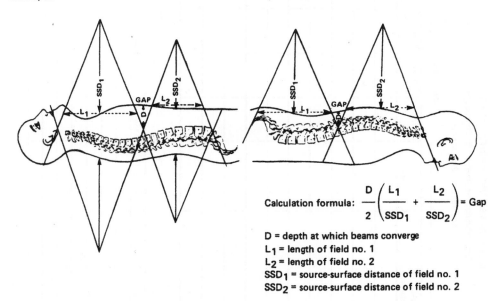

Calculation formula: $\dfrac{D}{2}\left(\dfrac{L_1}{SSD_1} + \dfrac{L_2}{SSD_2}\right) = Gap$

D = depth at which beams converge
L_1 = length of field no. 1
L_2 = length of field no. 2
SSD_1 = source-surface distance of field no. 1
SSD_2 = source-surface distance of field no. 2

* *

1. Measure the patient's thickness at the gap.
2. Assume a 2 cm gap.
3. Using this gap, determine the length of field no. 2.
4. Calculate the gap using this field length. Round out calculation up to the nearest 1/2 cm.
5. Shift field no. 2 based on the final result.

* *

$$\frac{\quad}{2}\left(\frac{\quad}{\quad} + \frac{\quad}{\quad}\right) = \underline{\quad} \text{ cm gap}$$

Actual gap on the patient's skin surface _____ cm. (rounded off to the nearest 1/2 cm. larger.)

_____
Signature

(For more than one gap calculation on the same patient use another sheet.)

Figure 8.25 A gap-calculation page.

Patient Name: _____

History #: _____

𝔓𝔥𝔬𝔱𝔬𝔫 Monitor Unit Calculation

Date:				
Field Number:				
Field Description:				
Treatment Unit:				
Energy (MV)/Technique:	/	/	/	/
Collimator—W x L:				
FS = 2WL/(W + L):				
SSD = :				
Patient Thickness:				
Depth of calculation = d:				
Calculation distance; SSD + d:				
ESQ = treatment eq. sq. at SSD+d:				
Wedge Angle:				
Off Axis Distance:				
Prescription Dose:				
TPR (d, ESQ) (from Table 1):				
S_c (FS) (from Table 2):				
S_p (ESQ) (from Table 3):				
CF (from Table 4):				
Isodose line—IDL (if from plan):				
Tray Factor—TF (from Table 4):				
Misc. Factor—MF (from Table 4):				
Wedge Factor—WF (from Table 4):				
Inverse Square Factor—INV: Note: INV $=\left(\dfrac{SAD}{SSD+d}\right)^2$	REMEMBER: INV. SQ MUST ALWAYS BE CALCULATED FOR SSD SETUPS			
Off axis ratio—OAR (from Table 5):				
M.U.:				
Initials:				

$$MU = \frac{\text{Prescription Dose}}{TPR \times S_c \times S_p \times CF \times IDL/100 \times TF \times WF \times MF \times INV \times OAR}$$

Figure 8.26 A monitor unit or treatment time-calculation page.

Patient's name:_____   #_____

A2 B2 ▨ B1 A1	Bolus:					
	Wedge:					
	Block:					

Beam Energy assigned:
x = x-rays   e=electrons

19....... Month Date	Elap. days	Tx. No.	Alternate energy or field size Change	Field # ____ Size:_____ A1: A2: B1: B2: Field descr.:		Field # ____ Size:_____ A1: A2: B1: B2: Field descr.:		Field # ____ Size:_____ A1: A2: B1: B2: Field descr.:		Field # ____ Size:_____ A1: A2: B1: B2: Field descr.:		Field # ____ Size:_____ A1: A2: B1: B2: Field descr.:		Field # ____ Size:_____ A1: A2: B1: B2: Field descr.:	
				MU	Tissue Dose	MU	Tissue Dose	MU	Tissue Dose	MU	Tissue Dose	MU	Tissue Dose	MU	Tissue Dose

Figure 8.27   A page of the daily treatment log.

Patient's name:_____   #_____

ACCUMULATED TISSUE DOSE												Technologist's reminders:			
Field #:		Field #:		Field #:		Field #:		Field #:		Field #:		Lab:			
												Port Film:			
												Bolus:			
Site:		Site:		Site:		Site:		Site:		Site:		Gap:			
												Alpha Cradle Headholder Cast			
												Simple Interm. Complex			
Depth or isodoseline:		Depth or isodoseline:		Depth or isodoseline:		Depth or isodoseline:		Depth or isodoseline:		Depth or isodoseline:		Other:			
Prev. dose:		Prev. dose:		Prev. dose:		Prev. dose:		Prev. dose:		Prev. dose:					
Daily Dose	Total Dose	Daily Dose	Total Dose	Daily Dose	Total Dose	Daily Dose	Total Dose	Daily Dose	Total Dose	Daily Dose	Total Dose	Tech	MD	Phys. QI	Notes

Figure 8.28   Daily dose-accumulation page.

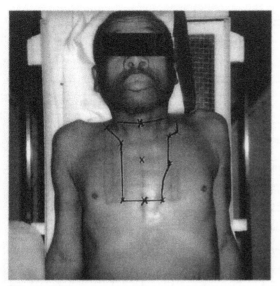

Figure 8.29   Polaroid picture of patient in treatment position and with the field clearly marked. Inclusion of areas surrounding the treatment field provides reference marks.

previous treatment fields when further radiation therapy was contemplated. With the high-energy beams now being used, there is very little if any skin reaction inside the treatment field, and other means of documenting the field location have become necessary.

Photographs of the treatment field outlined on the patient's skin are now used routinely for future reference and for new technologists treating the patient (Fig. 8.29). Such photographs should also show surrounding areas of the patient's skin, so that reference points can be used later on to determine where the fields were located. These photographs should, of course, also be labeled with the patient's name and date along with the identifying field numbers that they represent.

TATTOO

Tattoos indicating treatment fields can be very helpful in determining where previous treatment fields may have been located. Tattoos alone cannot be used to determine what tissues have been irradiated because—although the field may have entered in a

certain area on the skin—the beam angle may not be known. Even when the beam orientation is known, tattoos may be misleading because skin tends to move over rigid underlying structures; thus, the tattoos may not necessarily indicate the deep tissues within the treatment area. It is also important to realize that as patients lose or gain weight, the skin will move with respect to underlying tissues. Changes in tumor size, swelling, and—in the case of a child—growth will also change the relative position of the tattoos and the underlying anatomy. Tattoos should therefore be used with caution when the location of previously treated areas must be identified, particularly if some time has passed between the placement of the tattoos and the subsequent treatment.

As previously mentioned, most fields nowadays have very irregular shapes; therefore, even if pertinent corners are tattooed, these will not precisely show the area treated. Tattoos made on patients should always be indicated on the photograph of the field (Fig. 8.29). With both sets of information, the treatment field can be outlined by connecting the tattoos, as shown on the photograph. As a minimum, a tattoo should be made on the skin to indicate the segment of spinal cord that lies within the treated field (Fig. 8.30). However, tattoos must never be the only parameter by which to determine the location of a previously treated area; instead, they should be used along with radiographs of the field.

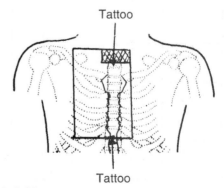

Figure 8.30   Tattoos should always be made indicating the length of the spinal cord actually treated—not the length within the collimator setting.

RADIOGRAPHIC DOCUMENTATION

Probably the most important documentation of a treatment field is a port film. A port film is a radiograph exposed with the treatment beam while the treatment geometry is maintained and with the patient in treatment position.[131,132] The cassette holding the film must be placed near the patient in the exit beam. The patient should never be lifted to place the cassette under the body. Instead, the cassette should be placed under the couch. This may not always be easy to accomplish, but when the patient is moved between the treatment and the port film exposure, the relationship between the radiation beam and the patient's anatomy is disturbed and the port film no longer represents the true treatment situation. Introducing a cassette under the patient causes the curvature of the spine to change in a similar fashion to that described when rolls of clothing are present under the patient's body.

Port films should always be obtained on the first day of treatment of every field to verify the shape and location of the treatment field. Port films are then compared with the simulation film (prescription or reference image) of the particular field. Any correction that may be needed should also be documented by a follow-up film of the change on the next treatment. Errors in cutting or mounting of the blocks in the beam may be observed on the first set of films and can be corrected prior to the second treatment. When treatment fields with small tumor margins are treated or the dose fraction is unusually high, the treatment fields are often verified prior to delivering any treatment. It is highly recommended that, prior to any treatment, all new customized beam-shaping blocks be carefully inspected for shape and directions while viewing the radiograph from which they were cut. Major errors—such as a block being reversed in the beam or a left and right block tray being mislabeled—could then be noted and corrected prior to any treatment. Some authors suggest that port films be obtained more frequently in the beginning of each treatment course so as to reduce the number of systematic errors.[133,134]

Another method of portal imaging is one in which a radiograph is left in the exit beam during the entire treatment. The image quality of these verification films is usually poor and they are therefore rarely used. High-energy x-ray beams used in radiation therapy produce low-contrast films; therefore, the port films are often difficult to interpret. Film-screen combination, which results in an improved image quality, has been published,[135–138] but each clinic must determine the combination that is best for the beam energies available to it. A digital enhancement technique for port films has been described.[132]

It is not unusual to find small discrepancies between laser alignment systems in the simulation room and the treatment room.[139] Some couches also sag more than others, and such differences may also be noticeable on the first set of port films. A mathematical method to determine discrepancies in patient position between simulation films and port films has been described by Balter et al.[140]

ELECTRONIC PORTAL IMAGING

Many electronic portal imaging devices (EPIDs) have been developed to replace radiographic portal imaging.[141–147] Electronic imaging systems operate on different principles. In the optical approach, the distribution of radiation intensity is converted into a visible light image via a metal sheet–fluorescent screen combination. The data are captured via a mirror with a camera located outside the radiation beam. In the scanning devices, either straight arrays or a matrix of radiation detectors scan the intensity of the exit beam sequentially with predetermined intervals. The data are then manipulated to provide a digital portal image. In all systems, the image is displayed instantaneously on a video monitor near the linear accelerator control panel (Fig. 8.31). Assessment of the portal image, a task traditionally carried out by the radiation oncologist by reviewing weekly port films at some time after the first treatment has been delivered, must now be made daily by viewing the image on the monitor. Although the image quality generally is good, the evaluation of the image can be difficult, since the surrounding anatomy, visible in radiographic portal films through a second exposure with a larger collimator opening, is not visible in most on-line portal images. It is particularly difficult

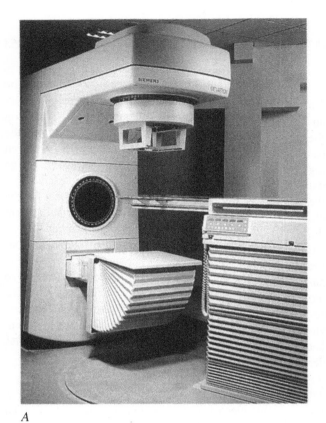

A

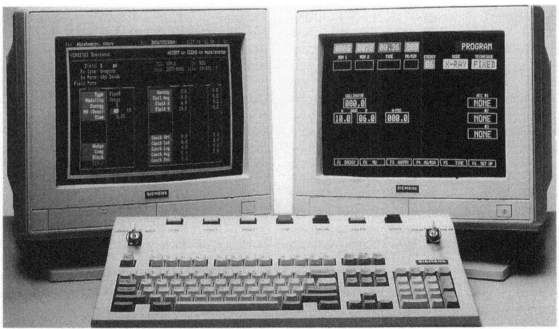

B

Figure 8.31 *A* and *B*. A real-time portal imaging device on the gantry can be retracted while the patient is being set up in the room. Before the treatment is delivered, the field alignment can be determined at the control console. (Courtesy of Siemens Medical Systems, Inc.)

to assess images where bony anatomy is absent within the field. Electronic methods for detecting differences in patient positioning between the simulation or "prescription" radiograph and the portal image have been described.[142,144,145,148-156]

Through the use of digital image processing techniques, the patient setup can be checked after only a few monitor units have been delivered. The patient's position can be adjusted before further treatment is delivered and multiple images can be obtained during the treatment to assess patient motion. Other advantages are the elimination of the need to reenter the treatment room to place the cassette, to change the collimator setting, or to retrieve the image, considerably reducing the time during which the patient must remain motionless. There is also a considerable savings in terms of cost, time, and space because there is no need to purchase films, no image to develop, and the electronic images are stored on diskettes requiring very little space.

RECORD AND VERIFY SYSTEMS

The various treatment parameters (field size, gantry, collimator and couch angles, block tray codes, wedge codes, dose, and so on) can be recorded in a computer system that will allow the treatment to be delivered only when all user-defined parameters have been met during the setup. As long as all parameters are correctly entered in the computer, the treatment is delivered correctly. It obviously cannot prevent the wrong patient or the wrong part of the body from being treated. In the near future one may, however, be able to also enter the coordinates of the isocenter position as recorded during the three-dimensional treatment-planning process in such a record-and-verify system. Following reposition of the patient so that the isocenter is at the origin of the spatial coordinate system (determined during the data acquisition procedure), the couch is moved via computer-control so that the isocenter is at the planned location for the treatment. The challenge will then be for the technologists to position the patient correctly on the couch.

Record-and-verify systems are also very reliable tools in documenting the treatment; they add to the confidence with which the treatment is delivered.

GENERAL RECOMMENDATIONS

The label of a treatment field should include the beam direction and the area where the beam enters the patient (anterior right oblique lung, right lateral pelvis, and so on). In addition, each field should have a unique number, so that similar but different fields are not confused. In the description of the field, it is also important to state whether the field includes the *right* or the *left* femur, for example. Frequently, a boost is delivered to the parametria through anterior and posterior fields following an intracavitary insertion. It is very important to describe whether the boost is to the left, right, or bilateral parametria. In head-and-neck treatment, it is also important to describe whether an anterior supraclavicular field includes the right, left, or bilateral supraclavicular area.

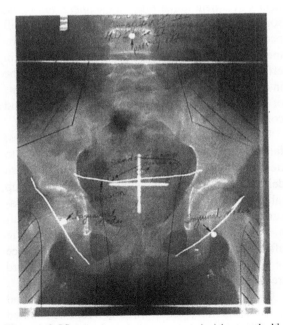

Figure 8.32 Lead markers on scars, incisions, palpable lymph nodes, and other important reference points during the simulation procedure are very useful for later reference. Each lead marker should be labeled to indicate what it represents. A statement of the diagnosis and a short note about the patient on the simulation film are also very helpful when port films are reviewed.

Port films are often reviewed without the treatment chart or other details of the patient's history nearby. A short note on the simulation film, giving the patient's diagnosis and any particular information about surgical margins and so forth, would be helpful to a reviewer who is unfamiliar with the case. It is also good practice to mark incisions, palpable nodes, and so on with lead markers during the simulation procedure and to label them on the radiograph (Fig. 8.32).

TREATMENT ERRORS

The delivery of radiation therapy is a very complex process and requires highly trained and dedicated technical staff who carefully use detailed documentation during every step of the treatment.

This section focuses on *errors* that sometimes occur in dose calculations or in the setup of a patient's treatment rather than on the *uncertainties* associated with treatment delivery. Human errors will occasionally occur in every radiation therapy department and a system to deal with such errors must be in effect. A rigid quality-assurance program should be in effect in all radiation therapy facilities. The focus of such a program should be to prevent errors and correct problems.

Treatment errors can be divided into two groups; failure to deliver the prescribed dose and failure to treat the intended volume of tissue. Errors in dose delivery can be caused by (1) error in looking up tables, (2) error in dose calculation, (3) error in measurements of the patient's dimensions, or (4) treatment machine malfunction. Errors of these types are often small and, through a rigid quality-assurance program, can be detected before a second or third treatment is delivered.

More serious errors, both in terms of dose and dose distribution, occur when a wedge is omitted from the beam or is inserted in the wrong orientation. In Chaps. 3 and 6, we learned that wedges, while altering the shape of the isodose curves, also attenuate the beam. The attenuation depends on the wedge angle and beam energy but can be as high as 50 percent. For example, if a wedge with 50 percent

attenuation is inadvertently omitted, then not only is the dose distribution altered but the *amount* of dose on the central axis is doubled. The changes in the dose distribution caused by the omission of a wedge with a steep angle are more severe than if a wedge with a smaller angle were omitted. When a wedge is inserted but the orientation is reversed, the dose on the central axis is unchanged, but the error in the dose distribution is obviously significant.

Errors in wedge orientation may be counteracted by using a wedge with a steeper angle in the correct orientation during the next few treatments, but that will, of course, deliver a somewhat different dose distribution; consideration must therefore be given to the effect that this will have on the tissues within the field. A good rule of thumb is that omission of a 30° wedge during only 1 of 30 treatments results in approximately 1° change in the slope of the isodose curve in this field. The slope of the isodose curve is 30°, whether we give 1 or 30 treatments, so by leaving the wedge out during a single treatment, the effect will be one-thirtieth, or in this case 1° (about 3 percent). Similarly, the omission of a 30° wedge during 5 of 10 treatments will result in a 15° (or 50 percent) change in the slope of the isodose curve.

Another serious error occurs when a beam-shaping block is inadvertently omitted, inserted in the wrong orientation, or inserted in the wrong field. Unlike dose-delivery errors, these types of errors are usually not repeated during multiple treatments and are more difficult to detect unless portal films are taken during delivery of each dose fraction. The impact of field-placement errors is similar to that of errors in dose delivery in that some segment of the target may have been outside the irradiated area and thus have received no dose.

The course of action when an error is discovered should be based on the magnitude of the error and its relative proportion of the entire treatment course. For example, was 185 rather than the prescribed 180 cGy delivered, or was 300 rather than 150 cGy delivered? Did the error occur during 1 of 20 treatments or was it during 2 of 5? Consideration should also be given to the radiosensitivity of the normal tissues that received the wrong dose and to the resulting effect in these organs.

The philosophy of how to correct errors in dose varies among physicians. While some think that the error in dose should be corrected during the following one or two treatments, depending on the magnitude of the error, others think that unintentionally deviating from the prescribed dose one day does not justify making the same deviation in the opposite direction, now intentionally, on another day. Each situation must be considered individually, and modifications must be made by the physician only. The most important action when an error has occurred is that it be reported to the responsible physician immediately, so that appropriate action can be taken.

COMMUNICATION

One often-encountered problem concerns the differences in terminology among staff, even within the same department. Confusion and error can be reduced by proper use of the technical terms of radiation oncology; though these terms are inherently precise, careless use of terminology can lead to serious errors.

In treatment planning, for example, it is more important to outline the *target volume* (often symbolized by TV) than the *tumor volume* (also symbolized by TV), because the former is always larger than the latter. In most situations, it is necessary for the treatment-planning staff to know the size and location of the *target* so that it can be included in the final plan. For a subsequent boost, the target and tumor volumes may be synonymous. The dosimetrist is often presented with CT images or simulation films where TV is outlined. The dosimetrist plans the fields so that this volume will be covered, only to learn later that the physician also wanted to treat a large margin surrounding the area marked TV, now intended to signify the target volume. A new plan must now be made to include this TV (target volume). If everyone would agree on proper terminology, symbols, and abbreviations before a great deal of effort is spent on planning the treatment, everyone would benefit, including the patient, and embarrassments would be prevented.

The physician may sometimes use terminology unfamiliar to technologists. Occasionally, to avoid having to ask, other staff just guess at the physician's intentions, and the desired result may not be achieved. In radiation therapy as in other medical specialties, a certain level of jargon is used. For example, it used to be common practice to refer to a certain treatment field by its shape or something that it resembled. For example, a field often used to treat the paraaortic and inguinal lymph nodes with a central pelvic block is often referred to as an *inverted Y*. A field including the internal mammary and supraclavicular lymph nodes, which is no longer commonly utilized, was often referred to as a *hockey stick.* Treatment fields with these shapes can, of course, be used in many other sites. The words "hockey stick", for example, are also used by some to describe a craniospinal field or a field used to treat the paraaortic and hemipelvic lymph nodes. Prescribing the dose to a hockey stick or an inverted Y can lead to major errors. The prescription as well as the field identification should identify the treatment site anatomically rather than by the shape of the field. The term *mantle field,* generally used in the United States to describe treatment of all major lymph-node groups above the diaphragm, is also used in this text. A more appropriate description would probably be "supradiaphragmatic lymph nodes."

The term *given dose* was once in common use to describe surface or D_{max} doses. This expression is too vague and leads to ambiguities unacceptable in modern radiation oncology. Is the given dose delivered by one field on the surface, at a depth, at a depth on the central axis, at an isodose curve? Is it the minimum tumor dose or perhaps the maximum tumor dose? All of them are "given dose." With modern sophisticated methods of determining dose at practically any point in tissue, *given dose* has given way to terminology that describes dose more clearly. The reporting of doses must be accompanied by a description of where the dose was delivered, using current methods of determination. There must be no ambiguity as to what dose was delivered and where.

In describing simple anatomic landmarks, careless use of proper terminology can cause major errors in beam position. For example, giving instructions to the simulator technologist to place a lead marker on the "bony canthus" is ambiguous. The canthus is the angle at *either* end of the eyelid, so there are two canthi, distinguished as the temporal or outer canthus and the nasal or inner canthus.[157] Not only can the two canthi be confused with each other but the outer canthus is sometimes confused with the lateral bony ridge of the orbit, resulting in an error of as much as 0.75 cm in field placement, with obvious consequences (Fig. 8.33).

The abbreviation L. V., used to describe an area of a mantle field that was to have a 50 percent transmission block, could be interpreted to mean lung volume, when in fact the left ventricle of the heart is intended. Such a misinterpretation could have serious consequences.

In the treatment of a paraaortic and spleen field, a note to add a "spleen block at 2000 cGy" can be interpreted to mean that the spleen section of the field is to be blocked at 2000 cGy when in fact it means to block the kidney within the spleen section of the field.

A vertical beam direction is, to many individuals, synonymous with an anterior field because of the conventional supine patient position. However, when the patient's position is changed (prone or decubitus), the vertical beam direction becomes a posterior or lateral field (Fig. 8.34). The field positions are usually described with respect to the patient and not to the way the treatment machine happens to be positioned in the room. It is not unusual to hear someone refer to a vertical beam as an anterior field regardless of the patient's position. Such very simple misunderstandings can lead to serious errors in treatment delivery. In communicating the intended field arrangement among the staff, it is critical that everyone understand and carry out the prescribed treatment with proper patient-beam arrangement.

In a growing number of treatments, not only are the gantry and collimator angled but also the treatment couch. Gantry angles are customarily expressed from 0 to 360°, while collimator and couch angles are usually expressed from 0 to 90°. Gantry angles are not uniform between treatment machines, and different manufacturers may have different systems of defining gantry angles. Since there is little or no need to turn the collimator or couch more than 90° to either side, the problem of expressing these angles is simpler. However, there is a serious problem of defining in which direction these angles are; for example, whether the couch is turned 10° to the left or to the right, positive or negative, and is it with respect to the patient or to the gantry? The expression "kicking the couch out" is much too general in modern radiation therapy. Specific instructions as to the direction in which the couch is to be turned and documentation of the number of degrees are vital in safely relaying the information from the simulation room to the treatment room. To minimize errors and misinterpretations, one must be as specific as possible, use commonly accepted terminology, and avoid abbreviations when giving instructions. Speaking and writing clearly are also very important.

With the growing number of new modalities and the rapid development and application of three-dimensional treatment planning systems, a common language is essential. The conventions, for example, by which gantry, collimator, and couch angles are described vary among institutions and may even vary among the staff within one institution. As a result,

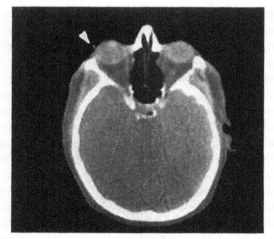

Figure 8.33 The lateral bony ridge of the orbit and the lateral canthus of the eye (*arrow*) are usually separated by approximately 0.75 cm in an adult.

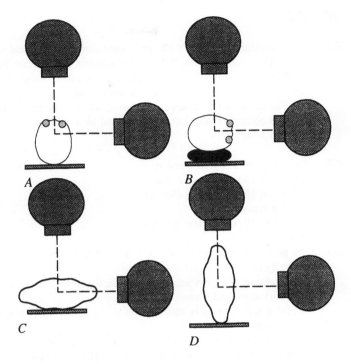

Figure 8.34 *A–D.* A vertical beam is not always an anterior field. Field descriptions should always be written with respect to the patient and not the machine or the room.

the confusion may lead to errors in treatment delivery. When discussions among the staff with reference to these ambiguities are carried on in front of the patient, as the case may be in the simulator room or treatment room, for example, the patient quickly loses confidence in the staff's abilities.

With the advent of three-dimensional treatment-planning capability and the ability to rotate and view CT and MR images in practically any plane, a common language becomes paramount to the communication and understanding among the many individuals involved in the planning and delivery of a course of treatments. Descriptions of different beam angles or the planes in which we view the patient's anatomy can be very confusing. The precision in delivering radiation therapy which we are capable of with the use of very sophisticated tools must not be compromised by misunderstandings or ambiguities. Many

treatment fields planned with the help of three-dimensional treatment-planning systems cannot be described using conventional terminology. Goitein and Sailer et al. have proposed a uniform language for describing such treatment fields.[158,159] The increasing use of computers both in planning and execution of the treatments require that the treatment parameters entered in the computer software be independently verified. Due to the large number of persons and different parameters involved from one step to the next, correct transfer of the treatment information is critical.[160] In many departments, setup and planning parameters are handled via computers; they are then transferred manually to another computer, which virtually "drives" the treatment delivery. The final treatment instructions (beam direction, field size, dose, etc.) should be independently verified prior to the first treatment.

PROBLEMS

8.1 When a linear accelerator with one independently moving leaf is used with a wedge in the beam, there is a chance that the independent jaw cannot be used because
  (*a*) It is impossible to use an independent jaw and a wedge at the same time
  (*b*) There is never a need to use an independent jaw when a wedge is used
  (*c*) The collimator must always be turned when a wedge is used
  (*d*) The collimator may have to be turned in a direction such that the independent jaw cannot be used

8.2 The attenuation of Cerrobend is
  (*a*) About 15 percent more than lead
  (*b*) About 15 percent less than lead
  (*c*) The same as lead
  (*d*) About 10 percent less than lead

8.3 The potential hazards of working in a mold room where alloy shields are made consists primarily of
  (*a*) Inhalation of vapors and dust particles, ingestion of small fragments of the metal, skin penetration, and burns
  (*b*) Inhalation of vapors and dust particles, skin penetration, and causing a fire when smoking
  (*c*) Inhalation of vapors, skin penetration, and causing a fire when smoking
  (*d*) Ingestion of small fragments of the metal, skin penetration, and eye irritation

8.4 To reduce the risks of ingestion of small fragments of the alloy in a block cutting room, the following precautions should be taken:
  (*a*) Have proper ventilation in the block cutting room, wear special goggles, and wear protective shoes
  (*b*) Practice good hygiene and wash hands before eating, drinking, and smoking
  (*c*) Wear gloves when handling the alloy, have proper ventilation in the room, and wear protective shoes
  (*d*) Wear special boots and gloves when handling the blocks and wash hands before taking the blocks to the treatment room

8.5 Multileaf collimators are different from custom-shaped blocks because
  (*a*) They produce steplike field edges, leakage can occur between leaves, and they can only be used with limited field sizes
  (*b*) They produce scalloped isodose distributions in the penumbra, are extremely heavy, and can produce any field shape or size
  (*c*) They are easy to set up, produce sharper penumbras, and can be used with any field size
  (*d*) They are easy to remove and replace between patients, produce sharper field edges, and can be used with any field size

8.6 Custom-made electron shields are different from custom blocks for photon beams because
  (*a*) They have no focused edges, are slightly thinner, and are mounted on a tray near the skin surface
  (*b*) They are much thinner and much bigger and they weigh more

(c) They have no focused edges, are much thinner, and usually weigh more

(d) They have no focused edges and are much thinner; also, the size of the opening is practically the same as the field on the skin surface

8.7   When a skin lesion is treated using an electron or orthovoltage beam, the shielding

(a) Should be placed inside the cone, so when the patient moves the shielding follows the motion of the patient

(b) Should be custom-made and the cutout should be made as small as possible so that it will not cause discomfort for the patient

(c) Should be placed directly on the patient, covering a large area surrounding the lesion

(d) Should be placed inside the mouth to protect the mucosa and absorb secondary scatter from the teeth

8.8   Secondary scatter in the metal-tissue interface

(a) Can cause decreased dose in the adjacent tissues, but this can be increased by using an electron beam

(b) Can cause lower dose in the mouth, and the patient should not be treated until a dentist has been consulted

(c) Can cause high dose in the adjacent tissues but can be reduced by placing 2 to 4 mm of tissue-equivalent material over the teeth

(d) Can cause high dose in the adjacent tissues, but this can be reduced by using lower-energy beams and asking patients to brush their teeth after the treatment

8.9   When a lip lesion is treated, it is possible to reduce the mucosal reaction by

(a) Placing an internal shield proximal to the tumor and coating the shield with wax

(b) Placing an internal shield distal to the tumor and covering the shield with wax

(c) Placing a large shield around the tumor and coating it with wax

(d) Placing a shield inside the cone and covering it with wax

8.10   When a missing tissue compensator is used in a photon beam, the compensator should be

(a) Placed at some distance from the skin surface

(b) Placed directly on the skin surface to be most effective

(c) Made the same size as the missing tissue volume and be placed at some distance from the skin surface

(d) Placed directly on the skin surface to take advantage of the skin-sparing properties of a compensator

8.11   The most practical material to use when making a compensator for photon beams is

(a) Cerrobend, lead, brass, or aluminum

(b) Cerrobend, brass, water, or rice bags

(c) Wax, brass, lead, or water

(d) Wax, paraffin, Lucite, brass, or aluminum

8.12   Bolus material is used to

(a) Compensate for surface irregularities when photon beams are used

(b) Compensate for surface irregularities when any beam energy is used

(c) Reduce the depth of the maximum dose when photon beams are used

(d) Reduce the percent depth dose when photon beams are used

8.13 The function of the Radiological Physics Center (RPC) is to
   (a) Review patient treatment records, dosimetry calibration of equipment used in the treatment of patients enrolled in clinical trials, and communicate instructive findings to the clinical study groups
   (b) Review patient treatment records, calibrate all radiation therapy equipment, and establish quality control procedures for all radiation therapy centers
   (c) Carry out dosimetry calibration of equipment used in the treatment of patients enrolled in clinical trials, advise study chairmen on proper quality procedures
   (d) Review patient treatment records, communicate instructive findings to the clinical study groups, and stage surprise site visits to departments participating in national clinical trials

8.14 Departmental weekly chart rounds should include verifying
   (a) Presence of diagnosis, histology, and stage; presence of consent for treatment; presence of pathology report; and evidence that the patient is making progress
   (b) Presence of diagnosis and histology, and stage; presence of consent for treatment; presence of pathology report; presence of dose prescription dated and signed; and weekly port films of each field approved, signed, and dated by the radiation oncologist
   (c) Presence of pathology report; presence of dose prescription dated and signed, and that at least one port film has been approved, is signed, and dated by the radiation oncologist
   (d) Presence of pathology report; presence of dose prescription dated and signed prior to the first treatment; presence of dose prescription dated and signed by the radiation oncologist prior to the first treatment, and evidence that the patient has been seen by a resident each week

8.15 The frequency of port films varies, but they
   (a) Should be taken at the first possible opportunity
   (b) Should be taken at least in the first week of treatment
   (c) Should always be taken on the first day of treatment
   (d) Should be taken of at least one field each week

8.16 Electronic portal imaging is a method whereby the patient/beam alignment is checked
   (a) After the entire first treatment has been delivered
   (b) By the physician in his office when everyone else has gone home
   (c) After just a few monitor units have been delivered
   (d) By the technologist at the end of the day

8.17 Various methods of documenting the treatment parameters include
   (a) Tattoo, photograph of each field, recording of the dose, and a fingerprint
   (b) Tattoo, photograph of each treatment field, and a port film of each field
   (c) Photograph of the patient taken on the first visit and a port film of each field
   (d) Tattoo, sending a copy of the chart to the medical record room, photograph of each field, and recording of the dose

8.18 If a 30° wedge is left out of the treatment during two of five treatments,
   (a) The central axis dose is decreased and the isodose distribution is affected
   (b) The central axis dose is decreased and the isodose distribution is not affected
   (c) The central axis dose is increased and the isodose distribution is not affected
   (d) The central axis dose is increased and the isodose distribution is affected

8.19 When an error in dose delivery is discovered,
(*a*) The attending radiation oncologist should be notified
(*b*) No action need be taken until at the end of the day
(*c*) What action should be taken is based on where the treatment was given
(*d*) The patient should be told that a mistake was made and that it can be made up on the next treatment

8.20 Treatment fields should be labeled in the chart with reference to
(*a*) Whatever shape it resembles, and it should have a unique number
(*b*) An anatomic description, and it should have a unique number
(*c*) An anatomic description with abbreviations, so that the patient cannot understand it
(*d*) An anatomic description and any number

REFERENCES

1. Chui C, Mohan R, Fontanela D: Dose computation for asymmetric fields defined by independent jaws. *Med Phys* 15:92, 1986.
2. Loshek DD, Parker TT: Dose calculation in static or dynamic off-axis fields. *Med Phys* 21:401, 1994.
3. Khan FM, Gerbi BJ, Diebel FC: Dosimetry of asymmetric x-ray collimators. *Med Phys* 13:936, 1986.
4. Khan F: Dosimetry of wedged fields with asymmetric collimation. *Med Phys* 20:1447, 1993.
5. Marinello G, Dutreix A: A general method to perform dose calculations along the axis of symmetrical and asymmetrical photon beams. *Med Phys* 19:275, 1992.
6. Woo MK, Fung A, O'Broen P: Treatment planning for asymmetric jaws on a commercial TP system. *Med Phys* 19:1273, 1992.
7. Palta JR, Ayyanger KM, Suntharalingum N: Dosimetric characteristics of a 6 MV photon beam from a linear accelerator with asymmetric collimator jaws. *Int J Radiat Oncol Biol Phys* 14:383, 1988.
8. Earl JD, Bagshaw MA: A rapid method for preparation of complex field shapes. *Radiology* 88:1162, 1967.
9. Edland RW, Hansen H: Irregular field-shaping for ^{60}Co teletherapy. *Radiology* 92:1567, 1969.
10. Jones D: A method for the accurate manufacture of lead shields. *Br J Radiol* 44:398, 1971.
11. Karzmark CJ, Huisman PA: Melting, casting and shaping of lead shielding blocks: Method and toxicity aspects. *Am J Radiol* 114:636, 1972.
12. Kuisk H: New method to facilitate radiotherapy planning and treatment, including a method for fast production of solid lead blocks with diverging walls for cobalt 60 beam. *AJR* 117:161, 1973.
13. Maruyama YM, Moore VC, Burns D, Hilger MTJ: Individualized lung shields constructed from lead shots embedded in plastic. *Radiology* 92:634, 1969.
14. Parfitt H: Manufacture of lead shields. *Br J Radiol* 44:895, 1971.
15. Powers WE, Kinzie JJ, Demidecki AJ, Bradfield JS, Feldman A: A new system of field shaping for external-beam radiation therapy. *Radiology* 108:407, 1973.
16. Purdy JA, Sorenson A, Eisenhoffer J: A combination styrofoam cutter/block checker for fabricating field shaping blocks. *Int J Radiat Oncol Biol Phys* 2:1209, 1977.
17. Paliwal BR, Asp L: A technique to evaluate styrofoam cutouts used in irregular field shaping. *Int J Radiat Oncol Biol Phys* 1:791, 1976.
18. Chu JCH, Stafford PM, Hanks GE, Peters L: Use of computerized hot wire block cutter in radiation therapy. *Med Dosim* 17:11, 1992.
19. DeMeyer CL, Whitehead LW, Jacobson AD, Brown DG: Potential exposure to metal fumes, particulates, and organic vapors during radiotherapy shielding fabrication. *Med Phys* 13:748, 1986.
20. Glasgow GP: The safety of low melting point bismuth/ lead alloys: A review. *Med Dosim* 16:13, 1991.
21. McCullough EC, Senjem DH: Airborne concentrations of toxic metals resulting from the use of low melting point lead alloys to construct radiotherapy shielding. *Med Phys* 8:111, 1981.
22. Occupational Safety and Health Administration, OSHA: *Code of Federal Regulation,* Type § 1910.1027, Report #29, 1993.
23. Occupational Safety and Health Administration, OSHA: *Code of Federal Regulation,* Type § 1910.1025, Report #29, 1992.
24. Keus R, Noach P, deBoer R, Lebesque J: The effect of customized beam shaping on normal tissue complications in radiation therapy of parotid tumors. *Radiother Oncol* 21:211, 1991.
25. Douglas K, Wilson WP, Bridge LR: A simple shift technique for the production of shielding blocks at extended distances. *Br J Radiol* 57:273, 1984.
26. Nair TKM, Sadeghi A: Simulation of extended mantle field by tray shift technique. *Br J Radiol* 53:1088, 1980.
27. Boyer AL, Ochran TG, Nyerick CE, et al: Clinical dosim-

etry or implementation of a multileaf collimator. *Med Phys* 19:1255, 1992.

28. Brahme A: Optimal setting of multileaf collimators in stationary beam radiation therapy. *Strahlenth Onkol* 164:343, 1988.

29. Galvin JM, Smith AR, Lally B: Characterization of a multileaf collimator system. *Int J Radiat Oncol Biol Phys* 25:181, 1993.

30. LoSasso T, Chui CS, Kutcher GJ, et al: The use of multileaf collimator for conformal radiotherapy of carcinomas of the prostate and nasopharynx. *Int J Radiat Oncol Biol Phys* 25:161, 1993.

31. Powlis WD, Smith AR, Cheng E, et al: Initiation of multileaf collimator conformal radiation therapy. *Int J Radiat Oncol Biol Phys* 25:171, 1993.

32. Lichter AS, Fraass BA, McShan DL: Recent advances in radiotherapy treatment planning. *Oncology* 2:43, 1988.

33. Goede MR, Gooden DS, Ellis RG, Brickner TJ: A versatile electron collimation system to be used with electron cones supplied with Varian Clinac 18. *Int J Radiat Oncol Biol Phys* 2:791, 1977.

34. Purdy JA, Chot MC, Feldman A: Lipowitz metal shielding thickness for dose reduction of 6-20 MeV electrons. *Med Phys* 7:251, 1980.

35. Gosselin M, Podgorsak EB, Evans MDC: Dosimetry of centrally shielded electron beams. *Med Phys* 21:1245, 1994.

36. Gibbs FA, Palos B, Goffinet DR: The metal/tissue interface effect in irradiation of the oral cavity. *Radiology* 119:705, 1976.

37. Thambi V, Murthy AK, Alder G, Kartha PK: Dose perturbation resulting from gold fillings in patients with head and neck cancers. *Int J Radiat Oncol Biol Phys* 5:581, 1979.

38. Gagnon WF, Cundiff JH: Dose enhancement from backscattered radiation at tissue-metal interfaces irradiated with high energy electrons. *Br J Radiol* 53:466, 1980.

39. Khan FM, Moore VC, Levitt SH: Field shaping in electron beam therapy. *Br J Radiol* 49:833, 1976.

40. Klevenhagen SC, Lambert GD, Arbari A: Backscattering in electron beam therapy for energies between 3 and 35 MeV. *Phys Med Biol* 27:363, 1982.

41. Saunders JE, Peters BG: Back-scattering from metals in superficial therapy with high energy electrons. *Br J Radiol* 47:467, 1974.

42. Khan FM: *The Physics of Radiation Therapy,* 2d ed. Baltimore-London: Williams & Wilkins, 1994.

43. Arora VR, Weeks KJ: Characterization of gypsum attenuators for radiotherapy dose modification. *Med Phys* 21:77, 1994.

44. Weeks KJ, Fraass BA, Hutchins KM: Gypsum mixture for compensator construction. *Med Phys* 15:410, 1988.

45. Beck GG, McGonnagle WJ, Sullivan CA: Use of a styrofoam block cutter to make tissue-equivalent compensators. *Radiology* 100:694, 1971.

46. Boge RJ, Edland RW, Matthes DC: Tissue compensators for megavoltage radiotherapy fabricated from hollowed styrofoam filled with wax. *Radiology* 111:193, 1974.

47. Feaster GR, Agarwal SK, Huddleston AL, Friesen EJ: A missing tissue compensator. *Int J Radiat Oncol Biol Phys* 5:277, 1979.

48. Khan FM, Moore VC, Burns DJ: An apparatus for the construction of irregular surface compensators for use in radiotherapy. *Radiology* 90:593, 1968.

49. Khan FM, Moore VC, Burns DJ: The construction of compensators for cobalt teletherapy. *Int J Radiat Oncol Biol Phys* 6:745, 1970.

50. Purdy JA, Keys DJ, Zivnuska F: A compensation filter for chest portals. *Int J Radiat Oncol Biol Phys* 2:1213, 1977.

51. Renner WD, O'Connor TP, Amtey SR, et al: The use of photogrammetry in tissue compensator design: Part I. Photogrammetric determination of patient topography. *Radiology* 125:505, 1977.

52. Renner WD, O'Connor TP, Amtey SR, et al: The use of photogrammetry in tissue compensator design Part II. Experimental verification of compensator design. *Radiology* 125:511, 1977.

53. Renner WD, O'Connor TP, Bermudez NM: An algorithm for design of beam compensators. *Int J Radiat Oncol Biol Phys* 17:227, 1989.

54 Faw FL, Johnson RE, Warren CA, Glenn DW: A standard set of "individualized" compensating filters for mantle field radiotherapy of Hodgkin's disease. *Am J Roentgenol* 111:376, 1971.

55. Leung PMK, Van Dyk J, Robins J: A method for large irregular field compensation. *Br J Radiol* 47:805, 1974.

56. Dixon RL, Ekstrand KE, Ferree C: Compensating filter design using megavoltage radiography. *Int J Radiat Oncol Biol Phys* 5:281, 1979.

57. Ekstrand KE, Ferree CR, Dixon RL, Raben M: The inverse compensating filter. *Radiology* 132:201, 1979.

58. Ansbacher W, Robinson DM, Scrimger JW: Missing tissue compensators: Evaluation and optimization of a commercial system. *Med Phys* 19:1267, 1992.

59. Kutcher GJ, Burman C, Mohan R: Compensation in three-dimensional non-coplanar treatment planning. *Int J Radiat Oncol Biol Phys* 20:127, 1991.

60. Mageras GS, Mohan R, Burman C, et al: Compensators for three-dimensional treatment planning. *Med Phys* 18:133, 1991.

61. Shragge PC, Patterson MS: Improved method for the design of tissue compensators. *Med Phys* 8:885, 1981.

62. Ellis F, Hall EJ, Oliver R: A compensator for variations in tissue thickness for high energy beam. *Br J Radiol* 32:421, 1959.

63. Hall EJ, Oliver R: The use of standard isodose distributions with high energy radiation beams—The accuracy of a compensator technique in correcting for body contours. *Br J Radiol* 34:43, 1961.

64. Sewchand W, Bautro N, Scott RM: Basic data of tissue-equivalent compensators for 4 MV x-rays. *Int J Radiat Oncol Biol Phys* 6:327, 1980.

65. Sundblom L: Individually designed filters in cobalt-60 teletherapy. *Acta Radiol Ther Biol Phys* 2:189, 1964.

66. van de Geijn J: The construction of individualized intensity modifying filters in cobalt-60 teletherapy. *Br J Radiol* 38:865, 1965.

67. Ellis F, Feldman A, Oliver R: Compensation for tissue inhomogeneity in cobalt 60 therapy. *Br J Radiol* 37:795, 1964.

68. Ellis F, Lescrenier C: Combined compensation for contours and heterogeneity. *Radiology* 106:191, 1973.

69. Jursinic PA, Podgorsak MB, Paliwal BR: Implementation of a three-dimensional compensation system based on computed tomography generated surface contours and tissue inhomogeneities. *Med Phys* 21:357, 1994.

70. Khan FM, Williamson JF, Sewchand W, Kim TH: Basic data for dosage calculation and compensation. *Int J Radiat Oncol Biol Phys* 6:745, 1980.

71. Boge RJ, Tolbert DD, Edland RW: Accuracy beam flattening filter for the Varian Clinac-4 linear accelerator. *Radiology* 115:475, 1975.

72. Lebesque JV, Keus R: The simultaneous boost technique: The concept of relative normalized dose. *Radiother Oncol* 22:45, 1991.

73. Weeks KJ, Arora VR, Leopold KA, et al: Clinical use of a concomitant boost technique using a gypsum compensator. *Int J Radiat Oncol Biol Phys* 30:693, 1994.

74. Gladstone DJ, van Herk M, Chin LM: Verification of lung attenuator positioning before total body irradiation using an electronic imaging device. *Int J Radial Oncol Biol Phys* 27:449, 1993.

75. Barth NH: An inverse problem in radiation therapy. *Int J Radiat Oncol Biol Phys* 18:425, 1990.

76. Brahme A: Optimization of stationary and moving beam radiation therapy techniques. *Radiother Oncol* 12:129, 1988.

77. Bortfield TR, Kahler DL, Waldron TJ, Boyer AL: X-ray field compensation with multileaf collimators. *Int J Radiat Oncol Biol Phys* 28:723, 1994.

78. Bortfield T, Boyer AL, Schlegel W, Kahler DL, Waldron TJ: Realization and verification of three-dimensional conformal radiotherapy with modulated fields. *Int J Radiat Oncol Biol Phys* 30:899, 1994.

79. Goitein M: The inverse problem (Editorial). *Int J Radiat Oncol Biol Phys* 18:489, 1990.

80. Gokhale P, Hussein EMA, Kulkami N: Determination of beam orientation in radiotherapy planning. *Med Phys* 21:393, 1994.

81. Gustafsson A, Lind BK, Brahme A: A generalized pencil beam algorithm for optimization of radiation therapy. *Med Phys* 21:343, 1994.

82. Källman P, Lind B, Eklöf A, Brahme A: Shaping of arbitrary dose distributions by computer-controlled collimator motion. *Phys Med Biol* 33:1291, 1988.

83. Lind BK, Källman P: Experimental verification of an algorithm for inverse radiation therapy planning. *Radiother Oncol* 17:359, 1990.

84. Mackie TR, Holmes T, Swerdloff S, et al: Tomotherapy: A new concept for the delivery of dynamic conformal radiotherapy. *Med Phys* 20:1709, 1993.

85. Mohan R, Mageras GS, Baldwin B, et al: Clinically relevant optimization of 3-D conformal treatments. *Med Phys* 19:933, 1992.

86. Morrill SM, Rosen II, Lane RG, Belli JA: The influence of dose constraint point placement on optimized radiation therapy treatment planning. *Int J Radiat Oncol Biol Phys* 19:129, 1990.

87. Morrill SM, Lane RG, Jacobson G, Rosen II: Treatment planning optimization using constrained simulated annealing. *Phys Med Biol* 36:1341, 1991.

88. Raphael C: Mathematical modelling of objectives in radiation therapy planning. *Phys Med Biol* 37:1293, 1992.

89. Webb S: Optimisation of conformal radiotherapy dose distributions by simulated annealing. *Phys. Med Biol* 34:1349, 1989.

90. Chui CS, LoSasso T, Spirou S: Dose calculation for photon beams with intensity modulation generated by dynamic jaw or multileaf collimators. *Med Phys* 21:1237, 1994.

91. Spirou SV, Chui CS: Generation of arbitrary intensity profiles by dynamic jaws or multileaf collimators. *Med Phys* 21:1031, 1994.

92. Proimos BS: Synchronous field shaping in rotational megavolt therapy. *Radiology* 74:753, 1960.

93. Proimos BS: Synchronous protection and fieldshaping in cyclotherapy. *Radiology* 77:591, 1961.

94. Proimos BS: New accessories for precise teletherapy with cobalt-60 units. *Radiology* 81:307, 1963.

95. Proimos BS: Beam shapers oriented by gravity in rotational therapy. *Radiology* 87:928, 1966.

96. Proimos BS: Shaping the dose distribution through a tumor model. *Radiology* 92:130, 1969.

97. Proimos BS, Goldson AL: Dynamic dose-shaping by gravity-oriented absorbers for total lymph node irradiation. *Int J Radiat Oncol Biol Phys* 7:973, 1981.

98. Rawlinson JA, Cunningham JR: An examination of synchronous shielding in Co-60 rotational therapy. *Radiology* 102:667, 1972.

99. Engler MJ, Herskovic AM, Proimos BS: Dosimetry of rotational photon fields with gravity-oriented eye blocks. *Int J Radiat Oncol Biol Phys* 10:431, 1984.

100. Levene MB, Kijewski PK, Chin LM, et al: Computer-controlled radiation therapy. *Radiology* 129:769, 1978.

101. Mantel J, Perry H, Weinkam JJ: Automatic variation of field size and dose rate in rotation therapy. *Int J Radiat Oncol Biol Phys* 2:697, 1977.

102. Takahashi S, Kitabatake T, Morita K, et al: Methoden zur besseren Anpassung der dosisverteilung an tiefliegende Krankheitsherde bei Bewegungsbestrahlung. *Strahlenth* 115:478, 1961.

103. Takahashi S: Conformation radiotherapy rotation techniques as applied to radiography and radiotherapy of cancer. *Acta Radiol* 242:57, 1962.

104. Takahashi K, Purdy JA, Liu YY: Treatment planning system for conformational radiotherapy. *Radiology* 147:567, 1983.

105. Sharma SC, Derbel FC, Khan RM: Tissue-equivalence of bolus materials for electron beam. *Radiology* 146:854, 1983.

106. American College of Radiology: *Draft Standards for Radiation Oncology*. Chicago: American College of Radiology, 1990.

107. Kutcher GJ, Coia L, Gillin M, et al: Comprehensive QA for radiation oncology: Report of AAPM Radiation Therapy Task Group 40. *Med Phys* 21:581, 1994.

108. Reinstein LE, McShan D, Glicksman AS: A dosimetry review system for cooperative group research. *Med Phys* 9:240, 1982.

109. Hansen WF, Shalek RJ, Kirby TH: *Information That Should Be Included in Every Patient's Radiotherapy Treatment Record*. Houston: Radiological Physics Center, 1985.

110. Suntharalingam N, Johansson KA: Quality assurance: Physics/dosimetry. *Int J Radiat Oncol Biol Phys* 14:521, 1988.

111. Bush RS: Quality assurance past and present in Canada. *Int J Radiat Oncol Biol Phys* 10(suppl 1):19, 1984.

112. Chaffey JT: Quality assurance in radiation therapy: Clinical considerations. *Int J Radiat Oncol Biol Phys* 10(suppl 1):15, 1984.

113. Cunningham JR: Quality assurance in dosimetry and treatment planning. *Int J Radiat Oncol Biol Phys* 10(suppl 1):105, 1984.

114. Laughlin JS: Development of quality assurance in radiation therapy in North America. *Int J Radiat Oncol Biol Phys* 10(suppl 1):9, 1984.

115. Littbrand B: Quality assurance in radiation therapy: Multidisciplinary considerations-European experience. *Int J Radiat Oncol Biol Phys* 10(suppl 1):67, 1984.

116. Perez CA, Gardner P, Glasgow GP: Radiotherapy quality assurance in clinical trials. *Int J Radiat Oncol Biol Phys* 10(suppl 1):119, 1984.

117. Perez CA: The U.S. perspective. *Int J Radiat Oncol Biol Phys* 10:151, 1984.

118. Purdy JA: Dosimetry and treatment planning. *Int J Radiat Oncol Biol Phys* 10:139, 1984.

119. Suntharalingam N: Quality assurance in radiation therapy: Future plans in physics. *Int J Radiat Oncol Biol Phys* 10:43, 1984.

120. Svensson GK: Quality assurance in radiation therapy: Physics efforts. *Int J Radiat Oncol Biol Phys* 10(suppl 1):23, 1984.

121. Svensson H: Quality assurance in radiation therapy: Physical aspects. *Int J Radiat Oncol Biol Phys* 10:59, 1984.

122. Wambersie A: Quality assurance in radiation therapy with special reference to the situation in Europe. *Int J Radiat Oncol Biol Phys* 10(suppl 1):153, 1984.

123. McCullough EC, Earle JD: The selection, acceptance testing and quality control of radiation therapy simulators. *Radiology* 131:221, 1979.

124. McCullough EC, Krueger AM: Performance evaluation of computerized treatment planning systems for radiotherapy: External photon beams. *Int J Radiat Oncol Biol Phys* 6:1599, 1980.

125. ICRU: *Dose Specification for Reporting External Beam Therapy with Photons and Electrons*. Washington DC: International Commission on Radiation Units and Measurements, 1978.

126. ICRU: *Prescribing, Recording, and Reporting Photon Beam Therapy*. Washington DC: International Commission on Radiation Units and Measurements, 1993.

127. Bynum S, McMurray H: The development and organization format of a radiotherapy patient treatment chart. *Med Dosim* 14:193, 1989.

128. Nair RP: A typical patient simulation and dosimetry data sheet. *Med Dosim* 14:79, 1989.

129. Thompson RW, Rosemark PJ, Greenberg SH, et al: A daily radiation therapy record form. *Med Dosim* 14:75, 1989.

130. Maciá M, Rubio AM, DeBlas R, et al: Treatment charts in radiation therapy: An analysis of European treatment records. *Radiother Oncol* 26:147, 1993.

131. Byhardt RW, Cox JD, Hornburg A, Liermann G: Weekly localization films and detection of field placement errors. *Int J Radiat Oncol Biol Phys.* 4:881, 1978.

132. Rosenman J, Roe CA, Cromartie R, et al: Portal film enhancement: Technique and clinical utility. *Int J Radiat Oncol Biol Phys* 25:333, 1993.

133. Denham JW, Dally MJ, Hunter K, Wheat J, Fahey PP, Hamilton CS: Objective decision making following a portal film: The results of a pilot study. *Int J Radiat Oncol Biol Phys* 26:869, 1993.

134. Valicenti RK, Michalski JM, Bosch WR et al: Is weekly port filming adequate for verifying patient position in modern radiation therapy? *Int J Radiat Oncol Biol Phys* 30:431, 1994.

135. Galkin B, Wu R, Suntharalingam N: Improved techniques for obtaining teletherapy portal radiographs with high energy photons. *Radiology* 127:828, 1978.

136. AAPM: *AAPM Report No. 24: Radiotherapy Portal Imaging Quality*. New York: American Institute of Physics, 1987.

137. Faerman S, Krutman Y: Generation of portal film charts for 10-MV x-rays. *Med Phys* 19:351, 1992.

138. Reinstein LE, Orton CG: Contrast enhancement of high-energy radiotherapy films. *Br J Radiol* 52:880, 1979.

139. McCullough EC, McCullough KP: Improving agreement between radiation-delineated field edges on simulation and portal films: The edge tolerance test tool. *Med Phys* 20:375, 1993.

140. Balter JM, Pelizzari CA, Chen TY: Correlation of projection radiographs in radiation therapy using open curve segments and points. *Med Phys* 19:329: 1992.

141. Boyer AL, Antonuk L, Fenster A, et al: A review of electronic portal imaging devices (EPIDs). *Med Phys* 19:1, 1992.

142. DeNeve W, Van den Heuvel F, Coghe M, et al: Interactive use of on-line portal imaging in pelvic radiation. *Int J Radiat Oncol Biol Phys* 25:517, 1993.

143. Lam KS, Partowmah M, Lam WC: An on-line electronic portal imaging system for external beam radiotherapy. *Br J Radiol* 59:1007, 1986.

144. Meertens H, Van Herk M, Bijhold J, Bartelink H: First clinical experience with a newly developed electronic portal imaging device. *Int J Radiat Oncol Biol Phys* 18:1173, 1990.

145. Reinstein LE, Pai S, Meek AG: Assessment of geometric treatment accuracy using time-lapse display of electronic portal images. *Int J Radiat Oncol Biol Phys* 22:1139, 1992.

146. Van Herk M, Bijhold J, Hoogervorst B, Meertens H: Sampling methods for a matrix ionization chamber system. *Med Phys* 19:409, 1992.

147. Wong JW, Binns WR, Cheng AY, et al: On-line radiotherapy imaging with an array of fiber-optic image reducers. *Int J Radiat Oncol Biol Phys* 18:1477, 1990.

148. DeNeve W, Van den Heuvel F, DeBeukeleer N, et al: Routine clinical on-line portal imaging followed by immediate field adjustment using a telecontrolled patient couch. *Radiother Oncol* 24:45, 1992.

149. El-Gayed AAH, Bel A, Vijbrief R, et al: Time trend of patient setup deviations during pelvic irradiation using electronic portal imaging. *Radiother Oncol* 26:162, 1993.

150. Ezz A, Munro P, Porter AT, et al: Daily monitoring and correction of radiation field placement using a video-based portal imaging system: A pilot study. *Int J Radiat Oncol Biol Phys* 22:159, 1992.

151. Gilhuijs KGA, van Herk M: Automatic on-line inspection of patient setup in radiation therapy using digital portal images. *Med Phys* 20:667, 1993.

152. Jones SM, Boyer AL: Investigation of an FFT-based correlation technique for verification of radiation treatment setup. *Med Phys* 18:1116, 1991.

153. Lam KS, Partowmah M, Loo DJ, Wharam MD: On line measurements of field placement errors in extended beam radiotherapy. *Br J Radiol* 60:361, 1987.

154. Lam WC, Herman MG, Lam KS, Lee DJ: On-line portal imaging: Computer assisted error measurement. *Radiology* 179:871, 1991.

155. Meertens H, Bijhold J, Struckee J: A method for the measurement of field placement errors in digital portal images. *Phys. Med Biol* 35:299, 1990.

156. Reinstein LE, Pai S, Meek AG: Assessment of geometric treatment accuracy using time-lapse on-line portal imaging. *Int J Radiat Oncol Biol Phys* 19:171, 1990.

157. Friel JP: *Dorland's Illustrated Medical Dictionary,* 26th ed. Philadelphia: Saunders, 1985.

158. Goiten M: Oblique sections need 3-D names also. *Int J Radiat Oncol Biol Phys* 19:821, 1990.

159. Sailer SL, Bourland D, Rosenman JG, et al: 3-D beams need 3-D names. *Int J Radiat Oncol Biol Phys* 19:797, 1990.

160. Leunens G, Verstraete J, Van den Bogaert W, et al. Human errors in data transfer during preparation and delivery of radiation treatment affecting the final result: "garbage in, garbage out." *Radiother Oncol* 23:217, 1992.

Treatment Planning—Head and Neck Region

The upper aerodigestive tract is a common site for many malignant neoplasms. These include lesions arising in the mucous membranes, salivary glands, and lymphatics. Cancers can originate in a large number of sites within the head and neck region and each one represents a unique set of characteristics (history, anatomy, and pattern of spread). Appropriate treatment decisions therefore require a thorough knowledge of the anatomy, specifically with respect to the lymph node distribution in this region. This text is limited to discussion of the most common tumors.

The general principle for management of localized head and neck malignancies is that most small lesions can be equally well treated by surgery or radiation therapy, while more advanced disease is often treated with a combination of surgery, radiation therapy, and sometimes chemotherapy. Selection of treatment modality depends upon site and size of the disease, whether cervical lymph nodes are involved, cosmesis and functional outcome, patient reliability, sequelae of treatment, and patient preference. Preoperative radiation therapy is delivered to attempt to improve resectability and reduce the risks of tumor spread at surgery.

Head and neck tumors requiring radiation therapy are most commonly treated using cobalt-60 beams and 4- to 6-MV photon beams. Electron beams are sometimes used in the treatment of lip cancer, cervical lymph nodes, and laterally located tumors (parotid, buccal mucosa). Electron or orthovoltage beams are sometimes used to deliver a boost dose via an intraoral cone in tumors that are small, visible, and accessible to the cone.[1-4] This includes tumors in the soft palate, retromolar trigone, floor of mouth, and anterior tongue. Interstitial implants are also used to boost the dose to the primary lesion when accessible. An intracavitary implant is sometimes used to boost the dose to tumors originating in the nasopharynx. A boost can also be delivered to lesions in the floor of the mouth via a submental field using photon or electron beams. Boost doses delivered via a submental field, intraoral cone, interstitial or intracavitary implants are used in an effort to spare the salivary glands and the mandible, thus reducing the risks of xerostomia and injury to the mandible (osteoradionecrosis).

A majority of lesions originating in the upper aerodigestive tract are squamous cell carcinoma. Doses ranging from 5000 to 5500 cGy are generally considered adequate to sterilize microscopic or occult disease.[5] For larger tumors, 6500 to 7000 cGy is required for control of gross disease. For advanced tumors, 7500 to 8000 cGy is required, but delivery of this dose is difficult because of mucosal toxicity. The fields are progressively reduced so that these high doses are delivered only to a very small volume. If field reductions cannot be made without compromising tumor coverage, dose reductions may be necessary. Irradiation schemes consisting of multiple daily fractions are used in an attempt to improve the local tumor control rate for advanced lesions and to improve long-term normal-tissue tolerance.[6–13]

Radiation therapy of malignancies in the head and neck region often unavoidably includes large volumes of normal tissues within the fields. Irradiation of oral mucosa to high doses will cause mucositis, which may prevent the patient from continuing oral intake of nourishment. It is therefore important to try to design the treatment fields so that the volume of oral mucosa within the fields is limited to either the upper or lower half of the mouth. A bite block inserted between the teeth helps the patient keep his or her mouth open during the treatment. With the mouth open, it is often possible to include the target with adequate margins while shielding a large volume of oral mucosa. In other situations, it may be possible to spare either the right or left side of the mouth, thus reducing the volume of oral mucosa within the radiation field. It is also important to avoid

unnecessary irradiation of the salivary glands. Saliva is a necessary ingredient in the swallowing process. It moistens the food and is also necessary for digestion and prevention of tooth decay. When the dose to the salivary glands is in excess of about 2000 cGy, the production of saliva decreases, and it may cease with doses of 4000 to 4500 cGy. It is often impossible to spare all salivary glands; however, if one can limit the dose to the salivary glands, use shrinking fields, or treat ipsilaterally, xerostomia may be prevented or be less severe.

When treatment fields for head and neck malignancies are designed, special attention should be given to the possibility of avoiding the cervical spinal cord, eyes, lacrimal glands, optic nerve, optic chiasm, pituitary gland, brain, and brainstem. The addition of electron beams, changes in field size, or changes in beam orientations should be considered at appropriate dose levels to reduce the morbidity.

Radiation therapy of malignancies in the head and neck region requires careful selection of beam energies, since, in the majority of patients, shallow regional lymph nodes often must be irradiated also. The beam orientations for treatment of many tumor sites are straightforward. Field junctions are often necessary, however, and must be accomplished so that no overlap occurs in critical tissues. In many situations, complex field arrangements are needed to treat the target adequately while avoiding radiosensitive organs in the region. In the following pages, several treatment techniques are presented. An important aspect of head and neck irradiation which first must be discussed is patient immobilization.

POSITIONING AND IMMOBILIZATION

Immobilization techniques described for treatments in the head and neck area also include those for intracranial tumors. The proximity of the eyes, optic chiasm, spinal cord, and brain requires very precise reproducibility of the setup, particularly when the prescribed dose to the target area exceeds the tolerance of these neighboring organs. The frequency and magnitude of treatment field misalignment in the irradiation of head and neck malignancies has been studied by several authors.[14-20]

As in all sites, the two most important factors in reproducing and maintaining the patient's position are comfort and immobility. Other concerns for patients treated to this area are unsightly setup marks on the patient's skin. These marks can have a detrimental psychological effect on the average patient. Most cancer patients suffer under a heavy burden without having to worry about stares, questions, and perhaps loss of friends because of these unsightly marks. Many modern immobilization devices include a mask of some type on which setup marks can

be made, obviating skin marks altogether. In the head and neck area, where field margins around the tumor must often be small in order to avoid adjacent radiosensitive organs, effective immobilization techniques are particularly important.

Even very cooperative patients find it difficult to maintain the head position for any length of time and require some type of stabilization. Swallowing, respiration, coughing, and sneezing can cause significant changes in the position, and the patient needs some type of restraint to prevent motion. The simplest but now outdated method of "immobilizing" head and neck patients is a tape stretched across the

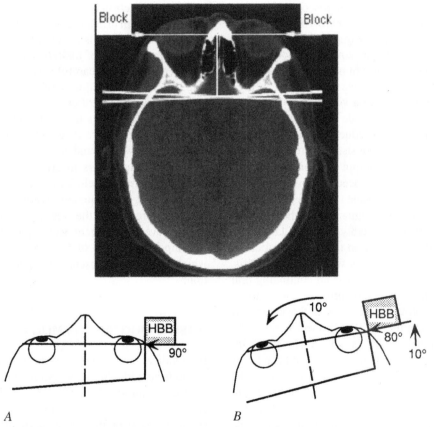

Figure 9.1   *A.* To exclude them both, the lenses must be on a line parallel with the beam direction. *B.* When the immobilized head is at an angle, the gantry must be angled until the two lenses are on a line parallel with the beam direction. *C* and *D.* In patients with proptosis, a gantry angle may be necessary even when the head is straight, because the two eyes no longer lie on a horizontal line.

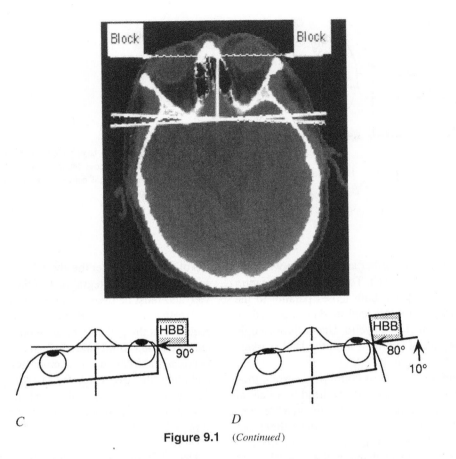

Figure 9.1 (*Continued*)

forehead and attached to each side of the couch. A large number of more modern and effective head and neck immobilization techniques consisting of bite block systems or different casting materials have been described.[18,20–32] Routine implementation of some of these techniques requires a special mold room and mold room technologist, while others are quite simple and can be implemented in practically any small department with modest resources.

HEAD AND NECK POSITIONING

The choice of head position for the treatment of head and neck malignancies (including intracranial tumors) is very important and can have an effect on the ability to reproduce the position daily.

The angle at which the radiation beam impinges on the patient's surface is defined either by the angles of the machine or by the position of the patient. For example, a true anterior field implies that the beam axis is parallel with the patient's sagittal plane. If the patient's head is rotated 10°, the gantry of the machine must also be rotated 10° in order to achieve a true anterior field. In the head and neck area, this becomes more of a problem than in any other site because it may be difficult to position the patient's head precisely "straight." Since the head is immobilized prior to tumor localization or simulation procedures, the desired beam orientation with respect to the patient can be achieved by changing the gantry angle. When lateral fields are used to treat tumors near the eyes, it is particularly important that the two lenses be parallel to the beam direction (Fig. 9.1*A*). If the head is immobilized at an angle, the gantry must be turned the same number of degrees as the head is rotated (Fig. 9.1*B*). In patients with prop-

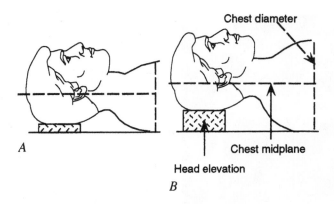

Figure 9.2 In a large patient where the midplane of the chest lies higher above the couch than in a thin patient, a higher head support is needed to position the head in a neutral position.

tosis, one lens can be farther anterior even when the head is straight (Fig. 9.1*C*). To determine the gantry angle necessary to have both lenses parallel to the beam orientation, a small lead marker is placed on the center of each closed eyelid. Under fluoroscopic viewing, the gantry is turned until the lead markers are superimposed (Fig. 9.1*D*).

Patients are usually most comfortable when they are in the supine position with the head in a neutral position (i.e., the forehead and chin lie on a horizontal line). The beam with respect to the patient can then be directed by rotating the couch, gantry, and collimator rather than by changing the patient's head position. In the absence of three-dimensional treatment-planning capabilities, it can be difficult to determine the exact setting of such compound angles, and the patient's head position is therefore often modified. The head elevation required to produce a neutral position varies from patient to patient and depends to a great extent on the size of the patient's chest (Fig. 9.2). In a large patient, the midplane of the torso is elevated higher above the couch than in a small patient. To elevate the head so that its midplane lies on the same plane as the torso, a higher support is required under the head of the larger patient (Fig. 9.2*B*). In some patients, particularly children, it might even be necessary to elevate the chest to achieve a comfortable position. A flat piece of Styrofoam®* of adequate thickness can be placed on

* Registered by Dow Chemical, Midland, MI.

top of the couch under the chest. This piece of Styrofoam becomes an integral part of the positioning device and must be used during each treatment.

Treatment of a maxillary antrum lesion usually require that the patient's head be positioned with the chin extended to include the cephalad extent of the maxillary antrum in an anterior field without also including the eye (Fig. 9.3*A*). Alternatively, this field can be treated with the head in a neutral position, using a combination of couch and gantry angle (Fig. 9.3*B* and *C*).

Dental Impression. It is crucial to minimize the volume of oral mucosa within the treatment field. In certain situations, however, it is necessary to include some of the oral cavity, particularly when tumors in the maxillary antrum, tongue, or floor of the mouth are treated. By using a tongue blade and keeping the patient's mouth open during the treatment of a maxillary antrum tumor, the tongue and the lower half of the mouth can be excluded from the radiation field. Likewise, when a tumor in the tongue or the floor of the mouth is treated, the upper half of the mouth can be excluded by keeping the patient's mouth open. The patient's mouth can be kept open by inserting a bite block made from dental impression material. A tongue blade and a plastic tube made from a 10- or 20-mL syringe is inserted in the softened dental impression material to make breathing easier (Fig. 9.4). An impression of the patient's teeth (or gums in an edentulous patient) is made in the softened dental

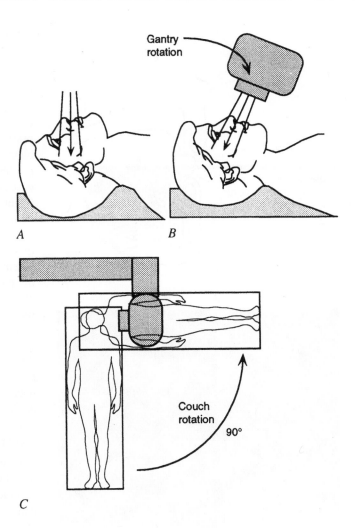

Figure 9.3 *A.* To include the apex of the maxillary antrum while excluding the eye, the beam can be vertical with the chin extended or (*B* and *C*) the head position can be neutral and the couch rotated 90°. The gantry is then turned to the appropriate angle.

material, and within approximately 5 min, the material becomes hard. Using this bite block during each treatment helps in reproducing the opening of the mouth.

Head Supports. A comfortable head support is one that fits tightly to the posterior surface of the head and neck and helps the patient maintain the position without straining (Fig. 9.5A). When the head is extended so much that only the neck and not the head is resting on the support, there is room for motion of the head and, furthermore, the patient is not comfortable (Fig. 9.5B). Elevating the chest helps the patient tilt the head back farther without

increasing the strain on the neck (Fig. 9.6A). The curvature of the patient's cervical spine can also be altered by changing the support under the head (Fig. 9.6B).

Standard head supports are often uncomfortable and do not fit tightly to the posterior surface of the head and neck, leaving room for motion (Fig. 9.5B). A customized head support, on the other hand, fits tightly and leaves no room for motion (Fig. 9.5A). Customized supports are made from a set of foaming agents* that swell up and form a mold around the patient's head and shoulders while the patient is in

* Smithers Medical Products, Inc., Akron, OH.

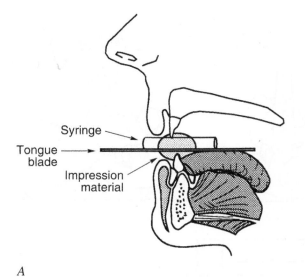

A

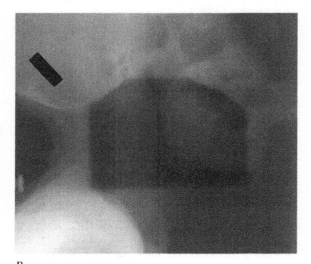

B

Figure 9.4   *A*. A bite block to keep the patient's mouth open during the treatments must have indentations of the teeth so it can be repositioned correctly during each treatment. *B*. Keeping the mouth open allows exclusion of the oral mucosa. In this field, a large portion of the mouth can be shielded.

the desired position (Fig. 9.7). The patient's head is then immobilized in this position by strips of radiolucent material or a thermoplastic sheet fastened to a base plate, which in turn is fastened to the treatment couch.

HEAD IMMOBILIZATION SYSTEMS

Facial Mask Systems.   One elaborate head immobilization system consists of a thin, transparent plastic material that can be formed to the shape of the patient's face through a vacuum process on an industrial machine. This method requires that an impression of the patient's head, using plaster-of-Paris bandages, be made first. From this impression, a plaster model of the head is produced. This procedure is quite elaborate and its use is therefore limited. Other face mask systems use strips of Scotchcast®* or a thermoplastic material called Aquaplast.®† Aquaplast can be purchased in either strips or sheets, in solids, or in perforated form. It becomes pliable when softened in hot water. When it is placed over the patient's face and gentle pressure is applied, the material conforms snugly to the prominences of the face. The material hardens again within approximately 5 min, and the facial mask is finished. This type of facial mask is easy to make, requires very little time, effort, and equipment, and can therefore be used in practically any radiation therapy department. Another, more elaborate head immobilization device, developed for stereotactic radiotherapy, consists of a head cast, where the entire head with the exception of the tip of the nose is encased.[33]

Bite Block Systems.   Many head and neck immobilization devices consist of a bite block system or a facial mask that is fixed to a base plate under the patient's head which in turn is attached to the treatment couch. A bite block system, shown in Fig. 9.8, usually consists of two vertical rods and one horizontal one (graduated in centimeters) and a piece of dental impression material (the bite block). The dental material is softened in hot water and placed in the patient's mouth. The patient is asked to bite down into the material loosely and the three rods are adjusted until the desired position is achieved. The position of each of these rods is recorded in the patient's chart so that the position can be reproduced precisely for each treatment. When the material hardens, usually within a couple of minutes, the impression of the patient's teeth remains.

* Registered by 3M Corp., St. Paul, MN.
† Registered by WFR Aquaplast Corp., Wyckoff, NJ.

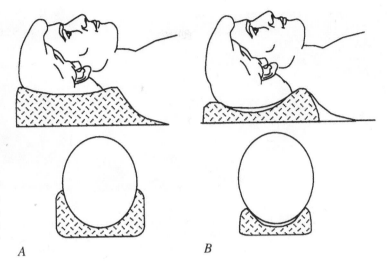

Figure 9.5   *A.* A head support that follows the head's posterior contour and also supports the sides and superior portion of the head is comfortable and leaves no room for motion. *B.* Standard head supports often do not match the posterior contour of the head. When the support under the neck is too high, the posterior aspect of the head may not be supported at all, causing the position to be uncomfortable and leaving room for motion.

A   *B*

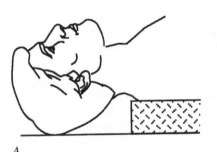

A

Figure 9.6   *A.* Elevation of the chest often helps in tilting the head back without patient discomfort. *B* and *C.* Changing the support under the patient's head also changes the curvature or angle of the spine. The radiograph on the left was taken with a larger support and the corner of the beam is in the spinal canal, making any subsequent field matching practically impossible. The radiograph on the right was taken with a smaller head support. Here the spine is straight and well inside the field. Note also the absence of lead markers at the eyes *(left).*

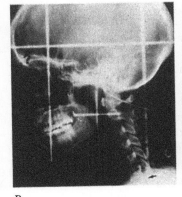

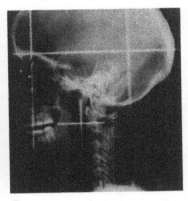

B   *C*

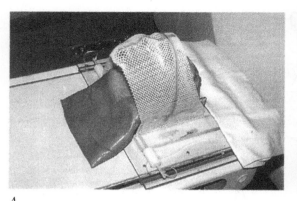
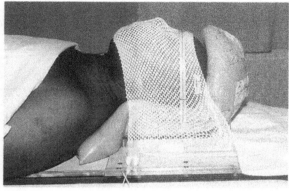

A   *B*

Figure 9.7   *A.* A customized head support and a thermoplastic mask used in head and neck immobilization are fixed to a base plate under the head. The base plate is then fixed to the couch. *B.* A patient
immobilized with a customized head support and a thermoplastic mask. All setup marks are made on the
mask.

**A Customized Head and Neck Immobilization
System.**   An effective head immobilization system
should adhere to the patient's skin surface—
anteriorly, posteriorly, and on the sides—and leave
no room for motion. Efforts to make a tight-fitting
facial immobilization mask or a reproducible bite
block system becomes fruitless when they are used
with an ill-fitting head support that leaves room for
motion.

A customized head and neck immobilization system, routinely used at Duke University Medical
Center, consists of a customized support under the
patient's head, neck, and shoulders and a perforated
thermoplastic sheet draped over the face (Fig. 9.7).
Both the head rest and face mask are rigidly fixed to
a base plate,[34,35] which in turn is fixed reproducibly
to the treatment couch.

The height above the couch that is required for the
head to be in the neutral position is determined first.
Small pieces of Styrofoam are placed under the head
until the desired position is achieved. A plastic bag,
approximately 10 in. wide and 18 in. long, containing about 100 mL of a foaming agent is placed under
the patient's head, neck, and shoulders. The piece(s)
of Styrofoam used to determine the head elevation
are taped together and placed inside the bag to maintain the head elevation while the support is being
made. Within a few minutes, the foam expands and

fills the space under the patient and conforms to the
repositioning guides of the head holder base plate.
While the foam is expanding, the patient's head is
held straight while the foam is simultaneously
guided up on the sides and around the top of the
head. The foam, which is very light, expands in the
direction of least resistance and therefore must be
constrained to remain in contact with the patient as it
expands and sets. Constraining the foam causes the
support to conform to the posterior contour of the

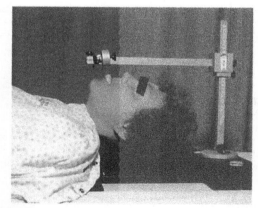

Figure 9.8   An immobilization device consisting of a bite
block attached to an arm with centimeter markers used for patient
repositioning.

head, neck, and shoulders and also to form an elevated ridge around the head.

The dimensions of the plastic bag are important, since it must be large enough to allow the foam to expand and fill the space behind and around the head. If the bag is too small, the head support may not conform to the shape of the head but instead may assume the shape of an inflated bag and displace the head. The opening of the plastic bag should be superior of the head and should not be sealed, allowing excess foam to escape if necessary. In general, less foam is required for a large patient because there is less empty space to fill conversely; more foam is needed for a small patient.

Within approximately 10 min, when the foam is firm, a perforated thermoplastic sheet (Aquaplast), which is softened in hot water, is draped over the patient's face from the middle of the forehead to below the chin. The thermoplastic sheet should be molded closely to the patient's facial prominences without distorting, for example, the tip of the nose. The use of excessive pressure during the forming of the mask may make it so tight that it will cause discomfort or pain during future use. It is particularly important that the mask conform well to the bridge of the nose, where there is a very thin layer of soft tissue over the bony prominences; this is a reliable reference point for the mask. To make an effective face mask, the thermoplastic sheet should be pulled straight back to the anchor points on the base plate. Any deflection of the sheet due to slack, manipulation during placement, or bulges in the foam head support will result in a mask that has a springlike flexibility and so does not immobilize the patient rigidly.

When a bite block, nasogastric tube, or anesthesia is used, a small hole may be made in the thermoplastic sheet prior to the softening. The bite block, nasogastric tube, or anesthesia tube is then threaded through the hole as the mask is placed over the face. In situations where lead markers must be placed on a particular surface structure during the simulation procedure (lymph node, canthus, etc.), these can be placed prior to making the mask, or a small opening can be made in the thermoplastic sheet following hardening of the mask. It is important to recognize

that when openings are cut in the mask or when it is stretched, it becomes weaker and thus less effective. Openings in the mask should therefore be minimal.

In this immobilization system, the patient's head is "sandwiched" between the customized head support and the facial mask, leaving no room for motion. The support and the mask are fastened to a base plate under the head, which fits tightly over and is secured to the treatment couch to prevent slipping or skewing. Since this immobilization device conforms very tightly to the patient's anatomy, a difference in clothing can cause the mask to be too tight or too loose from one day to the next. All clothes above the waist are therefore routinely removed prior to making the mask as well as prior to each treatment.

All setup marks are made on the mask, thus eliminating the risks of the marks being washed off or inadvertently changed during remarking. Consequently, the patient will have no unsightly skin marks. Another important consideration in head and neck immobilization is to facilitate a quick-release mechanism in the event of an emergency. In this system, the face mask is secured to the base plate via a clamp and pin on each side of the head.[34,35] In our experience of treating several hundred patients using this system, the need for a quick release has never arisen. The device is used in small children as well as in adults without any difficulty.

Another important consideration when a face mask is used is its effect on the radiation beam, both in terms of attenuation and possible reduction of the skin-sparing effect.[29,36–39]

TREATMENT TECHNIQUES

BASIC TREATMENT TECHNIQUE

Regional lymphatic irradiation is often necessary in the treatment of most head and neck tumors (Fig. 9.9). This is usually accomplished via opposed lateral fields including the primary tumor site and cervical lymph nodes. A third anterior field covering the lower neck and bilateral supraclavicular lymph nodes may also be used. Following the delivery of a dose lower than the spinal cord tolerance, (approximately 4500 cGy), the lateral fields are reduced off

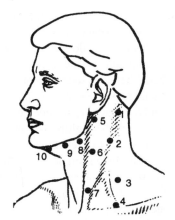

Figure 9.9 Diagram of the major lymphatic groups in the head and neck region. 1 = Upper posterior cervical; 2 = mid posterior cervical; 3 = low posterior cervical; 4 = supraclavicular; 5 = deep superior jugular; 6 = mid jugular; 7 = low jugular; 8 = subdigastric; 9 = submandibular; 10 = submental.

the spinal cord, and the anterior neck along with the primary tumor is treated to a higher dose. The anterior field is discontinued at this dose if only prophylactic nodal irradiation is being given. In those patients where the posterior cervical lymphatics overlying the spinal cord must be treated to a higher dose, lateral electron fields are used. If the field reduction off the spinal cord is accomplished without moving the central axis of the beam but rather through changing of the customized blocks, almost one-half of the field is blocked (Fig. 9.10). In this way, as much as possible of the cervical lymphatic area is included without beam divergence into the spinal cord. This also results in a sharper field edge than if the margin were defined by the collimator. A second field reduction is often made to direct higher doses to the primary tumor site.

Whenever lateral head and neck fields are used in conjunction with a low anterior supraclavicular field, there is potential for field overlap in the spinal cord. The lateral fields diverge caudally into the anterior supraclavicular field, and the anterior supraclavicular field diverges cephalad into the lateral fields (Fig. 9.11).[40-43] This field-matching problem is similar to the problem of matching lateral cranial fields with a posterior spine field and the matching of tangential breast fields with an anterior supraclavicular field.

(These field-matching problems are also discussed in Chaps. 10 and 11.)

In the treatment of head and neck tumors, several methods can be used to eliminate this three-field overlap. A midline spinal cord block can be used in the anterior supraclavicular field (Fig. 9.12), or, alternatively, a small spinal cord block can be placed over the spinal cord in the caudal portion of the lateral fields (Fig. 9.13). This prevents an overlap in the spinal cord, but there is still an overlap in the lateral and anterior soft tissues. This overlap can be reduced by turning the collimator of the lateral fields until the caudal margins become parallel with the diverging cephalad margin of the anterior supraclavicular field (Fig. 9.14). To avoid an overlap from the diverging lateral fields, the foot of the treatment couch can be turned away from the collimator of the machine (Fig. 9.15).

Another method to reduce the risks of overlap is to set the central axis of each field at the junction between the fields and use a half-beam block or close the independent jaw to the central axis (Fig. 9.15).[40,41] This will eliminate all beam divergence at the junction. However, due to small variations in the setup, penumbra of the beam, and involuntary patient motion, a small anterior or lateral spinal cord block should be used as a precaution (Fig. 9.16). In another field-matching technique, small junctional wedges are used to make the penumbra of each beam wider and thus reduce the risks of hot spots.[43]

The location of the field junction is often chosen with a view to shielding the spinal cord without also blocking potential tumor. For example, a spinal cord block in the anterior field may not be feasible in patients with centrally located tumors such as those of the pyriform sinus or larynx. Conversely, gross cervical adenopathy or high risk of tumor involvement in the posterior lymph nodes may prevent the use of a spinal cord shield in the lateral fields. An anterior spinal cord block will also shield the uninvolved laryngeal and hypopharyngeal tissues; thus, mucositis and laryngitis caused by unnecessary irradiation in these tissues is avoided.[46] Lateral blocks are preferable for large primary laryngeal and hypopharyngeal lesions. The width of the anterior spinal cord shield must be designed so that it casts a

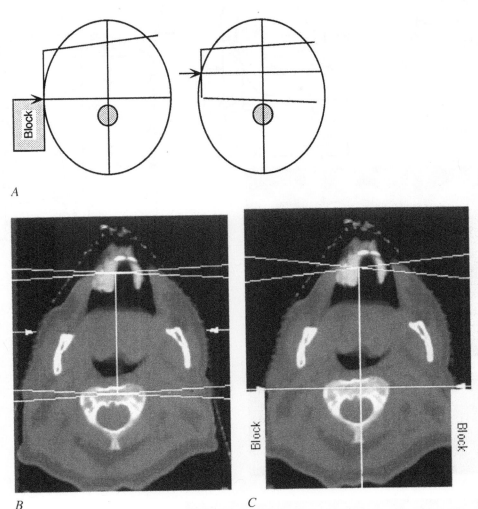

Figure 9.10 *A–C.* Reducing lateral head and neck fields to exclude the spinal cord is usually accomplished by inserting a block, causing the beam to be practically half-beam blocked. This results in a sharper beam edge and includes more of the lateral neck than if the central axis were shifted and the collimator size reduced.

shadow that is approximately 3 cm wide at the depth of the spinal cord. The width of the block can be tapered so that it is narrower near the suprasternal notch, where the low jugular lymph nodes lie close to the midline.

Another difficulty with field matching in external beam radiation therapy of head and neck malignancies is the junction between lateral photon and electron fields.[44] It is often difficult to place the electron cone directly on the skin surface because of the patient's shoulders. When the source-surface distance (SSD) is extended for an electron beam, the dose inhomogeneity along the junction line is accentuated.[44] The dose delivered through these lateral boost fields is relatively low and—with some daily variations in the reproducibility of the electron field—adverse effects are rare.

The electron beam energy used when these fields

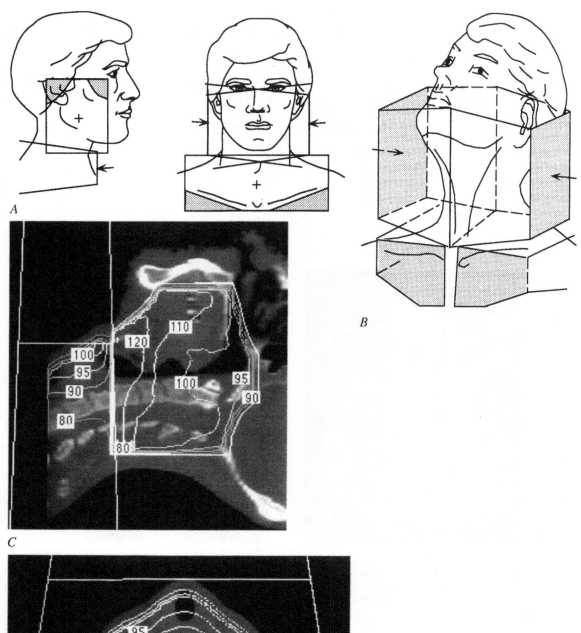

Figure 9.11 *A.* The caudal margin of lateral head and neck fields diverges into the anterior supraclavicular field and the cephalad margin of the anterior field diverges into the lateral fields, causing an overlap. *B.* Diagram illustrating the beam divergence when the beam direction of adjacent fields is orthogonal. *C.* A sagittal dose distribution shows an overlap in the spinal cord. The dose is also high anteriorly because of the smaller transverse diameter of the neck. *D.* The dose distribution in the anterior lower neck and supraclavicular area.

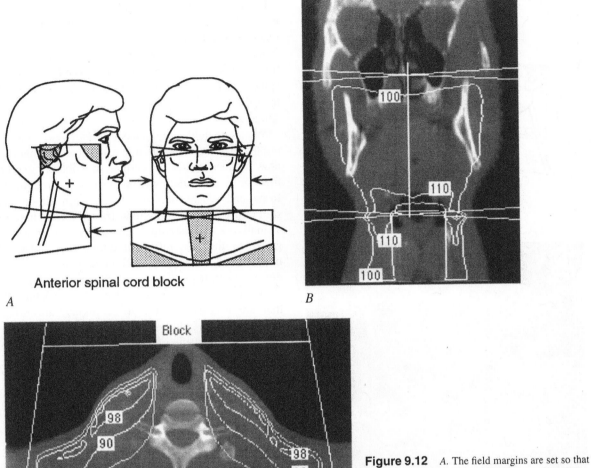

Anterior spinal cord block

A

B

C

Figure 9.12   *A.* The field margins are set so that they are adjacent on the skin surface, and a midline spinal cord shield is used in the anterior field. This avoids an overlap in the spinal cord, but there is an overlap in the lateral aspect of the neck. *B.* Isodose distribution in the coronal plane with an anterior spinal cord block in place. *C.* Isodose distribution in the anterior field with a spinal cord block in place.

are treated should be selected so that there is no further irradiation of the spinal cord. The depth of the spinal cord and the percent depth dose (%DD) of the electron beam must be known. The most accurate method to find the depth of the spinal cord is to obtain computed tomography (CT) scans of the neck. In the absence of a CT scan, the depth can be estimated by measuring the transverse diameter of the neck over the spinal cord where the neck is thinnest

and assume that the spinal cord is in the midline. Caution should be used when the measurements are obtained in patients where the neck is asymmetrical due to surgery, there are large neck nodes, and so on, because in that situation, the spinal cord may not be in the midplane. Also, the thickness of the spinal cord is about 2 cm, so at least 1 cm should be subtracted from the midplane depth (Fig. 9.17).

In a few patients with advanced disease, it is

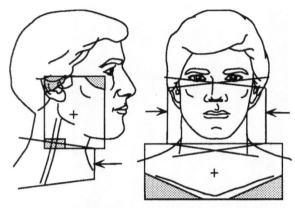

Lateral spinal cord block

A

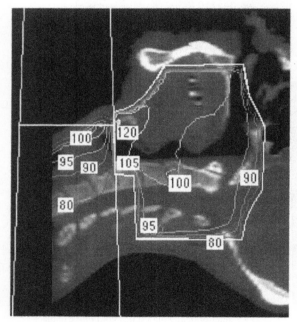

B

Figure 9.13 *A.* A small spinal cord shield can be used in the lateral fields where the overlap occurs. *B.* Isodose distribution in the sagittal plane with bilateral spinal cord shields in the lateral fields.

sometimes impossible to set the field junction where there is no gross tumor. In these cases, opposed anterior and posterior fields may be used without any field junction and without spinal cord shielding (Fig.

9.18). If possible, portions of the oral mucosa should be shielded. When spinal cord tolerance has been reached, the technique is changed to the field arrangement described previously, where lateral photon fields are used to treat the tissues anterior to the spinal cord and lateral electron beams are used to treat the posterior lateral lymph nodes overlying the spinal cord.

When the fields are reduced, 4 to 5 weeks following the initial simulation, it is recommended that the new reduced fields be verified by obtaining port films or by resimulating the fields prior to treatment. In patients where the setup marks are made on the skin rather than on an immobilization mask, there is a small risk that the initial skin marks may have migrated as they are refreshed during the course of treatment. The patient's weight may also change during this time period, causing the overlying skin to shift with respect to the target. Head and neck tumors that are accessible through the mouth are often marked with a gold seed, so that inclusion of the tumor can be verified on simulation and port films. These seed markers may also migrate during the course of treatment, making them obsolete for tumor

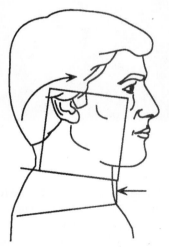

Figure 9.14 To reduce the overlap in the lateral aspects of the neck, the collimator can be rotated on the lateral fields until the caudal margin is parallel with the cephalad margin of the anterior field. The spinal cord shield must also be used to prevent an overlap in the spinal cord.

localization purposes. The position of the marking seed must be verified and, if the tumor is still visible or palpable, it may be necessary to place a new gold seed in the tumor. Boost fields are usually designed with small margins, which is another reason to resimulate these fields prior to treatment.

A difficult dilemma occurs with patients where the entire anterior neck needs to be treated through spinal-cord-sparing lateral fields without a field junction or where the disease is potentially below the level of the shoulders. In this scenario, long lateral fields with a table angle can be used. With the patient

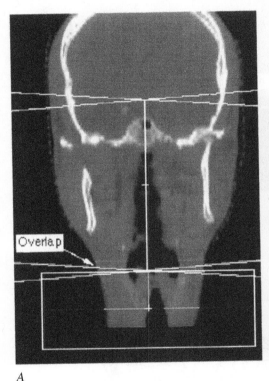

A

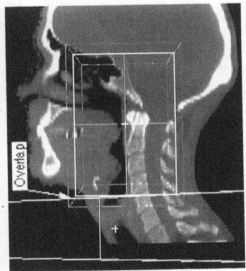

B

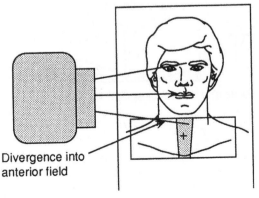

Divergence into anterior field

C

Figure 9.15   *A* to *C*. The caudal margin of the lateral fields diverges into the anterior field and the anterior field diverges into the lateral fields. (The clear white line indicates the lateral fields in the patient's midline, the weaker line inside indicates the field at the entrance point, and the weaker line outside indicates the lateral field at the exit point.) *D* to *F*. To achieve a geometric field match, both the collimator and the couch must be tuned when the lateral fields are treated. The collimator is turned until the caudal margin is parallel with the diverging cephalad margin of the anterior field. The couch is then turned until the diverging caudal margin of the lateral fields becomes parallel and crosses the patient in a straight line—that is, perpendicular to the sagittal axis of the patient, and also matches the cephalad margin of the anterior field. *G*. A geometric field match can also be achieved by setting the central axis at the field junction and then using half-beam blocking on all three fields.

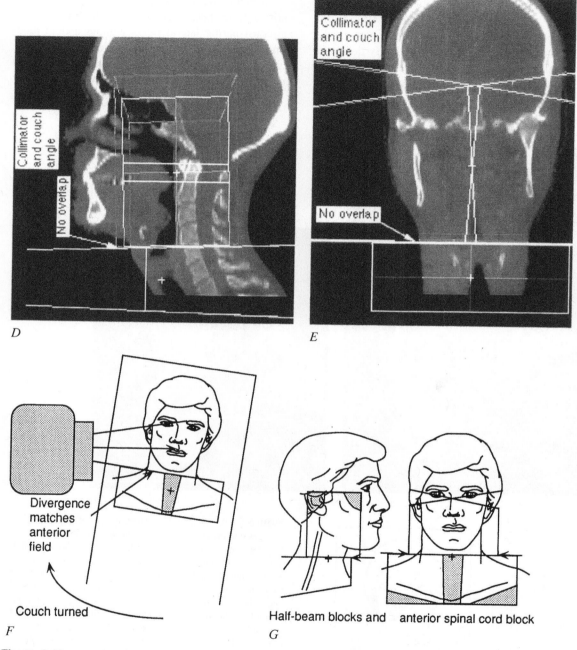

Figure 9.15   (*Continued*)

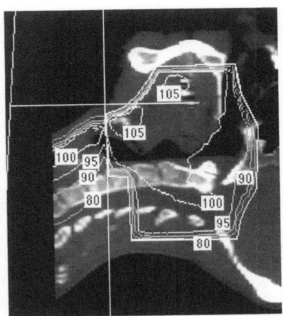

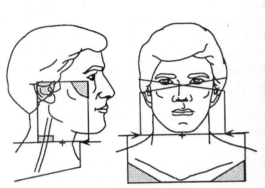

Half-beam blocks and lateral spinal cord block

A

B

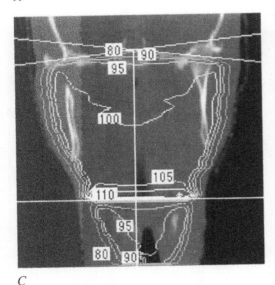

C

Figure 9.16 *A.* In addition to using half-beam blocking on all three fields, a small junction block should be used. Isodose distribution in the sagittal *(B)* and coronal *(C)* plane (anterior of the spinal cord block) with all fields half-beam blocked and a small junction block in each of the lateral fields.

in the supine position and the gantry turned 90°, the foot of the couch can be turned away from the collimator by about 10 to 15° (Fig. 9.19).[45] This will cause the beam to be angled caudally into the upper mediastinum. This technique is usually employed during a portion of the treatment course.

Treatment Simulation. The field arrangements described above usually require a treatment-simulation procedure to determine field margins with respect to bony anatomy. Palpable disease that is to be included and normal anatomy that should be avoided can be indicated by radiopaque markers. This is very

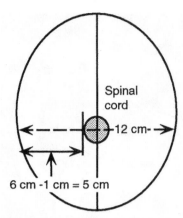

Figure 9.17 In determining the depth of the spinal cord, the transverse diameter of the patient's neck is measured at the spinal cord. At least 1 cm is subtracted from half of the neck diameter for the thickness of the spinal cord.

rior, posterior, cephalad, and caudal margins are determined. If a half-beam block technique is used in these fields, the isocenter is set at the caudal margin and the lower half of these fields is then shielded, either via a half-beam block or by closing in the independent jaw. If a half-beam block is not used in the anterior field, a collimator angle is necessary to make the caudal margin follow the diverging cephalad margin of the anterior field. If a half-beam block is used in all three fields, the isocenter is left at the caudal margin of the lateral fields and, after both the lateral radiographs have been obtained, the gantry is turned to the vertical position. The SSD is adjusted so that the anterior beam is at the desired SSD (usually 100 cm) and the field margins are set in the usual manner. A radiograph of the anterior field is also obtained.

In some patients, where the field junction is relatively low, it is sometimes necessary to have the pa-

helpful when the customized shielding blocks are subsequently designed on the simulation radiographs.

Before the simulation procedure begins, it is important to make sure that the physician has made a decision about where the junction between the lateral and the anterior fields should be. In patients with primary lesions in the nasopharynx, oropharynx, or oral cavity, the junction should be made above the thyroid notch[46]; thus, the anterior spinal cord block will also shield the larynx. As a matter of principle, field junctions are not usually made where there is gross disease. In a few situations, this might be impossible, particularly in patients with large cervical lymph node disease. It is usually preferable to have a "hot spot" rather than a "cold spot" in the lateral aspect of the neck near the field junction. Various field-matching techniques have been described above.

The patient's position should also be determined prior to the immobilization procedure. With the patient immobilized as described above, the lateral fields are usually simulated first. The isocenter is set such that it is in the patient's midline, and the ante-

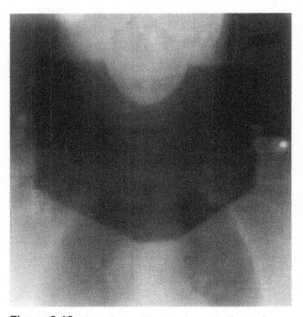

Figure 9.18 In patients with extensive neck disease, it may be an advantage to use opposed anterior and posterior fields, at least during a portion of the treatment, to avoid a field junction in gross tumor.

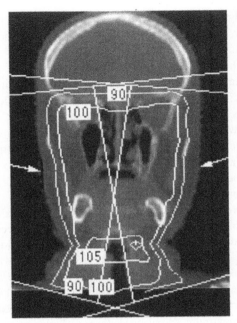

Figure 9.19 When the lower neck and superior mediastinum must be treated without further spinal cord irradiation, the couch can be turned 10 to 15° so that the beam is angled caudally into the mediastinum.

tient pull the shoulders down. This can be accomplished by having the patient pull with both hands on elastic straps attached to the sides of the couch. It is important to see that the patient's head position does not change while he or she is pulling on the straps.

In the treatment of head and neck disease, many variables play a role in the selection of a suitable treatment technique. It would be an impossible task to try to describe every aspect of every situation here; however, it must be emphasized that in each particular case, the procedure that best suits the situation should be used.

DOSE CALCULATION

The dose prescription is routinely made on the central axis at the midplane of the patient, as is done in many other areas where opposed fields are used. In the treatment of head and neck tumors, it is not un-

usual for the central axis to be moved once or twice during the course of the treatment. It is important to recognize that the dose calculated on the central axis of one set of opposed fields cannot be added to the dose calculated on the central axis of another set of opposed fields (i.e., at different points). Unless compensators are used, the dose inhomogeneity within lateral head and neck fields can be significant. For example, lateral opposed fields used to treat a supraglottic larynx tumor usually include the cervical lymph nodes (Fig. 9.20). The central axis of such a field is usually located where the transverse diameter is about 12 to 14 cm, and the prescribed dose is calculated at middepth (6 to 7 cm). Because the neck is thinner in the anterior aspect where the larynx is located, the dose at this point will be higher than the prescribed central-axis dose. Off-axis dose calculations are helpful to assess the actual laryngeal dose and adjust the dose prescription accordingly, if necessary. Overflattening of the beams from most linear accelerators also causes the dose at this point to be higher than at the central axis. When the fields are reduced and the central axis is moved to the larynx, the dose is calculated at middepth (usually on the order of 3 to 4 cm) at this level.

The dose distribution shown in Fig. 9.21 was cal-

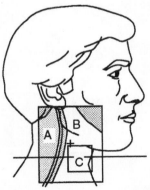

Figure 9.20 The large lateral field (A) is usually treated until spinal cord tolerance is reached, after which the field is reduced off the spinal cord (B). A boost is then often delivered to the site of the primary tumor (C). A = 4400 cGy; B = 6000 cGy; C = 6800 cGy.

culated for a patient who received 4500 cGy at the central axis of the large opposed fields and then an additional 1000 cGy with shielding of the spinal cord, followed by an additional 1500 cGy to the larynx through small boost fields. The dose in the larynx is well over 8000 cGy, rather than the intended 7000 cGy. The maximum dose to a small volume anteriorly was 8350 cGy. Delivering 7000 cGy in 35 fractions of 200 cGy each, the daily fraction to the area receiving 8000 cGy is 228.5 cGy; to the area receiving 8350, the daily fraction is 238.5 cGy. In this case, not only is the total dose high but the daily fraction size is also higher than prescribed. This dose, which is more than 20 percent higher than the prescribed dose, should be calculated and recorded in the patient's chart on a daily basis. Compensators can be used to improve dose uniformity. Wedges in the larger fields may be a disadvantage, since these fields also include areas more cephalad and anterior, where the patient's head has a transverse diameter similar to that at the central axis; thus, at this plane, a

wedge may be disadvantageous. Wedges may, however, be used in the smaller field to reduce the hot spot.

The practice of prescribing the dose at the midplane depth on the central axis probably originates with the complexities of performing hand calculations of the dose at off-axis points. However, with the widely accepted use of computer algorithms capable of calculating dose at practically any point in just a few seconds, it may be more practical to prescribe the dose at a point in the primary tumor site rather than on the central axis of the beam.

Even when the dose is prescribed and calculated on the central axis of the beam, it is highly recommended that it also be calculated and recorded in at least two sites in head and neck treatments where shrinking opposed lateral fields are used. One suggested site is the primary tumor where the final boost will be delivered. It is also a good practice to record the maximum spinal cord dose. Calculation of the dose in off-axis sites is recommended for radiation

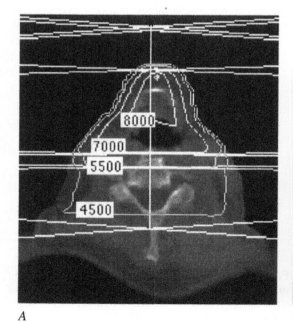

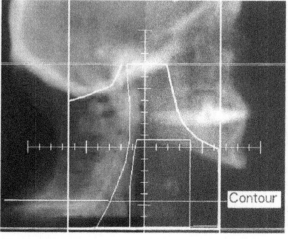

A   *B*

Figure 9.21   *A.* In a patient where the dose prescription is made at middepth on the central axis, the dose anteriorly can be very high. *B* demonstrates the fields and the plane of the dose distribution shown in *A*.

treatment in any area. In the head and neck region, where the surface topography is irregular and radio-sensitive critical structures necessarily are included in the fields, it is particularly important.

When the opposed lateral and anterior fields are half-beam blocked, the central axis of the fields is under the block or outside the irradiated area. In these situations, it is necessary to select an off-axis point for the dose prescription and calculation (Fig. 9.22). To perform the dose calculation when a source-axis distance (SAD) treatment technique is used, the off-axis distance and the patient's thickness in the beam direction must be known. When an SSD treatment technique is used, it is necessary to also know the SSD at the dose calculation point. When the fields are defined using independent jaws, the collimator scatter factor is found by using the size of the collimator setting (i.e., if the open field is 10 × 20 cm and one jaw is closed to make the field 10 × 10, the smaller field is used to find the collimator scatter factor). This approximation is correct to within about 2 percent. Dose calculations at off-axis points were described in Chap. 5.

Since the anterior field is usually not opposed, it is

treated via an SSD technique and the dose is often prescribed at a small depth or at d_{max} on the central axis. When bilateral lower neck and supraclavicular lymph nodes are treated, the central axis is in the patient's midline. The prescription point on the central axis, therefore, does not represent the location of either of the treated lymph node groups and is often shielded by an anterior spinal cord block. The stated dose to these lymph node groups is thus different from the dose actually delivered. The dose calculation therefore must be made at an off-axis point. It is important to recognize that when a near cylinder-shaped object (the neck) is treated via a single anterior field or by opposed anterior and posterior fields, the dose increases laterally where the neck is thinner (Fig. 9.23A). Thus, the dose inhomogeneity across the neck can be marked. Selection of the dose prescription point plays a role in the magnitude of the hot spots laterally—i.e., if the dose is prescribed at middepth near the spinal cord block, the dose in the lateral aspect of the neck is higher than if the prescription point is 2 to 3 cm lateral of the spinal cord block (Fig. 9.23B). The dose gradient is improved slightly and, by prescribing the dose in the mid-section of the neck, the hot spot in the lateral aspect of the neck is decreased.

In patients with a postlaryngectomy tracheostomy, the risk of tumor recurrence at the site of a tracheostomy is relatively high (about 10 percent). Predisposing factors include subglottic extension of tumor, positive surgical margins, positive lymph nodes, and vascular invasion. The risk of recurrence can be reduced by including the stoma in the irradiation field in these patients. A full-length midline spinal cord block in the anterior supraclavicular field would also shield the stoma; consideration should therefore be given to inserting a shorter block to shield the larynx and spinal cord near the field junction only. Bolus material, placed on the tissues surrounding the stoma, will increase the dose to the tissues that are at risk for recurrence. This bolus can be doughnut-shaped to allow breathing through the tracheostomy during the treatment. Consideration should be given to the possibility of an increased dose in the spinal cord as a result of the absence of tissue and the presence of an air column in front of the spinal cord in

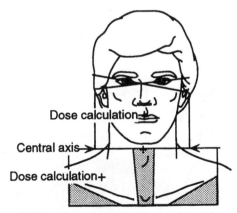

Figure 9.22 When a half-beam block technique is used, the dose prescription cannot be made on the central axis, since it is effectively under the block. Instead, the dose should be calculated at a representative point inside the irradiated area—for example, at middepth in the center of the lateral fields and in the supraclavicular region of the anterior field.

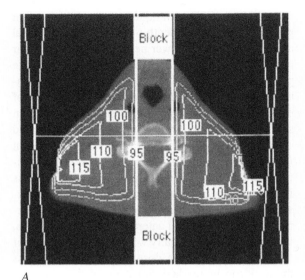

A

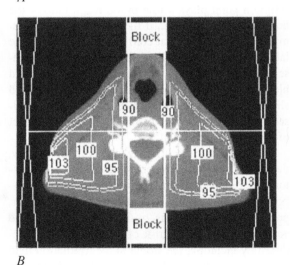

B

Figure 9.23 When the dose prescription is made near the midline spinal cord block in opposed neck fields, the dose in the lateral aspect, where the neck is thinner, can be very high. *B.* When the dose is prescribed farther from the block, the dose in the lateral aspect is reduced and the dose gradient throughout the neck is slightly improved.

patients with a tracheostomy (Fig. 9.24). If an electron beam is used to boost the stoma dose, the air space in front of the spinal cord may be of less concern, as the bone in the vertebral body attenuates much of the electron beam. The effect on the electron

beam of the tissue between each vertebral body is more complex. In most patients, the cervical spine is curved; thus, the anterior beam is rarely perpendicular to the vertebral bodies but passes through any given vertebral body at an angle (Fig. 9.24). The beam must therefore pass through some thickness of bone at all levels before reaching the spinal cord.

Sometimes it is necessary to treat through a posterior field. This field will often be intercepted by either a Plexiglas support in the treatment couch or a head immobilization device (Fig. 9.25). A transmission factor for the device is then used in the calculation of monitor units (MU), as shown in Chaps. 4 and 5. Sometimes only a portion of the posterior treatment field is intercepted by the base plate holding the immobilization device. In these situations, a question often arises as to whether the transmission factor should or should not be included in the MU calculation. Where the neck, in the direction of the beam, is thinnest, the spinal cord dose is usually highest. If this point lies outside the base plate, inclusion of the transmission factor for the base plate in the MU calculation only further increases the dose in the spinal cord (Fig. 9.25*A*). If this portion of the neck lies within the base plate, it is probably best to include the transmission factor in the MU calculation (Fig. 9.25*B*). These suggestions should be considered, but the decision as to whether the transmission factor should be included or not in the MU calculation should be made for each individual situation.

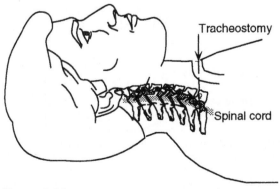

Figure 9.24 An air column caused by a tracheostomy can result in increased dose in the spinal cord.

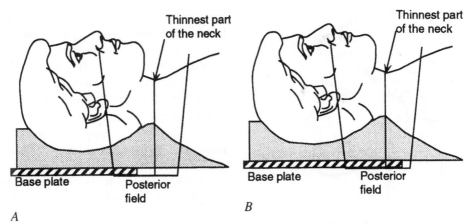

Figure 9.25 *A.* A posterior beam does not transect the base plate where the neck is thinnest. *B.* The posterior beam transects the base plate where the neck is thinnest.

TREATMENT

ORAL CAVITY

The treatment technique described above is often used for the treatment of tumors arising in many sites, including the oral cavity, oropharynx, hypopharynx, larynx, and nasopharynx. Small squamous cell carcinomas originating in the oral cavity are generally resected if the functional and cosmetic result is satisfactory. Otherwise radiation therapy is employed. For larger tumors, a combined approach is employed because more extensive tumors are rarely cured by either modality alone.

Anterior Tongue. Small tumors arising in the anterior two-thirds of the tongue (mobile portion of the tongue) are usually resected. Radiation therapy is used in patients who are medically inoperable. Postoperative radiation therapy to the primary site and the cervical lymph nodes is used for many reasons: positive margins, extensive primary tumor with bone or skin invasion, and multiple positive lymph nodes. Radiation therapy can also be used for larger, unresectable tumors because it yields superior cosmetic and functional results.

The lymphatic drainage from the tongue should be considered when the treatment fields are designed. The anterior portion of the tongue drains into the submandibular lymph nodes, while the posterior portion drains more to the jugulodigastric, posterior pharyngeal, and upper cervical lymph nodes (Fig. 9.26). The primary lesion and the first echelon of lymph nodes are given approximately 4600 cGy in 4.5 weeks. The lateral fields are then reduced off the spinal cord and are treated to approximately 6000 cGy. The posterior cervical lymph nodes can be treated using lateral electron beams. In large primary lesions, the final boost can be delivered via a submental field using electron or photon beams (Fig. 9.27). In small primary lesions, a boost can be delivered via an intraoral cone or an implant to approximately 7500 cGy following 4500 cGy to the primary lesion and the first echelon of lymph nodes. The intraoral cone boost is often given first because painful mucositis, caused by the dose to the large fields, may prevent the patient from holding the cone in the mouth.

Floor of Mouth. Small tumors arising in the floor of mouth can be treated via external beam therapy and an intraoral cone or an interstitial implant. If the tumor is well circumscribed, the boost treatment may be delivered first. If the tumor is not well appreciated, external beam therapy, including the primary lesion and the cervical lymph nodes, can be given first (Fig. 9.28). At a dose of approximately

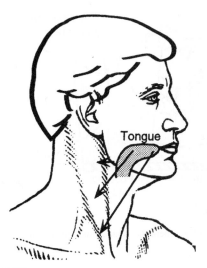

Figure 9.26   The lymphatic drainage from the anterior portion of the tongue is primarily to the submandibular lymph nodes, while the posterior portion drains primarily to the jugulodigastric, posterior pharyngeal, and upper cervical lymph nodes.

2000 cGy, ''tumoritis'' (redness of the tumor) usually develops and thus helps to define the tumor extent. The boost treatment can then proceed. If the mucositis resulting from high-dose external beam irradiation is severe, insertion of an intraoral cone may be too painful; it is therefore preferably done prior to the external beam treatment. Eight treatments of 300 cGy are given via the intraoral cone, followed by external beam to bring the dose to the primary lesion to approximately 7000 cGy. In large lesions, the boost can be delivered via a submental field. Sparing as much of the mandible as possible is critical to reducing the risk of osteoradionecrosis.

Small floor-of-mouth lesions that are infiltrating and fixed to the mandible are often treated with surgical excision followed by radiation therapy. The preferred treatment of large lesions with extensive infiltration consists of surgery and postoperative radiation therapy. Small lesions adhering to the mandible can be excised surgically with removal of a small section of the mandible. This is followed by postoperative radiation therapy to approximately 6000 cGy in 6 weeks.

Comprehensive treatment of positive cervical

lymph nodes in oral cavity lesions consists of parallel opposed lateral fields to the upper neck and an anterior field including the lower neck and supraclavicular fossa (Fig. 9.29). This is followed by a radical neck dissection or limited nodal resection, depending on the extent of the disease.

Lip.   Most lip cancers are found on the lower lip, but they can occur on either lip. Small lesions originating in the lip are often treated via orthovoltage or electron beams using a lead cutout to protect the surrounding tissues. In many patients, an intraoral lead shield can be used to protect the underlying mucosa. More advanced disease is treated by photon beams with a boost delivered via an interstitial implant (Chap. 16) or by using an electron or orthovoltage beam. Bolus may be necessary to bring the maximum dose to the surface. For small lesions, a dose of 4500 to 5000 cGy in 3 weeks may be adequate. A large lesion may be treated to 4500 cGy by an external beam followed by a boost via an implant delivering 2000 to 2500 cGy, for a total dose of 6500 to 7000 cGy. The cervical lymph nodes are usually not treated if the primary lesion is small. The submental, submandibular, and subdigastric lymph nodes are usually treated if the primary lesion is large. These can be treated using opposed lateral fields only.

Retromolar Trigone and Anterior Faucial Pillar.   The treatment of tumors in the retromolar trigone usually involves surgical resection or radiation therapy. In early lesions, radiation therapy is the pre-

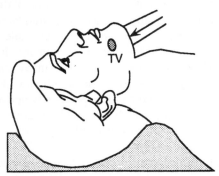

Figure 9.27   Diagram illustrating the setup of a submental boost field.

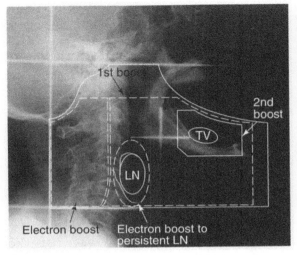

A

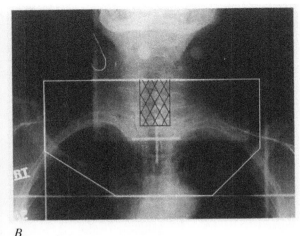

B

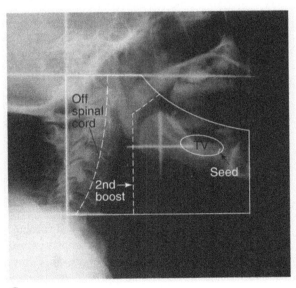

C

Figure 9.28   Typical treatment fields for floor-of-mouth lesions. A lead wire marks a palpable lymph node (*A* and *B*). A gold seed marks the anterior extent of the tumor (*C*).

ferred treatment, with surgery being reserved for the salvage of radiation therapy failures. Approximately 2000 cGy is delivered to develop tumoritis, which will help to determine the extent of the disease. If the tumor is laterally located, this can be followed by 4500 cGy delivered through anterior and lateral fields using wedges or anterior and posterior oblique fields using wedges. Small, well-defined lesions in cooperative patients may be boosted via an intraoral cone using an electron beam. Large retromolar trigone lesions sometimes also involve the base of tongue, and they tend to invade bone. Radiation therapy is usually the primary treatment; it is delivered via opposed lateral fields to the primary lesion

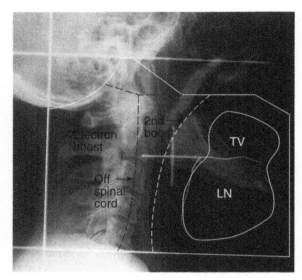

A

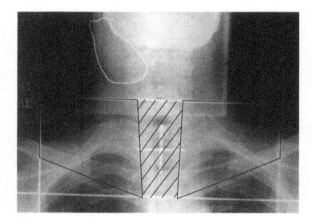

B

Figure 9.29   *A* and *B*. Treatment fields for an extensive oral cavity tumor. A lead wire marks a large lymph node.

and cervical lymph nodes and via an anterior field including the lower cervical lymph nodes and bilateral supraclavicular fossa.

Buccal Mucosa.   Small, well-defined lesions can be treated via surgical resection or external beam therapy combining photon and electron beams.[47] Some lesions may be suitable for an implant or intraoral cone treatment to deliver a boost. In interme-

diate lesions, radiation therapy is preferred because it yields superior cosmetic and functional results and a high cure rate. Radiation therapy usually consists of 5500 to 6000 cGy delivered in 6 weeks, followed by a boost of 2000 cGy sparing the mandible. In advanced tumors, radiation therapy is followed by surgical resection of the primary lesion and regional lymph nodes.

Gingival Ridge.   The choice of treatment modality depends on the extent of the tumor, nodal involvement, and presence or absence of bone involvement. Small lesions without bone involvement can be managed with external beam treatment alone. The treatment can be delivered via lateral and anterior wedged fields. Large lesions require high-dose irradiation, and the treatment can result in osteoradionecrosis. The local control rate is poor and surgery is therefore generally preferred. Pre- or postoperative radiation therapy may be given in an attempt to eradicate microscopic disease in the surgical margins. The preoperative dose is usually approximately 4500 to 5000 cGy in 5 weeks. Postoperative irradiation in patients with positive margins is usually 6000 cGy.

OROPHARYNX

The oropharynx consists of the tonsils, base of tongue, and the oropharyngeal wall. Tumors arising in this area present with a high incidence of regional lymph node involvement irrespective of the stage and size of the tumor. Whereas oral cavity carcinomas are more often treated surgically, oropharyngeal carcinoma is usually treated by radiation therapy. Tumors arising in the oropharynx are also usually treated via lateral opposed fields, including the primary lesion and bilateral upper cervical lymph nodes, matched with an anterior field at the thyroid notch to treat the lower neck and bilateral supraclavicular lymph nodes. The spinal cord block placed on the anterior field will also shield the larynx and avoid its unnecessary irradiation.

Tonsil.   Early lesions (T1 and small T2) are usually treated with once-daily radiation therapy, while more advanced tumors are usually treated with radiation therapy given in twice-daily fractions (bid). Some institutions still employ surgery and postoperative radiation therapy. Radiation therapy in the treatment of tonsillar carcinoma consists of large fields including adjacent structures such as the base of tongue, the inferior nasopharynx, pharynx, and regional lymph nodes. If the base of tongue or the soft palate is involved, the cervical lymph nodes are at risk bilaterally. All of the radiation therapy should instead be delivered via opposed lateral fields. Very large tumors are usually treated to 7400 to 7600 cGy if a regimen of 120 to 125 cGy bid with shrinking fields is used. Large parallel opposed fields are used to 4500 cGy and then the fields are reduced off the spinal cord. An additional 2000 to 2500 cGy is delivered via smaller boost fields, and bilateral electron fields are used to boost the dose in the posterior cervical lymph nodes. The lower cervical lymph nodes and supraclavicular fossae are treated to 5000 cGy in 5 weeks.

Base of Tongue.   Radiation therapy is the treatment of choice for carcinoma of the base of tongue, since surgical resection is mutilating and the patient often loses the ability to speak and swallow. Large parallel opposed fields are used to 4500 cGy and then the fields are reduced off the spinal cord. An additional 2000 to 2500 cGy is delivered via smaller boost fields, and bilateral electron fields are used to boost the dose in the posterior cervical lymph nodes. The field junction is set above the thyroid notch so that the anterior spinal cord block also will shield the larynx. Some institutions use an interstitial implant to deliver the boost (Chap. 16). The lower cervical and bilateral supraclavicular lymph nodes are treated 4500 to 5000 cGy in 5 weeks. Persistent tumor following completion of radiation therapy requires a comprehensive resection. Cervical lymph node disease is usually treated with combined irradiation and a neck dissection.

Lateral Pharyngeal Wall.   Tumors arising in the oropharynx are often quite large at presentation. The lymphatic drainage is primarily to the subdigastric, midjugular, and retropharyngeal lymph nodes. The retropharyngeal lymph nodes are also referred to as Rouviere's nodes and are located posterior and

lateral of the pharyngeal space at C1 and C2 (cervical vertebral body). Early lesions in the lateral pharyngeal wall are often treated with radiation therapy or surgery and large tumors are treated with combined-modality therapy or radiation therapy alone. Radiation therapy requires large fields, including the entire pharynx from the nasopharynx to the pyriform sinus. When the fields are reduced off the spinal cord, sharp field edges are necessary in order to include the primary tumor site and Rouviere's nodes while also shielding the spinal cord (Fig. 9.10).

Soft Palate and Uvula.   Small lesions of 1 cm or less can be treated either with surgery alone or radiation therapy delivered via external beam therapy to approximately 2000 cGy in 2 weeks, followed by intraoral cone treatment using an electron beam in edentulous patients. Larger lesions are usually treated by radiation therapy followed by surgical resection of residual disease. The treatment technique consists of opposed lateral fields, which are reduced as described above. A dose of approximately 6500 to 7000 cGy in 7 weeks is delivered to the primary lesion. Except in patients with very early lesions, the low cervical and bilateral supraclavicular lymph nodes are treated via an anterior field to approximately 5000 cGy in 5 weeks. Extensive tumors may involve the oropharynx, base of tongue, and tonsils and are often associated with bilateral cervical lymph node disease.

HYPOPHARYNX

The hypopharynx extends from the plane of the hyoid bone and the pharyngeoepiglottic fold to the plane of the lower border of the cricoid cartilage inferiorly. The lymphatic drainage is primarily to the subdigastric, superior, deep- and midjugular and para- and retropharyngeal (Rouviere's) lymph nodes.

Pyriform Sinus.   Early lesions arising in the pyriform sinus are usually treated with radiation therapy, with surgery reserved for salvage of radiation failures. For more advanced tumors, combined-modality therapy may yield higher local control rates. Radiation therapy requires large fields with the inferior margin including the subglottic area and upper trachea. Opposed lateral fields are used to 4500 cGy and then the fields are reduced off the spinal cord. If once-a-day treatment is used, the dose to the primary lesion is approximately 6500 cGy in 6.5 weeks and the posterior cervical lymph nodes are boosted via bilateral electron fields using 6- to 10-MeV electrons. When preoperative radiation therapy is employed, approximately 4500 to 5000 cGy is given, which is followed by laryngopharyngectomy. When postoperative radiation therapy is employed, the dose is approximately 5000 cGy in 6 weeks delivered via lateral fields. An additional 1000 to 2000 cGy may be delivered to the stoma if the surgical margins were not clear.

Posterior Pharyngeal Wall. Tumors arising in the posterior pharyngeal wall are usually considered unresectable. Radiation therapy consists of large fields, including the entire pharynx and upper cervical esophagus and extending superiorly to include the nasopharyngeal vault; superior deep, middle, and low jugular; and Rouviere's lymph nodes (Fig. 9.30). These large fields are treated to 4500 cGy and are then reduced off the spinal cord. The smaller

fields are continued to 6500 to 7000 cGy if once-a-day radiation therapy is used or 7500 cGy with a bid regimen. Sharp field edges are necessary posteriorly in order to include the primary and Rouviere's lymph nodes while at the same time shielding the spinal cord (Figs. 9.10 and 9.30).

LARYNX

The larynx consists of the supraglottis, glottis, and subglottis. The most common route of spread from supraglottis is to the subdigastric, superior deep, and midjugular lymph nodes. Occasionally, these tumors also spread to Rouviere's lymph nodes. The glottis (true vocal cord) is practically void of lymphatics; thus the incidence of lymph node involvement in very early (T1) lesions is 0 to 5 percent.

Glottis. Early vocal cord lesions with normal vocal cord mobility are cured by radiation therapy alone in about 90 percent of cases.[48,49] Radiation therapy is delivered through small (5 × 5 or 6 × 6 cm) opposed lateral fields (Fig. 9.31). Due to the slope of the patient's surface contour, the dose increases anteriorly. Wedges of 15 or 30° can be used

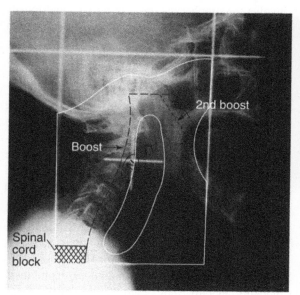

A

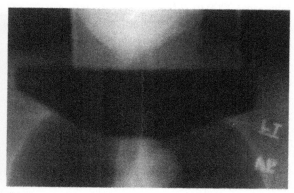

B

Figure 9.30 *A* and *B*. Treatment fields used in a patient with a large posterior pharyngeal wall lesion. Node of Rouviere is indicated. A small spinal cord block is placed in the lateral fields rather than in the anterior field. An anterior midline block could possibly also shield tumor, since determination of the caudal tumor extent is difficult.

to compensate for the sloping skin surface and to produce a uniform dose distribution (Fig. 9.32). Alternatively, the first half of the treatment can be delivered through open fields with wedges inserted for the remainder of the treatment. The fields are centered on the vocal cords and there is flash over the anterior skin surface to prevent underdosage of the anterior commissure. The cephalad margin is usually at the caudal aspect of the hyoid bone and the caudal margin at the inferior border of the cricoid. Those margins should be determined for each patient, as the individual anatomy may vary. In many older patients, it is possible to observe the vocal cords on a lateral radiograph. The posterior margin usually extends to the anterior aspect of the vertebral body. Some authors advocate giving 6000 cGy and, with a subsequent reduction of the posterior border off the posterior arytenoids and the esophagus, continuing to 6400 to 6600 cGy. If the wedge angles are not chosen carefully, the dose in the anterior commissure can be compromised due to overcompensation. The beam energy should preferably be cobalt-60 or 4-MV photons, as higher-energy beams may provide an inadequate dose distribution.[50] There has also been some concern about the effect on the dose in the surface layers of lesions located in the air-tumor tissue interface with higher beam energies.[51] If a 6-MV photon beam is used, beam spoilers or some bolusing should be used to allow adequate dose buildup.

Glottic lesions with supraglottic or subglottic extension with impaired vocal cord mobility may have lymph node involvement. Treatment fields should therefore include the primary lesion and the subdigastric and midjugular lymph nodes to 4500 cGy. A boost is then often delivered to the glottis. For larger lesions, the fields are tailored to the disease. If subglottic extension is present, the lower cervical lymph nodes, bilateral supraclavicular lymph nodes, and upper mediastinum should be considered in the target volume (Fig. 9.33). This can be accomplished by using lateral fields, with the foot of the treatment couch turned away from the collimator (Fig. 9.15). A boost can then be delivered through lateral opposed fields to the primary lesion. Wedges may be necessary in these fields to compensate for the slope of the skin surface.[52]

Supraglottis. Tumors arising in the supraglottis carry a poorer prognosis than true glottic tumors because they have a higher propensity for lymph node involvement. The treatment is controversial and

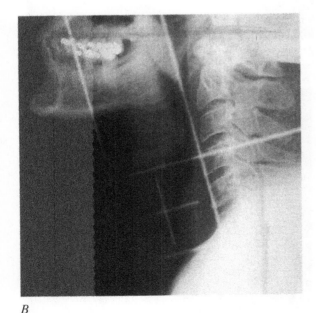

A

B

Figure 9.31   A typical treatment field for vocal cord lesions.

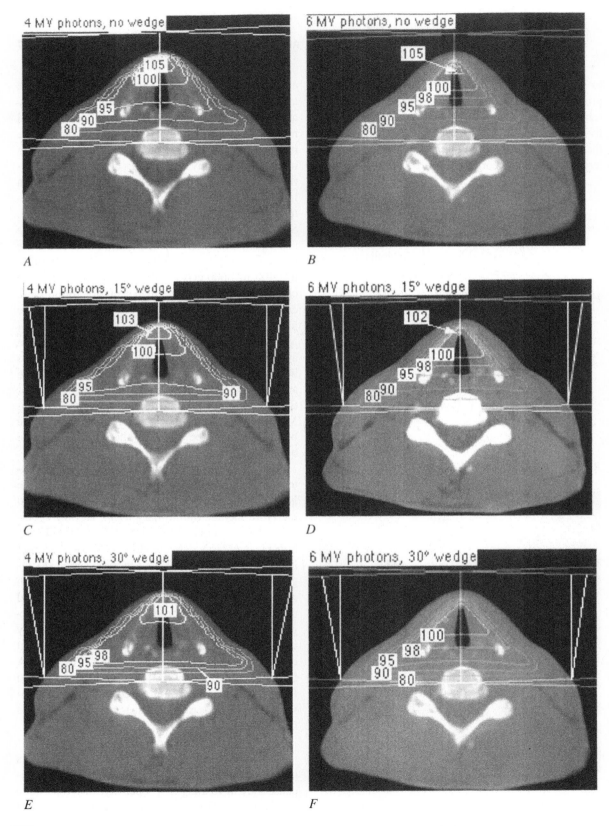

298

while some advocate a laryngectomy, others advocate a partial supraglottic laryngectomy or radical radiation therapy. The choice of treatment depends on the extent of the disease, location of the tumor, growth pattern, physical condition of the patient, and patient's preference. Radiation therapy is considered the initial treatment of early superficial tumors. For more advanced disease, surgery with pre- or postoperative radiation therapy is considered the preferred treatment (Fig. 9.33). Radical radiation therapy is often given with bid treatment in order to deliver higher tumor dose without higher complication rates. Typical doses would be 120 to 125 cGy bid and shrinking fields to 7440 to 7500 cGy. Postoperative radiation therapy can be delivered via opposed lateral fields to 4000 to 4500 cGy, followed by an electron boost for an additional 1000 cGy to the stoma.

Subglottis. Subglottic tumors represent less than 1 percent of all larynx cancer. Most subglottic tumors are probably glottic lesions with subglottic extension. Early lesions can be successfully treated by radiation therapy alone; thus the voice is preserved. More advanced lesions are treated with laryngectomy followed by radiation therapy. The treatment fields should include the primary lesion, upper trachea, and the inferior jugular and upper mediastinal lymph nodes using anterior and posterior fields to 4000 cGy. The larynx and the upper trachea are treated further through lateral fields to 6500 cGy. Residual lymph nodes are usually removed through a neck dissection.

NASOPHARYNX

The nasopharynx is a very difficult area to examine and tumors arising in this location are therefore often not detected on routine examination. Patients presenting with metastatic disease in cervical lymph nodes from an unknown primary site are often found to have a tumor in the nasopharynx. Due to the rich lymphatic supply in the nasopharynx and because many tumors are not found until after they have metastasized to the cervical lymph nodes, the majority of patients with carcinoma of the nasopharynx present with cervical lymphadenopathy.[53] Surgical resection with adequate margins is often impossible due to the adjacent base of the skull, hence radiation therapy is the primary treatment for carcinoma of the nasopharynx. Prior to irradiation, careful determina-

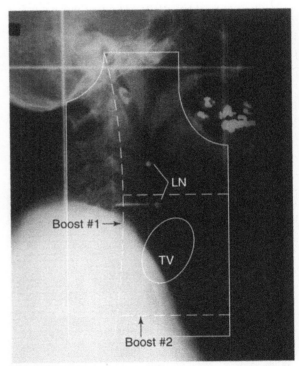

Figure 9.33 Typical lateral treatment field for supraglottic carcinoma. Palpable lymph nodes are indicated by lead shots. The foot of the couch is turned 10° away from the collimator so that the beam is angled caudally. The shoulder on the exit side is in the beam.

◀ **Figure 9.32** Isodose distributions using opposed lateral fields to treat a vocal cord lesion. The dose distributions on the left are calculated using 4-MV and on the right 6-MV photon beams. *A* and *B*. The dose distribution using open beams. *C* and *D*. The dose distribution using 15° wedges. *E* and *F*. The dose distribution using 30° wedges.

tion of the tumor extent, preferably with magnetic resonance imaging, is critical to prevent underdosage of the tumor as the fields are being reduced.[54] Irradiation is delivered via opposed lateral fields (Fig. 9.34), including the nasopharynx, base of the skull, and bilateral cervical lymph nodes. The anterior margin of the field should include the posterior ethmoids, the posterior third of the maxillary antrum, and the nasal cavity. A matching anterior field is also used to treat lower neck and bilateral supraclavicular lymph nodes. After 4500 cGy, the fields are reduced off the spinal cord and an additional 1500 cGy is delivered. Rouviere's node is a common route of spread and should be included when the fields are reduced off the spinal cord. The posterior cervical lymph nodes are treated via bilateral electron beams. The lower neck and bilateral supraclavicular lymph nodes are treated to 5000 cGy in 5 weeks.

A final boost can be delivered through a variety of techniques. Anterior oblique fields or an arc technique can be used to reduce the dose to the temporal lobes (Fig. 9.35). When an arc technique is used, the

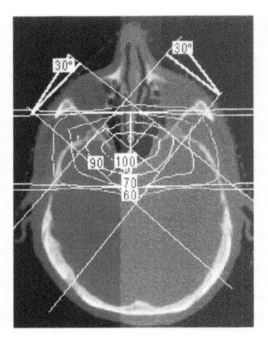

A

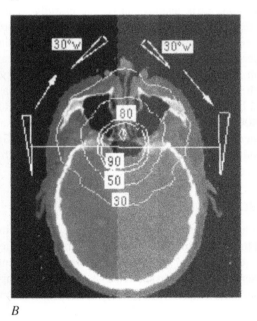

B

Figure 9.35 *A.* Isodose distribution resulting from opposed lateral and anterior oblique wedged fields equally weighted to boost the nasopharynx. *B.* Isodose distribution resulting from a 180° arc with wedges that are reversed midway through the arc to prevent a hot spot anteriorly.

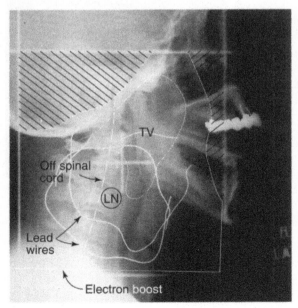

Figure 9.34 Typical lateral treatment field for carcinoma of the nasopharynx. Lead wires outline large bilateral cervical lymphadenopathy.

patient's head is tilted back so that the beam remains below the eyes (Fig. 9.3). A 180 or 270° arc with wedges that are reversed midway through the arc (Chap. 6) will deliver a cylinder-shaped, uniform high-dose volume with rapid dose fall-off in the surrounding tissue (Fig. 9.35*B*). If the cervical lymph nodes also require a boost dose, opposed anterior and posterior fields with a midline block can be used (Fig. 9.36). It is crucial to avoid excessive irradiation of the spinal cord, brain, brainstem, optic

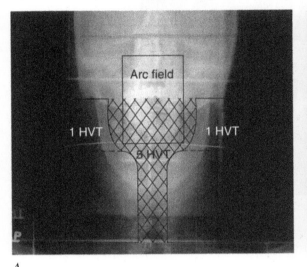

A

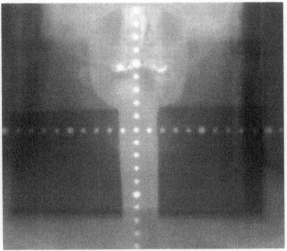

B

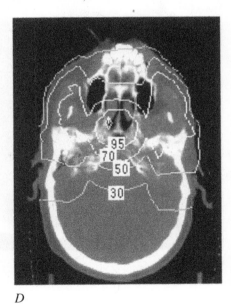

C   *D*

Figure 9.36   *A* and *B*. Bilateral cervical lymph nodes can be boosted via opposed anterior and posterior fields using a midline spinal cord block and a wider midline block shielding the high-dose area created by the arc treatment. A 1-HVT block can be used in the lateral aspect of the neck, where the dose from the arc treatment is lower. *C*. A diagram illustrating the field arrangement for the boost to the primary tumor site and to the cervical lymph nodes. *D*. Isodose distribution through the plane where the arc and the opposed anterior/posterior fields overlap.

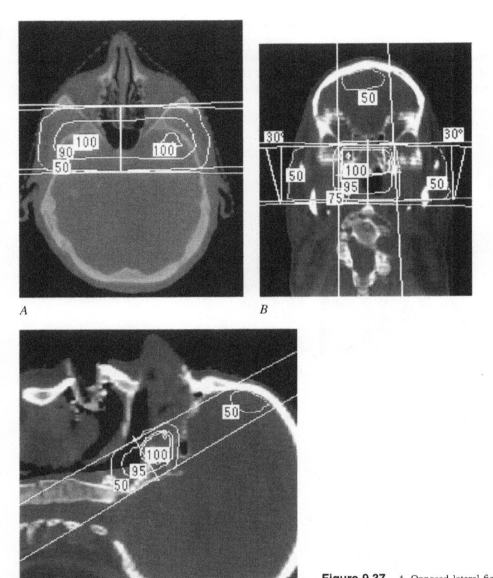

A

B

C

Figure 9.37   *A.* Opposed lateral fields using 15-MV photon beams to deliver a boost to the nasopharynx. Isodose distributions in coronal (*B*) and sagittal (*C*) planes resulting from using opposed lateral wedged fields and an unwedged vertex field duplication to deliver a boost to the nasopharynx.

chiasm, eye, and oral mucosa. Alternatively, the boost to the nasopharynx can be delivered using small lateral fields and high-energy beam providing an additional 500 to 800 cGy (Fig. 9.37*A*) or a three-field technique using opposed lateral and vertex fields treated with high-energy beams (Fig. 9.37*B* and *C*). A final boost can also be delivered via an intracavitary implant using cesium 137 sources, as described in Chap. 16.

Carcinoma of the nasopharynx has a propens-

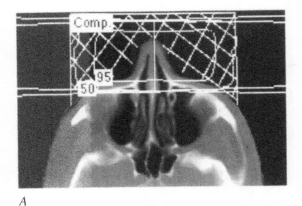

A

B

Figure 9.38   *A.* Parallel opposed lateral fields used in treating a small lesion in the nose yield uniform dose distribution when a compensator is used. *B.* To increase the depth, the lateral fields can be angled slightly and an anterior field can be added. Wedges are then needed in the lateral fields. In this plan, the fields are weighted equally.

ity for local recurrence even following high-dose irradiation; occasionally, reirradiation is considered.[55-60] Retreatment requires very careful treatment planning and small fields. Localized treatment using external beams and one or two intracavitary implants can result in reasonably good survival.[59] The risk of brain stem and temporal lobe necrosis is high, but this must be weighed against the risk of destruction by progressive disease.

NASAL CAVITY

Tumors arising in the anterior nasal cavity and septum can be treated via opposed lateral fields (Fig. 9.38A) or fields that are angled posteriorly to improve the depth in the posterior direction. The beam energy is preferably 4- to 6-MV photons. For tumors near the surface, bolus may be necessary, and in many situations tissue-equivalent material can be used directly on the surface to achieve both bolusing and compensating effect (Fig. 9.38). A dose of approximately 6000 cGy in 6 weeks followed by an interstitial or intracavitary implant to bring the dose to 7000 cGy is usually given. Large tumors extending to a greater posterior depth are often treated to 6500 cGy in 6 to 7 weeks. A treatment technique that consists of an anterior field in addition to right and left anterior oblique wedged fields may yield a superior dose distribution (Fig. 9.38B). Care must be taken to respect tolerance of critical structures such as the optic nerve, pituitary gland, and brain tissue. Because of the unpredictable nature of electrons traversing air cavities in the nasal cavity and paranasal sinuses, anterior electron fields are not recommended.

Extensive carcinoma of the nasal cavity often requires a complex field arrangement to include the tumor while avoiding adjacent normal tissues, particularly the lenses of the eyes. Figure 9.39A and B illustrates a large tumor invading the nasal cavity, the ethmoids, and the frontal sinus. With a three-dimensional treatment-planning system, a field arrangement consisting of an anterior and a right anterior oblique vertex field was designed (Figs. 9.39A, B, and C). The resulting isodose distribution is also shown in Figs. 9.39D and 9.40A, B, and C.

Port films of vertex fields are difficult to obtain because it is not possible to place a cassette in the exit beam. A technique in which an image of the field in the anterior/posterior direction can be obtained is, however, possible (Fig. 9.41).[61,62] A cassette should be placed horizontally on the treatment couch and as close to the patient's head as possible. First, a lateral port film is taken, using the appropriate field size and isocenter. A second exposure is then made with the beam wide open to include the

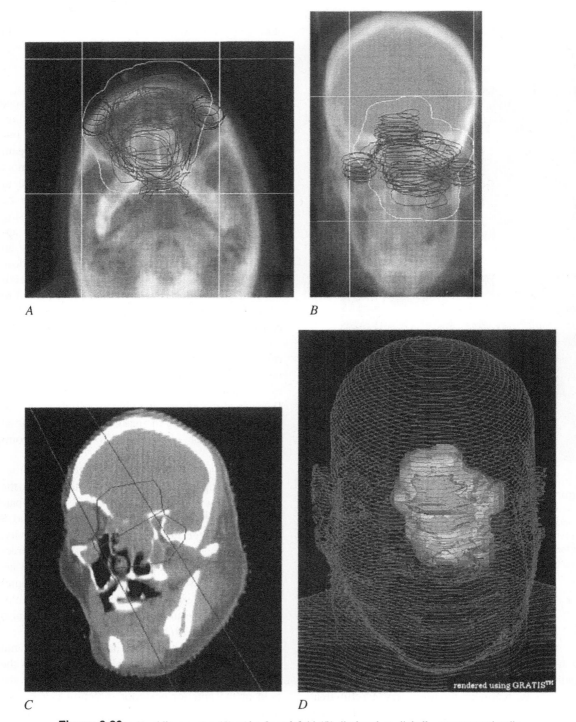

Figure 9.39 An oblique vertex (*A*) and a frontal field (*B*) displayed on digitally reconstructed radiographs (DRR) used in treating an extensive carcinoma of the nasal cavity. *C.* The two treatment fields displayed on an oblique CT image. *D.* Surface-rendered tumor volume *(red)* and 98 percent isodose surface *(yellow).* The 98 percent isodose line does not totally enclose the tumor, which is seen outside the isodose surface. (See color illustration 2, which appears between pages 532 and 533.) (The Virtual Simulator, Sherouse Systems, Inc.™)

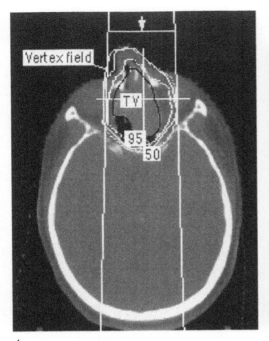

A

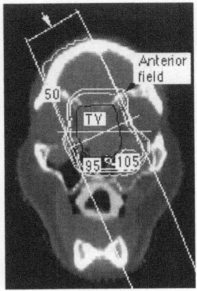

B

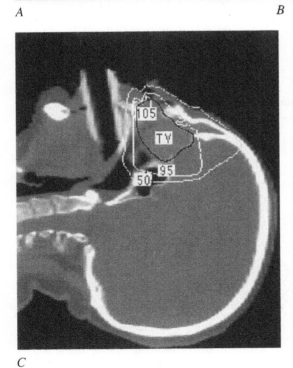

C

Figure 9.40 Isodose distribution in the transverse *(A)*, coronal *(B)*, and sagittal *(C)* planes resulting from the treatment of the tumor in Fig. 9.39.

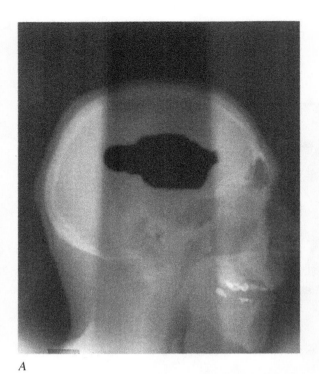

A

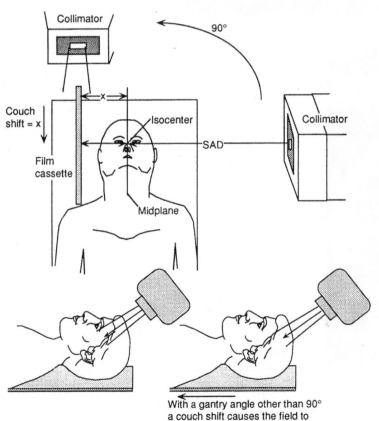

B

Figure 9.41 *A.* A port film of a vertex field can be obtained; however, only the anterior and posterior extent of the field can be determined. *B.* The port film is obtained by placing a cassette on the couch as close as possible to the patient's head. If a lateral field is also being treated, an exposure of this field is made first and then the collimator is opened to include the entire head. The distance from the isocenter to the cassette (x) is measured. Without changing anything else, the couch is turned 90° so that the top of the head is toward the collimator. The appropriate field size is set and the couch is then moved longitudinally a distance that equals x, so as to maintain the same TFD for all fields. The couch is then shifted laterally until the beam intercepts the cassette. If there is a gantry angle other than 90° for the vertex field, the appropriate gantry angle must be set before the couch is moved. After the couch has been shifted longitudinally, the height of the couch is adjusted until the field is returned to the marks on the head.

entire head, providing anatomic details. To ensure the same magnification of all ports, the target-to-film distance (TFD) must remain constant. For the lateral exposures, the distance is measured from the midsagittal plane, or isocenter, to the cassette. This distance, indicated by x in Fig. 9.41*B* is often 15 to 20 cm. With the gantry still in the lateral position, the couch is turned 90°, as shown in Fig. 9.41*B*. The couch is then shifted laterally until the central axis of the beam intercepts the cassette. Alternatively, since it is only the anterior/posterior field dimension that will be projected on the film, the width can be opened until it catches the film. The couch is also shifted away from the collimator (i.e., in the longitudinal direction) by the same distance as x, to achieve the proper TFD. After the proper field size has been set, a third exposure is made, which projects the vertex field on the lateral film (Fig. 9.41*A*). If the treatment plan does not include a lateral field, only one lateral exposure, including the entire head, is necessary.

MAXILLARY ANTRUM

Complete surgical resection of tumors in the maxillary antrum is often not possible. Radiation therapy is therefore often recommended postoperatively or for palliation. Tumors are usually limited to one maxillary antrum, but the sphenoid sinus and ethmoids are also at risk for involvement. Extensive tumors may also involve the orbit and the opposite maxillary antrum. It is necessary to include the entire maxillary antrum in the fields, and since the apex of the sinus extend behind the orbit,[63] it is difficult to irradiate the superior portion without also irradiating the eye (Fig. 9.42). The field arrangement usually consists of anterior and lateral wedged fields (Fig. 9.43).[64] If the tumor involves the orbit, shielding of the eye may not be possible (Fig. 9.44). The lacrimal glands, situated in the lateral aspect of the upper eyelid, should be shielded if this can be accomplished without also shielding tumor (Fig. 9.45). If the orbit is not involved, the superior portion of the maxillary antrum can be included in the anterior field without also including the eye if the patient's head is tilted back or the gantry is angled so the beam enters from a caudal angle (Fig. 9.3). The anterior margin

of the lateral field should be placed at the lateral orbital rim and be angled approximately 10° posteriorly to avoid irradiating the opposite eye.[65] This leaves the most anterior aspect of the tumor out of the lateral field and more weight is therefore needed on the anterior field in order to irradiate the entire target adequately (Fig. 9.46). Loss of vision is a potential complication of irradiation of paranasal sinus tumors.[66-68] Careful field shaping to spare the lens of the eye, the optic nerves and the optic chiasm is therefore critical. Calculation of isodose distributions in multiple levels is recommended, since the dose can vary significantly within the treated volume.[64]

A sophisticated treatment technique that offers eye protection while the adjacent tissues are irradiated involves using synchronized eye shields; this has been described in Chap. 8.[69,70] Other eye-sparing treatment techniques for the treatment of maxillary antrum and nasal cavity tumors have also been described.[71-73]

Treatment Simulation. In treating maxillary antrum tumors with anterior and lateral wedged fields, a contralateral field is sometimes necessary to improve the uniformity of the dose distribution. The lateral field must enter posterior to the eye on the involved side and be angled posteriorly away from the contralateral eye (Fig. 9.43). The patient's position has already been discussed. It is usually advantageous to treat the patient with a bite block to maintain an open mouth, since the caudal margin is usually at the vermilion line. With the mouth open and the tongue under a bite block, the tongue and much of the mucosa in the floor of the mouth can be excluded from the radiation fields. With the patient in an immobilization mask, the anterior field is first centered in the cephalad-caudal direction and from left to right (Fig. 9.43). The cephalad margin is usually about 1 cm above the eyebrows and the caudal margin is at the vermilion line. The width of the field usually extends from the medial canthus of the contralateral eye and flashes over the surfaces of the involved side; however, these borders are variable, depending on extent of disease. The gantry is then turned to the appropriate angle for the lateral field (usually 80°) to accomplish a 10° posterior angle off

A

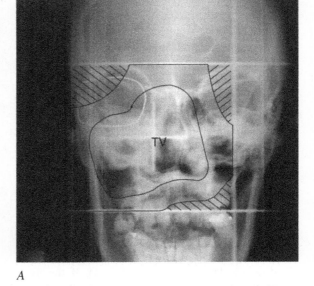

A

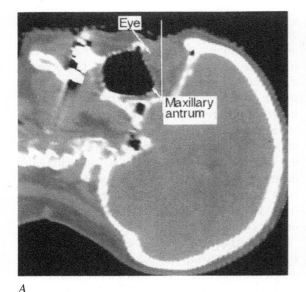

B

Figure 9.42 Sagittal view through the maxillary antrum. *A.* A vertical field including the entire maxillary antrum would also include the eye. *B.* When the chin is raised so that the beam enters from a caudal angle, the maxillary antrum can be included without also including the eye.

B

Figure 9.43 *A* and *B.* Typical fields used in treatment of carcinoma of the maxillary antrum. The lateral field is angled posteriorly about 10° to avoid the contralateral eye. The entire tumor volume cannot be included within the lateral fields without also including the eyes. The weighting on the anterior field is therefore increased.

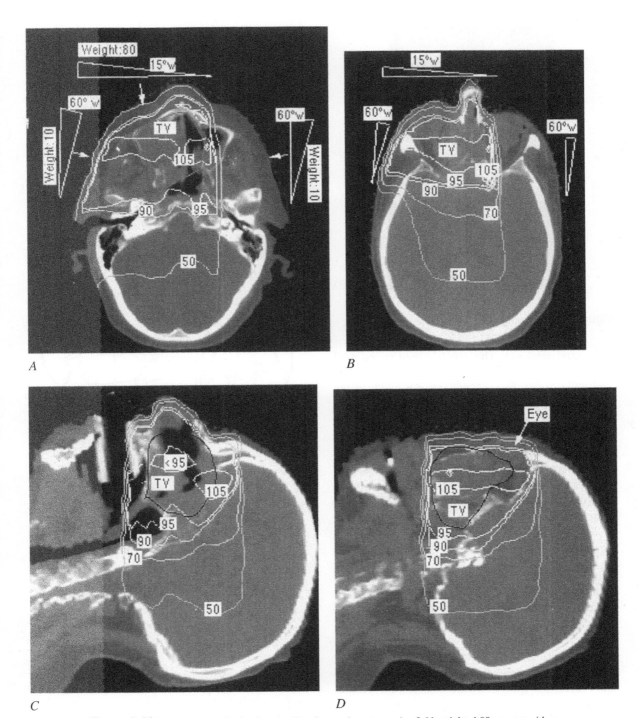

Figure 9.44   The isodose distribution resulting from using an anterior field weighted 80 percent with a 15° wedge and bilateral fields angled 10° posteriorly with 60° wedges and weighted 10 percent each superimposed on a transverse plane below the eyes *(A)*, transverse plane at the level of the eyes with no eye shielding because the tumor involves the orbit *(B)*, sagittal plane in the midline *(C)*, sagittal plane at the ipsilateral eye *(D)*, and coronal plane through the eye *(E)*.

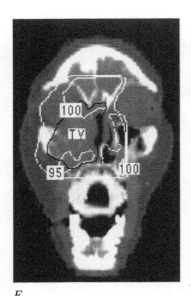

E

Figure 9.44 *(Continued)*

the contralateral eye. The couch is then raised until the anterior margin is at the palpable lateral bony orbit (Fig. 9.43). In most patients the width of the lateral field is about 7 to 9 cm. Radiographs are taken of each field—with the aid of CT scans obtained in the treatment position—isodose distributions can be produced to determine coverage of the target volume and appropriate shielding. It is always important to mark critical structures such as the eyes and palpable disease with radiopaque markers so as to facilitate beam shaping.

SALIVARY GLANDS

The major salivary glands are the parotid, submandibular, and sublingual glands. Of these, the parotid gland is the most common site of malignancy. Surgical removal is the treatment of choice; in patients where the surgical margins are microscopically or grossly positive, there is nerve involvement, or the tumor is of high-grade histology, postoperative radiation therapy is given. In unresectable cases, radiation therapy can be used as a sole treatment modality. Treatment with neutrons is superior to treatment with photons in terms of normal tissue sparing for unresectable disease.[74]

In treating the parotid gland postoperatively, the treatment can be delivered via a unilateral field using a mixed photon and electron beam (Fig. 9.47).[47,75,76] The field should include the entire incision and parotid bed with a margin (Fig. 9.48), and the dose should be prescribed at the deep lobe of the parotid gland or approximately 4 cm. When an electron beam is used, it is important to consider the attenuation by bone that may occur within the field.[47,75,76] Elective irradiation of the ipsilateral cervical lymph nodes can be given in patients with an incomplete resection or those with high-grade lesions and the positive neck dissection. The dose should be approximately 5000 cGy in 5 weeks. For gross disease, higher doses with shrinking fields are used. When

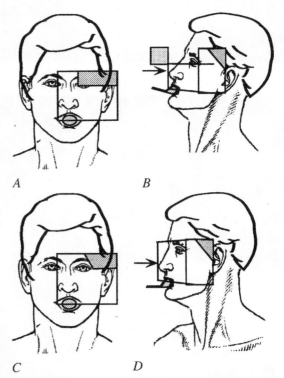

A *B*

C *D*

Figure 9.45 *A* and *B.* If possible, the eye should be shielded in the anterior field and the lateral field is placed posterior of the eye. *C* and *D.* If the orbit is involved, it may not be possible to shield the eye; however, the lacrimal gland in the superior lateral aspect of the eye lid may be shielded. If the eye cannot be excluded, the dose in the lens can be reduced by treating with an open eye, taking advantage of the build-up.

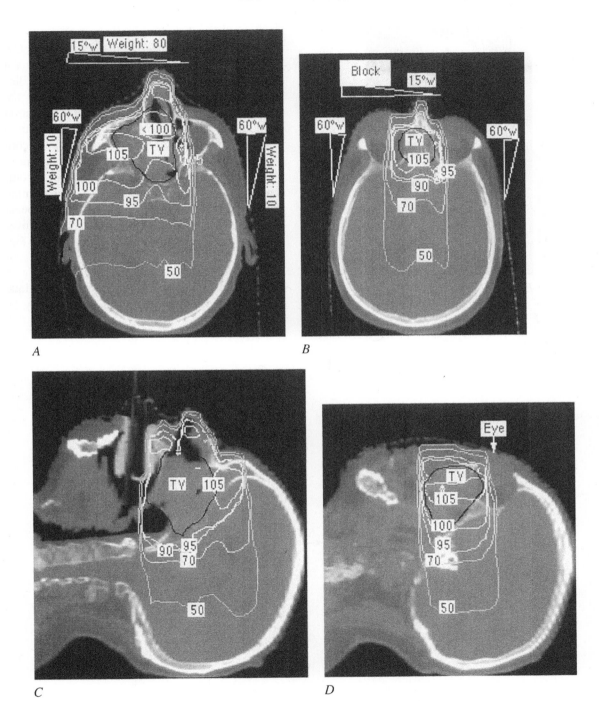

Figure 9.46   The isodose distribution resulting from using an anterior field weighted 80 percent with a 15° wedge and bilateral fields angled 10° posteriorly with 60° wedges and weighted 10 percent each superimposed on a transverse plane below the eyes *(A)*, transvere plane at the level of the eyes with the eye shielded *(B)*, sagittal plane in the midline *(C)*, sagittal plane at the ipsilateral eye *(D)*, and coronal plane through the eye *(E)*.

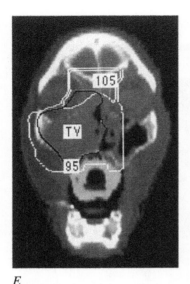

E

Figure 9.46   *(Continued)*

the cervical lymph nodes are involved, the treatment field may be reduced only minimally after 5000 cGy. The ipsilateral lymph nodes can be treated via a matching anterior field. If the spinal cord still lies within the treatment field, a larger fraction of the dose may be delivered via an 8- to 10-MeV electron beam or a wedge can be used in the photon beam to avoid delivering an excessive dose to the spinal cord (Fig. 9.49A). If a higher-energy electron beam is necessary in order to treat the primary tumor, a compensator may be placed in the electron beam over the spinal cord to reduce the depth of the effective beam (Fig. 9.49B). A wedge, with the thick portion over the spinal cord, can be used in the photon beam (Fig. 9.49B).

In the absence of electrons, a wedged pair of oblique fields can be used (Fig. 9.50). When oblique fields are used, the patient's chin must usually be

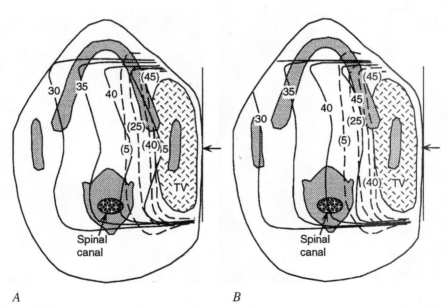

A   *B*

Figure 9.47   *A*. Isodose distribution resulting from using 4-MV photon (50 percent) and a 14-MeV electron (50 percent) beams to treat a parotid tumor. The solid lines represent the dose from the photon beam and the hatched line the electron beam. *B*. The same field arrangement using 6-MV photon (50 percent) and 14-MeV electron (50 percent) beams.

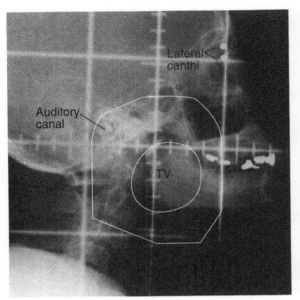

Figure 9.48   A typical field for the treatment of a parotid tumor.

raised so that the beam direction is caudal of the eyes (Fig. 9.51). Alternatively, a combination of couch and gantry angles can be used to cause the beam to enter and exit below the eyes. Such compound angles should not be attempted without the use of three-dimensional treatment planning capabilities.

AUDITORY CANAL AND MIDDLE EAR

Other than skin cancer, tumors arising in the ear are rare. A benign, highly vascular tumor called glomus jugulare, or carotid body tumor, can arise in various areas of the head and neck but usually grows along the course of the tympanic nerve or along blood vessels in the neck. Complete resection is often not possible due to bone invasion and the nature of the tumor. Radiation therapy is therefore often given alone or postoperatively.[77] The dose is often 4500 to 5000 cGy in 5 weeks. The treatment technique consists of a pair of anterior and posterior oblique wedged fields (Fig. 9.52). The beam direction must be such that the radiation beams enter and exit below the eyes. Alternatively, the beam orientation can be

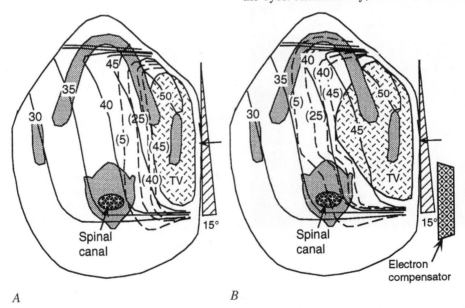

A   *B*

Figure 9.49   *A.* Isodose distribution resulting from using 4-MV photon (15° wedge), 50 percent, and 14-MeV electron (50 percent) beams to treat a parotid tumor. The solid lines represent the dose from the photon beam and the hatched line the electron beam. A wedge is used in the photon beam to reduce the spinal cord dose. *B.* The same field arrangement using 6-MV photon (50 percent) and 18-MeV electron (50 percent) beams with a compensator over the spinal cord to reduce the depth of the electron beam in a parotid tumor that extends to a greater depth.

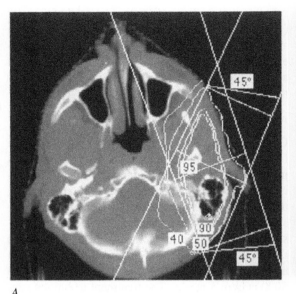

A

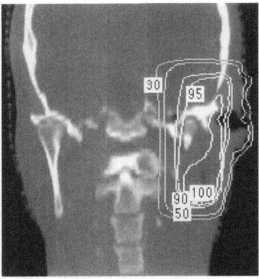

B

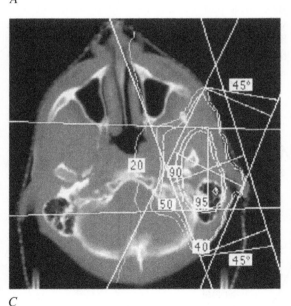

C

Figure 9.50   Isodose distribution resulting from using anterior and posterior oblique fields with 45° wedges to treat a parotid tumor using 6-MV photon beams *(A)* in a transverse plane and *(B)* in a coronal plane. *C.* A lateral field is added to reduce the dose anteriorly and posteriorly. The beam energy is 6-MV photons and the beams are equally weighted.

cephalad/caudal oblique with wedges (Fig. 9.53*A*). The addition of an ipsilateral field reduces the dose under the thin portion of the wedges (Fig. 9.53*B*).

EYE AND ORBIT

Basal cell carcinoma in the eyelids is a relatively common disease. These lesions are preferably treated via a superficial x-ray beam. A lead cutout placed directly on the skin is usually used to form the radiation field and to shield the surrounding structures, including the contralateral eye. An internal eye shield can be placed under the eyelid to shield the underlying eye. The total dose and the fractionation scheme vary widely but, as a rule, better cosmesis result with a more protracted dose fractionation scheme.

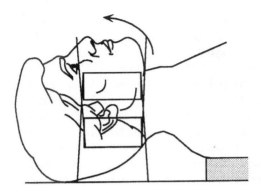

Figure 9.51 When oblique fields are used to treat a parotid tumor, the chin must be extended so that the beams remain caudal of the eyes.

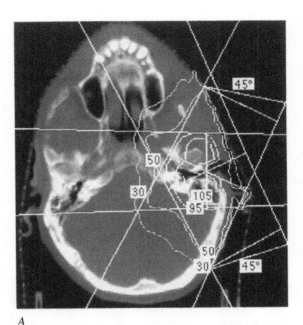

A

B

Figure 9.52 Isodose distribution resulting from using lateral and anterior-posterior oblique fields with 45° wedges to treat a glomus jugulare tumor: a transverse plane (*A*) and a coronal plane (*B*). The beam energy is 6-MV photons and the beams are equally weighted.

Many different tumors arise in the eye and orbit, including carcinoma of the lacrimal gland, lymphoma, rhabdomyosarcoma, retinoblastoma, malignant melanoma, and optic glioma. The treatment techniques for rhabdomyosarcoma, lymphoma, and optic glioma are quite similar and consist of an anterior and a lateral wedged field. The anterior margin of the lateral field is usually placed at the lateral bony orbit and is angled approximately 10° posteriorly to avoid the contralateral eye (Fig. 9.54). Since disease anterior to this field is irradiated only by the anterior field, preference must be given to the weighting of this field (Fig. 9.54). If the orbit is exenterated, it is essential that the orbital cavity be filled with tissue-equivalent material to avoid a very hot spot in the brain tissue behind the orbit (Fig. 9.55). Omission of this can lead to fatal brain necrosis. The dose delivered for rhabdomyosarcoma and optic glioma is approximately 5000 to 6000 cGy in 6 weeks while the dose for lymphoma is approximately 3000 cGy in 3 to 4 weeks.

Choroidal Melanoma. The optimal treatment of choroidal melanoma is unclear. Small choroidal melanoma tumors are usually treated by a radioactive plaque, described in Chaps. 15 and 16, while large tumors are often treated by enucleation. Preenucleation radiation therapy, delivering 2000 cGy in five fractions, is also used. The target consists of the posterior half of the globe with a 1-cm margin (Fig.

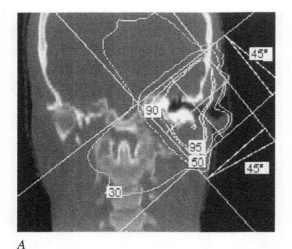

A

B

Figure 9.53   *A.* Isodose distribution in the coronal plane resulting from using a cephalad and caudal oblique fields with 45° wedges to treat a glomus jugulare tumor. *B.* The same fields as in *A,* with a lateral field added. The beam energy is 6-MV photons and the beams are equally weighted.

9.56). A commonly used treatment technique consists of anterior and anterior oblique wedged fields (Fig. 9.57). Bolus may be necessary to bring the high-dose region closer to the surface in the periphery of the globe. Helium ion–charged particle therapy[78] or proton beams[79] have been used in the treatment of choroidal melanomas in an effort to spare the surrounding normal tissues, including the lens of

the eye and the optic nerve. Metastatic lesions in the choroid are often treated by external beam radiation therapy. An electron beam can also be used to treat tumors in the globe of the eye.[80–83]

Retinoblastoma.   Retinoblastoma usually occurs at a very young age (weeks to months after birth). Approximately 80 percent of the tumors are unilateral and 20 percent bilateral. Enucleation is recommended if the eye is blind or the chance of vision after therapy is small. Efforts must be made to preserve vision in the remaining eye. For small single lesions, an eye plaque can be used; however, for most cases, external beam therapy to 4000 to 4500 cGy in 4 to 5 weeks is usually employed. Different treatment techniques have been proposed.[80,82,84–87] Treatment of retinoblastoma is very difficult because the distance between the lens of the eye, which must be spared, and the retina, which must be treated, is very small even in an adult. Considering the penumbra of the beam, total sparing of the lens while including the retina is impossible. The patients are usually treated supine in a positioning device and under general anesthesia (Fig. 9.58*A*). A lateral field using a 4-MV photon beam is frequently used. The central axis of the field is set midway between the bony orbital rim and the limbus and the anterior half of the beam is blocked to reduce the penumbra and prevent beam divergence into the lens. In unilateral disease, the lateral beam must be angled posteriorly 2 to 5° to avoid the contralateral lens (Fig. 9.58*B*). The beam is shaped to encompass the entire retina, with a 1.5 cm margin posteriorly, superiorly, and inferiorly and to minimize irradiation in the pituitary gland and the teeth buds (Fig. 9.59). An anterior field is also used; however, the weighting on this field is very small (10 to 15 percent). This field is also shaped to minimize irradiation of adjacent normal tissues. A 60° wedge is used to accomplish a uniform dose distribution and a 2-HVT central lens block can be used to reduce the dose in the lens (Fig. 9.60). This lens block also shields part of the posterior retina[88]; thus a 5-HVT shield should not be used. Bilateral disease is treated in a similar fashion, but the lateral field is opposed and the unwedged anterior field includes both eyes with a midline shield (Fig. 9.61). The weight is often increased on the

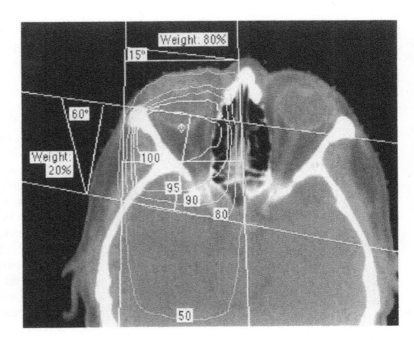

Figure 9.54   Isodose distribution resulting from an anterior field with a 15° wedge weighted 80 percent and a lateral field with 60° wedge and weighted 20 percent to treat an orbital tumor. The anterior margin of the lateral field is angled 10° posteriorly to avoid the contralateral eye. The beam energy is 6-MV photons.

anterior and decreased on the lateral fields. Wedges are usually needed in the lateral fields. Although these children are always treated under general anesthesia, motion of the lens is not arrested. The setup of these fields is extremely critical and should therefore be monitored daily by the treating physician.

Graves' Ophthalmopathy.   Radiation therapy is also sometimes used in the treatment of a benign condition called *Graves' ophthalmopathy.* This condition, sometimes seen in patients with hyperthyroidism, is characterized by exophthalmos secondary to swelling of the muscles in the orbit. Opposed lateral fields, centered behind the lens and with a half-beam block to produce a sharp beam edge and prevent divergence into the contralateral lens, are used (Fig. 9.62).[89] A dose of 1800 to 2000 cGy in 2 weeks is usually sufficient to relieve the symptoms.

When opposed lateral fields are used in treating the orbital contents, it is important to realize that the patient's head may not have been positioned so that the lenses lie on a horizontal line, as discussed earlier. A half-beam blocked horizontal beam centered

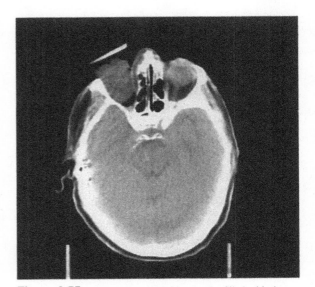

Figure 9.55   An exenterated orbit must be filled with tissue-equivalent material to avoid a hot spot in the brain behind the orbit. A water balloon was used in this patient.

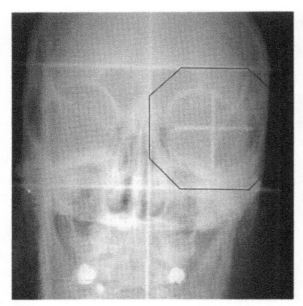

A

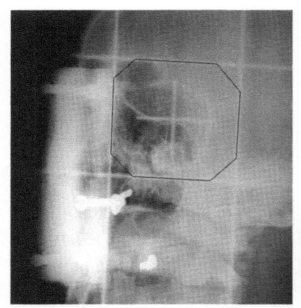

B

Figure 9.56 Typical fields to treat a choroidal melanoma. An anterior left eye field (*A*) and a left anterior oblique field (*B*).

behind the lens of one eye may therefore include the lens of the contralateral eye (Fig. 9.1). It is important to recognize this and instead turn the gantry until

both beams exclude the lens bilaterally. The procedure to accomplish this was discussed earlier.

SCALP

Superficial malignancies sometime occur in the scalp. When the tumor infiltrates the underlying brain or when the depth of the tumor is uncertain, tangential fields across the skull using photon fields are usually an acceptable treatment technique. When the lesion is superficial and is not involving the skull, electron beam treatment should be considered in order to spare the brain. When the entire scalp requires treatment, there is a difficult problem of matching multiple electron fields. One technique uses opposed lateral 4-MV photon fields to treat the outer areas of the scalp (Fig. 9.63) while the brain is blocked. Low-energy (6-MeV) electron fields are then used to treat the scalp overlying the brain. The same beam-central axis is used in an effort to reproduce the geometry of the photon fields. Bolus is used in both the photon and the electron fields to increase the surface dose. For the photon beams, it also used as a compensator for the curvature of the skull.[90]

THYROID GLAND

Tumors originating in the thyroid gland are usually not considered as head and neck malignancies but are included here rather than in the thorax section.

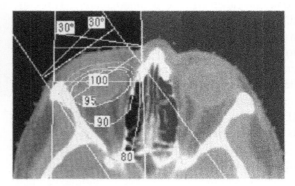

Figure 9.57 Isodose distribution resulting from using an anterior and a right anterior oblique field to treat a choroidal melanoma. The beam energy is 6-MV photons and 30° wedges are used in both fields.

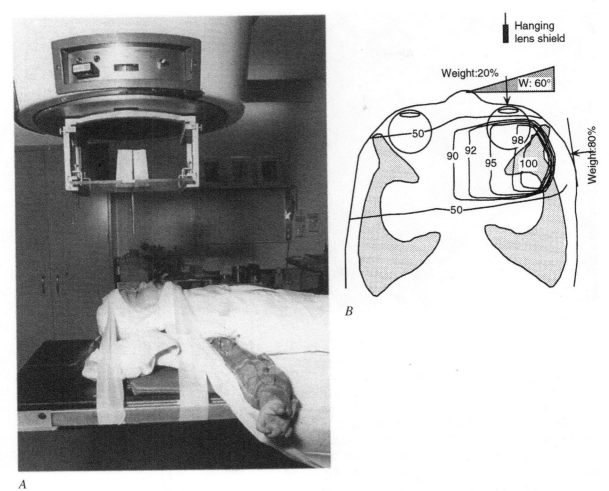

Figure 9.58 *A.* A child treated in the supine position in a positioning cast. A hanging lens block is used in the anterior field. *B.* Isodose distribution resulting from treating a retinoblastoma using a half-beam blocked lateral field angled 3° posteriorly to avoid the contralateral eye and an anterior field with a 60° wedge. The beam energy is 4-MV photons; the lateral field is weighted 80 percent and the anterior 20 percent. A 2-HVT hanging lens shield is used in the anterior field (not shown in the dose distribution).

The thyroid gland, which consists of two lobes joined by an isthmus, is situated anterior to the trachea and larynx, with the superior poles at the inferior half of the thyroid cartilage. Surgical resection is frequently required and radiation therapy is used for inoperable, residual, recurrent, or metastatic disease.

The target volume includes the thyroid gland as well as the bilateral cervical and superior mediastinal lymph nodes. A treatment technique consisting of

opposed anterior and posterior fields weighted with preference to the anterior field and a midline block in the posterior field delivers a dose distribution with some sparing of the spinal cord (Figs. 9.18 and 9.64). A boost to the primary site can then be delivered via anterior oblique wedged fields or an anterior electron field.

Similar treatment options are available when patients with cervical lymphadenopathy with an un-

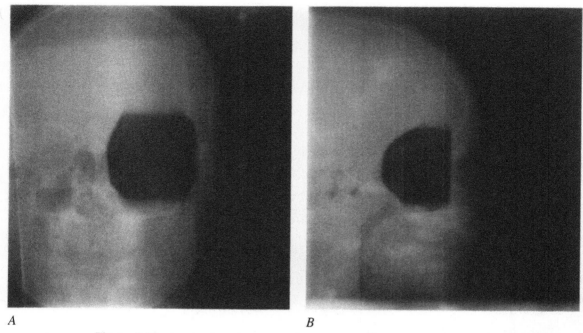

A   *B*

Figure 9.59 *A* and *B*. Port films of anterior and lateral fields used to treat retinoblastoma.

known primary tumor site or with metastic disease require lymph node irradiation. A moving-beam treatment technique using wedges and a spinal-cord block in the cervical segment of the treatment field has also been described.[91] The dose required for the treatment of thyroid malignancies depends on the tumor type but is approximately 6000 to 7000 cGy in 7 to 8 weeks to the primary site. Iodine 131 can also be used in the treatment of thyroid carcinoma (Chap. 15).

MORBIDITY

Efforts should be made to keep the adverse effects of high-dose irradiation of head and neck cancer to a minimum, although *some* effect is unavoidable. The incidence of morbidity is related to the treatment technique employed, the size of the irradiated volume, the time/dose fractionation scheme used, the location and the extent of the disease, and the patient's age and nutritional status. The incidence is also higher when radiation therapy and surgery are combined, particularly when curvative doses are

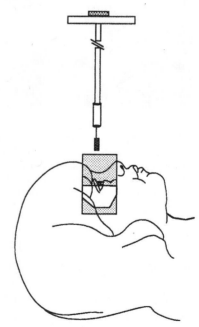

Figure 9.60 A hanging lens shield is placed with the help of a removable plumb bob. The shadow of the block cannot be seen on the patient since the Lucite button securing the block to the tray casts a larger shadow.

given prior to radical surgery. Specifically, the difficulties consist of delayed wound healing due to impaired blood supply and infection.

The main culprit for many sequelae of radiation therapy in the adult is salivary dysfunction. The saliva has several functions: (1) it serves as a protective barrier for the teeth, (2) it lubricates food for mastication and swallowing, and (3) it contributes to taste function. When irradiated, the salivary function decreases[92]; therefore the mouth becomes acutely dry and taste is altered. With meticulous dental care, regular dental cleaning, daily flossing, and use of fluoride trays, the teeth can be maintained without caries.[93-95] However, without care, the teeth rapidly

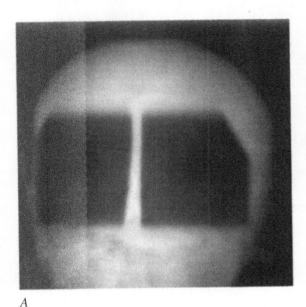

A

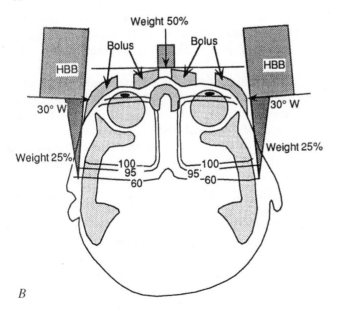

B

Figure 9.61 In a child with bilateral retinoblastoma, the field arrangement is the same with the exception of the anterior unwedged field, which includes both eyes with a midline block. Wedges are used instead in the lateral fields.

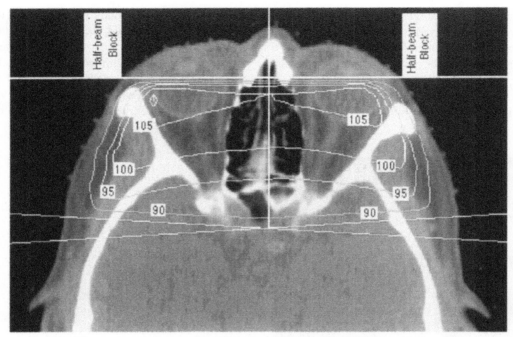

Figure 9.62 Isodose distribution resulting from using 6-MV photon beams to treat both orbits via parallel opposed half-beam blocked lateral fields.

develop severe periodontal disease and caries. Extraction of carious teeth after radiation therapy is not recommended if the bone has received significant

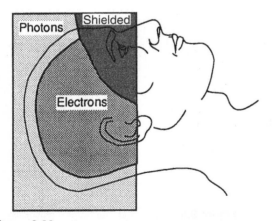

Figure 9.63 When the entire scalp must be treated, opposed lateral photon fields can be used to treat the periphery of the head while the brain is shielded. Electron fields are then used to treat the scalp overlying the brain.

doses, since healing is poor after treatment. Aggressive extractions after high-dose radiation therapy can lead to osteoradionecrosis. If a patient has carious teeth prior to treatment, the teeth should be extracted before radiation therapy begins. Oral pilorcapine has recently been introduced and helps to reduce the severity of postirradiation xerostomia in many patients.[96]

Mucositis of the oral mucosa usually occurs after approximately 2000 to 3000 cGy and becomes more severe with higher doses. Patients need careful evaluation of nutritional intake because mucositis may be severe enough to prevent oral intake. Intravenous hydration or nasogastric feeding may be necessary in severe cases. Very high radiation dose can occur on the lingual and buccal mucosa adjacent to amalgam fillings or gold teeth due to secondary scatter observed in the metal-tissue interface. Local mucosal doses can be as high as 120 percent of the prescribed midplane dose. A 2- to 4-mm tissue-equivalent absorber over the teeth is sufficient to reduce the secondary scatter.[97] Separating the mucosa and the fill-

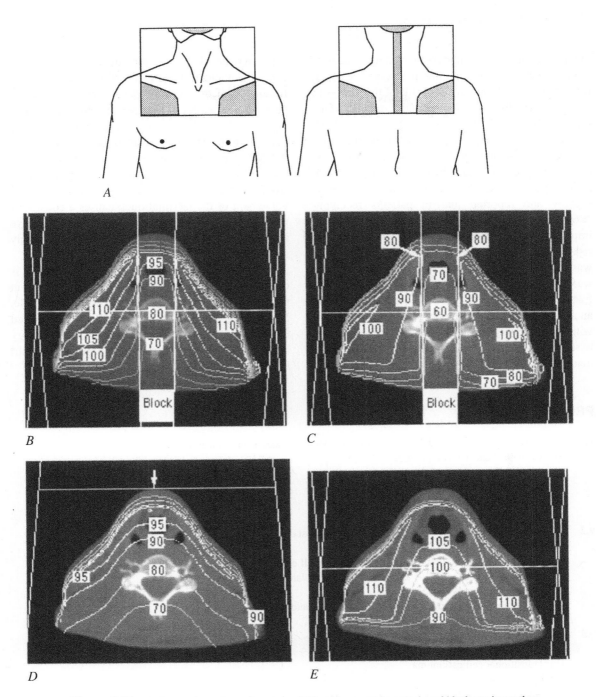

Figure 9.64 *A.* Opposed anterior and posterior fields with a posterior spinal-cord block can be used to treat thyroid carcinoma. *B.* When the anterior field is weighted 80 percent and the posterior 20 percent, a higher dose is achieved in the anterior portion of the neck with some spinal-cord sparing. *C.* The same field arrangement but with a 2-to-1 weighting favoring the anterior field results in a lower dose in the midline of the anterior neck. *D.* A single anterior field also delivers a high dose in the anterior neck with some spinal-cord sparing. *E.* Opposed anterior and posterior fields without a spinal-cord block and weighted 2 to 1 favoring the anterior field offers only about a 5 percent lower dose in the spinal cord than in the anterior neck.

323

ings by a couple of millimeters by placing a cap over the teeth can also eliminate the problem.[98] A dental roll can also be placed on either side of the fillings to increase the distance. The metal-tissue interface issue has been studied by several other authors.[99–102]

Radiation doses in excess of 4500 cGy to the retina and 5500–6000 cGy to the optic nerve and optic chiasm may cause visual loss.[103,104] Parsons et al. also studied the risk of radiation-induced optic neuropathy and reported that in patients receiving ≥ 6000 cGy, the fraction size appeared to be more important than the total dose. The 15-year actuarial risk of optic neuropathy after doses of ≥ 6000 cGy was reported as 11 percent when the fraction size was < 190 cGy, compared with 47 percent when the fraction size was ≥ 190 cGy.[105] There appears to be an increased risk of developing optic nerve injury with increasing age. One of the most radiosensitive tissue in the head and neck area is the lens, and formation of cataracts, which can be removed surgi-

cally, may develop following doses lower than 1000 cGy. The incidence increases with increased dose. Irradiation of the lacrimal gland, situated in the superior-lateral aspect of the upper eyelid, may cause a dry painful eye. Parsons et al. reported severe dry-eye syndrome in 100 percent of patients receiving ≥ 5700 cGy and in only 19 percent of patients who received ≤ 4500 cGy.[106] Obstruction of the tear duct, which is rare and usually associated with tumor involvement of the lacrimal duct, causes a constantly wet eye. The effects of radiation therapy on the eye and the optic nerve have been studied by many authors.[103–114]

A late sequela of high-dose radiation therapy is osteroradionecrosis.[115,116] The bone particularly at risk in the head and neck region is the mandible. Minimizing mandibular dose can be accomplished through the use of shrinking fields, high-energy beams, intraoral cone, interstitial implant, or a submental field when the boost is delivered.

PROBLEMS

9.1 The most commonly used beam energy to treat head and neck cancer is
  (a) Cobalt-60 and 10-MV photons
  (b) 10-MV photons and 12-MeV electrons
  (c) 4-MV photons and 5-MeV electrons
  (d) Cobalt-60 and 4-MV photons

9.2 The following techniques can be used to deliver a boost dose in the treatment of carcinoma of the base of tongue:
  (a) Intracavitary implant, an intraoral cone, and small external beam fields
  (b) Small external beam fields and an interstitial implant
  (c) An interstitial implant and an intraoral cone
  (d) An intraoral cone and a small external electron field

9.3 The majority of cancer in the head and neck region is
  (a) Adenocarcinoma
  (b) Transitional cell carcinoma
  (c) Lymphoma
  (d) Squamous cell carcinoma

9.4 A bite block is sometimes inserted between the patient's teeth because
  (a) It helps the patient keep his or her mouth open during the treatment for easier breathing
  (b) It helps the patient keep his or her mouth open during the treatment so more of the oral mucosa can be excluded from the radiation field

(c) It is part of the immobilization system and it keeps the patient from talking while being treated

(d) It helps in extending the patient's chin more so an anterior field can enter inferior of the eyes

9.5   To make patients more comfortable during treatment, it is a good idea to
(a) Have them lie in the prone position
(b) Provide supports under the head, knees, and arms
(c) Place a soft pillow under the back
(d) Have them lie in the supine position with arms raised above the head

9.6   Xerostomia is caused by irradiation of the
(a) Salivary glands
(b) Tonsils
(c) Floor of mouth
(d) Base of tongue

9.7   The functions of saliva are to
(a) Prevent tooth decay and improve taste
(b) Promote swallowing and improve taste
(c) Moisten food and promote digestion
(d) Moisten food, promote swallowing, and prevent tooth decay

9.8   In the treatment of head and neck cancer, immobilization is particularly important because
(a) These patients are often uncooperative and some of them are abusing alcohol
(b) Fields are often very large and could include radiosensitive organs
(c) The proximity of several radiosensitive organs and often small tumor margins
(d) Immobilizing the head is very easy

9.9   When carcinoma of the oropharynx is treated, the field junction between opposed lateral and an inferior field should be set
(a) Cephalad of the thyroid notch
(b) Caudal of the thyroid notch
(c) It does not matter where it is set as long as it is not where there is palpable tumor
(d) Caudal of the larynx

9.10 When a patient, immobilized in the supine position, is treated for Graves' ophthalmopathy, half-beam blocked opposed lateral fields centered on the lateral canthus are usually used. Both lenses of the eyes are excluded from the beam when rotating the gantry to
(a) The lateral position (90°)
(b) An angle when both lead markers placed on the eyelids of the closed eyes are superimposed
(c) The lateral position (90°), and then the patient's head is turned 10° to the right
(d) 80° to each side and then the patient's head is turned until both lead markers placed on the eyelids of the closed eyes are superimposed

9.11 To place a large patient so that the head is in a neutral position
(a) A very low support is needed under the head
(b) A low support is needed under the chest
(c) A high support is needed under the head
(d) A high support is needed under the chest

9.12 To include the entire maxillary antrum without also including the eye when a patient is treated for a maxillary antrum tumor,
  (*a*) The head is in a neutral position and a large, comfortable support is under the head
  (*b*) The chin is extended and the head is tilted back
  (*c*) The neck is flexed and the chin is tucked down on the chest
  (*d*) The head position is not important

9.13 To avoid overlap between the opposed lateral and anterior fields used in treatment of head and neck cancer
  (*a*) A small anterior block can be placed in the cephalad margin of the lateral fields over the spinal cord
  (*b*) A small block can be used in the caudal margin of the anterior field over the spinal cord
  (*c*) A full-length midline block can be used over the spinal cord in the anterior field
  (*d*) A gap should be calculated between the lateral and anterior fields

9.14 The junction between the lateral and anterior fields is chosen so that, when a full-length spinal cord block is used, the larynx is also blocked in an effort to
  (*a*) Avoid oral mucositis
  (*b*) Avoid laryngitis
  (*c*) Avoid cataracts
  (*d*) Avoid xerostomia

9.15 Prior to starting the treatment of boost fields, it is a good idea to take port films because
  (*a*) Skin and seed markers may have shifted and margins are small
  (*b*) Seed markers placed when the treatments started are reliable and should always be used to verify the position of the field with respect to the tumor
  (*c*) Skin marks may have shifted and the patient may be less cooperative
  (*d*) Margins are small and the tumor may no longer be visible

9.16 When the final boost is given and the central axis is moved
  (*a*) The dose in the midplane on the central axis of the boost field is added to the midplane dose on the central axis of the previous fields
  (*b*) The dose in the midplane on the central axis of the boost field is added to the dose received at the same point from the previous fields
  (*c*) The dose in the midplane on the central axis of the boost field is not added into the previous dose at all
  (*d*) The dose in the midplane on the central axis of the boost field is added to the maximum dose within the previous fields

9.17 When true vocal cord tumors are treated
  (*a*) A wedge is never needed, because using 1-cm bolus will make the dose uniform
  (*b*) A 30° wedge is always used so the dose in the anterior commissure will not be excessive
  (*c*) Wedges are never needed because a higher dose posteriorly is an advantage
  (*d*) A 15 or 30° wedge is often used, but the dose in the anterior commissure could be compromised

9.18 Early vocal cord cancers with normal cord mobility are cured by radiation therapy alone in
  (*a*) About 90 percent of cases
  (*b*) About 50 percent of cases

(c) About 100 percent of cases

(d) About 75 percent of cases

9.19 Retinoblastoma is a tumor of the eye that usually occurs in

  (a) Adults

  (b) Very young female patients

  (c) Small children

  (d) Teenagers

9.20 Parotid tumors are often treated using

  (a) A proton beam

  (b) An electron beam alone

  (c) A single ipsilateral 6-MV photon beam

  (d) Mixed electron and photon beams

REFERENCES

1. Biggs PJ, Wang CC: An intraoral cone for an 18 MeV linear accelerator. *Int J Radiat Oncol Biol Phys* 8:1251, 1982.

2. Biggs PJ, Wang CC: Breakaway safety feature for an intraoral cone system. *Int J Radiat Oncol Biol Phys* 10:1117, 1984.

3. Hudson FR, Samarasekara MG: Techniques for intraoral electron treatments. *Int J Radiat Oncol Biol Phys* 11:1731, 1985.

4. Wexler MC, Tobochnik N, Spiegler P, Herman MW: Characteristics of an intraoral cone for electron beam therapy with an 18 MeV linear accelerator. *Int J Radiat Oncol Biol Phys* 8:2001, 1982.

5. Fletcher GH: Elective irradiation of subclinical disease in cancers of the head and neck. *Cancer* 29:1450, 1972.

6. Brizel DM, Leopold KA, Fisher SR, et al: A phase I/II trial of twice daily irradiation and concurrent chemotherapy for locally advanced squamous cell carcinoma of the head and neck. *Int J Radiat Oncol Biol Phys* 28:213, 1993.

7. Horiot JC, LeFur R, N'Guyen T, et al: Hyperfractionated compared with conventional radiotherapy in oropharyngeal carcinoma: An EORTC randomized trail. *Eur J Cancer* 26:779, 1990.

8. Parsons JT, Cassisi NJ, Million RR: Results of twice-a-day irradiation of squamous cell carcinomas of the head and neck. *Int J Radiat Oncol Biol Phys* 10:2041, 1984.

9. Parsons JT, Mendenhall WM, Cassisi NJ, et al: Hyperfractionation for head and neck cancer. *Int J Radiat Oncol Biol Phys* 14:649, 1988.

10. Parsons JT, Mendenhall WM, Cassisi NJ, et al: Neck dissection after twice-a-day radiotherapy: Morbidity and recurrence rates. *Head Neck* 11:400, 1989.

11. Sailer SL, Weissler MC, Melin SA, et al: Toxicity and preliminary results from a trial of hyperfractionation radiation with or without simultaneous 5-flourouracil-cisplatin in advanced head and neck squamous cell carcinomas. *Semin Radiat Oncol* 2:38, 1992.

12. Saunders MI, Dische S: Continuous hyperfractionated, accelerated radiotherapy (CHART). *Semin Radiat Oncol* 2:41, 1992.

13. Wang CC, Suit HD, Phil D, Blitzers PH: Twice-a-day radiation therapy for supraglottic carcinoma. *Int J Radiat Oncol Biol Phys* 12:3, 1986.

14. Byhardt RW, Cox JD, Hornburg A, Liermann G: Weekly localization films and detection of field placement errors. *Int J Radiat Oncol Biol Phys* 4:881, 1978.

15. Halverson KJ, Leung TC, Pellet JB, et al: Study of treatment variation in the radiotherapy of head and neck tumors using a fiberoptic on-line radiotherapy imaging system. *Int J Radiat Oncol Biol Phys* 21:1327, 1991.

16. Huizenga H, Levendag PC, DePorre PMZR: Accuracy in radiation field alignment in head and neck cancers: A prospective study. *Radiother Oncol* 11:181, 1988.

17. Hunt MA, Kutcher GJ, Burman C, et al: The effect of setup uncertainties on the treatment of nasopharynx cancer. *Int J Radiat Oncol Biol Phys* 27:437, 1993.

18. Marks JE, Haus AG: The effect of immobilization on localization error in the radiotherapy of head and neck cancer. *Clin Radiol* 27:175, 1976.

19. Mitine C, Leunens G, Verstatete J, et al: Is it necessary to repeat quality control procedures for head and neck patients? *Radiother Oncol* 21:201, 1991.

20. Verhey LJ, Goitein M, McNulty P, et al: Precise positioning of patients for radiation therapy. *Int J Radiat Oncol Biol Phys* 2:289, 1982.

21. Barish RJ, Lerch IA: Patient immobilization with low-temperature splint/brace material. *Radiology* 127:548, 1978.

22. Bentel GC, Marks LB, Sherouse GW, Spencer DP: Customized head immobilization system. *Int J Radiat Oncol Biol Phys* 32:245, 1995.

23. Devereux C, Grundy G, Littman P: Plastic molds for patient immobilization. *Int J Radiat Oncol Biol Phys* 1:553, 1976.

24. Gerber RL, Marks JE, Purdy JA: The use of thermal plastics for immobilization of patients during radiotherapy. *Int J Radiat Oncol Biol Phys* 8:1461, 1982.

25. Goldson AL, Young J, Espinoza MC, Henschke UK: Simple but sophisticated immobilization casts. *Int J Radiat Oncol Biol Phys* 4:1105, 1978.

26. Hauskins LA, Thompson RW: Patient positioning device for external-beam radiation therapy of the head and neck. *Radiology* 106:706, 1973.

27. Jones D, Hafermann MD: A radiolucent bite-block apparatus. *Int J Radiat Oncol Biol Phys* 13:129, 1987.

28. Lewinsky BS, Walton R: Lightcast: An aid to planning, treatment and immobilization in radiotherapy and research. *Int J Radiat Oncol Biol Phys* 1:1011, 1976.

29. Niewald M, Lehman W, Uhlmann U, et al: Plastic material used to optimize radiotherapy of head and neck tumors and the mammary carcinoma. *Radiother Oncol* 11:55, 1988.

30. Sherouse GW, Bourland JD, Reynolds K, et al: Virtual simulator in the clinical setting: some practical considerations. *Int J Radiat Oncol Biol Phys* 19:1059, 1990.

31. Sørenson NE, Sell A: Immobilization, compensation and field shaping in megavoltage therapy. *Acta Radiol Ther Biol Phys* 11:129, 1972.

32. Wang CC, Boyer A, Dosoretz D: A head holder for treatment of head and neck cancers. *Int J Radiat Oncol Biol Phys* 6:95, 1980.

33. Schlegel W, Pastyr O, Bortfeld T, et al: Computer systems and mechanical tools for stereotactically guided conformation therapy with linear accelerators. *Int J Radiat Oncol Biol Phys* 24:781, 1992.

34. Thornton AF, TenHaken RK, Weeks KJ, et al: A head immobilization system for radiation simulation, CT, MRI, and PET imaging. *Med Dosim* 16:51, 1991.

35. Thornton AF, TenHaken RK, Gerhardsson A, Corell M: Three-dimensional motion analysis of an improved head immobilization system for simulation, CT, MRI, and PET imaging. *Radiother Oncol* 20:224, 1991.

36. Fiorino C, Cattaneo GM, del Vecchio A, et al: Skin dose measurements for head and neck radiotherapy. *Med Phys* 19:1263, 1992.

37. Fiorino C, Cattaneo GM, del Vecchio A, et al: Skin-sparing reduction effects of thermoplastics used for patient immobilization in head and neck radiotherapy. *Radiother Oncol* 30:267, 1994.

38. Fontenla DP, Napoli JJ, Hunt M, et al: Effects of beam modifiers and immobilization devices on the dose in the build-up region. *Int J Radiat Oncol Biol Phys* 30:211, 1994.

39. Niewald M, Lehmann W, Tkoez H-J, et al: Moulagen der karzinoms mit schnellen Electronen: Vergleichende Tes-

tung verschiedener Materialen. *Strahlenth Onkol* 162:448, 1986.

40. Chiang TC, Culbert H, Wyman B, et al: The half field technique of radiation therapy for the cancers of head and neck. *Int J Radiat Oncol Biol Phys* 5:1899, 1979.

41. Datta R, Mira JG, Pomeroy TC, Datta S: Dosimetry study of split beam technique using megavoltage beams and its clinical implications—I. *Int J Radiat Oncol Biol Phys* 5:565, 1979.

42. Gillin MT, Kline RW: Field separation between lateral and anterior fields on a 6 MV linear accelerator. *Int J Radiat Oncol Biol Phys* 6:233, 1980.

43. Slessinger E, Haenschen M, Nalesnik WJ, Giri PGS: The utilization of junctional filters in head and neck treatment. *Treatment Planning; Journal of American Association of Medical Dosimetrists* 6:9, 1981.

44. Johnson JM, Khan FM: Dosimetric effects of abutting extended source to surface distance electron fields with photon fields in the treatment of head and neck cancers. *Int J Radiat Oncol Biol Phys* 28:741, 1994.

45. Sailer SL, Sherouse GW, Chaney EL, et al: A comparison of postoperative techniques for carcinomas of the larynx and hypopharynx using 3-D dose distributions. *Int J Radiat Oncol Biol Phys* 21:767, 1991.

46. Mendenhall WM, Parsons JT, Million RR: Unnecessary irradiation of the normal larynx. *Int J Radiat Oncol Biol Phys* 18:1531, 1990.

47. Richaud P, Tapley ND: Lateralized lesion of the oral cavity and oropharynx treated in part with the electron beam. *Int J Radiat Oncol Biol Phys* 5:461, 1979.

48. Johansen LV, Overgaard J, Hjelm-Hansen M, Gadeberg CC: Primary radiotherapy of T1 squamous cell carcinoma of the larynx: analysis of 478 patients treated from 1963 to 1985. *Int J Radiat Oncol Biol Phys* 18:1307, 1990.

49. Terhaard CHJ, Snippe K, Ravasz LA, et al: Radiotherapy in T1 laryngeal cancer: Prognostic factors for locoregional control and survival, uni- and multivariate analysis. *Int J Radiat Oncol Biol Phys* 21:1179, 1991.

50. Devineni VR, King K, Perez C, et al: Early glottic carcinoma treated with radiotherapy: Impact of treatment on success rate (abstr). *Int J Radiat Oncol Biol Phys* 24(suppl 1):186, 1992.

51. Niroomand-Rad A, Harter KW, Thobejane A, Bertrand K: Air cavity effects on the radiation dose to the larynx using Co-60, 6 MV, and 10 MV photon beams. *Int J Radiat Oncol Biol Phys* 29:1139, 1994.

52. Teshima T, Chatani M, Inoue T: Radiation therapy for early glottic cancer (T1NOMO): II. Prospective randomized study concerning radiation field. *Int J Radiat Oncol Biol Phys* 18:119, 1990.

53. Wang CC, Meyer JE: Radiotherapeutic management of carcinoma of the nasopharynx: Analysis of 170 patients. *Cancer* 28:566, 1971.

54. Kuchnir FT, Heffron J, Myrianthopoulos LC, Haraf DJ: Beam's-eye-view aided treatment planning for a naso-

pharyngeal lesion: A case report. *Med Dosim* 14:231, 1989.

55. Fu KK, Newman H, Philips TL: Treatment of locally recurrent carcinoma of the nasopharynx. *Radiology* 117:425, 1975.

56. McNeese MD, Fletcher GH: Re-treatment of recurrent nasopharyngeal carcinoma. *Radiology* 138:191, 1981.

57. Pryzant RM, Wendt CD, Delclos L, Peters LJ: Re-treatment of nasopharyngeal carcinoma in 53 patients. *Int J Radiat Oncol Biol Phys* 22:941, 1992.

58. Wang CC, Schultz MD: Management of locally recurrent carcinoma of the nasopharynx. *Radiology* 86:900, 1966.

59. Wang CC: Re-irradiation of recurrent nasopharyngeal carcinoma—Treatment techniques and results. *Int J Radiat Oncol Biol Phys* 13:953, 1987.

60. Yan JH, Hu YH, Gu XZ: Radiation therapy of recurrent nasopharyngeal carcinoma—Report on 219 patients. *Acta Radiol Oncol* 22:23, 1983.

61. Orr KY, Miller RW, Wersto N, Glatstein E: A simple method for indirectly verifying noncoplanar treatment fields in radiotherapy. *Med Dosim* 17:213, 1993.

62. Reisinger SA, Palta J, Tupchong L: Vertex field verification in the treatment of central nervous system neoplasms. *Int J Radiat Oncol Biol Phys* 23:429, 1992.

63. Bunting JS: The anatomical influence in megavoltage radiotherapy of carcinoma of the maxillary antrum. *Br J Radiol* 38:255, 1965.

64. Parsons JT, Mendenhall WM, Mancuso AA, et al: Malignant tumors of the nasal cavity and ethmoid sinuses. *Int J Radiat Oncol Biol Phys* 14:11, 1988.

65. Million RR, Cassisi NJ, Hamlin DJ: Nasal vestibule, nasal cavity, and paranasal sinuses, in Million RR, Cassisi NJ (eds): *Management of Head and Neck Cancer: A Multidisciplinary Approach,* Philadelphia: Lippincott, 1984.

66. Ellingwood KE, Milton RR: Cancer of the nasal cavity and ethmoid/sphenoid sinuses. *Cancer* 43:1517, 1979.

67. Morita K, Kawabe Y: Late effects on the eye of conformation radiotherapy for carcinoma of the paranasal sinuses and nasal cavity. *Radiology* 130:227, 1979.

68. Nakissa N, Rubin P, Strohl R, Keys H: Ocular and orbital complications following radiation therapy of paranasal malignancies and review of literature. *Cancer* 51:980, 1983.

69. Engler MJ, Herskovic AM, Proimos BS: Dosimetry of rotational photon fields with gravity-oriented eye blocks. *Int J Radiat Oncol Biol Phys* 10:431, 1984.

70. Proimos BS: Synchronous protection and fieldshaping in cyclotherapy. *Radiology* 77:591, 1961.

71. Bataini JP, Ennuyer A: Advanced carcinoma of the maxillary antrum treated by cobalt teletherapy and electron beam irradiation. *Br J Radiol* 44:590, 1971.

72. Galbraith DM, Aget H, Leung PMK, Rider WD: Eye sparing in high energy x-ray beam. *Int J Radiat Oncol Biol Phys* 11:591, 1985.

73. Hancock SL: Anterior eye protection with orbital neoplasia. *Int J Radiat Oncol Biol Phys* 12:123, 1986.

74. Griffin TW, Wambersie A, Laramore G, Castro J: High LET; heavy particle trials. *Int J Radiat Oncol Biol Phys* 14:S83, 1988.

75. Prasad SC, Ames TE, Howard TB, et al: Dose enhancement in bone in electron beam therapy. *Radiology* 151:513, 1984.

76. Tapley N: *Clinical Application of the Electron Beam.* New York: Wiley, 1976.

77. Lederman M, Jones CH, Mould RF: Cancer of the middle ear; technique of radiation treatment. *Br J Radiol* 38:895, 1965.

78. Char DH, Castro JR, Quivey JM, et al: Helium ion charged particle therapy for choroidal melanoma. *Ophthalmology* 87:565, 1980.

79. Gragoudas ES, Goitein M, Verhey L, et al: Proton beam irradiation: An alternative to enucleation for intraocular melanomas. *Ophthalmology* 87:571, 1980.

80. Armstrong DI: The use of 4–6 MeV electrons for the conservative treatment of retinoblastoma. *Br J Radiol* 47:326, 1974.

81. Chu FCH, Huh SH, Nisce LZ, Simpson LD: Radiation therapy of choroid metastasis from breast cancer. *Int J Radiat Oncol Biol Phys* 2:273, 1977.

82. Griem ML, Ernest JT, Rozenfeld ML, Newell FW: Eye lens protection in the treatment of retinoblastoma with high energy electrons. *Radiology* 90:351, 1968.

83. Hultberg S, Walstam R, Asard PE: Two special applications of high energy electron beams. *Acta Radiol Ther Phys Biol* 3:287, 1965.

84. Cassady JR, Sagerman RH, Tretter P, Ellsworth RM: Radiation therapy in retinoblastoma. *Radiology* 93:405, 1969.

85. Cassady JR: Retinoblastoma: Questions in management, in Carter SK, Glatstein E, Livingston RB (eds): *Principles of Cancer Management,* New York: McGraw Hill, 1982.

86. Gagnon JD, Ware CM, Moss WT, Stevens KR: Radiation management of bilateral retinoblastoma: The need to preserve vision. *Int J Radiat Oncol Biol Phys* 6:669, 1980.

87. Weiss DR, Cassady JR, Petersen R: Retinoblastoma: A modification in radiation therapy technique. *Radiology* 14:705, 1975.

88. Chenery SC, Leung MK: Dosimetry under pencil eye shields for cobalt-60 radiation. *Int J Radiat Oncol Biol Phys* 7:661, 1981.

89. Donaldson S, Bagshaw M, Kriss J: Supervoltage orbital radiotherapy for Graves' ophthalmopathy. *J Clin Endocrinol Metab* 37:276, 1973.

90. Akazawa C: Treatment of the scalp using photon and electron beams. *Med Dosim* 14:129, 1989.

91. Thambi V, Pedapatti PJ, Murphy A, Kartha PK: A radiotherapy technique for thyroid cancer. *Int J Radiat Oncol Biol Phys* 6:239, 1980.

92. Wescott WB, Mira JG, Starcke EN, et al: Alteration in whole saliva flow rate induced by fractionated radiotherapy. *Am J Roentgenol* 130:145, 1978.

93. Rogezi JA, Courtney RM, Kerr DA: Dental management of patients radiated for oral cancer. *Cancer* 38:994, 1976.

94. Horiot JC, Bone MC, Ibrahim E, Castro JR: Systematic dental management in head and neck irradiation. *Int J Radiat Oncol Biol Phys* 7:1025, 1981.

95. Wescott WB, Starcke EN, Shannon IL: Chemical protection against postirradiation dental caries. *Oral Surg Oral Med Oral Pathol* 40:709, 1975.

96. Joensuu H, Boström P, Makkonen T: Pilocarpine and carbacholine in treatment of radiation-induced xerostomia. *Radiother Oncol* 26:33, 1993.

97. Gibbs FA, Palos B, Goffinet DR: The metal/tissue interface effect in irradiation of the oral cavity. *Radiology* 119:705, 1976.

98. Thambi V, Murthy AK, Alder G, Kartha PK: Dose perturbation resulting from gold fillings in patients with head and neck cancers. *Int J Radiat Oncol Biol Phys* 5:581, 1979.

99. Gagnon WF, Cundiff JH: Dose enhancement from backscattered radiation at tissue-metal interfaces irradiated with high energy electrons. *Br J Radiol* 53:466, 1980.

100. Khan FM, Moore VC, Levitt SH: Field shaping in electron beam therapy. *Br J Radiol* 49:833, 1976.

101. Klevenhagen SC, Lambert GD, Arbari A: Backscattering in electron beam therapy for energies between 3 and 35 MeV. *Phys Med Biol* 27:363, 1982.

102. Saunders JE, Peters BG: Back-scattering from metals in superficial therapy with high energy electrons. *Br J Radiol* 47:467, 1974.

103. Parsons JT, Fitzgerald CR, Hood CI, et al: The effect of irradiation on the eye and optic nerve. *Int J Radiat Oncol Biol Phys* 9:609, 1983.

104. Parsons JT, Bova FJ, Fitzgerald CR, et al: Radiation retinopathy after external-beam irradiation: Analysis of time-dose factors. *Int J Radiat Oncol Biol Phys* 30:765, 1994.

105. Parsons JT, Bova FJ, Fitzgerald CR, et al: Radiation optic neuropathy after megavoltage external-beam irradiation: Analysis of time-dose factors. *Int J Radiat Oncol Biol Phys* 30:755, 1994.

106. Parsons JT, Bova FJ, Fitzgerald CR, et al: Severe dry-eye syndrome following external beam irradiation. *Int J Radiat Oncol Biol Phys* 30:775, 1994.

107. Britten JA, Halnan KE, Meredith WJ: Radiation cataract —New evidence on radiation dosage to the lens. *Br J Radiol* 39:612, 1966.

108. Chan RC, Shukovsky LJ: Effects of irradiation on the eye. *Radiology* 120:673, 1976.

109. Egbert PR, Donaldson SS, Moazed K, Rosenthal AR: Visual results and ocular complications following radiotherapy for retinoblastoma. *Arch Ophthalmol* 96:1826, 1978.

110. Harris JR, Levene MB: Visual complications following irradiation for pituitary adenomas and craniopharyngiomas. *Radiology* 120:167, 1976.

111. Merriam JGR, Focht EF: A clinical study of radiation cataracts and the relationship to dose. *Am J Roentgenol* 77:759, 1957.

112. Merriam JGR, Szechter A, Focht EF: The effects of ionizing radiation on the eye. *Front Radiat Ther Oncol* 6:346, 1972.

113. Parker RG, Burnett LL, Wooton P, McIntyre DJ: Radiation cataract in clinical therapeutic radiology. *Radiology* 82:794, 1964.

114. Shukovsky LJ, Fletcher GH: Retinal and optic nerve complications in a high dose irradiation technique of ethmoid sinus and nasal cavity. *Radiology* 104:629, 1972.

115. Bedwinek JM, Shukowsky LJ, Fletcher GH, Daley TE: Osteonecrosis in patients treated with definitive radiotherapy for squamous cell carcinomas of the oral cavity and naso- and oropharynx. *Radiology* 119:665, 1976.

116. Cheng VST, Wang CC: Osteoradionecrosis of the mandible resulting from external megavoltage radiation therapy. *Radiology* 112:685, 1974.

Treatment Planning—Central Nervous System and Pituitary Gland

CENTRAL NERVOUS SYSTEM

It is estimated that approximately 17,200 new cases of primary malignant central nervous system (CNS) tumors would be diagnosed and 13,300 deaths from primary CNS malignancies would occur in 1995 in the United States.[1] The 5-year survival rate for all malignant tumors arising in the CNS above the foramen mangum is about 20 percent and the median survival is only a few years. The distressing fact is that many pediatric solid neoplasms arise in the CNS.

Many imaging techniques to diagnose brain tumors have emerged over recent years. Simultaneously, many new treatment approaches have been tried, including immunotoxins, intraarterial chemotherapy, interstitial chemotherapy, radiolabeled antibodies, radiosensitizers, radiosurgery, brachytherapy, hyperthermia, and multiple fractions per day of external beam radiotherapy. Despite these approaches, survival after a diagnosis of malignant brain tumor has not changed significantly in the last 30 to 35 years. The most important prognostic factors are age, with better prognosis for younger patients; Karnofsky performance status; and tumor size.

The most common intracranial malignancy is metastatic disease from elsewhere in the body (melanoma, breast, lung, and so on). Of all primary CNS malignancies, gliomas represent approximately 40 to 45 percent. Gliomas can be divided into several subclassifications, including astrocytoma, oligodendroglioma, and ependymoma. Other intracranial malignancies include medulloblastoma, meningioma, lymphoma, germ cell tumors (germinoma, embryonal carcinoma, choriocarcinoma, teratoma, and mixed germ cell tumors), pineal cell tumors, and craniopharyngioma. This list of CNS tumors is by no

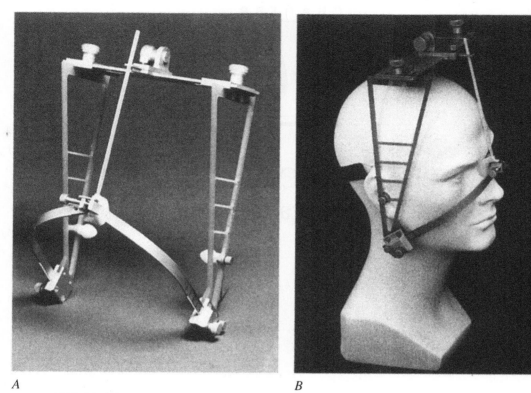

A

B

Figure 10.1 *A* and *B*. Relocatable head immobilization device for stereotactic radiotherapy. (Courtesy of Sandström Trade & Technology Inc.)

means complete; treatment planning for only a few of these is discussed here, since the treatment techniques are similar for many such tumors.

POSITIONING AND IMMOBILIZATION

Positioning and immobilization of patients being treated for brain tumors is similar to that for patients with tumors of the head and neck (Chap. 9) and are therefore not described again here. For patients treated by a technique called *stereotactic radiosurgery* and for patients receiving craniospinal irradiation (CSI), the immobilization is different, and it is therefore described below.

Stereotactic Radiosurgery. The immobilization systems used in stereotactic radiosurgery, where the precision required is greater than in any other treatment, consist of a stereotactic frame. This is bolted to the patient's head prior to the target-localization procedure and remains attached until the

treatment has been completed. Fiducial markers for three-dimensional target localization and image correlation are present on a variety of attachments that are rigidly fixed to the frame. This stereotactic frame, which remains in place from the beginning of the localization procedure until the treatment is completed, is uncomfortable for the patient and is generally used in single-fraction treatments. As this bolted system is impractical for fractionated treatment, relocatable fixation systems have been developed.

One system has the patient's head, with the exception of the nostrils, totally encased in a cast, which in turn is rigidly fixed to the treatment couch.[2] A photogrammetric method to measure the accuracy of this system has also been described.[3] In a second system, the head is immobilized by a frame that is held in place by a rod in each external auditory canal and a clip molded to the bridge of the nose (Fig. 10.1).[4,5] A third device consists of a frame that is

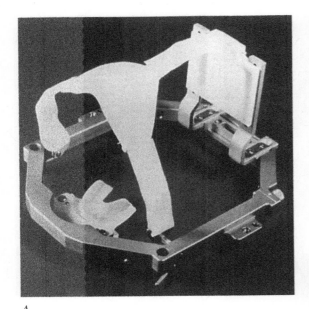

A

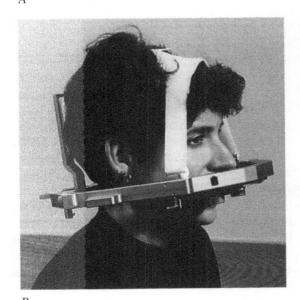

B

Figure 10.2 *A* and *B*. Relocatable head immobilization device for stereotactic radiotherapy. (Courtesy of Radionics.)

is fixed to the head and treatment couch in a reproducible fashion during the treatment to facilitate accurate treatment delivery.

Craniospinal Irradiation. Patients receiving CSI are often children. Many have neurological deficits making it difficult for them to remain motionless for any length of time. More than any other patients, they require stabilization to prevent them from falling off the treatment couch. The field arrangement, which usually consists of opposed lateral brain fields and a posterior spinal axis field, all of which are matched in the cervical spine area—usually re-

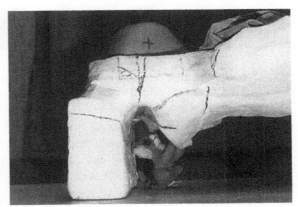

A

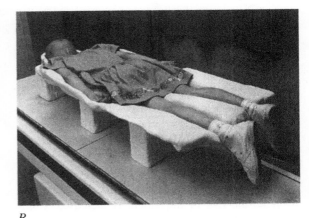

B

Figure 10.3 Total-body cast used for craniospinal irradiation. *A*. The patient's eye is visible and the nose and mouth are free for administration of anesthesia. A favorite toy helps to keep the child calm. *B*. Supports are used to level the cast. (Clothing is removed prior to treatment).

secured to the head by an impression of the upper teeth, an occipital tray with an impression of the occiput, and a strap that forcibly holds the dental and occipital impressions against the head (Fig. 10.2).[6,7] A fourth device is based on a thermoplastic facial mask.[8] For each of these fixation systems, the device

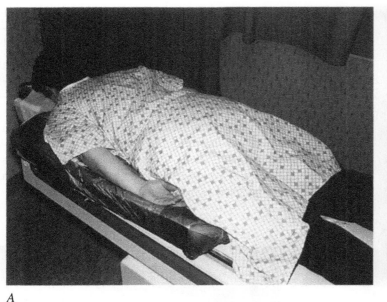
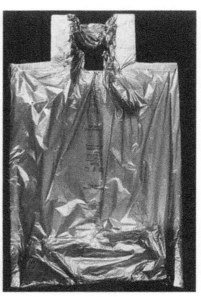

A   *B*

Figure 10.4 *A*. Alpha Cradle used for craniospinal irradiation. (Clothing is removed prior to treatment.) *B*. The form is covered by a polyvinyl sheet under which the foam is poured before the patient lies down.

quires that the patient be placed in the prone position. To achieve a perfect match between these fields, rotation of the collimator, couch, and gantry is required. This field matching, which is extremely difficult with beams arranged in an orthogonal fashion, requires a relatively motionless patient and satisfactory repositioning. The devastating result of overdosage in the spinal cord serves as an impetus for achieving a perfect match. It is important to emphasize that in matching these field margins, as in all field matching, *achieving a perfect match of field margins during a given treatment* is much more important than precisely reproducing the *location* of this field match from treatment to treatment.

For most patients, the prone position is less comfortable than the supine, and it is therefore less likely to be maintained throughout a treatment session unless the patient is positioned in a body shell. Children often move unintentionally, and if they are uncomfortable, the risk of movement is increased. Comfortable and effective immobilization techniques are therefore needed.

Small children requiring anesthesia present a problem because the anesthesiologist requires access

to the nose and mouth. These patients are usually treated in an inverted full-body plaster cast where the facial area is open, with access for anesthesia, suction, and so on (Fig. 10.3). The cast is made with the patient in the supine position and includes the anterior half of the body from the head except for the eyes, nose and mouth to below the knees. When the cast is removed, supports are added anterior to the forehead, chest, and thighs in such a way that when the cast is inverted and the patient is treated in the prone position, the dorsal surface is more or less horizontal. These casts are usually made with the child under anesthesia, and the size of the facial opening can be determined with the assistance of the anesthesiologist.

Total-body plaster shells have been used at Duke University Medical Center for many years. Plaster shells built for larger patients require approximately 1 h for fabrication (by three persons) and 2 days to dry. They are also quite heavy, and, for elderly and neurologically compromised patients, somewhat difficult to get in and out of.

Patients requiring CSI are often treated on an emergent basis to relieve neurological symptoms.

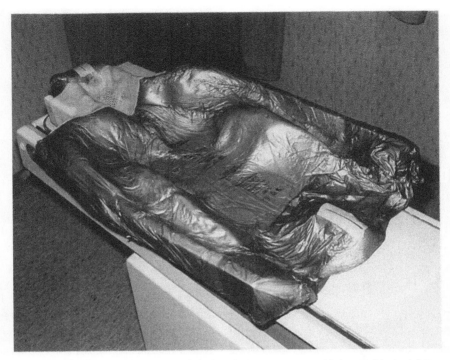

Figure 10.5   A thermoplastic sheet, molded to the facial prominences, aids in repositioning of the patient.

For them, a device that allows the treatments to begin immediately and makes it easier for patients to get in and out of has been developed. Known as an Alpha Cradle®*, it provides support and aids in the repositioning of the head, torso, and thighs (Fig. 10.4A).

The Alpha Cradle consists of a Styrofoam form that roughly fits the shape of the patient's head and torso and is covered by a polyvinyl sheet (Fig. 10.4B). The polyvinyl sheet is taped around the periphery of the head support, forming a channel around the patient's face. Foaming agents are mixed and prepared as directed by the supplier and are poured into the form. The patient lies down in the prone position on the polyvinyl sheet. Within a few minutes, the foam expands and fills the space between the patient and the walls of the Styrofoam form. The patient's head rests on the channel where the foam has been poured. The foam swells up around the patient's face, leaving an opening for the eyes, nose, and mouth. The polyvinyl sheet covering

the body part of the Alpha Cradle is pulled up between the patient's arms and the torso so that the foam can rise and form a mold of the arms as well as the torso. In some patients, it is necessary to elevate the torso so that the head and the torso are on a horizontal line. This can be accomplished by placing a large piece of Styrofoam of appropriate thickness in the body part of the Alpha Cradle prior to pouring the foaming agents.

When the foam has hardened, the patient lifts up his or her head from the facial support formed by the foam and a softened thermoplastic sheet is placed across the head support. When the patient resumes the position, the head is supported by a staff member who places one hand on each side, so that the head is straight and the chin extended to prevent the posterior spinal field from exiting through the oral cavity. The thermoplastic sheet is then gently contoured to the facial prominences to form a tight mask, into which the head is repositioned for each treatment (Fig. 10.5).

The Alpha Cradle requires approximately 30 min

---

* Smithers Medical Products, Inc., Akron, OH.

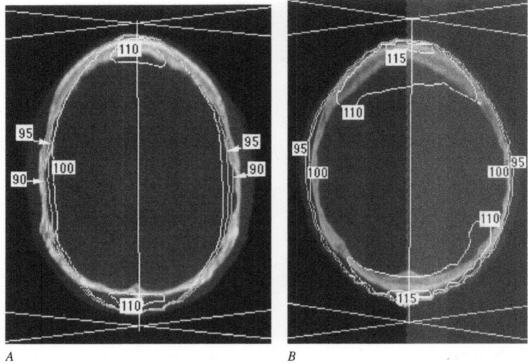

A　　　　　　　　　　　　　　　　　　　　　*B*

Figure 10.6　*A* and *B*. Dose distribution resulting from using opposed whole-brain fields using 15-MV photons *(A)* and 4-MV photons *(B)*.

for fabrication (by two persons), and the treatment simulation procedure can be carried out immediately following fabrication. Other benefits are that patients can more easily be repositioned in the Alpha Cradle because they can brace themselves on the sides as they lie prone. The face fits tightly in the thermoplastic face mask which is secured to the cast; thus, the head position can be reproduced and maintained.

During the simulation procedure, openings are made in the Styrofoam and the thermoplastic sheet such that the patient's eyes can be visualized. Radiopaque markers are placed on each lateral canthus during the simulation procedure. The position of the treatment field relative to the eyes is usually checked daily.

TREATMENT TECHNIQUES —WHOLE BRAIN

The condition most frequently requiring whole-brain radiation therapy is metastatic disease.[9] Since meta-static disease is frequently multifocal, whole-brain irradiation is generally used. Beams of relatively low energy (cobalt-60, 4-MV photons) should be used to avoid underdosage in the lateral aspect of the brain, where the skin-sparing effects of higher-energy beams may actually be a disadvantage (Fig. 10.6).[10] Whole-brain irradiation in the management of brain metastasis is often initiated without simulation of the treatment fields. The treatment fields are set up so that the beam flashes over the entire head in three directions and only the caudal margin is defined by the collimator of the treatment machine. This caudal margin is at times inappropriately set up, so that it follows a line drawn from the eyebrow through the external auditory canal to the posterior aspect of the skull (Fig. 10.7). However, as shown in Fig. 10.8, in order to include the entire cranial contents, the caudal margin must be farther caudal, as indicated by the sagittal and coronal magnetic resonance imaging (MRI) scans. Isodose distributions in sagittal planes through the midplane of the brain and through the

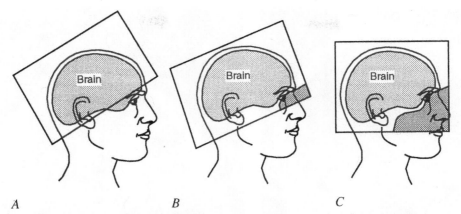

Figure 10.7   *A*. Whole-brain treatment fields are often set up without simulation and sometimes the inferior margin is set too far superior; consequently, part of the brain is untreated. *B*. The inferior margin must be set caudal of the eye and the earlobe with a small eye block over the anterior half of the eye. *C*. Alternatively, a large field is set with the help of a simulator and a customized block is used to define the caudal margin.

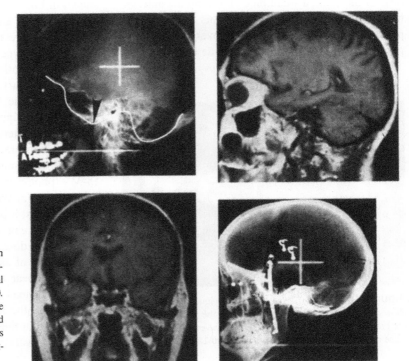

Figure 10.8 A lateral radiograph *(upper left)* demonstrating the lower margin of the brain as traced from the sagittal MRI image through the eye *(upper right)*. The coronal image *(lower left)* shows the caudal margins of the temporal lobes and the lateral radiograph *(lower right)* shows lead markers placed in the cranium indicating the lower aspect of the brain.

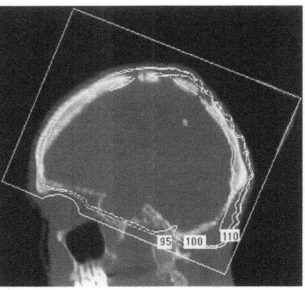

A   *B*

Figure 10.9 *A* and *B*. Sagittal dose distribution using opposed whole brain fields with a small eye block showing inadequate coverage of the brain *(A)* in the midline and *(B)* through the eye.

eye show that portions of the brain are missed (Fig. 10.9). When the collimator is turned to follow the base of the skull, a small block to shield the anterior half of the eye may be necessary. This block must be placed carefully and should not cover the posterior portion of the eye in order to include the portion of

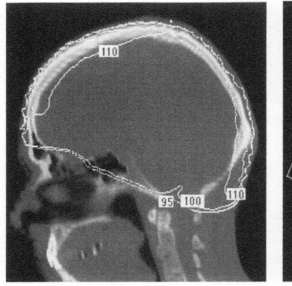

Figure 10.10 Axial and coronal MRI images of the brain show the proximity of the eyes. Inclusion of the entire contents of the brain in lateral fields while excluding the eyes requires very close margins. (This is also shown in Fig. 10.24*E*.)

the brain that extends inferiorly, between the posterior aspect of the eyes (Fig. 10.10). (This is also shown in Fig. 10.24*E*.) Alternatively, the collimator is not rotated and a larger customized block is formed to spare the eye and the facial area (Fig. 10.7*C*). This type of field will, in most situations, require a simulation procedure (Fig. 10.11).

Due to the curvature of the skull, dose heterogeneities within the brain volume are often observed when parallel opposed lateral fields are used (Fig. 10.6). This heterogeneity is greater when lower-energy beams are used (Fig. 10.12). In this illustration, the maximum dose within the brain, using 15-MV photon beams, is about 15 percent higher than the central axis midplane dose, while for 4-MV photon beams, it is about 20 percent higher. Using a high-energy photon beam, on the other hand, compromises the dose in the lateral aspect of the brain. The amount of beam extension beyond the scalp does not appear to have any effect on these high doses but instead depends on the beam energy and the shape of the head.[10] To improve the dose uniformity within the brain, a compensating filter consisting of several aluminum plates can be used.[11]

However, this is generally not used in most clinical situations where the dose heterogeneity is not clinically relevant.

As with any other patient being treated near the eyes, a radiopaque marker should be placed on each lateral canthus to document radiographically where the eyes are with respect to the beam. This helps guide the physician in shaping the treatment field and it also helps document the exclusion of the eyes from the radiation beam. An explanation of precisely what the marker represents should be written on the radiograph—that is, whether it represents the lateral canthus, the lateral aspect of the bony orbit, or anything else. Labeling on radiographs is also discussed in Chap. 8. Divergence of the lateral beam into the eye on the opposite side is always a problem if the entire cranial contents are to be treated (Fig. 10.13). The proximity of the eyes to the brain is demonstrated in Figs. 10.10 and 10.24E. To avoid beam divergence into the opposite eye, the beam can be angled posteriorly (right and left anterior oblique

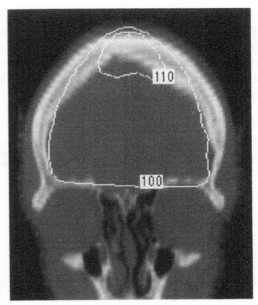

A

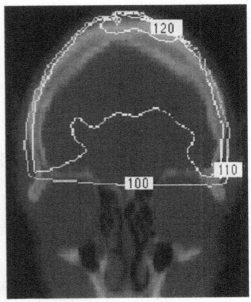

B

Figure 10.12 High-dose areas occur in the brain a result of the curvature of the head; isodose distributions in the coronal plane showing the highest dose to be approximately 115 percent using 15-MV photons (*A*) and 120 percent using 4-MV photons (*B*).

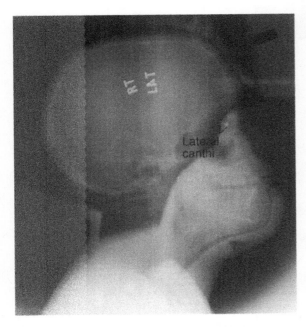

Figure 10.11 Port film showing a whole-brain field with a customized block defining an appropriate inferior margin. (In this patient, the first cervical vertebra was also included.)

fields). This usually requires approximately 2 to 3°, depending on the setup geometry (i.e., where the central axis is set with respect to the eyes, field size, and treatment distance and whether the eyes lie on a horizontal line). If the eyes are not on a horizontal line, the angle of the two fields may be different (Chap. 9, Fig. 9.1). The necessary angle is best determined by viewing in fluoroscopy and turning the gantry until the two lead markers are superimposed. Alternatively, the central axis of the beam can be set

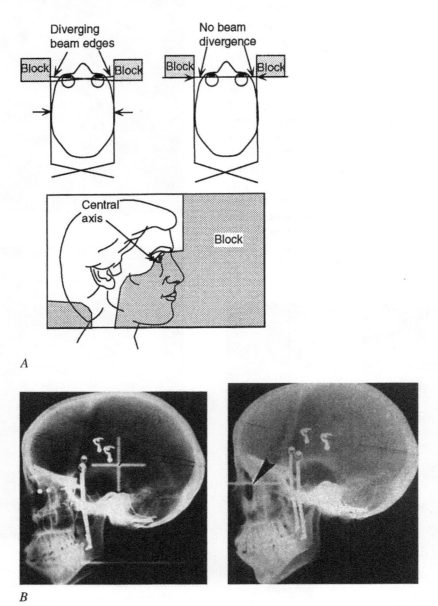

Figure 10.13 *A.* To minimize beam divergence into the contralateral eye, the central axis of the field of the eye can be placed behind the lens and the field is then shaped using a customized block. Such fields can be very large. *B.* In the radiograph on the left, where the field is centered on the brain, the bony orbits are not aligned. In the radiograph on the right, where the central axis is set at the eye, the bony orbits are aligned, indicating no beam divergence.

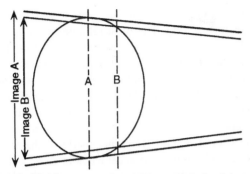

Figure 10.14   On a lateral radiograph of the head the maximal sagittal dimensions are shown *(image A),* while a sagittal CT or MRI may represent a smaller dimension on either side of the midline *(image B).* These images therefore cannot be enlarged to the same size and superimposed for the purpose of transposing the tumor volume. Image A = simulation film; image B = CT or MRI.

very near the eyes so as to minimize beam divergence, but this requires very large fields (Fig. 10.13).

Treatment Simulation—Whole Brain. Whole-brain treatment often does not require a simulation procedure; however, in some cases, simulation is necessary to produce customized beam-shaping blocks. In those situations where a simulation procedure is needed, the patient is placed in the supine position with appropriate immobilization. A lead marker should be placed on the lateral canthus

of each eye. This facilitates design of the shielding blocks so that the anterior portions of the eyes are protected. When an isocentric treatment technique is used, the patient's midline is aligned with the sagittal laser alignment line. The gantry of the simulator is then turned 90° to either side. Alternatively, the gantry is turned 87 to 88° to eliminate beam divergence into the opposite eye, as noted in the previous section. The exact angle can be determined in fluoroscopy by rotating the gantry until the markers on each eye become superimposed. Without moving the patient from left to right, the couch is then moved until the whole brain, with adequate flash over the skull, lies within the beam-defining wires of the simulator. In situations where the central axis is set at the lateral canthus, the field size is opened until the entire cranial contents are included and the beam flashes over the skull in all directions. After a radiograph is taken of each field, the laser alignment lines are marked on the patient and/or the immobilization device to facilitate reproducibility in the treatment room.

TREATMENT TECHNIQUES—LIMITED VOLUME

Recent advances in diagnostic imaging—computed tomography (CT), MRI, and so on—have improved our ability to localize brain tumors and facilitated the use of limited radiation fields. Generally, tumors that tend not to infiltrate beyond radiologically identifi-

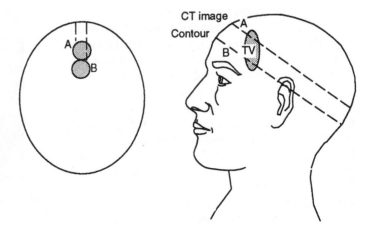

Figure 10.15   A transverse CT or MRI image may be parallel with the contour plane, but—due to the curvature of the head—using measurements off the image to transpose the tumor may cause a displacement. Distance A, measured from the anterior surface to the tumor on a CT image, is much shorter than the same measurement on the contour *(distance B).* Localization of the tumor from this CT image onto the contour would result in a serious displacement of the tumor.

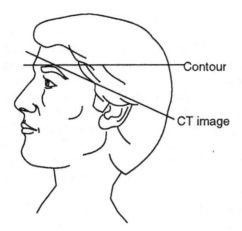

Figure 10.16 A transverse CT or MRI image may not represent the same plane as a contour.

able tumor margins—such as benign meningiomas, pituitary adenomas, craniopharyngiomas, and acoustic neurilemmomas—may be treated with narrow margins. Conversely, malignant tumors, such as glioblastoma multiforme, are often treated with generous margins, since they tend to infiltrate beyond apparent tumor margins[12,13]

It is helpful to use a scout view, a sagittally reconstructed CT image, or a sagittal MRI as a surrogate for a simulation film. At times, tumor volumes may inappropriately be transferred from a sagittal MRI or reconstructed CT image to the simulation film. Caution should be exercised, because while the lateral simulation radiograph represents the largest dimension of the patient's head in the sagittal plane (midline), the MRI or reconstructed CT, also in the sagittal plane, may represent the smaller dimension of the head on either side of the midline (Fig. 10.14). Similarly, when a target volume is transposed from a transverse CT or MRI image to a transverse contour that is *parallel* to the plane of the CT or MRI image but taken at a slightly *different plane,* the target can be inadvertently displaced (Fig. 10.15). It is also important to recognize that when information is transferred from transverse CT images to a transverse contour of the head, the plane of the CT image *may not be parallel* to the plane of the contour (Fig. 10.16).

Overlooking this discrepancy can lead to errors in tumor localization. The most reliable method of localizing the target on the transverse contour is to ensure that the plane of the CT scans is the same as the contour. In radiation therapy departments where CT scanning is available, a treatment-planning CT should be obtained in treatment position and with reference marks made on the patient's head (or immobilization device). Reference marks on the patient and/or the immobilization device help in the transfer of information from the CT scan into the simulation procedure, as described in Chap. 7.

When a limited volume of the brain requires treatment (astrocytoma, craniopharyngioma, brainstem tumors, boost fields, and so on), the treatment can be delivered via a variety of multiple-field techniques as well as through opposed lateral fields (Fig. 10.17). Dose-limiting tissues are the optic chiasm, retina, the lens of the eye, and brain tissue. The beam direction and position of the patient must be such that the dose tolerance in these organs is respected. Deep-seated tumors can be treated using high-energy photon

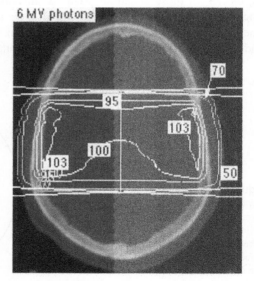

Figure 10.17 Opposed lateral fields can be used to treat a brain tumor. Using 6-MV photon beams results in a fairly uniform dose throughout the irradiated area but does not provide lateral sparing of brain tissue.

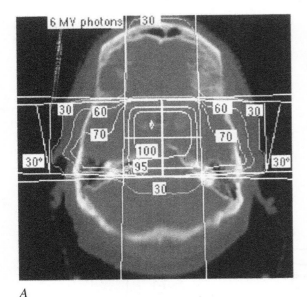

A

B

beams to limit the dose to lateral brain tissue. Anterior and posterior fields may be used in addition to lateral opposed fields, depending on the location of the tumor and the patient's ability to flex or extend the neck, so that irradiation of the eyes can be avoided. Such a four-field technique would deliver approximately 50 percent of the target dose to the nontarget tissue within the entrance and exit regions of the beams. Alternatively, the patient's position can be neutral, with beam directions determined through compound angles of the collimator, couch, and gantry.

A three-field technique, using lateral opposed wedged fields and a third field (vertex, anterior, or posterior), can be used if the patient's position permits (Fig. 10.18). Such a field arrangement is often used to treat pituitary gland lesions and is described later in this chapter. Wedges are necessary in the lateral fields to prevent a hot spot near the intersection of the third field. The vertex field is treated either by having the patient tilt the head forward (Fig. 10.19) or by turning the couch 90°, so that the sagittal plane is parallel to the gantry rotation. The

Figure 10.18 *A*. A three-field technique, using opposed lateral fields and a vertex (or an anterior or posterior field) provides sparing of lateral brain tissue. When these fields are equally weighted, the dose in the temporal lobes is high due to the entrance/exit doses. Anteriorly, the dose is lower because there is no exit dose from an opposing field. *B*. Increasing the weight on the anterior field and decreasing it on the lateral fields reduce the dose in the temporal lobes. Here the vertex field is weighted 40 percent, while the opposed lateral fields are weighted 30 percent each. The surrounding normal brain in the lateral entrance/exit regions and anteriorly receives approximately 50 percent of the prescribed dose.

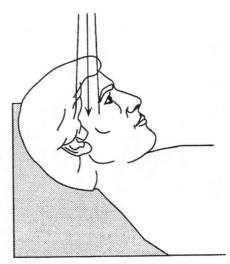

Figure 10.19 When a frontal or vertex field is used, the patient must flex the neck so the beam remains superior and posterior of the eyes.

gantry is then rotated so that the beam enters the patient's head at the desired angle (Fig. 10.20). When the lateral fields are treated, the collimator must be angled until the wedge direction becomes parallel to the central axis of the vertex field (Fig. 10.21). The disadvantage of this technique is that the vertex field, depending on the size and the angle at which it is directed, often exits in the pharynx or neck or follows the axis of the spinal cord. Another

disadvantage is the inability to obtain verification radiographs of the field position. An alternative method of obtaining confirmation of the field position is a vertex field superimposed on a lateral port film of the head, as described in Chap. 9 (Fig. 9.41).[14,15]

Another technique that can be used to treat tumors in the lateral aspect of the brain and that minimizes irradiation of the opposite hemisphere is using op-

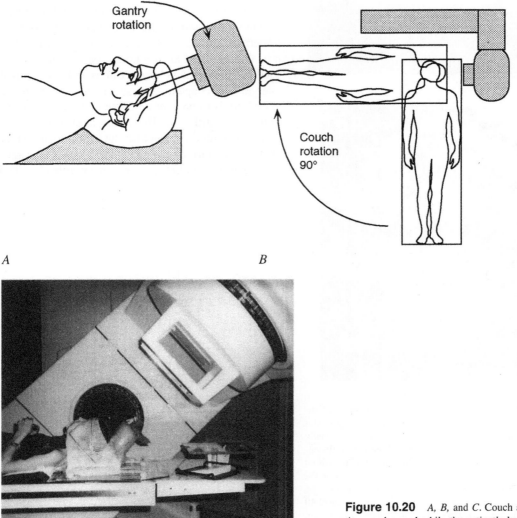

A

B

C

Figure 10.20 *A, B,* and *C.* Couch and gantry rotation can be used while the patient's head remains in a neutral position.

posed anterior and posterior wedged fields and an ipsilateral unwedged field (Fig. 10.22A). The weighting and wedge angles can be modified to achieve an acceptable dose distribution. Tumors located either anteriorly or posteriorly in one hemisphere can also be treated using a wedged pair of beams (Fig. 10.22B).

Small brain tumors are also well suited for treatment by rotation and arc techniques. The use of a small field and a high-energy photon beam will result in excellent sparing of the unaffected brain tissues. A full rotation (360°) usually means that the beam must traverse the head immobilization device and sometimes a segment of the treatment couch. Uncertainties in the dose distribution and the need for calculation of the beam attenuation are then introduced. These problems can be eliminated by omitting the posterior arc directions and using an anterior arc limited to 180 or 270°. A wedge is needed in such an arc to avoid a higher dose anterior to the axis of rotation. The wedge must be reversed midway through the rotation, so that the thick part of

the wedge is always directed anteriorly (see similar plan in Chap. 9, Fig. 9.35, and Chap. 6, Fig. 6.34).

Reirradiating patients with recurrent brain tumors poses a certain degree of hazard and generally should not be undertaken without clear documentation of previous treatment. Because some brain tumors, especially craniopharyngioma, are very slow-growing, patients with recurrent tumor may return many years after the initial irradiation. Logistical issues sometimes make review of prior records difficult; the documentation of the treatment fields may be poor, the dose delivery may be poorly reported, machine data are sometimes unavailable, treatment records may have been lost or destroyed, or some combination of these difficulties may exist. Some patients may have been treated during an era when deep-seated tumors were treated with orthovoltage beams. Because of the increased dose in the entrance/exit regions resulting from parallel opposed low-energy beams, sparing of these areas becomes paramount when reirradiation is necessary. Techniques that avoid or minimize the dose to these high-dose areas

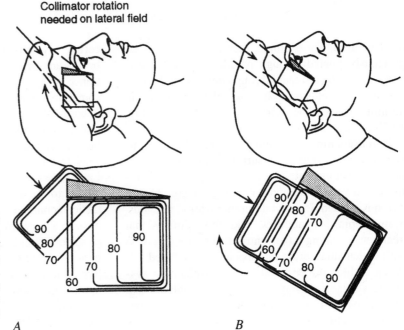

Figure 10.21 *A* and *B*. The wedge orientation must always be such that the isodose tilt is parallel to the direction of the vertex field. The wedge orientation in the left diagram requires a collimator rotation to make the tilt of the isodose curves parallel to the intersection of the vertex field. The arrangement in the right-hand diagram is correct.   *A*   *B*

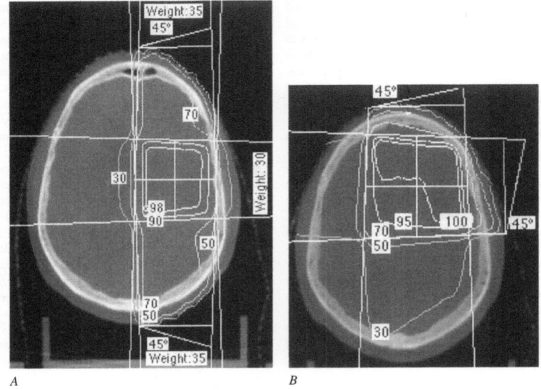

A   *B*

Figure 10.22   *A.* A three-field technique can also be used when the tumor is located in one hemisphere. This provides sparing of the contralateral hemisphere. *B.* A wedged pair of fields can also be used when the tumor is located either anteriorly or posteriorly.

must be used. For example, recurrent brain tumors, previously treated through parallel opposed lateral fields, might be retreated through anterior and posterior opposed fields or with a sagittal arc technique to minimize dose in the lateral aspect of the brain (Fig. 10.23).

In reirradiating brain tumors where the previous dose was high, sparing of surrounding normal brain tissues is paramount. The tumor margins are therefore often very small and a very high degree of precision is needed. Improved immobilization methods, beam-shaping capabilities, and three-dimensional treatment planning have contributed to the precision with which small brain tumors can be irradiated.[16,17] When a three-dimensional treatment-planning system is available, complex treatment techniques can be employed. For example, multiple noncoplanar beams or radiosurgery result in a uniform high dose in the tumor, while the surrounding brain tissue re-

ceives a relatively low dose (Fig. 10.24). These beams are unopposed so as to avoid cumulative entrance and exit doses. Recurrent brain tumors are sometimes also considered for interstitial implants (Chap. 16).

A newer and more complex treatment technique, briefly discussed above, is stereotactic radiosurgery. This technique, developed in 1951 in Sweden by Lars Leksell, a neurosurgeon, was originally intended to obviate invasive procedures.[18,19] A stereotactic technique allows one to focus the radiation dose to a very small volume, with excellent sparing of surrounding brain tissue. Very high doses (on the order of 1000 to 3000 cGy) of radiation can be delivered to a small volume (4 to 50 mm in diameter) in a single fraction. Although this technique is usually employed in the treatment of arteriovenous malformation (AVM—a congenital abnormality of the blood vessels in the brain),[20] it is also used for the treatment or retreatment of patients with small tumors.

Stereotactic treatments can be delivered using either a gamma knife or a modified linear accelerator.[21] The gamma knife consists of a large lead sphere that holds 201 well-collimated individual cobalt 60 sources.[22,23] The radiation from these sources converges at a common point referred to as the *isocenter*. The beams from the cobalt 60 sources enter an area covering approximately half of the upper hemisphere of the skull. The shape of the isodose distribution can be altered by selectively blocking some of these sources or by using multiple isocenters.[24] As an alternative, linear accelerators have been modified in many centers to achieve a similar treatment plan.[25-27] By taking advantage of the

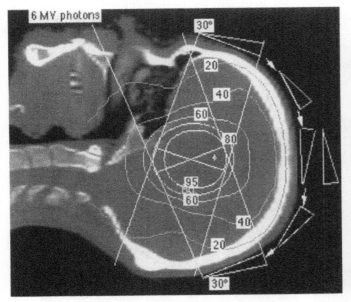

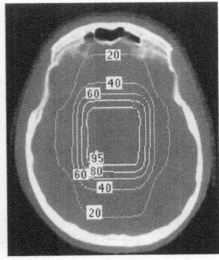

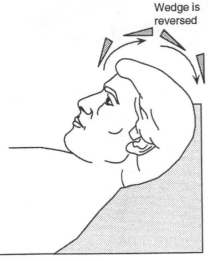

Figure 10.23 Retreatment of centrally located brain tumors can be accomplished via a sagittal arc with reversed wedges. An isodose distribution in the sagittal plane using 30° wedges *(A)* and another in a transverse plane showing excellent sparing laterally, anteriorly, and posteriorly *(B)*. A diagram illustrating the direction of the arc treatment *(C)*.

gantry and couch rotations, isodose distributions that conform to the target can be achieved. The couch is turned to several positions (≥ 4) and then the gantry rotates over an arc ($100°$) at each of the couch positions (Fig. 10.25). In the gamma knife, the collimators are from 4 to 18 mm in diameter, while in the linear accelerator, special collimators (circular cones) are available with diameters from 10 to 50 mm. The actually treated volume can be enlarged by using more than one isocenter. Precise localization of intracranial targets and treatment planning must precede each treatment.[28,29] Stereotactic treatment techniques are labor-intensive and costly.

More recently, fractionated radiosurgery has been used, delivering several smaller fractions to exploit the potential radiobiologic advantages of fractionation. This type of treatment might also be termed fractionated stereotactic (or conformal) radiotherapy.

Treatment Simulation—Limited Volume. Target localization should be made via imaging studies such as CT or MRI, with the patient firmly immobilized in the treatment position. From the CT scans, the target volume is transposed to a contour of the head and the field arrangement is then determined. In the simulator room, the patient's position is reproduced and the isocenter is positioned with respect to the reference marks made on the immobilization device. Lead markers should be placed on

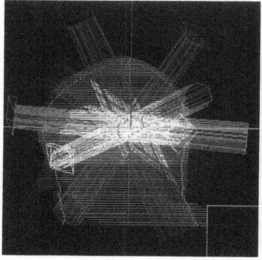
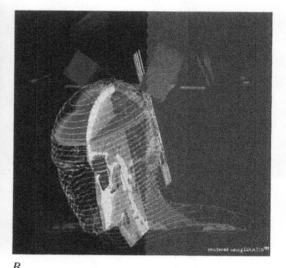

A   *B*

Figure 10.24 Retreatment of small brain tumors can also be delivered through a large number of conformal beams, none of which are opposed, to limit the dose in the entrance/exit regions. *A.* A "bouquet" of beams is aimed at a small brain tumor. The wedges are oriented in an unconventional fashion to deliver a uniform dose in the tumor. *B.* A color display of the CT images in sagittal, coronal, and transverse planes and the location of the tumor *(red)* and the eyes *(green)*. Beam and wedge orientations are also shown in green. The resulting isodose distribution without wedges *(C)* and with wedges *(D)*. The maximum dose with wedges is 100.4 percent and the target is covered by the 98 percent isodose line. *E.* The wire outline of the brain *(blue)* and the eyes *(red)* shows that the posterior superior portions of the eye and the brain are superimposed in the lateral beam's-eye view. *F.* A color wash of a patient with two small lesions treated through opposed fields angled such that the lesions are superimposed in the beam's-eye view. A third right anterior field was designed such that it included only the lesions with small margins, and the area between the tumors was blocked. (See color illustration 3, which appears between pages 532 and 533.) Neither of these plans could be carried out without three-dimensional treatment planning tools. (The Virtual Simulator™, Sherouse Systems, Inc.)

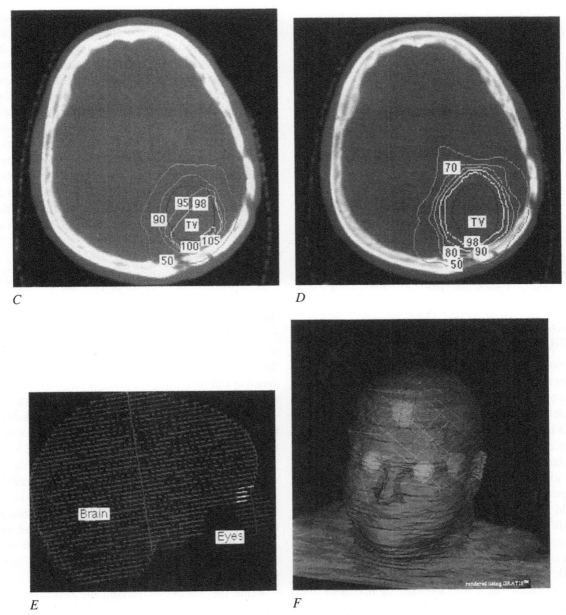

Figure 10.24 (*Continued*)

each lateral canthus to facilitate beam shaping so as to protect the anterior half of the eyes. The gantry is then turned to the appropriate position and the field size is set on the machine. The position of the fields with respect to relevant bony anatomy is verified in fluoroscopy. A radiograph is obtained of each field and the three laser alignment lines are marked on the immobilization device or on the patient's skin.

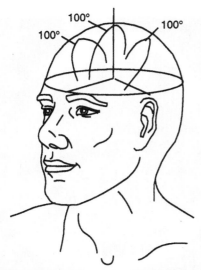

Figure 10.25 Stereotactic radiosurgery is usually carried out via three or more arcs of about 100°.

TREATMENT TECHNIQUES —CRANIOSPINAL IRRADIATION

In many patients, such as those with medulloblastoma and primitive neuroectodermal tumor, it is necessary to treat the entire CNS. Different techniques to deliver this treatment have been described.[30-42] This treatment is complicated by the fact that several adjacent fields must be used. Typically, the brain is treated through lateral opposed fields while the spinal axis is treated via one or two posterior fields (depending on the length of the spine) (Fig. 10.26). Field matching between the two posterior spinal fields is usually accomplished by calculating the separation between the two fields on the skin surface in a manner identical to that used for typical adjacent fields (Chap. 6). Matching the inferior border of the lateral cranial fields with the superior border of the most cephalad posterior field is more complicated, since the cephalad aspect of the posterior spine field is diverging cephalad and the caudal aspect of the brain fields is diverging caudal and posteriorly. The first step is to rotate the collimator of the lateral fields so that its inferior border is parallel to the divergence of the superior aspect of the spinal field (Fig. 10.27). This prevents the superior aspect of the spine field from exiting into the anterior-superior aspect of the brain fields. In effect, it moves this

anterior portion of the lateral brain fields cephalad and out of the path of the spine field. Second, to avoid overlap resulting from inferior divergence of the caudal border of the lateral fields into the cephalad aspect of the posterior spinal field, the foot of the couch is rotated toward the collimator so that the caudal field margins of the two fields become parallel and cross the patient's neck in a straight line—that is, perpendicular to the patient's sagittal axis (Fig. 10.28). The number of degrees by which the couch must be turned depends on the length of the lateral cranial fields in the direction of the gap and the distance at which the field size is defined. The appropriate number of degrees can be found from a graph in Chap. 6, Fig. 6.43 or from the following:

$$\text{Tan } \theta = \frac{\text{half-field length}}{\text{SSD}} \qquad (10.1)$$

The locations of these field junctions are usually moved two or three times during a course of treatment to blur out the dose inhomogeneities at the junction. The field junctions are often shifted by increasing and decreasing the sizes of the two fields on either side of the junctions (Fig. 10.29).[43,44] The caudal spine field, which is usually shortened to move the junction, should therefore be set up farther caudal than the intended treatment and then be defined by a block. Thus, the caudal border of the spine field is unchanged when the collimator size is decreased. Alternatively, asymmetrical jaws can be used to keep the caudal margin fixed. Likewise, the lateral brain fields need to flash over the vertex of the head by several centimeters, so that when these fields are decreased in the gap-shifting process, there is still sufficient flash over the skull.

While the practice of turning the couch for the lateral cranial fields solves the field-matching problem, depending on the location of the cranial field central axes, it may cause the most inferior aspect of the opposite temporal fossa to be missed (Fig. 10.30). The caudal field margins, usually defined by a customized block, may therefore need to be more generous when the couch is rotated.

Another note of caution should be added here, because when the foot of the couch is rotated toward the collimator for treatment of each of the lateral

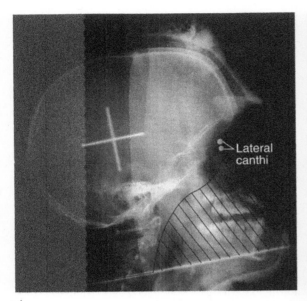

Lateral canthi

A

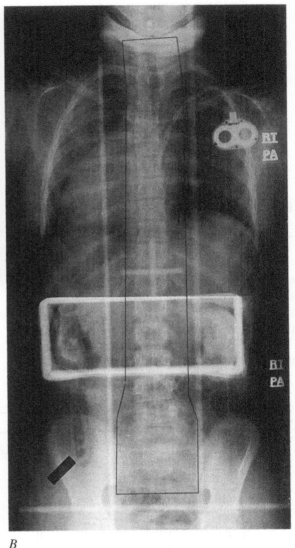

B

Figure 10.26 Craniospinal irradiation usually consists of lateral cranial fields *(A)* and a posterior spinal field *(B)*.

brain fields, the treatment distance (SSD) in the caudal half of the lateral brain field is effectively decreased while in the cephalad half is increased (Fig. 10.31). The change in SSD becomes larger as the distance from the isocenter increases. The SSD is usually shorter by 1 to 2 cm in the cervical spine, depending on the couch angle and the location of the central axis of the lateral fields. The length by which the distance is decreased, which must be measured at an appropriate distance from the isocenter, can be found by measuring the distance between the sagittal

laser line when the couch is set on 0° versus where it is when the couch is rotated to the treatment position. It is important to recognize that this change in SSD is in the same direction for both of the lateral fields (i.e., one does not offset the other but, instead, there is a cumulative effect).

The shorter SSD causes the dose in the cervical spine to increase. The dose here is also higher than in the midbrain due to the smaller thickness of the neck. It is important always to calculate and record the cervical spine dose in the daily treatment record,

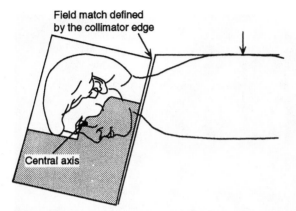

Figure 10.27 The collimator of the lateral cranial fields is turned until the caudal margin is parallel with the diverging cephalad margin of the posterior spinal field.

taking into account both the reduced separation and the shorter SSD. A field reduction may be required to keep the dose in the cervical spine within tolerance limits, recognizing that the dose fractions are larger. The same issues that apply to the cervical spine also apply to the posterior fossa. This area is also moved

toward the collimator when the couch is rotated, but this is of lesser consequence than in the cervical spine because it is closer to the isocenter and therefore the change in SSD is smaller. The transverse separation is usually larger here than in the cervical spine, thus excessive dose is less likely.

It is difficult to treat the entire brain without having divergence into the eye on the opposite side. The solution previously described for whole-brain irradiation was to set the central axis of the beam at the lateral canthus of the eye, thereby eliminating the beam divergence. While the practice of fixing the central axis of the field at the lateral canthus reduces eye irradiation, this technique usually cannot be used when the CSI technique is used. In this technique, where the couch is rotated to eliminate the caudal beam divergence of the lateral cranial fields, the opposite eye is projected more cephalad and cannot be shielded without also blocking brain tissue. A gantry angle here will not solve the problem, because that motion causes both eyes to move posteriorly with respect to the beam. While the anterior/posterior motion can be changed only by a gantry angle, the

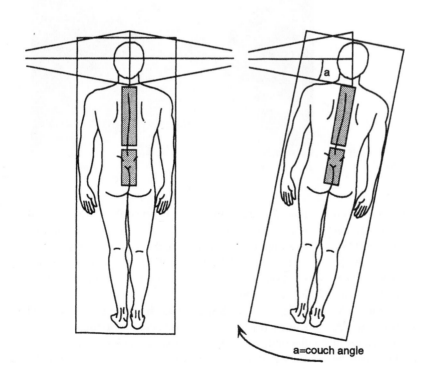

a=couch angle

Figure 10.28 The foot of the couch is turned toward the collimator such that the caudal margin of the lateral cranial fields become parallel and crosses the patient's neck in a straight line (i.e., perpendicular to the sagittal axis of the patient).

cephalad/caudal motion can be changed only by a couch rotation (Fig. 10.32).

The precise depth of the spinal cord along its axis is sometimes difficult to determine. Lateral radiographs with the patient in treatment position and a lead wire along the posterior surface can be obtained without difficulty. It is, however, sometimes very difficult to see the vertebral column on a lateral radiograph, particularly at the level of the shoulders. A scout view from a CT scanner, with the patient in the treatment position and a radiopaque marker along the skin surface over the spine, produces a much better image (Fig. 10.33). After appropriate enlargement, such scout views can be used to determine the depth of the spine for gap calculation between the spinal fields and for a contour on which to calculate an isodose distribution from the posterior spinal fields in the sagittal plane.

The dose along the spinal axis varies due to vary-

ing depth and SSD and also because of the overflattening of the beam from linear accelerators, which usually is most noticeable near the surface and in large fields. An isodose distribution calculated on the patient's sagittal midline contour provides an estimate of the dose heterogeneity along the spinal axis (Fig. 10.34). Obtaining a sagittal contour and the depth of the spinal cord may not always be possible. The dose may then be prescribed on the central axis at an estimated depth, or, if the depth can be determined from diagnostic CT or MRI images, at an average of depths measured at several points along the spinal cord.

As an example of the dose variations along the spinal axis, the dose in the patient seen in Fig. 10.34A varies from about 80 to 95 percent. Some patients treated for metastatic disease in the spine in the prone position may be unable to lie prone without propping the chest up on the arms. This can cause the

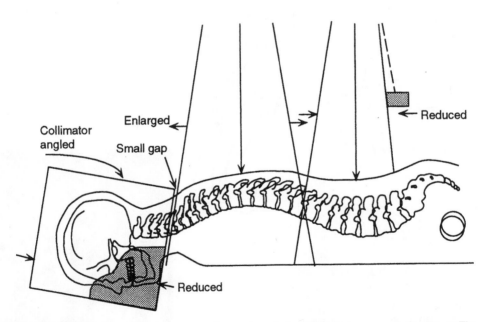

Figure 10.29 The field junctions are moved approximately three times during a course of treatment. The shift is accomplished by decreasing and increasing the field lengths, as indicated by the arrows. The original field sizes must be set with this in mind, so that there is still room to make the fields longer without exceeding the field-length limitation of the machine. Since the caudal spine field is usually decreased in length, the caudal margin of this field should be set farther inferior than the intended treatment area. A block is then inserted to the appropriate treatment level. As the field length is decreased in the gap-shifting process, the beam treatment area remains unchanged.

SSD to vary along the spinal axis, and thus the dose heterogeneity is exacerbated (Fig. 10.34*B*). Here the dose varies from about 75 percent in the lumbar spine to 100 percent in the thoracic spine. In this patient, the SSD, which is shorter in the thoracic spine where the spinal cord usually is shallow, can be reduced by positioning the patient flat with the arms raised above the head.

An attempt to improve the dose uniformity in the spinal axis and also to eliminate field junctions through the use of conformation therapy has been described.[37] In this technique, the patient is moved through the beam by computer-driven motion of the couch. The dose at the various segments of the spine is monitored by varying the speed with which the couch moves. An alternative technique to treat the spinal axis is using electron beams.[32,45] While this technique offers normal tissue sparing in the more anteriorly located anatomic structures, it raises uncertainties due to attenuation by the spinal skeleton.

In summary, an attempt should be made to keep the patient's posterior surface horizontal, an isodose distribution should be calculated on a sagittal contour, and the dose gradient within the spinal canal should be considered when the dose prescription is formulated. Problems associated with matching of adjacent fields in the spinal cord are discussed in Chap. 6.

Treatment Simulation—Craniospinal Irradiation.   The patient is placed prone in the immobilization cast or Alpha Cradle. Lead markers are placed on the lateral canthus of each eye to facilitate design of beam-shaping blocks such that the anterior aspect

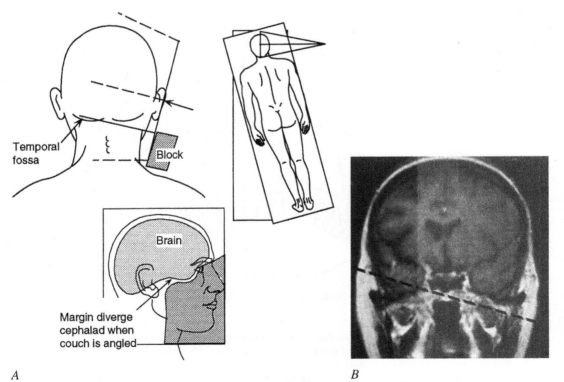

A   *B*

Figure 10.30   *A*. A couch angle on the lateral brain fields can cause the contralateral temporal lobe to be missed. *B*. The sagittal MRI shows the position of the temporal fossa. The line across the image indicates the blocked edge in the diagram.

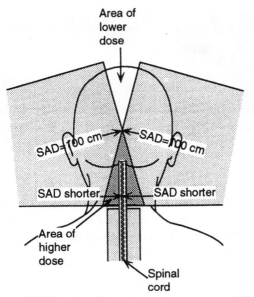

Figure 10.31 When the couch is turned to accomplish the field match, the treatment distance is decreased in the posterior fossa and the cervical spine while, in the cephalad portion of the brain, the opposite occurs.

of the eyes is spared. In fluoroscopy, the patient's midline is aligned with the central axis of the beam. This requires moving the couch in and out from the gantry to see that the central axis indicator of the simulation unit always lies in the center of the patient's spine, from the cervical spine to the sacrum. Several adjustments must be made until this has been achieved. The sagittal laser alignment line is then marked on the immobilization device both cephalad of the head and between the legs. Reproducing this alignment in the treatment room prior to the treatment is vital to accurate treatment delivery (Chap. 7). As in all other treatments and simulations, the gantry, couch, and collimator angles should be set on 0° prior to the procedure.

A cross-table lateral radiograph with a lead wire on the skin along the spine will help determine the depth of the spinal cord and also the depth at which the beams should converge without causing an overlap in the spinal canal. Alternatively, a scout view can be obtained using a CT unit. The two posterior spine fields are set up using an SSD technique, and a

Figure 10.32 While the anterior/posterior motion of the beam edge can be changed only by a gantry angle (A), the cephalad/caudal motion can be changed only with a couch rotation (B). The difficulties are synonymous with the displacement of the contralateral temporal fossa when the couch is turned.

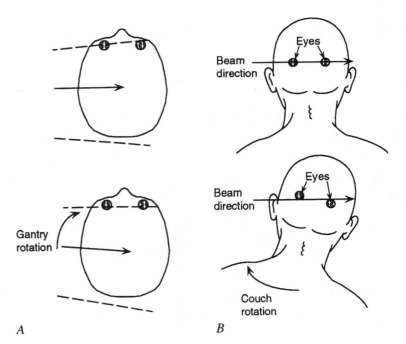

gap is calculated between the fields in the usual manner (Chap. 6). Since the field junction is shifted during the course of treatment by increasing and decreasing the length of these fields, the initial length must be set such that the length can be increased by 4 to 6 cm without exceeding the maximum field length possible on the particular treatment machine. For setting up the lateral brain fields, it is also helpful to mark the projection of the posterior spine field on the lateral aspect of the neck. This can be accomplished by widening the spine field such that the cephalad field margin flashes over the sides of the neck.

The lateral brain fields are then simulated. The patient's position on the simulation couch must not be changed between the simulation of the spinal axis and the lateral brain fields. If it is, the geometric relationship between the posterior fields and the diverging lateral fields has been disturbed, preventing a ''perfect'' field match. If the patient's head was straight (i.e., not turned right or left or rolled from side to side during the production of the immobilization device), the sagittal laser line should now be in the midplane of the head. Without moving the simulation couch, the gantry is turned 90° to either side and the couch is then moved until the entire brain lies within the field-defining wires of the simulator and there is adequate flash over the skull in all directions. The collimator is turned until the caudal margin is

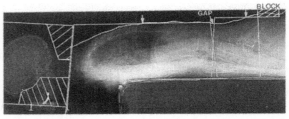

Figure 10.33   A sagittal scout view with a plastic marker on the skin surface in the patient's midline can be used to obtain a contour for calculating the dose distribution for CSI.

parallel with the diverging posterior field. The necessary degree of collimator rotation depends on the length and the SSD of the superior posterior field and can be found from Eq. (10.1).

The foot of the couch is then turned toward the collimator to prevent the lateral field from diverging into the superior aspect of the posterior spine field. The necessary degree of couch rotation depends on the length of the lateral field in the direction of the gap (distance from the central axis to the caudal margin), and the SAD and can be found from Eq. (10.1). A visual check should be made to verify that the caudal margin of the lateral fields in fact match the cephalad margin of the posterior spine field. When the opposite lateral field is simulated, the couch and collimator angels are in the opposite di-

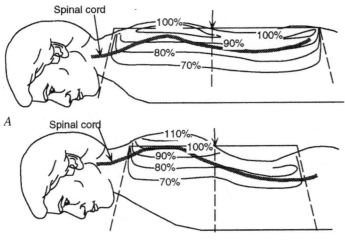

Figure 10.34   Isodose distributions in the sagittal plane in a patient with a horizontal skin surface *(A)* and in a patient where the posterior surface is not horizontal *(B)*.

rection. In addition to shifting the location of the gaps during the treatment course, it is also recommended that a small gap (~ 0.5 cm) be set between these fields. A radiograph should be taken of each of the two lateral fields. The central axis of each field is marked on the patient or, alternatively, on the immobilization device. It is recommended that the laser alignment lines also be marked, but in another color, to prevent confusion about what each mark indicates.

TREATMENT—CENTRAL NERVOUS SYSTEM

GENERAL CONSIDERATIONS

Most primary brain tumors are unifocal and can be irradiated with limited fields. Since many tumors tend to infiltrate for a considerable distance into surrounding normal-appearing brain tissue and/or their borders are poorly demarcated on imaging studies, generous margins are usually added beyond demonstrable tumor. The large volume of normal brain tissue that then lies within the target volume and receives the same dose as the target becomes a dose-limiting factor.

Surgical management of CNS tumors, in addition to partial or total excision (which is often curative) establishes histologic diagnosis. In patients with evidence of tumor-induced hydrocephalus, surgical decompression is usually indicated, either by a shunt or tumor resection. Hydrocephalus is a condition in which there is a blockage of the ventricular system, preventing cerebrospinal fluid from draining into the spinal canal. Conditions of increased intracranial pressure usually constitute an oncologic emergency. Decompressive surgery and the initiation of steroids generally precedes radiation therapy, since the response time is usually much faster. The goal of surgery is primarily to remove the tumor. If this is not possible, due to either tumor location or size, partial resection may be useful. For totally unresectable lesions, a stereotactically guided needle biopsy is usually performed to obtain a histologic diagnosis. In some instances, patients are irradiated without a firm histologic diagnosis.

Radiation therapy is usually delivered via exter-

nal-beam treatments, and sometimes interstitial implants are used (Chap. 16). In recent years, stereotactic radiosurgery has become more popular in the treatment of small intracranial lesions. The use of radiation therapy in young children with brain tumors raises some special considerations. Since children are likely to experience significant radiation-induced normal-tissue reactions, aggressive immobilization and field shaping are usually used to minimize irradiation of nontarget normal tissues. Due to the often disastrous normal-tissue reactions in very young children, radiation is frequently withheld. Treatment is often with surgery alone with or without chemotherapy, with radiation therapy reserved for salvage.

Gliomas. Tumors of glial origin can be oligodendrogliomas, ependymomas, or most commonly astrocytomas. They represent approximately 45 percent of all intracranial tumors. A low-grade astrocytoma is slower-growing and less aggressive than a high-grade or malignant astrocytoma, which grows more rapidly. In patients with low-grade astrocytomas that are totally resected, no further therapy is generally necessary. In patients with a subtotal resection, the need for radiation therapy is uncertain. The value of postoperative radiation therapy in incompletely resected malignant astrocytomas, is clearer.[46] The dose is somewhat controversial but is often 5500 to 6000 cGy delivered at 180 to 200 cGy per fraction. Boost doses are sometimes delivered using an interstitial implant. Chemotherapy is also often administered.

Complete resection of gliomas is sometimes not possible due to the tumor location—for example, in the brainstem. A stereotactically guided needle biopsy is usually performed to establish the diagnosis. Radiation therapy is the primary treatment of these tumors. The treatment is usually given via opposed lateral fields, which should encompass the tumor with approximately 2 cm margins. The dose is usually 5000 to 6000 cGy at conventional fractionation. Due to the relatively poor results with conventional dose fractionation schedules, hyperfractionated treatment schedules are being investigated. The treatment is delivered twice daily (bid), in fractions of 100 to 120 cGy each, 5 days per week, to 7020 to 7200 cGy. Ependymomas can arise in the brain or the spinal cord and may require postoperative CSI irradiation.

Medulloblastoma. Medulloblastoma represents about 20 percent of all childhood brain tumors, with the peak age of incidence of at approximately 5 years. It can also occur in older children and adults. The primary lesion is usually found in the posterior fossa, and it may cause hydrocephalus secondary to obstruction of the fourth ventricle. In patients with increased pressure, a shunt may be necessary. The shunt is often ventricular-peritoneal, and malignant cells can possibly spread to the peritoneal cavity through the shunt. Patients with medulloblastoma require radiation therapy to the entire craniospinal axis due to the marked propensity for cerebrospinal fluid (CSF) seeding. The dose is usually approximately 3600 cGy to the whole brain and spinal axis at 150 to 180 cGy per fraction. A boost of an additional 1000 to 2000 cGy is then delivered to the posterior fossa. Chemotherapy is often used in addition to radiation therapy. In very young children, it is given to delay tumor growth, with radiation therapy reserved for use at a later date.

Craniopharyngioma. Craniopharyngioma, which primarily occurs in children, originates in remnants of Rathke's pouch* at the junction between the infundibular stalk and the pituitary gland. It is usually located superior to the sella turcica and may cause pressure on the surrounding structures, such as the hypothalamus, optic chiasm, pituitary stalk, and cavernous sinus. Pressure on the optic chiasm or the optic nerve may cause diminished visual acuity and produce visual field deficits. Pressure on the pituitary gland may cause diabetes insipidus. These tumors are usually cystic and can be drained to relieve pressure. Total removal is usually attempted through a frontal craniotomy; however, total exci-

* Rathke's pouch, named for the German anatomist Martin Heinrich Rathke (1793–1860), is a diverticulum from the embryonic buccal cavity, from which the anterior lobe of the pituitary gland is developed. The lumen persists in adults as a small colloid-filled cyst.

sion is often not possible due to the location. Subtotal surgical resection is usually followed by radiation therapy. Postoperative external beam radiation therapy is usually employed to the site of the remaining tumor plus a small margin, delivering approximately 4500 to 5500 cGy in 5 1/2 to 6 weeks. Instillation of colloidal yttrium 90 has been used in the treatment of cystic craniopharyngiomas (Chap. 15).[47]

Meningioma. Meningiomas, which represent approximately 20 percent of all primary brain tumors, arise from the lining of the CNS. They are most commonly found in the convexity of the skull, the falx, the sphenoid ridge, posterior fossa, parasellar region, olfactory groove, and sometimes the spine. Most meningiomas are considered benign because they have low proliferative capacity and limited invasiveness. They are "locally malignant" because they cause mechanical pressure. These tumors are usually well circumscribed and do not invade the adjacent brain. Occasionally, meningiomas are more anaplastic, have a higher proliferative capacity, and are invasive into the adjacent brain and/or bone. Surgical resection is the treatment of choice for meningiomas, and radiation therapy is used in inoperable cases, following incomplete resection, and for management of recurrences. The need for adjunctive radiation therapy is determined on the basis of surgical resection and histologic features. For completely resected benign meningiomas, radiation therapy is usually not recommended; in incompletely resected patients, however, there is an apparent benefit of postoperative radiation therapy.[48] It is not clear whether postoperative radiation therapy should be given in the immediate postoperative period following an incomplete resection or when disease progression occurs. Patients with benign meningioma appear to do fairly well with either scenario.[49] The treatment volume should include the site of residual disease or the tumor site, with a margin of at least 2 cm. More generous margins may be necessary in areas where it is difficult to be certain of the remaining tumor. A dose of 5000 to 5400 cGy with conventional fractionation is recommended. Radiation therapy is usually used in patients with malignant meningiomas due to their more aggressive behavior.

Lymphoma of the Central Nervous System.
Primary CNS lymphoma has increased in frequency as a result of the AIDS epidemic. Because AIDS-related lymphomas occur in a younger population (usually male), the age for the peak incidence is decreasing. Since primary CNS lymphoma is usually aggressive, invasive, and multifocal, whole-brain irradiation is generally recommended. Due to the risk of ocular involvement, the posterior orbits should be included in the treatment fields. The prognosis for patients with CNS lymphoma is poor. For AIDS-related CNS lymphoma, the prognosis is worse, and these patients are often treated with a shorter course of irradiation.

PITUITARY GLAND

The pituitary gland is a hormone-producing gland situated in the sella turcica, inferior to the brain. The sphenoid sinus is anterior-inferior while the optic chiasm lies above and anterior of the sella turcica. Pituitary tumors often secrete hormones, and the presenting symptoms are usually referable to excess hormone levels (hyperthyroidism from excess thyroid-stimulating hormone production, acromegaly from excess growth hormone, galacturia, impotence,

and so on). These tumors, often termed microadenomas, are usually small. Nonfunctioning tumors usually present as larger masses with symptoms caused by compression of the gland or the optic chiasm, leading to changes in hormone production and visual loss. The tumors can grow fairly large and extend into the temporal fossa, causing headaches and other neurologic symptoms. For small tumors, surgical resection is usually performed via a transsphenoidal approach. This procedure is usually safer and better tolerated than a frontal craniotomy. For large tumors, craniotomy may be necessary. With either approach, complete resection is not always possible, and the addition of postoperative radiation therapy may prevent recurrence.[50] Radiation therapy alone is also an effective alternative. A dose of 4500 to 5000 cGy with conventional fractionation appears to provide tumor control in most patients.

POSITIONING AND IMMOBILIZATION

Positioning and immobilization for pituitary gland tumors is difficult and usually requires a modification of the conventional immobilization used for head and neck irradiation. In the treatment of pituitary lesions and intracranial tumors near the sella

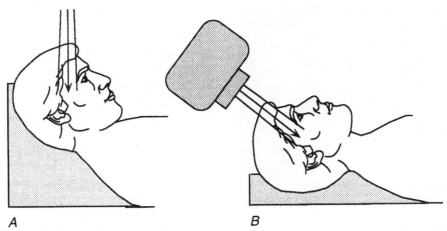

A   *B*

Figure 10.35 For a vertex field used in the treatment of pituitary lesions, the neck must be flexed *(A)* or, alternatively, the patient's head remains in a neutral position and the couch is turned 90° and then the gantry is turned to the appropriate angle *(B)*.

through a three-field or arc technique, the head is often tilted forward, with the chin tucked down on the chest (Fig. 10.35A) to allow an anterior (or fron-

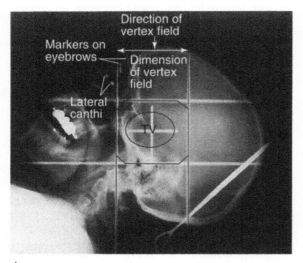

A

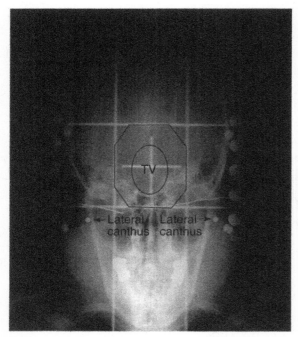

B

Figure 10.36 *A* and *B*. The caudal field-defining wire must be superior and posterior of the eye to prevent the vertex field from including the eyes. Typical vertex and lateral fields used in the treatment of pituitary lesions are shown.

tal) field to enter in a plane posterior and superior to the eyes. To verify that the head position is acceptable, a radiopaque marker should be placed on each lateral canthus. With the patient's head tilted forward and the gantry of the simulator turned to 90° (to the lateral), the isocenter is placed in the center of the target. The lateral fields are usually posterior and cephalad to the eyes, but if the patient's neck is not flexed enough, the vertex field may not clear the eyes. To test if the head position is acceptable, the field size is first set with the gantry in the lateral position. In fluoroscopy, the position of the anterior vertical field-defining wire, which indicates the caudal border of the vertex field, is determined with respect to the eye marker. When it is posterior and cephalad of the marker, the vertex field will project posterior and superior to the eyes (Fig. 10.36). If this is not the case, the neck must be flexed more. This method of testing the amount of needed head flexion should precede the head-immobilization procedure.

A customized support should be provided under the patient's head and shoulders to fix the patient properly in the flexed position. A large triangular-shaped Styrofoam block, produced from leftover pieces of Styrofoam from the block-cutting room, can be placed under the head and shoulders as a support. The dimensions of this support depend on the amount of neck flexion required and should be tested prior to immobilization. The dimensions are usually on the order of 8 to 10 in. on each of the three sides and the width is approximately 3 in. The support is then placed in a plastic bag on top of the head holder base plate so that it extends down to the shoulders. Foaming agents* (approximately 250 to 300 mL) are then poured inside the bag and, with the air squeezed out of the bag, the patient is returned to the head support. The foam will expand in the direction of least resistance and will therefore have to be constrained to remain in contact with the patient as it expands and sets. It is important to minimize the width of this mold on either side of the head where the face mask later will be pulled down. Excess foam should therefore be allowed to expand superior to the patient's head rather than laterally. When the foam has hardened, a thermoplastic mask is made, as de-

* Smithers Medical Products, Inc., Akron, OH.

scribed in Chap. 9. This position, with the head flexed, is sometimes uncomfortable for the patient and difficult for the patient and the technologist to maintain. Some patients tend to slide down on the treatment couch. A board fastened to the treatment couch below the feet may eliminate this problem. An alternate technique is to leave the head in a neutral position and then turn the treatment couch 90° with respect to its normal position and rotate the gantry until the frontal field enters posterior-superior to the eyes (Figs. 10.35*B*, 10.19, and 10.20). Leaving the patient's head in a neutral position and arranging the beam orientations through the motions of the machine cannot, in most departments, be used in moving-beam treatments (rotation or arcs), since it requires simultaneous collimator, gantry, and couch motions.

Treatment Techniques and Simulation. For small tumors, an arc technique using wedges that are reversed midway through the arc can be used, as shown in Chap. 9, Fig. 9.35, for a nasopharynx tumor. This technique delivers a cylinder-shaped high-dose area with a fairly rapid fall-off in the periphery. The wedge angle needed for the arc depends on the number of degrees of the rotation and the beam energy used. Using 6-MV photons and a 180° arc usually requires a 30° to 45° wedge, while higher photon energy beams (15-MV) or larger arcs require a smaller wedge angle. Alternatively, a three-field technique, consisting of anterior and opposed lateral wedged fields can be used in an effort to spare the temporal lobes (Fig. 10.18). A sagittal arc, as described earlier, can also be performed (Fig. 10.23). In patients with large pituitary lesions, the width of the anterior field may have to be so wide that very little sparing occurs laterally. In those patients, it may be adequate to treat only opposed lateral fields (Fig. 10.17). If the field extends close to the skull laterally, low-energy beams may have to be used.

MORBIDITY

A dose of 6000 cGy over 6 to 7 weeks can usually be given to all or part of the brain without significant acute or late consequences in an adult patient. Hy-

perfractionated and accelerated irradiation schedules delivering higher doses have also been used.

Acute reactions to irradiation are thought to be caused by radiation-induced edema, which causes symptoms of increased intracranial pressure, such as headaches. This can usually be successfully treated with steroids. Several weeks to months following radiation therapy, patients may experience some intermediate increase of the preexisting symptoms and fatigue. Administration of steroids may be necessary to alleviate the symptoms.

The late sequelae of brain irradiation can be severe and vary in appearance. The most severe injury is probably necrosis, which can be fatal. The risk of adverse effects depends on both the fraction size and total dose. Other factors, such as chemotherapy, may affect the tolerance of the brain. Children under the age of 3 years are thought to be more susceptible to injuries due to the brain's incomplete development. Decreased IQ, learning disabilities, and behavioral difficulties have been attributed to brain irradiation.[51] Brain irradiation may also cause hypothalmic-pituitary dysfunction; therefore children in whom the pituitary gland is irradiated probably should be evaluated for pituitary function before and periodically after radiation therapy. Another late sequela of brain and spine irradiation in children is retarded growth. Decreased levels of intellectual function have been observed in adults following brain irradiation.[13,52]

Acute radiation-induced spinal injury has been termed *Lhermitte's sign.** It is manifest as sudden, transient, electric-shock-like paresthesias or numbness radiating from the neck to the extremities when the patient flexes the head. The syndrome usually develops several weeks to months following radiation therapy and usually resolves gradually over the following 3 to 6 months without intervention.

Radiation-induced transverse myelitis is one of the most dreaded complications of radiation therapy. The fear makes radiation oncologists uncomfortable using high doses near the spinal cord. The symptoms of myelitis, which are irreversible, may be partial in some patients; in others, there is progressive loss of

---

* Named after Jean Lhermitte (1877–1959), a French neurologist.

function that becomes complete over a several-month period. Approximately 50 percent of the patients die of secondary complications. Less commonly, radiation-induced myelopathy is manifest by the acute onset of paraplegia or quadriplegia that evolves over several hours or days. This is thought to be caused by an infarction of the spinal cord. Other spinal cord lesions may simulate radiation myelopathy, and it can be difficult to distinguish them from radiation myelopathy. The risk of myelopathy following 5000 cGy in 25 fractions is less than 0.5 percent.[53] The spinal cord's tolerance has been studied by many authors.[54–62]

PROBLEMS

10.1 The most common of all intracranial malignancies is
(*a*) Glioblastoma multiforme
(*b*) Astrocytoma
(*c*) Pituitary adenoma
(*d*) Metastatic disease

10.2 A stereotactic frame is intended for use in
(*a*) Multifraction large-field treatments
(*b*) Single-fraction treatments
(*c*) Any brain treatment
(*d*) Retreatment of brain tumors

10.3 When adjacent fields are matched, it is more important to
(*a*) Reproduce the *location* of the gap during the entire treatment course than to match the fields correctly on a given day
(*b*) Match the fields precisely in the same *location* every treatment than to have a perfect match in a slightly different place
(*c*) It does not matter where the gap is as long as the beams do not overlap
(*d*) Match the fields precisely during a given treatment than to reproduce the *location*

10.4 To appreciate the position of the eyes relative to the beam
(*a*) A visual check is made before taking the simulation film
(*b*) A radiopaque marker is placed on the lateral canthus of each eye
(*c*) A radiopaque marker is placed on the bridge of the nose between the eyes
(*d*) A 3 to 4° couch angle is always necessary

10.5 Dose heterogeneities within the brain when opposed lateral fields are used
(*a*) Are increased when higher-energy photon beams are used
(*b*) Are of no concern when photon beams are used
(*c*) Are increased when lower-energy photon beams are used
(*d*) Can be avoided by increasing the weighting on one beam

10.6 To minimize beam divergence into the eye on the opposite side, when treating a brain through opposed lateral fields
(*a*) The collimator is rotated so there is no divergence
(*b*) The beam is centered at the lateral canthus of the eye

(*c*) The patient's head is turned when each field is treated so that the beam exits behind the eyes

(*d*) The couch is rotated so that the beam exits behind the eyes

10.7   A vertex field is difficult to treat because
   (*a*) The patient is usually not comfortable
   (*b*) The collimator and the gantry must both be turned
   (*c*) The couch and the gantry must be turned
   (*d*) There is no way of obtaining a port film

10.8   When the entire spinal axis must be treated, the patient's posterior surface should be as flat as possible
   (*a*) To make the gap between the spinal fields smaller
   (*b*) To make the dose more uniform
   (*c*) So the patient's position can be reproduced
   (*d*) So the patient is comfortable

10.9   Lateral brain fields and a posterior spinal field are matched by
   (*a*) Turning the collimator when treating the lateral fields and turning the couch when treating the posterior spinal field
   (*b*) Turning the couch when treating the lateral fields and turning the collimator when treating the posterior spinal field
   (*c*) Turning the collimator and the couch when treating the lateral fields
   (*d*) Turning the couch and the collimator when treating the posterior spinal field

10.10   To trace the tumor volume onto a lateral simulation film, a sagittally reconstructed CT or MRI image of the patient's head
   (*a*) Can be enlarged to the size of the head on the lateral simulation film
   (*b*) Can be used if they are enlarged to twice the size
   (*c*) Cannot be used because they may not represent the midsagittal plane
   (*d*) Cannot be used because the plane of the reconstruction may be tilted

10.11   When a three-field technique (vertex and opposed lateral) is used to treat a pituitary lesion
   (*a*) Wedges are used in the lateral fields
   (*b*) Wedges are used in all three fields
   (*c*) A wedge is used in the vertex field and this is weighted most
   (*d*) All fields are unwedged and equally weighted

10.12   When a 6-MV photon beam is used in a 180° arc technique to treat a pituitary lesion
   (*a*) A 45° wedge is used and the direction does not matter
   (*b*) No wedges are necessary
   (*c*) A 30° wedge is used in the same direction during one treatment and during the next treatment the direction is reversed
   (*d*) A wedge is used and is reversed midway in the arc

10.13   The disadvantages of a vertex field is that
   (*a*) It often exits through the brain and the chest
   (*b*) It often exits in the pharynx and the spinal cord

(*c*) It often exits in the eyes
(*d*) It often exits on the chest

10.14 Field gaps are often shifted two or three times during a course of treatment to
(*a*) Reduce the risk of nausea and vomiting
(*b*) Reduce the risk of overdosage in the spinal cord
(*c*) Change the exit point of the overlap
(*d*) Make the gap larger

10.15 When the lateral cranial fields are treated and the couch is turned to facilitate the gap with the posterior spinal field

(*a*) The SSD becomes shorter in the cervical spine segment when both lateral fields are treated
(*b*) The SSD becomes longer in the cervical spine segment when the right field is treated and shorter when the left field is treated
(*c*) The SSD in the cervical spine segment of the lateral fields is unchanged
(*d*) The SSD becomes longer in the cervical spine segment when both fields are treated

10.16 In a typical CSI setup, to avoid having the caudal margin of the lateral brain fields diverge into the cephalad aspect of the posterior spinal field, the foot of the couch is turned

(*a*) Away from the collimator
(*b*) There is no couch rotation
(*c*) In toward the collimator

10.17 To determine the depth of the spinal cord
(*a*) Measure the depth on a lateral radiograph taken with a lead wire over the spine
(*b*) Measure the depth on a recent MRI
(*c*) Measure the depth in an anatomy book
(*d*) Measure the depth on the myelogram

10.18 A sagittal contour to calculate a dose distribution from the posterior spine fields can be obtained
(*a*) From the lateral simulation films of the brain
(*b*) Using a lead wire
(*c*) Using a sagittal MRI image
(*d*) From a lateral scout view on the CT with radiopaque wire over the spine

10.19 Of all childhood brain tumors, medulloblastoma represents about
(*a*) 70 percent
(*b*) 20 percent
(*c*) 10 percent
(*d*) 50 percent

10.20 Symptoms of myelopathy
(*a*) Are reversible
(*b*) Start within a few weeks following radiation therapy
(*c*) Cause no harm
(*d*) Are irreversible

REFERENCES

1. Wingo AP, Tong T, Bolden S: Cancer statistics. *CA* 45:8, 1995.
2. Schlegel W, Pastyr O, Bortfeld T, et al: Computer systems and mechanical tools for stereotactically guided conformation therapy with linear accelerators. *Int J Radiat Oncol Biol Phys* 24:781, 1992.
3. Menke M, Hirschfield F, Mack T, et al: Photogrammetric accuracy measurements of head holder systems used for fractionated radiotherapy. *Int J Radiat Oncol Biol Phys* 29:1147, 1994.
4. Hariz MI, Eriksson AT: Reproducibility of repeated mountings of a noninvasive CT/MRI stereoadapter. *Appl Neurophysiol* 49:336, 1986.
5. Latinen LV: Noninvasive multipurpose stereoadapter. *Neurol Res* 9:137, 1987.
6. Gill SS, Thomas DGT, Warrington AP, Brada M: Relocatable frame for stereotactic external beam radiotherapy. *Int J Radiat Oncol Biol Phys* 20:599, 1991.
7. Kooy HM, Dunbar SF, Tarbell NJ, et al: Adaptation and verification of the relocatable Gill-Thomas-Cosman frame in stereotactic radiotherapy. *Int J Radiat Oncol Biol Phys* 30:685, 1994.
8. Delannes M, Daly NJ, Bonnet J, et al: Fractionated radiotherapy of small inoperable lesions of the brain using a non-invasive stereotactic frame. *Int J Radiat Oncol Biol Phys* 21:749, 1991.
9. Sheline GE, Brady LW: Radiation therapy for brain metastases. *J Neurooncol* 4:219, 1987.
10. Gillin MT, Kline RW, Kun LE: Cranial dose distribution. *Int J Radiat Oncol Biol Phys* 5:1903, 1979.
11. Lerch IA, Newall J: Adjustable compensators for whole brain irradiation. *Radiology* 130:529, 1979.
12. Halperin EC, Bentel G, Heinz ER, Burger PC: Radiation therapy treatment planning in supratentorial glioblastoma multiforme: An analysis based on post mortem topographic anatomy with CT correlations. *Int J Radiat Oncol Biol Phys* 17:1347, 1989.
13. Hochberg FH, Slotnick B: Neuropsychologic impairment in astrocytoma survivors. *Neurology* 30:172, 1980.
14. Orr KY, Miller RW, Wersto N, Glatstein E: A simple method for indirectly verifying noncoplanar treatment fields in radiotherapy. *Med Dosim* 17:213, 1993.
15. Reisinger SA, Palta J, Tupchong L: Vertex field verification in the treatment of central nervous system neoplasms. *Int J Radiat Oncol Biol Phys* 23:429, 1992.
16. Daftari I, Petti PL, Collier JM, et al: The effect of patient motion on dose uncertainty in charged particle irradiation for lesions encircling the brain stem and spinal cord. *Med Phys* 18:1105, 1991.
17. Tokuuye K, Akine Y, Tokita N, et al: Linac-based small-field radiotherapy for brain tumors. *Radiother Oncol* 27:55, 1993.
18. Leksell L: A stereotactic apparatus for intracerebral surgery. *Acta Chir Scand* 99:229, 1949.
19. Leksell L: The stereotaxic method and radiosurgery of the brain. *Acta Chir Scand* 102:316, 1951.
20. Souhami L, Oliver A, Podgorsak EB, et al: Radiosurgery of cerebral arteriovenous malformations with dynamic stereotactic irradiation. *Int J Radiat Oncol Biol Phys* 19:775, 1990.
21. Phillips MH, Frankel KA, Lyman JT, et al: Comparison of different radiation types and irradiation geometries in stereotactic radiosurgery. *Int J Radiat Oncol Biol Phys* 18:211, 1990.
22. Flickinger JC, Lunsford LD, Wu A, et al: Treatment planning for gamma knife radiosurgery with multiple isocenters. *Int J Radiat Oncol Biol Phys* 18:1495, 1990.
23. Lunsford LD, Flickinger J, Lindner G, Maitz A: Stereotactic radiosurgery of the brain using the first United States 201 cobalt-60 source gamma knife. *Neurosurgery* 24:151, 1989.
24. Flickinger JC, Maitz A, Kalend A, et al: Treatment volume shaping with selective beam blocking using the Leksell gamma unit. *Int J Radiat Oncol Biol Phys* 19:783, 1990.
25. Barish RJ, Barish SV: A new stereotactic X-ray knife. *Int J Radiat Oncol Biol Phys* 14:1295, 1988.
26. Lutz W, Winston KR, Maleki N: A system for stereotactic radiosurgery with a linear accelerator. *Int J Radiat Oncol Biol Phys* 14:373, 1988.
27. Saunders WM, Winston KR, Siddon RL, et al: Radiosurgery for arteriovenous malformations of the brain using a standard linear accelerator: Rationale and technique. *Int J Radiat Oncol Biol Phys* 15:441, 1988.
28. Gehring MA, Mackie TR, Kubsad SS, et al: A three-dimensional volume visualization package applied to stereotactic radiosurgery treatment planning. *Int J Radiat Oncol Biol Phys* 21:491, 1991.
29. Siddon RL, Barth NH: Stereotactic localization of intracranial targets. *Int J Radiat Oncol Biol Phys* 13:1241, 1987.
30. Bottrill DO, Rogers RT, Hope-Stone HF: A composite filter technique and special patient jig for the treatment of the whole brain and spinal cord. *Br J Radiol* 38:122, 1965.
31. Bukovitz AG, Deutsch M, Slayton R: Orthogonal fields: Variations in dose vs. gap size for treatment of the central nervous system. *Radiology* 126:795, 1978.
32. Dewit L, Van Dam J, Rijnders A, et al: A modified radiotherapy technique in the treatment of medulloblastoma. *Int J Radiat Oncol Biol Phys* 10:231, 1984.
33. Glasgow GP, Marks JE: The dosimetry of a single "hockey stick" portal for treatment of tumors of the cranio-spinal axis. *Med Phys* 10:672, 1983.
34. Griffin TW, Schumacher D, Berry HC: A technique for cranial-spinal irradiation *Br J Radiol* 49:887, 1976.
35. King GA, Sagerman RH: Late recurrence in medulloblastoma. *Am J Roentgenol* 123:7, 1975.
36. Landberg TG, Lindgren ML, Cavallin-Ståhl EK, et al: Im-

provements in the radiotherapy of medulloblastoma 1946–1975. *Cancer* 45:670, 1980.

37. Tate T, Shentall G: Conformation therapy to improve the irradiation of the spinal axis. *Int J Radiat Oncol Biol Phys* 16:505, 1989.

38. Thatcher M, Glicksman AS: Field matching considerations in craniospinal irradiation. *Int J Radiat Oncol Biol Phys* 17:865, 1989.

39. Tokars RP, Sutton HG, Griem ML: Cerebellar medulloblastoma: Results of a new method of radiation treatment. *Cancer* 43:129, 1979.

40. Van Dyk J, Jenkin RDT, Leung PMK, Cunningham JR: Medulloblastoma: Treatment technique and radiation dosimetry. *Int J Radiat Oncol Biol Phys* 2:993, 1977.

41. Werner BL, Khan FM, Sharma SC, et al: Border separation for adjacent orthogonal fields. *Med Dosim* 16:79, 1991.

42. Williamson TJ: A technique for matching orthogonal megavoltage fields. *Int J Radiat Oncol Biol Phys* 5:111, 1979.

43. Bentel GC, Halperin EC: High dose areas are unintentionally created as a result of gap shifts when the prescribed doses in the two adjacent areas are different. *Med Dosim* 15:179, 1990.

44. Haie C, Schlienger M, Constans JP, Meder JF, Reynaud A, Ghenim C: Results of radiation treatment of medulloblastoma in adults. *Int J Radiat Oncol Biol Phys* 11:2051, 1985.

45. Maor MH, Fields RS, Hogstrom KR, van Eys J: Improving the therapeutic ratio of craniospinal irradiation in medulloblastoma. *Int J Radiat Oncol Biol Phys* 11:687, 1985.

46. Leibel SA, Sheline GE, Wara WM, et al: The role of radiation therapy in the treatment of astrocytomas. *Cancer* 35:1551, 1975.

47. Coffey RJ, Lunsford LD: The role of stereotactic techniques in the management of craniopharyngiomas, in Rosenblum ML (ed): *The Role of Surgery in Brain Tumor Management,* Philadelphia: Saunders, 1991.

48. Graholm J, Bloom HJG, Crow JH: The role of radiotherapy in the management of intracranial meningiomas: The Royal Marsden Hospital experience with 186 patients. *Int J Radiat Oncol Biol Phys* 18:755, 1990.

49. Solan MJ, Kramer S: The role of radiation therapy in the management of intracranial meningiomas. *Int J Radiat Oncol Biol Phys* 11:675, 1985.

50. Tsang RW, Brierley JD, Panzarella T, et al: Radiation therapy for pituitary adenoma: Treatment outcome and prognostic factors. *Int J Radiat Oncol Biol Phys* 30:557, 1994.

51. Syndikus I, Tait D, Ashley S, Jannoun L: Long-term follow-up of young children with brain tumors after irradiation. *Int J Radiat Oncol Biol Phys* 30:781, 1994.

52. Eiser C: Intellectual abilities among survivors of childhood leukemia as a function of CNS irradiation. *Arch Dis Child* 53:391, 1978.

53. Marcus Jr RB, Million RR: The incidence of myelitis after irradiation of the cervical spinal cord. *Int J Radiat Oncol Biol Phys* 19:3, 1990.

54. Abbatucci JS, Delozier T, Quint R, et al: Radiation myelopathy of the cervical spinal cord: Time, dose and volume factors. *Int J Radiat Oncol Biol Phys* 4:239, 1978.

55. Jeremic BJ, Djuric L, Mijatovic L: Incidence of radiation myelitis in the cervical spinal cord at doses of 5500 cGy or greater. *Cancer* 68:2138, 1991.

56. Kim YH, Fayos JV: Radiation tolerance of the cervical spinal cord. *Radiology* 139:473, 1981.

57. Lambert PM: Radiation myelopathy of the thoracic spinal cord in long term survivors treated with radical radiotherapy using conventional fractionation. *Cancer* 41:1751, 1978.

58. McCunniff AJ, Liang MK: Radiation tolerance of the cervical spinal cord. *Int J Radiat Oncol Biol Phys* 16:675, 1989.

59. Reinhold HS, Kaalen JGAH, Unger-Gils K: Radiation myelopathy of the thoracic spinal cord. *Int J Radiat Oncol Biol Phys* 1:651, 1976.

60. Schultheiss TE: Spinal cord radiation "tolerance": Doctrine versus data (editorial). *Int J Radiat Oncol Biol Phys* 19:219, 1990.

61. Wara WM, Phillips TL, Sheline GE, Schwade JG: Radiation tolerance of the spinal cord. *Cancer* 35:1558, 1975.

62. Wong CS, Van Dyk J, Milosevic M, Laperriere NJ: Radiation myelopathy following single courses of radiotherapy and retreatment. *Int J Radiat Oncol Biol Phys* 30:575, 1994.

11

Treatment Planning—Thorax and Breast

TREATMENT PLANNING—THORAX

Malignant tumors occurring in the thorax include carcinoma of the esophagus, thymoma, germ-cell tumors, metastatic disease, and, most commonly, lung cancer. Lung cancer is the most common form of cancer in the United States, both in terms of incidence and mortality, with approximately 169,900 new cases and 157,400 deaths estimated to occur in 1995.[1] The most significant risk factor for the development of lung cancer is smoking; however, other risk factors include asbestos and radon exposure, air pollution, and occupation.

Esophageal cancer is relatively uncommon in the United States, with approximately 12,100 estimated new cases in 1995.[1] The incidence of esophageal cancer has the greatest variation in geographic distribution of any malignancy. For example, in one province in China (Hebi), the incidence is approximately 140 per 100,000 population, while in another Chinese province (Hunyuan), the incidence is only about 1.5 per 100,000 population.[2] Risk factors are thought to include tobacco and alcohol use; however, nutritional and environmental factors are also suspected of playing a role. The prognosis for patients with esophageal cancer is poor largely due to their frequently advanced stage at presentation. Advances in chemo/radiation therapy and surgical techniques appear to have modestly improved prognosis in recent years.

Thymomas, which arise from the thymus, are the most common primary tumor in the anterior mediastinum. Thymomas rarely metastasize but can become quite large and cause local symptoms. Some tumors are invasive into surrounding critical structures and may therefore not be completely resectable.

Mediastinal germ-cell tumors, most frequently located in the anterior-superior mediastinum, can originate in the mediastinum or be metastases from primary testicular tumors. Seminomas are highly curable with radiation therapy alone, while nonseminomatous germ-cell tumors—including teratomas, teratocarcinomas, embryonal carcinomas, and choriocarcinomas—are less radiosensitive and are frequently treated by surgery and chemotherapy.

PATIENT POSITIONING AND IMMOBILIZATION— INTRATHORACIC TUMORS

Treatment of many intrathoracic tumors requires doses higher than spinal cord tolerance; therefore, following anterior and posterior fields, some oblique or lateral field arrangement is needed. To make such a field arrangement possible, the patient's arms may have to be elevated above the head. Therefore, as in all situations, one must know the anticipated beam orientation to construct an appropriate position immobilization device.

Most patients are more comfortable and therefore more relaxed when they are in the supine position. This position is usually also more reproducible. Placing the patient in the prone position appears to cause a gravitational shift of the esophagus anteriorly in some patients, thus increasing the distance between the spinal cord and the esophagus.[3,4] This method, although more of an issue before linear accelerators with small penumbras and customized beam shaping were widely used, may be useful to facilitate delivery of radiation to an esophageal tumor while respecting spinal cord tolerance. In some patients, the prone position tends to exacerbate the curvature of the spinal cord, creating another

geometric disadvantage by causing the spinal cord to lie near or within the posterior corners of lateral or oblique fields (Fig. 11.1). When customized field-shaping capabilities are available, adequate shielding is usually possible with the patient in either position.

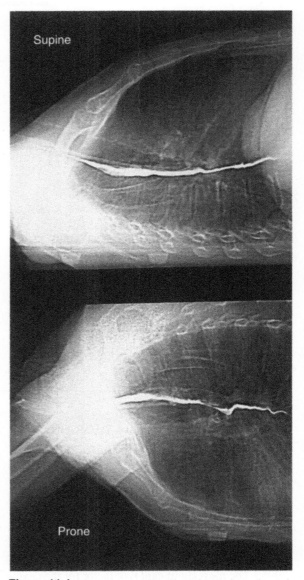

Figure 11.1   Lateral scout view of a patient in the supine and prone position with contrast in the esophagus. While the esophagus shifts anteriorly in the prone position, the curvature of the spine is increased.

The choice of position is therefore often an issue of reproducibility and the patient's ability to maintain the position during the treatment.

Traditionally, in all radiation therapy treatments, attempts have been made to position the patient "straight" on the couch. Although this is a desirable goal, more importantly, in order to treat the same volume as the simulation or "prescription" radiograph indicates, it is crucial to reposition the patient exactly as during the simulation procedure. That is, in order to deliver the "prescription treatment," the patient must be in the "prescription position." The ability to *reproduce* the position is more important than positioning the patient *straight*.

Immobilization devices for patients with intrathoracic tumors should generally extend to include the head, arms, torso, and thighs (Fig. 11.2). Such a device can be made using Alpha Cradles®*, which are described for other anatomic areas in this text. A Styrofoam form, which roughly matches the shape of the patient, is constructed to help confine the foam close to the patient's body. The Styrofoam form is placed inside a protective polyvinyl bag that is approximately 1 ft wider and 1 ft longer than the form. The foaming chemicals, prepared as recommended by the manufacturer, are evenly distributed within the form. With the patient on top of the bag, the foam expands within the bag and fills the space between the form and the patient's body. It is important that the bag be wider than the form to allow enough room for the foam to expand.

Masking tape, fastened to each side of the device and stretched across the patient, forces the foam in toward the body to form a tight-fitting mold (Fig. 11.2). Foam must also be forced up between the knees, where the sagittal alignment line is later marked. This elevation should be limited in height, since the patients must lift themselves over it to get in and out of the device. To produce a tight-fitting mold, it is important that the patient wear minimal or no clothing during its fabrication. Since patients usually wear different clothing each day during the course of treatment, the mold may be too large on some days and too tight on other days. Both situa-

tions could compromise the ability to reposition the patient correctly.

For patients in whom one or both arms need to be raised above the head, handles onto which the patient can hold can be added to the device.[5,6] Cylinder-shaped pieces of Styrofoam, small enough to hold in the hand, and about 30 to 50 mL of foaming chemicals are deposited inside a smaller bag, which is placed above the patient's head inside the larger bag. The purpose of the smaller bag is to contain some of the foam near the handles. With the required arm elevation, the cylinders are moved into the patient's

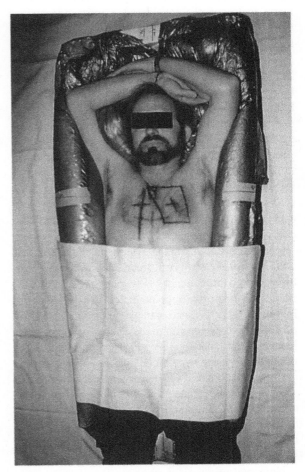

Figure 11.2 A patient repositioning is often improved by an immobilization device. Note the alignment marks on the device above the head and between the knees.

* Smithers Medical Products, Inc., Akron, OH.

hands; when the foam has hardened, these cylinders form handles. The addition of the handles appears to improve the reproducibility of the arm elevation, and it also relaxes the patient. The head elevation and degree of neck flexion can be modified by placing a piece of Styrofoam under the head or under the chest (Chap. 9, Figs. 9.2 and 9.6).

TREATMENT—LUNG CARCINOMA

Different histologic types of lung carcinoma include squamous cell (35 percent), adenocarcinoma (30 percent), large cell carcinoma (10 percent), and small cell carcinoma (20 to 25 percent). Small cell carcinoma is frequently considered a more aggressive subtype (because of early lymphatic and hematogenous spread), but all histologic types are quite aggressive and frequently fatal. Symptoms of lung cancer include cough, hemoptysis (blood in the sputum), and shortness of breath. Enlarged mediastinal lymph nodes or direct extension of the primary tumor can cause hoarseness (secondary to paralysis of the laryngeal nerve) or superior vena cava obstruction. The latter can cause edema of the upper torso and difficulty breathing; it is sometimes cause for semi-urgent radiation therapy intervention.

The primary treatment for early non-small cell cancer is usually surgical resection. The surgery can consist of pneumonectomy, lobectomy, or a wedge resection, depending on the extent and site of disease and the patient's overall medical condition. Although not without controversy, postoperative radiation therapy is often recommended in patients with involved hilar or mediastinal lymph nodes. The postoperative target volume is usually the centrally located hilar and mediastinal lymph nodes. The treatment is usually delivered via opposed anterior and posterior fields to a dose that does not exceed spinal cord tolerance, usually about 4500 cGy at conventional fractionation. This is usually followed by a boost of 1000 to 1500 cGy to the ipsilateral lymph nodes via a spinal cord–sparing technique, such as oblique or lateral fields.

Nonmetastatic limited-stage small cell carcinoma is usually treated with a combination of multiagent chemotherapy and thoracic radiation therapy. The dose is approximately 4500 to 6000 cGy delivered in fractions of 180 to 200 cGy. Hyperfractionated irradiation schedules have been used as well. To reduce the incidence of subsequent brain metastasis, prophylactic cranial irradiation is sometimes given in approximately 15 daily fractions of 200 cGy each.

Radiation therapy is also advocated as a curative mode of treatment in inoperable patients with lung cancer. The dose is approximately 6000 to 7000 cGy to sites of gross disease. These doses may have to be lowered, depending on the size of the treatment field, bearing in mind that a major risk factor for the development of radiation pneumonitis is field size. It is often impossible to deliver high doses to large targets that must include bilateral mediastinal lymph nodes because of concerns about spinal cord and lung tolerance. Due to the dose-limiting normal tissues in the chest, multiple daily fractions have been advocated in the irradiation of lung cancer. The rationale is to be able to deliver a higher target dose without increasing late normal-tissue morbidity. Radiation therapy can also be used to palliate hemoptysis, bronchial obstruction, and pain from metastasis.

TREATMENT TECHNIQUES—LUNG CARCINOMA

Patients with lung cancer usually require treatment of the primary tumor as well as the hilar, mediastinal and, in some cases, supraclavicular lymph nodes. This target volume is best covered by anterior and posterior fields (Fig. 11.3). The volume of irradiated lung parenchyma is smaller with anterior and posterior fields than with oblique fields, and the former should therefore be used until spinal cord tolerance is reached. When oblique fields are used, the angle should be minimized, since increasing the angle usually increases the volume of normal lung tissue (Fig. 11.4).

One disadvantage of using anterior and posterior fields is the dose gradient within the fields resulting from the slope of the chest in the caudal-cephalad direction. The dose in the spinal cord near the cephalad margin of the fields is therefore of particular concern because it is consistently higher than the calculated central-axis dose (Fig. 11.5). The dose

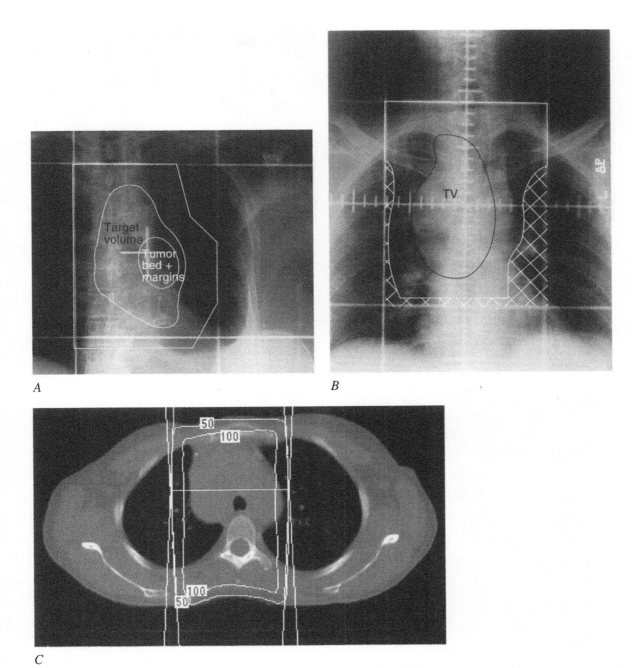

Figure 11.3 *A.* A typical lung field including the mediastinal and hilar lymph nodes. *B.* In some patients treated for lung cancer, the supraclavicular lymph nodes may have to be included bilaterally. *C.* Opposed anterior and posterior fields are usually used until spinal cord tolerance has been reached.

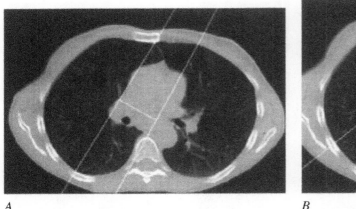 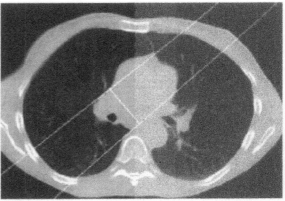

A   *B*

Figure 11.4 Increasing the angle off the vertical plane increases the volume of lung tissue within the boost fields. In *A*, 30° is used, and in *B*, the angle is increased to 50°.

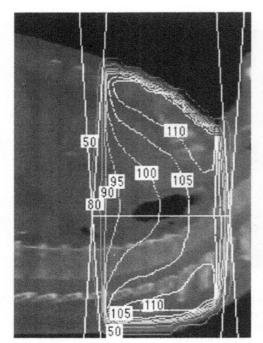

Figure 11.5 Isodose distribution in the sagittal plane from opposed anterior and posterior fields using 6-MV photon beams and showing increasing dose toward the cephalad margin.

differential depends on the steepness of the slope, the off-axis ratio, and the beam energy.

The boost is sometimes delivered via smaller anterior and posterior fields with a spinal cord block. Unfortunately, in many patients, the spinal cord block will also shield tumor, thus compromising target coverage (Fig. 11.6). Most frequently, however, the boost is delivered via oblique fields (Fig. 11.7*A*). These fields should be kept as small as possible. Figure 11.7*B* shows the combined dose distribution from delivering 4500 cGy via opposed anterior and posterior fields followed by 2000 cGy via opposed oblique fields. Figure 11.8 illustrates the same field arrangement in another patient, where 4000 cGy was delivered via opposed anterior and posterior fields, followed by opposed oblique fields delivering 1600 cGy. An additional 800 cGy was then delivered following further field reduction. The dose distributions in Fig. 11.8 show the actual dose corrected for lung inhomogeneity.

When parallel opposed fields are used and the isocenter lies at the same depth in both fields, the dose in the entrance/exit regions is usually higher (about 10 to 20 percent, depending on the overall separation and beam energy) than at the isocenter (Chap. 6, Fig. 6.23). When the oblique fields are simulated without a treatment plan, the depth of the isocenter can be different for the two opposed fields, leading to a very

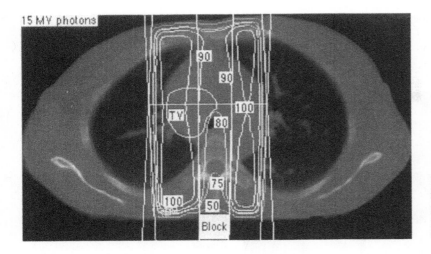

Figure 11.6 In delivering the boost in lung cancer via opposed anterior and posterior fields, a spinal cord block in the posterior field will often also block tumor.

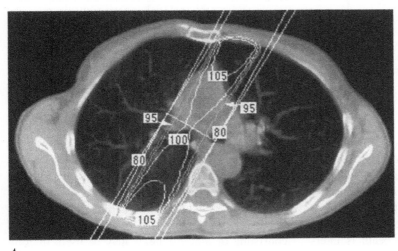

A

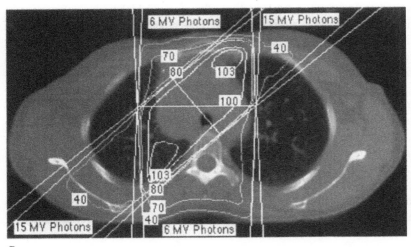

B

Figure 11.7 *A*. Dose distribution resulting from opposed oblique fields to deliver a boost to hilar and mediastinal lymph nodes. *B*. In another patient, combined dose distribution from delivering 4500 cGy via opposed anterior and posterior fields using 6-MV photon beams, followed by 2000 cGy via opposed oblique fields using 15-MV photon beams. A large hilar area receives full dose, while the dose in both the lung and spinal cord is below what is considered a tolerance dose.

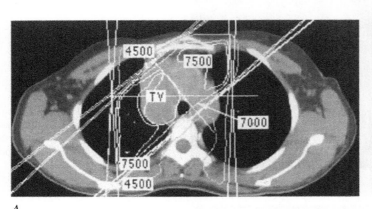
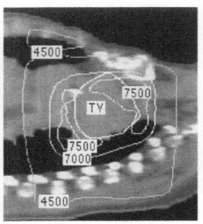

A   *B*

Figure 11.8   Combined dose distribution in the transverse *(A)* and the sagittal *(B)* planes in another patient but using the same field arrangement as in Fig. 11.7. This patient received 4000 cGy via opposed anterior and posterior fields and 1600 cGy via opposed oblique fields, followed by another field reduction delivering 800 cGy. Inhomogeneity correction has been applied to the doses in these plans.

high dose in the entrance/exit regions of the field with the greater depth. This high dose can be reduced by increasing the weighting of the field with the smaller isocenter depth. When oblique fields are used, it is sometimes difficult to determine the isocenter depth (source-surface distance, or SSD) of the posterior oblique field because the beam is intercepted by the couch, immobilization devices, and so on. Unless the isocenter is confirmed to be at the same depth in the two opposing fields, the appropriate weighting of the beams to minimize hot spots can be determined by obtaining a contour and calculating a treatment plan. Alternatively, the isocenter can be shifted to the middepth.

In some situations, usually when the target volume crosses the midline extensively, some or all of the boost is given via lateral fields. Since those fields usually include a large volume of normal lung tissue, the fields should be kept as small as possible and the dose limited (Fig. 11.9*A*). Higher-energy beams are useful due to the large lateral separation of most patients. Figure 11.9*B* and *C* illustrates the dose distribution resulting from delivering 4500 cGy via opposed anterior and posterior fields using 6-MV pho-

ton beams, followed by 1500 cGy via opposed oblique fields using 15-MV photon beams. An additional 800 cGy was then delivered via opposed lateral fields, also using 15-MV photon beams. Alternatively, a field arrangement similar to that illustrated for the treatment of esophageal cancer and consisting of multiple fields may be used. In complex multiple-field plans, additional dose to the spinal cord may be unavoidable. In these situations, it would therefore be advantageous to discontinue the large anterior and posterior fields before spinal cord tolerance has been reached.

Some very large lung tumors situated near the spinal cord cannot be adequately irradiated while respecting the spinal cord tolerance (Fig. 11.10). However, palliative treatment may be warranted. In other situations, the field arrangement can be designed to limit the volume of irradiated lung and also the dose to the spinal cord (Fig. 11.11).

There are some situations in the treatment of lung cancer that require special attention. A patient with superior vena cava obstruction, for example, may not be able to breathe while lying down and may have to be treated in an upright or reclining position. Until

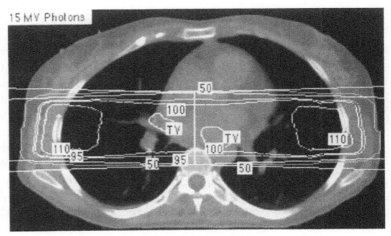

A

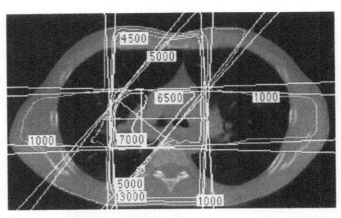

B

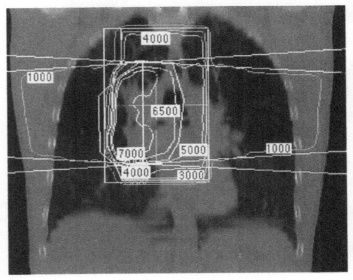

Figure 11.9 *A.* Opposed lateral fields using 15-MV photon beams often deliver higher doses in the entrance/exit regions than at the isocenter due to the large lateral separation. The composite dose distribution in *(B),* the transverse, and *(C),* the coronal plane, from using opposed anterior and posterior 6 MV-photon beams to deliver 4500 cGy, followed by opposed oblique fields using 15-MV photon beams to deliver 1500 cGy. An additional 800 cGy was then delivered via opposed lateral fields using 15-MV photon beams.

C

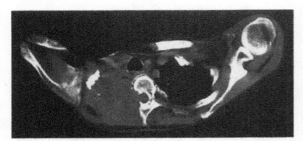

Figure 11.10 A very large lung tumor encroaching on the spinal cord cannot be treated without also irradiating the spinal cord. Irradiation may delay spinal cord compression by the tumor.

the patient's condition allows conventional positioning, treatment through a single anterior high-energy photon field may be necessary. Other conditions in which a patient may require treatment in an upright position include Hodgkin's disease with a large mediastinal mass. The upright position sometimes reduces the width of the mediastinum, and as a consequence, the volume of normal lung within the fields can be reduced.[7] Another difficult problem is posed by a kyphotic patient who is unable to lie flat on the treatment couch. These problems are also addressed in Chap. 7.

Design of treatment fields for lung tumors should

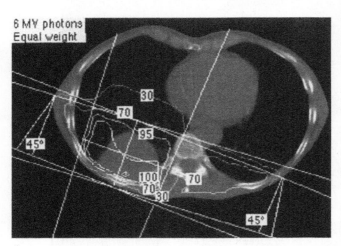

A

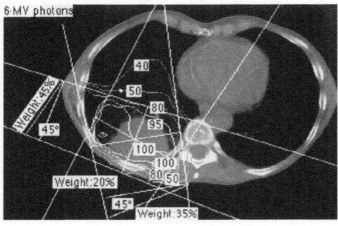

B

Figure 11.11 Treatment of a large tumor in the posterior aspect of the right lung, via *(A)* a three-field plan using equal weight, with wedges in two fields, results in approximately 75 percent of the dose in the spinal cord. *B.* The same field arrangement but with differential weights reduces the dose to the spinal cord, but the lung dose is increased.

be performed under fluoroscopy to permit observation of the motion of the target during respiration and to allow adequate margins for the motion. Customized field-shaping blocks should be used whenever possible in the irradiation of lung cancer so as to reduce the volume of normal lung tissue within the treatment fields. Because of the often complex field shapes that are needed, this is one of the major areas where customized field shaping is advantageous.

TREATMENT—ESOPHAGUS

Radiation therapy in the management of esophageal cancer is often given as definitive or preoperative treatment, usually in combination with chemotherapy or postoperatively in patients with involved surgical margins or regional lymph nodes. Palliative ra-

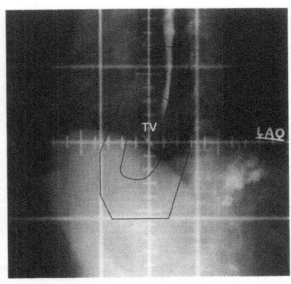

Figure 11.13 Simulation radiograph for the oblique boost fields in the same patient as in Fig. 11.12.

diation therapy is also used to relieve symptoms of obstruction and dysphagia.

For subclinical disease, approximately 5000 cGy in 5 weeks is often used, while for gross disease, approximately 6000 to 6500 cGy may be considered in fractions of 180 to 200 cGy. In patients receiving concurrent chemotherapy, slightly lower doses are sometimes used. If the tumor appears to infiltrate the tracheobronchial tree, with impending fistula development, a lower daily fraction is considered in the hope of avoiding rapid tumor regression and fistula formation. The dose used for palliation depends on the patient's general medical condition, but it is usually given in larger fractions (220 to 250 cGy) to a dose of approximately 4000 to 5000 cGy. Intraluminal brachytherapy can also be used as a palliative measure (Chap. 16).[8-11]

TREATMENT TECHNIQUES—ESOPHAGUS

Radiation therapy in the treatment of esophageal cancer generally requires relatively large fields. Be-

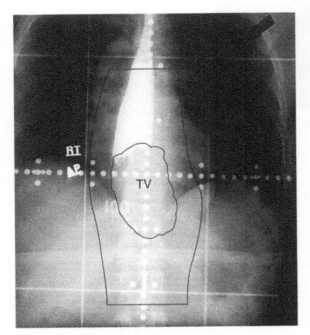

Figure 11.12 Simulation radiograph for the treatment of a large esophageal lesion causing complete blockage in the lower third of the esophagus.

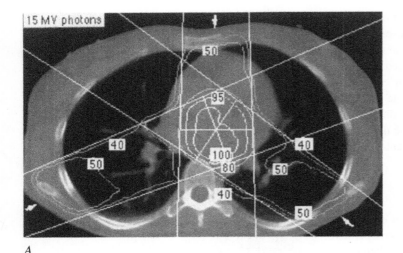

A

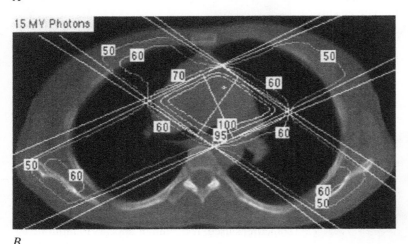

B

Figure 11.14   *A.* A three-field technique used to boost an esophageal lesion using an anterior and two posterior oblique fields. The anterior field includes the spinal cord, delivering approximately 40 percent of the boost dose. *B.* A four-field technique used to deliver a boost in the esophagus results in essentially no additional dose in the spinal cord.

cause of the pattern of spread along the mucosa of the esophagus, generous margins (5 to 6 cm) in the cephalad-caudal direction are commonly recommended.[12,13] The lateral margins should be 2 to 3 cm beyond demonstrable disease, bearing in mind that barium demonstrates only the lumen; therefore, the tumor size on CT imaging should be used when the margins are designed (Fig. 11.12). For carcinoma of the upper two-thirds of the esophagus, inclusion of bilateral supraclavicular lymph nodes should be considered.

Following approximately 4500 cGy via anterior

and posterior fields, additional dose is delivered via spinal cord–sparing techniques (Fig. 11.13). Localization of the target volume and surrounding normal radiosensitive structures such as the spinal cord is then required. A treatment-planning CT is highly recommended for planning the boost treatment. However, in the absence of CT capabilities, orthogonal radiographs obtained in the treatment position and with oral barium can also be used.

For lesions in the lower two-thirds of the esophagus, the boost is often delivered via a three- or four-field technique with customized beam shaping to

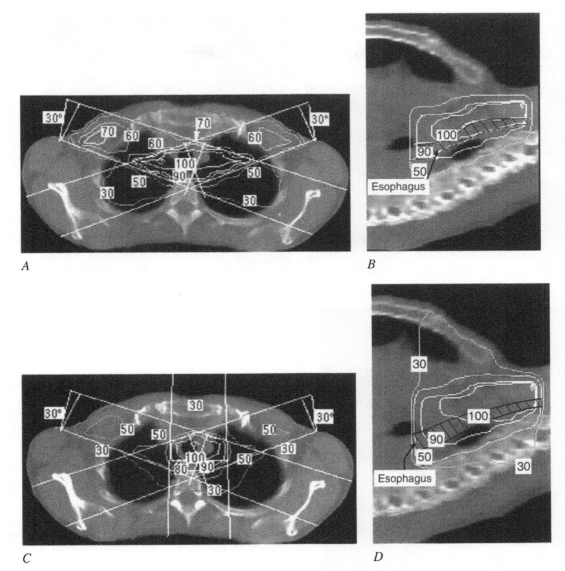

A

B

C

D

Figure 11.15 Isodose distribution shown in the transverse *(A)* and the sagittal *(B)* planes, resulting from using two anterior oblique wedged fields to boost the dose in an esophageal tumor. A large volume of lung tissue is being irradiated and the dose in the beam entrance region is relatively high. *C* and *D*. The addition of an anterior field reduces the dose in the beam entrance regions, but additional dose is delivered in the spinal cord via the anterior field.

minimize the volume of normal lung within the treatment fields. The three-field technique consists of an anterior and two posterior oblique fields, while the four-field arrangement usually consists of two anterior and two posterior oblique fields (Fig. 11.14). When the three-field technique is used, the anterior and posterior fields should be discontinued prior to reaching spinal cord tolerance, since the anterior field contributes additional dose to the spinal cord (Fig. 11.14*A*). The oblique fields used in the four-field technique can be angled so that minimal dose is delivered to the spinal cord. Since in both

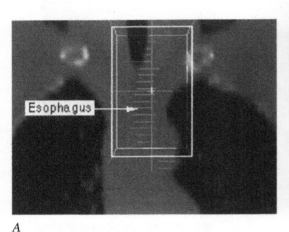

A

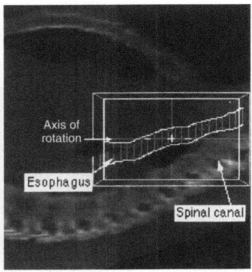

B

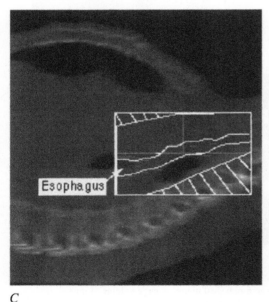

C

Figure 11.16 *A.* The esophagus, when "seen" in an anterior view, appears straight and is adequately covered by a rectangular field. *B.* In the lateral view, the field width must be increased to adequately cover the esophagus; the spinal cord is also unintentionally included. *C.* The field can be shaped to exclude the spinal cord and some other normal tissues at this beam orientation, but as the beam moves around the patient in an arc or rotation, the shape and relative position of the esophagus and the spinal cord change.

of these techniques the depth can be quite large, high-energy beams should be used to minimize the dose in the lung volume within these fields (Fig. 11.14*B*).

Delivering a boost in the upper third of the esophagus is more complicated. The difficulties are primarily due to the irregular topography of the patient's exterior contour, the curvature of the spinal canal, and the angle of the esophagus as it approaches the thoracic inlet. Anterior oblique wedged fields (Fig. 11.15) or moving-beam treatment techniques are sometimes used. In most patients, only

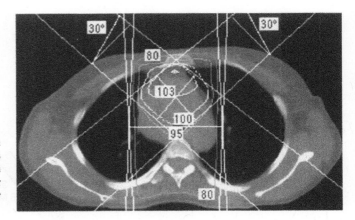

Figure 11.17 Anterior oblique wedged fields can be used to boost the dose in anterior mediastinal tumors such as thymomas. This dose distribution results from delivering 4500 cGy via opposed anterior and posterior fields followed by 1000 cGy delivered via anterior oblique fields with wedges.

moving-beam techniques with dynamic conformal beam-shaping capabilities are possible. Conventional moving-beam techniques, where the field size and shape remain unchanged as the beam moves around the patient, are frequently not possible in this region, since the esophagus and spinal cord lie at an angle with respect to the axis of the rotation (Fig. 11.16). In the anterior beam's-eye view, the esophagus appears fairly straight and a narrow rectangular field would be adequate (Fig. 11.16*A*). When the gantry is at the 90° or lateral position, the same field would be too narrow, because in this beam's-eye view, the esophagus and the spinal cord lie at an angle. If the field were to be set wide enough to include the esophagus in this view, a large volume of normal tissues, including the spinal cord, might also be irradiated (Fig. 11.16*B*). Beam shaping would protect the spinal cord at this particular beam orientation (Fig. 11.16*C*), but as the beam moves around the patient, the shape and position of the target and the spinal cord change in the beam's-eye view. The dose gradient caused by the difference in tumor depth in the neck portion as opposed to the chest portion of the fields is another disadvantage of rotational techniques. Anterior oblique field arrangements in the cervical esophagus are sometimes used but must be carefully planned to avoid inadvertent inclusion of the spinal cord. It is often difficult to appreciate the location of the spinal cord on oblique or lateral radiographs; thus the spinal cord exclusion is sometimes uncertain.

TREATMENT—MEDIASTINUM

Thymomas, which usually occur in relatively young patients, are frequently found on routine chest x-ray. The disease is often associated with myasthenia gravis, an autoimmune disease. Unlike benign thymomas, malignant thymomas grow invasively into adjacent mediastinal structures. Surgical removal is the treatment of choice. When complete resection is not possible, biopsy or partial resection is usually followed by postoperative radiation therapy (approximately 5000 to 5500 cGy at conventional fractionation). Spinal cord-sparing techniques such as anterior oblique wedged fields should be used for a boost after spinal cord tolerance has been reached (Fig. 11.17). Chemotherapy has also been used.

TREATMENT—TRACHEA

Tumors causing obstruction of the trachea sometimes constitute a radiation therapy emergency and, due to breathing difficulties, the treatment may need to be delivered with the patient in a sitting position. Delivering a few high-dose fractions (300 or 400 cGy per fraction) via an anterior field only will, it is hoped, relieve the obstruction. When the patient's condition is improved, tumor localization and treatment planning with the patient in treatment position can be carried out. A treatment technique consisting of a rotation or oblique fields can be used to minimize the dose to surrounding normal structures.

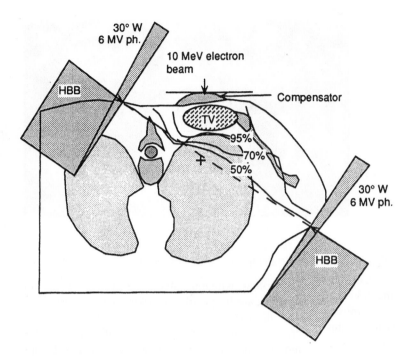

30° W
6 MV ph.

10 MeV electron
beam

HBB

Compensator

TV

95%
70%
50%

30° W
6 MV ph.

HBB

Figure 11.18 Isodose distribution resulting from using equally weighted opposed half-beam-blocked tangential fields with wedges and a 10-MeV electron beam to treat a posterior chest wall sarcoma.

TREATMENT—SOFT TISSUE TUMORS

Tumors usually occurring on the chest wall include recurrent breast cancer and connective tissue tumors such as desmoid tumors, Ewing's sarcoma, and soft tissue sarcoma. Treatment techniques for recurrent breast cancer are discussed in the section on breast cancer, below. Connective tissue tumors often present a difficult treatment problem because the necessary dose usually exceeds the tolerance of the spinal cord and the lung tissue in the vicinity. The size and location of the tumor play important roles in the choice of field arrangement. Tangential treatment fields, similar to those used in the treatment of breast cancer, can be used. When the tumor is localized but relatively large or extends to several centimeters in depth, tangential fields may include too much lung tissue or the spinal cord. The addition of an electron field may reduce the dose in a large volume of normal tissue (Fig. 11.18).

TREATMENT SIMULATION—THORAX

Prior to simulation procedures, it is necessary to have all machine settings (gantry, collimator, and couch angles) set to zero degrees. If an immobilization mold is used, the patient is repositioned in the device and the midline is aligned with the sagittal alignment line. This is determined under fluoroscopy by viewing the position of the patient's spinal column with respect to the central axis of the beam as the couch is moved along its longitudinal axis. The sagittal line is then marked on the patient's chest and on the Alpha Cradle both above the head and between the knees. Since alignment lines may not be accurate away from the isocenter, these lines are marked as close to the isocenter as possible by moving the couch along the longitudinal axis. The two alignment marks on the immobilization device are used in the daily repositioning of the patient on the couch (Fig. 11.2). Aligning two points separated by a long distance improves the accuracy of the setup. If no immobilization device is used, alignment marks are made on the patient's chest, bearing in mind that marks separated by a long distance are advantageous. These marks should preferably also be made at points where the skin tends to not move with respect to underlying structures (sternum, suprasternal notch, and so on).

When only anterior and posterior fields are used, the simulation is straightforward, with the four field-defining wires of the simulator set at the periphery of the target volume, with adequate margins, and with consideration given to respiratory motion. The isocenter should be set at the patient's midplane. Anterior and posterior radiographs should be taken for comparison with weekly port films obtained during the course of treatment. In the event that only an anterior simulation film is taken, a comparison with a posterior port film is possible, bearing in mind the differences due to beam divergence. When appropriate, oral barium should be given to patients with esophageal lesions immediately prior to the simulation procedure.

If a treatment-planning CT or orthogonal radiographs were obtained for target localization and determination of field arrangement, the patient should be realigned with reference marks made during that procedure. The position of the isocenter is then set with respect to these reference marks. The appropriateness of the isocenter position can be confirmed by viewing anterior and lateral images in fluoroscopy or by viewing the radiographs of these two beam orientations. This is accomplished by measuring the distance, both on the plan and on the radiograph, from the isocenter to a reliable reference point such as a vertebral body. When the isocenter position is satisfactory, the appropriate field size is set and the gantry is turned to the desired angle. Again, the appropriateness of these fields with respect to bony landmarks is verified. A radiograph is obtained of each treatment field for later design of beam-shaping blocks and subsequent comparison with port films. The particulars of each treatment field—such as date, field size, source-axis distance (SAD), beam angles, and so on—are recorded on each film. Both alignment lines and the treatment fields are marked on the immobilization device when possible. Experience from other treatment sites has indicated that marks made on the immobilization device are more reliable than skin marks.

In the event that the simulation of oblique fields is carried out without a treatment plan, it is customary to set the isocenter in the center of the tumor while viewing the image from the anterior direction. The gantry is then turned 90° to either side to adjust the height of the couch so that the isocenter is in the center of the tumor in this direction as well. The gantry is then turned to an angle that causes the beam to include the tumor while at the same time excluding the spinal cord. Caution should be used here, because when the isocenter for the oblique boost fields is set in the center of the tumor, the depth of the isocenter in the two fields is often not the same, and very high doses can result in the entrance/exit regions of the field with the greatest depth, as mentioned earlier. This is also discussed in detail in Chap. 6.

TREATMENT PLANNING— BREAST CARCINOMA

Breast cancer is the most commonly occurring cancer in women in the United States; approximately one in ten of all American women will develop it. It is estimated that 183,400 new cases will be diagnosed and 46,240 deaths from breast cancer will occur during 1995.[1] Breast tumors are found by the patient, on routine physical examination, or by mammography. With improved mammographic imaging techniques, tumors < 5 mm are often detected.

The first major use of radiation therapy in the treatment of primary breast cancer was to reduce locoregional recurrence rates following radical mastectomy. Radiation therapy is also used to treat locally advanced and metastatic disease. More recently, radiation therapy has been used in combination with conservative surgery as an option for patients who prefer breast-conserving treatment. The breast-conserving surgery consists of removal of the primary tumor with a margin and is referred to as *lumpectomy, tylectomy, tumorectomy*, and *segmental mastectomy*. An axillary dissection to determine the extent of regional disease is usually done as well. In appropriately selected patients, breast conservation with limited surgery and breast irradiation yields a good to excellent cosmetic result and survival rates equal to those obtained with total mastectomy.[14–17]

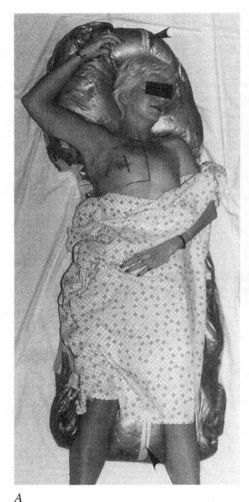

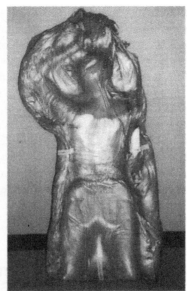

A

B

Figure 11.19 *A* and *B*. Patient positioning device for breast carcinoma. Note the alignment marks on the Alpha Cradle above the head and between the knees *(arrowheads)*. The mold is formed tightly to the patient's body *(B)*.

The regional lymph nodes are the axillary, supraclavicular, and internal mammary. The most important prognostic factor in breast cancer is the combination of the presence and extent of axillary metastasis. Patients with histologically negative axillary lymph nodes have a better likelihood of survival than patients with nodal involvement. The prognosis is inversely related to the number of involved axillary lymph nodes. While the axillary and supraclavicular lymph nodes can be palpated, the internal mammary nodes are difficult to detect. Lymphoscintigraphy can be used to localize the internal mammary lymph nodes, but this method may not always be available.[18-20] The importance of regional lymph node irradiation is uncertain.

Locally advanced disease is usually associated with axillary lymph node metastasis and occult distant disease. Systemic treatment (chemotherapy) is necessary in these situations, and this is usually combined with radiation therapy and/or surgery to treat the locoregional sites.

Hematogenous spread of breast cancer is usually

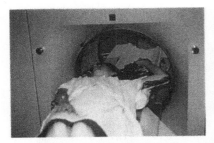

Figure 11.20   Most patients immobilized in an Álpha Cradle can be moved into the CT aperture with the arm on the involved side elevated.

to bones, lung, pleura, and liver, but it can spread anywhere, including the adrenals, ovaries, spleen, and eyes.[21]

PATIENT POSITIONING AND IMMOBILIZATION

Traditionally, breast patients are treated in the supine position, although a prone[22] or decubitus[23] position has also been proposed. The arm on the involved side is usually elevated above the head, with the face turned away from the involved side (Fig. 11.19). For several reasons, it may be advantageous, following the convention used in most other sites where the patient is placed in a symmetrical and basically straight position, to elevate both arms and keep the head straight.[24] Many patients are more comfortable with both rather than one arm elevated because they can clasp their hands together and therefore be more relaxed. Another potential advantage of a symmetrical position is the ability to match adjacent fields should the patient return for future treatment. The angle at which the arm on the involved side is elevated depends on several factors. Some of these are (1) the patient's ability to raise the arm without discomfort, (2) the ability to elevate the arm without skin folds forming in the supraclavicular area, and (3) with CT-based treatment planning, the ability to move the patient in the immobilization device through the aperture (Fig. 11.20).

To irradiate the breast, chest wall, and regional lymph nodes, several adjacent treatment fields are necessary. These are angled in different directions in an effort to spare underlying normal tissues. The

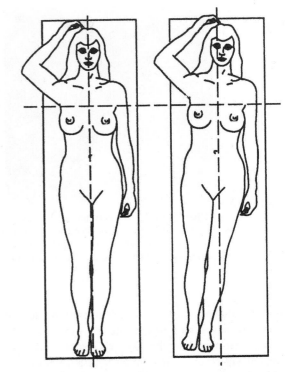

Figure 11.21   A small misalignment of the patient on the treatment couch will have the same effect as if the couch were angled.

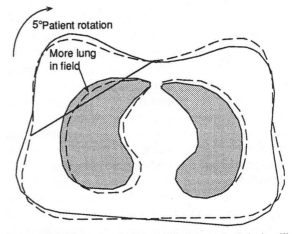

5°Patient rotation

More lung in field

Figure 11.22   A small rotation (5°) of the patient's body will have the same effect as if the gantry angle were changed by 5°. In tangential fields, the thickness of the lung tissue within the fields will be changed even when the field is set to the skin marks.

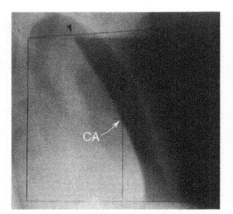 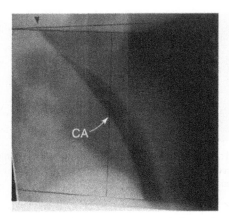

Figure 11.23 The curvature of the patient's chest wall in the beam's-eye view causes variation in the thickness of wedge material that the beam will pass through in the cephalad margin *(arrowhead, left)*. The dose is usually highest at this point unless compensators are used. In the patient on the right, the field extended farther into the thin segment of the wedge *(arrowhead)*; therefore the dose is higher than in the patient on the left.

breast and chest wall are most frequently treated via opposed tangential fields, while the supraclavicular and sometimes also the axillary lymph nodes are treated via an anterior oblique field adjacent to the tangential fields. The internal mammary lymph nodes are either included within the tangential fields or are treated in an anterior field adjacent to the medial tangential field. Matching of field margins between (1) the supraclavicular and tangential fields and (2) the internal mammary and tangential fields on the irregular chest surface is very difficult and requires rigid patient immobilization. A small misalignment of the patient with the sagittal alignment line will cause the beam orientations with respect to the patient to be changed (Fig. 11.21). A small rotation of the patient's body with respect to the lateral or horizontal alignment lines will also cause a change in beam angles with respect to the patient. For example, a tangential field that is planned to be angled 45° will actually be angled 40° (or 50°, depending on the direction of the rotation) if the patient's body is rotated 5°. When this field is set to the skin marks, it will include a larger volume of lung tissue than at the planned 45° angle (Fig. 11.22). This type of misalignment can occur even when the field edges match the skin marks correctly. To minimize these

misalignments, it is extremely important to reproduce the patient's position, and vigorous immobilization should be used.[24-27] At Duke University, an Alpha Cradle with a built-in handle—which helps in reproducing the arm elevation and is also comfortable for the patient—is used during computed tomography (CT), treatment simulation, and treatment (Fig. 11.19).[5]

The fabrication of this device is similar to that of other Alpha Cradles described for immobilization of patients with intrathoracic carcinoma and will therefore not be repeated here. There are, however, a few differences which will be addressed.

To prevent the foam from rising more than a couple of inches where the lateral tangential field is anticipated to enter, the polyvinyl bag, which covers the form, is usually taped down. With only a small barrier in this area, the lateral tangential beam is not intercepted by the foam, minimizing the loss of skin-sparing observed with high-energy beams. The skin sparing is already reduced in this region because the radiation beam enters the skin surface at a steep incline. Furthermore, the beam passes through a thinner portion of the wedge in the posterior-cephalad portion of the tangential fields than at the central axis, resulting in a higher dose in this area (Fig.

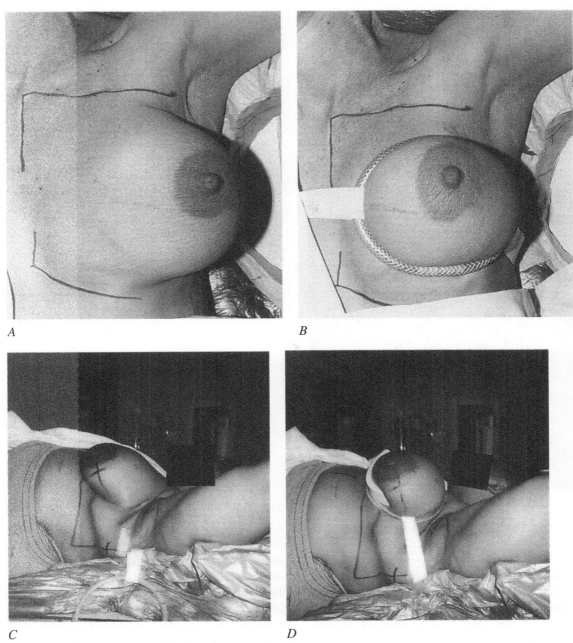

Figure 11.24 A breast positioning device is useful in shifting of the breast position on the chest. *A* and *B*. In the majority of patients with large breasts, the breast lies too far lateral and can be moved more anteriorly by using this ring. *C* and *D*. In a few patients, the breast is too far caudal and needs to be raised more cephalad. A piece of Styrofoam can be shaped to the breast and used as a barrier to elevate the breast. *E*. In some patients, a small shift of the breast medially may cause the lung volume within the tangential fields to be reduced. (The breast ring is visible in the lower image.) *F*. A port film of a patient with the breast ring in place.

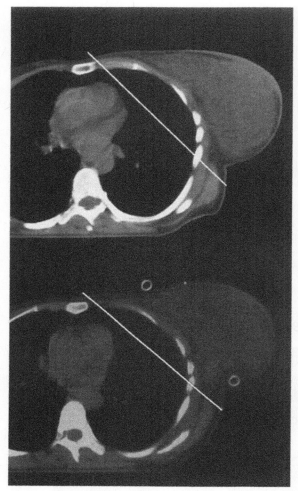

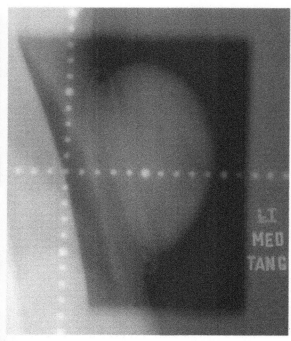

F

E

Figure 11.24   *(Continued.)*

11.23). This is also discussed in Chap. 6, Fig. 6.42. The small barrier also facilitates marking of the lateral tangential field on the Alpha Cradle. The finished Alpha Cradle must sometimes be trimmed on the uninvolved side in order to move the patient into the CT tunnel with the arm on the involved side elevated.

Alignment marks are made on the immobilization device and on the patient's skin surface during either the CT or simulation procedure, whichever is first. If the simulation procedure is first, the patient is aligned with the sagittal alignment laser under fluoroscopic visualization. Prior to aligning the patient, it

is necessary to have all machine settings (gantry, collimator, and couch angles) set to 0°. The sagittal line is then marked on the immobilization device above the head and between the knees (Fig. 11.19). Since alignment systems are frequently not accurate away from the isocenter, the lines should be marked as close to the isocenter as possible, which requires that the simulation couch be moved along the longitudinal axis (i.e., out from the gantry to mark above the head and in toward the gantry to mark between the knees). Marking the sagittal alignment line only within the treated segment—i.e., a short line on the chest—is insufficient, because a small rotation of

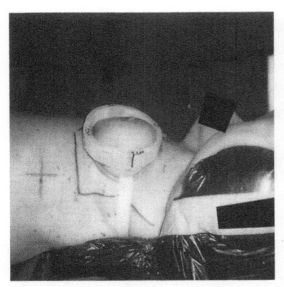

Figure 11.25 A circular barrier, made of Styrofoam, can be used in patients with flaccid breasts to prevent the breast from assuming a mushroomlike shape when the ring is used.

the patient's bony frame, though not appreciable externally, would likely lead to discrepancies when the port film was reviewed. The sagittal line is used to repeat the placement of the immobilization device with the patient during subsequent procedures, such as CT and treatment. When this line is not aligned correctly, it will have the same effect as a couch angle (Fig. 11.21). Such misalignment will also cause difficulty in repeating all other angles of these complicated treatments.

Patients with large or flaccid breasts are often difficult to treat,[28] particularly when the breast lies either too high, too low, or too far laterally for tangential fields to include it without also including a large volume of lung, axilla, or arm (Fig. 11.24). Repositioning of the breast on the anterior chest can be achieved by using a breast-positioning device* (Fig. 11.24). This consists of a polyvinyl tube formed to a ring and placed around the base of the breast. The ring is then fastened to a Velcro®† band placed

* Smithers Medical Products, Inc., Akron, OH.
† Velcro USA, Manchester, NH.

around the patient's chest. The breast is fixed in the desired position by tightening the Velcro band.[29] In the older patient with a flaccid breast, a barrier (made of Styrofoam) can be fastened to the ring to prevent the breast tissue from assuming a mushroomlike shape (Fig. 11.25).

TREATMENT TECHNIQUES

The difficulties involved in matching the fields used in breast treatment without causing over- or underdosage at the junctions has led to the development of the many breast treatment techniques described in the literature.[30–37] Most techniques address the problem of matching the tangential field with the supraclavicular field, and several solutions have been described.

Photon-Beam Techniques. The field-matching problem between the supraclavicular and tangential fields in breast treatment is similar to that described for craniospinal irradiation in Chap. 10. The primary difference in breast treatment is that the beam orientations are never vertical and horizontal; instead, they are oblique, further complicating the beam-matching problem, as discussed in the paragraphs following below.

The supraclavicular field—which is usually angled 15° to avoid inclusion of the trachea, esophagus, and the spinal cord—is set so that the central axis is on the cephalad margin of the tangential fields. A half-beam block is then used to shield the caudal half of the field that overlies the tangential fields. Thus, a transverse vertical match line with the tangential fields is created (Fig. 11.26). The cephalad margins of the two tangential fields, angled across the chest to minimize inclusion of lung tissue, diverge in opposite directions into the supraclavicular field (Fig. 11.27). To avoid this overlap, the foot of the couch is turned away from the collimator so that the two cephalad field margins become coplanar and cross the patient's chest in a straight line, that is, parallel with the caudal supraclavicular field margin (Fig. 11.28). The number of degrees by which the couch must be turned depends on the distance and the length of the tangential fields and can be found from a graph in Chap. 6 (Fig. 6.43) or from

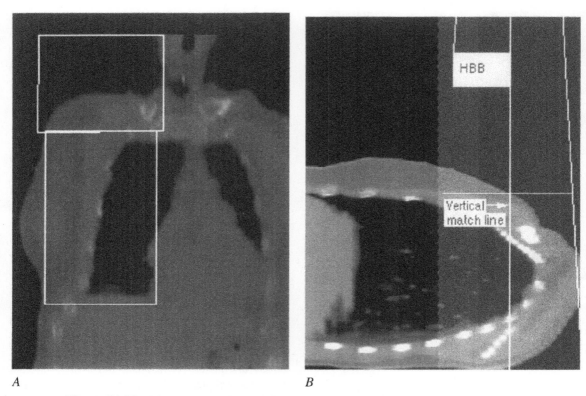

A   B

Figure 11.26 A half-beam block in the oblique supraclavicular field produces a transverse *(A)* and a vertical *(B)* match line for the tangential fields across the chest.

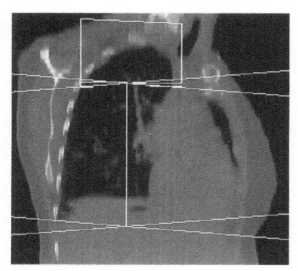

Figure 11.27 The opposed tangential fields diverge in opposite directions into the supraclavicular field.

$$\mathrm{Tan}\ \theta = \frac{\text{half-field length}}{\text{distance}} \qquad (11.1)$$

This field match would be perfect, but only if the gantry rotation for the supraclavicular and tangential fields were 0° and 90° respectively. The reason it is not perfect is that the direction of the tangential fields does not coincide with the couch motion (i.e., horizontal). Therefore, when the fields are matched on the skin surface, there is a small overlap at depth (Fig. 11.29). This overlap can be avoided by turning the collimator a few degrees.

The particular geometric problem described above is very difficult to understand and to explain, so we will go through it slowly one step at a time. We will examine the problem via the following example. The couch, gantry, and collimator angles are first set to 0°, and the vertical match line of the anterior supraclavicular field is transverse across the patient. We

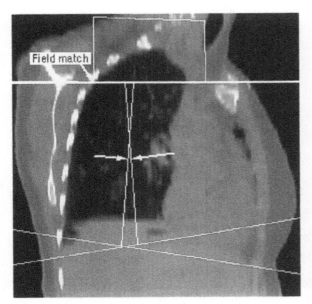

Figure 11.28   When the foot of the couch is turned away from the collimator, the tangential fields will cross the chest along the transverse vertical match line.

tangential field is angled, say 45°, to make the match perfect, the collimator must be turned half as many degrees as we have turned the couch. When the gantry was turned 90°, we had a match, and when we turned the gantry to 0°, we also had to turn the collimator the same number of degrees as the couch or return the couch to 0°. A mathematical formula to calculate the needed angles for a perfect match has been described.[38]

Another concern in breast treatment is how to prevent the "deep" margins of the tangential fields from diverging into the lung tissue (Fig. 11.31*A*). The tangential fields can be angled so that the central axes are not opposed but the deep field margins are. This requires that the cental axes of the two fields be separated by slightly more than 180° (Fig. 11.31*B*). The number of degrees depends on the field width and the distance. Another solution is to set the central axes where the deep treatment margin is desired and then use a half-beam block to shield the deep half of the field, eliminating the beam divergence.

will then set a rectangular (tangential) field so that the caphalad margin is parallel with and abuts the caudal margin of the supraclavicular field (Fig. 11.26*A*). The gantry is then turned 90° toward, for example, the right side, and the cephalad margin now diverges into the supraclavicular field (Fig. 11.30*A*). To prevent this, the foot of the couch is turned away from the collimator until the diverging beam margin becomes parallel with the vertical supraclavicular match line (Fig. 11.30*B*). Now there is a perfect match between these two fields. Without moving anything else, the gantry is returned to the vertical position or 0° (Fig. 11.30*C*). Obviously, the cephalad margin of the "tangential" field is now diverging into the supraclavicular field. We also note that, with the couch turned, the cephalad margin of the tangential field is no longer parallel to the caudal margin of the supraclavicular field (compare Fig. 11.26*A*). To make the two field edges parallel again, the collimator must be turned the same number of degrees as the couch (or the couch can be returned to 0°). From this exercise, we can deduce that when a

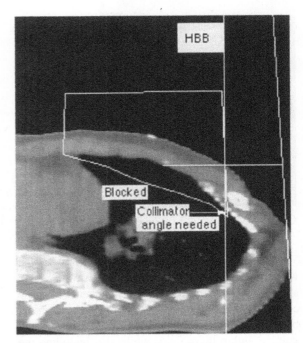

Figure 11.29   Because the beam direction of the tangential fields and the couch motion do not coincide, there is a small overlap at depth within the supraclavicular field.

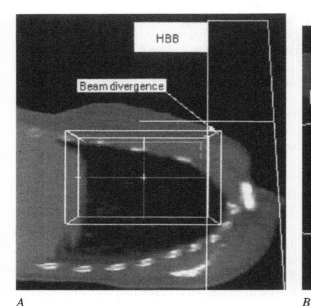

A

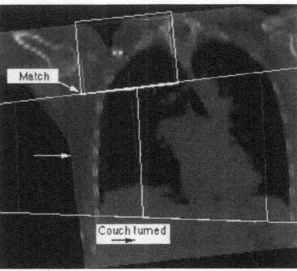

B

C

Figure 11.30 *A.* Without a couch angle, the lateral field diverges into the supra-clavicular field. *B.* To prevent this beam from diverging into the supraclavicular field, a couch angle is necessary. *C.* When the gantry angle is returned to the 0° or vertical position, the two fields no longer abut.

There is, however, yet another problem associated with breast treatment. That is, the chest wall, which also needs to be irradiated, slopes posteriorly in the cephalad direction when "seen" in the tangential beam's-eye view (Fig. 11.32). To minimize the lung volume within these fields while also including the chest wall, a collimator angle is necessary when the unblocked technique is used. The collimator angle should be such that the deep margin is more or less parallel with the slope of the chest wall (Fig. 11.32). When the half-beam block technique is used, the collimator position can remain and, instead, the block may be formed in such a way that it is parallel with the slope of the chest wall (Fig. 11.33). Each of these solutions introduces yet another problem. In the first scenario, the collimator rotation causes an

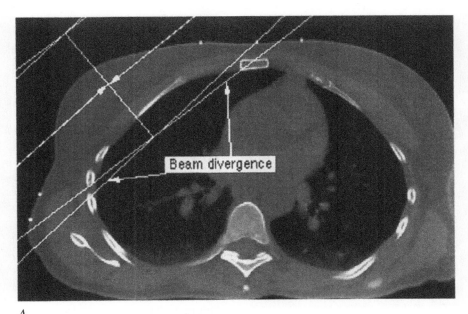

A

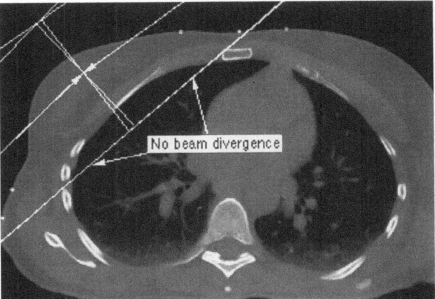

B

Figure 11.31   The ''deep'' field margins also diverge into the lung tissue *(A)*. To prevent this, the beams are angled so that the central axes are separated by slightly more than 180°, causing the ''deep'' margins to be parallel *(B)*.

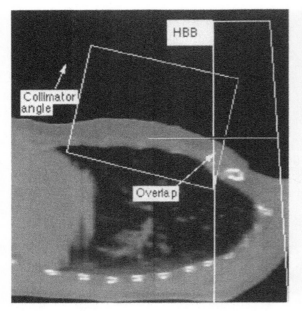

Figure 11.32 The chest wall usually slopes toward the cephalad margin. Therefore, to minimize the lung volume within the tangential fields, the collimator can be angled, so that the deep margin follows the slope of the chest wall.

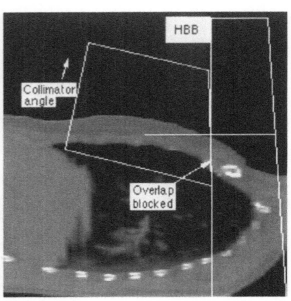

Figure 11.34 A corner block can be used to eliminate the overlap between the supraclavicular and tangential fields when the collimator is rotated in the tangential fields.

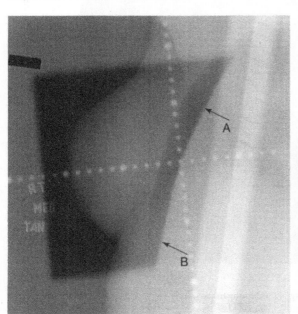

Figure 11.33 The tangential beams can also be shaped so that the field margin follows the slope of the chest wall. The beam is more or less half-beam blocked. At *A*, less than half of the field is blocked, and at *B*, more than half is blocked.

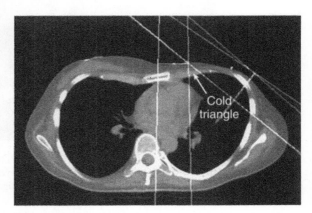

Figure 11.35 When an internal mammary lymph node field and the tangential fields are matched, there is a small triangle below and along the match line that is unirradiated.

overlap with the supraclavicular field (Fig. 11.32). This triangular overlap can be eliminated by using a corner block in the tangential fields (Fig. 11.34).[37] When the half-beam block technique is used, half of the beam is no longer blocked, but, instead, *less* than half of the field width is blocked near the cephalad margin and *more* than half of the field width is blocked near the caudal margin. Only at the central axis is half of the field width blocked (Fig. 11.33). This means that there is some divergence into the lung in the cephalad portion of the field while the divergence is slightly away from the lung in the caudal portion. The customized beam-shaping technique, offering simplicity and flexibility, has been used at Duke University since 1978.[30]

Another area where field margins must often be matched is between the internal mammary and the tangential fields. This field match is easier to understand than the problems already discussed. In this field match, there is an unirradiated triangle at depth between the fields due to the necessity of angling these fields in different directions (Fig. 11.35). To minimize the size of the "cold" area while at the same time avoiding an overlap on the skin surface, the deep margin of the tangential fields must match the ipsilateral margin of the internal mammary field. The internal mammary field, usually centered on the ipsilateral internal mammary lymph node chain, is rectangular (Fig. 11.36A). Since the chest slopes posteriorly in the cephalad direction, the field margin with which the tangential fields must be matched appears sloping in the beam's-eye view of the tangential fields (Fig. 11.36B).

As we did earlier, we will explain this in detail.

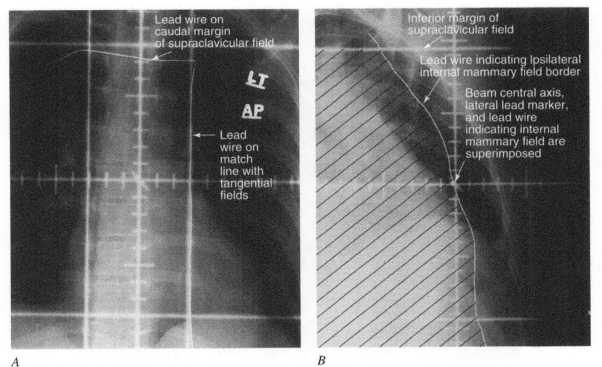

A

B

Figure 11.36   *A.* A lead wire is taped to the skin on the anterior chest where the tangential fields edge is desired. Usually, this is the match line between the internal mammary and the tangential fields, but it can also be the midline or across the midline if the internal mammary lymph nodes are to be treated in the tangential fields. *B.* The wire, although it appears straight in the anterior view, appears angled or curved when "seen" in the tangential beam's-eye view.

The field margin of the internal mammary field appears straight in the anterior view (Fig. 11.36A). When the gantry is turned to a lateral or 90° angle, it appears sloping, just as the chest slopes. Since the angle of the tangential fields lies somewhere between the anterior and lateral views just described, the slope, as seen in the tangential beam's-eye view, who have had surgery, the skin surface may even be quite irregular. Since it is the ipsilateral internal mammary field margin we must match, we need to know the exact shape of this line in the tangential beam's-eye views.

To achieve a perfect match on the skin surface, a thin lead wire is taped in place on the match line of the internal mammary field (Fig. 11.36A). In the tangential beam's-eye views, the posterior, or deep, side of the lead wire indicates the shape of the internal mammary match line on the skin surface. Customized blocks are formed to follow this line and shield the portion of the tangential fields which is deeper than the lead wire (Fig. 11.36B). In the method

where the tangential fields are defined by the straight collimator, the tangential and internal mammary field margins often do not match on the skin surface but, instead, depending on the shape of the chest surface, there are potential overlaps or gaps along the match line. In many patients, the internal mammary lymph nodes may not have to be treated, and sometimes they can be included within the tangential fields. In these situations, the field-matching problem just described is eliminated. However, it is often an advantage to maintain a straight line on the anterior chest surface to facilitate field matching in case the patient returns for additional treatment to an adjacent area later on.

In some patients there may be tumor in the unirradiated triangle along the border between the internal mammary and the tangential fields. If this area cannot be included within the tangential fields, the internal mammary field, treated primarily with an electron beam, can be angled so that its beam direction is more or less parallel to the tangential fields

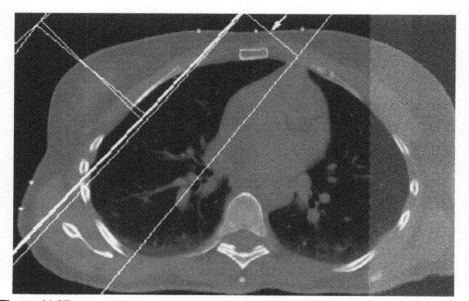

Figure 11.37 In some patients, there may be tumor present in the unirradiated triangle between the internal mammary and the tangential fields. When this area cannot be included within the tangential fields, the internal mammary field (using primarily an electron beam) can be angled along the medial tangential field. The angle should be slightly less than the tangential beam angle to account for beam divergence of the internal mammary field. (In this patient, used only for demonstration, there was no need to use this field arrangement.)

(Fig. 11.37). The portion of the dose that is delivered via photons should be kept low, since a large volume of lung tissue lies within this field. This field arrangement should be used only under extreme circumstances.

Since the position of either one of these breast fields depends on the position of its neighbor, misalignment of one field frequently results in the misalignment of all fields. One of the difficulties is that the skin surface in this area often moves with respect to deep-lying tissues, making setup marks quite unreliable. In obese patients or patients with large/flaccid breasts, the skin marks may move several centimeters with respect to underlying bony anatomy (Fig. 11.38). The degree of arm elevation on the involved side also plays a role in the position of the skin marks with respect to deeper, fixed tissues. Reproducible patient positioning and the ability to make setup marks peripheral to the breast itself as well as on a positioning device is crucial to successful radiation therapy of these patients.

A different solution to deal with the field-matching problem is to treat all fields using one isocenter that is set between the supraclavicular and tangential fields. The gantry is then turned to the appropriate angle and the areas of overlap are blocked—i.e.,

when the supraclavicular field is treated, the area irradiated by the tangential fields is blocked, and vice versa.[34,39,40] In this technique, the required field sizes are very large; for example, a typical tangential field is between 15 and 20 cm long, which means that in this technique, the collimator setting would have to be 30 to 40 cm. This may prevent wedges from being used, since most manufacturers supply wedges only for 20- to 30-cm fields. Alternatively, special wedges can be made so that they either wedge the maximum field length or can be mounted in the beam in such a way that they wedge only half of the beam in the longitudinal direction.

Electron-Beam Techniques. Use of electron beams to treat the chest wall requires very careful determination of the chest wall thickness within the entire treatment region. The electron energy is selected when one has ascertained the maximum depth within the treatment field. To prevent high doses in the underlying lung tissue, areas where the chest wall is thinner can be covered by a thickness of tissue-equivalent material (bolus), which equalizes the depth to the lung tissue within the entire field.

Treating the chest wall with multiple adjacent electron fields is difficult due to the problems of

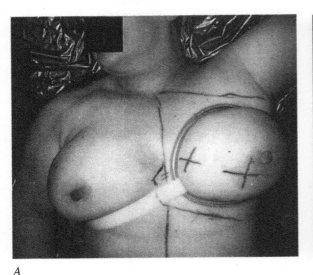 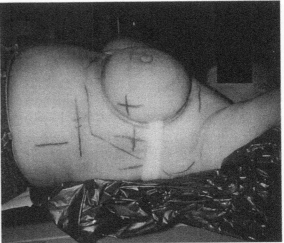

A   *B*

Figure 11.38 *A* and *B*. In many breast patients, skin marks made on the breast can shift several centimeters and should not be used for setting up the fields. In this patient, the breast was too high on the chest wall and the breast ring was used to shift the position caudally.

matching field edges and the varying thickness of the chest wall (Chap. 6, Figs. 6.57, 6.58, and 6.59). Unless the facility to build compensators and to verify the dose distribution carefully is available, multiple adjacent electron fields should be avoided. Electron-arc techniques, when carried out following careful planning, result in acceptable dose uniformity and eliminate field matching problems.[41–48] Compensating material is placed on the chest wall to provide uniform depth. Shielding of the surrounding area must be placed directly on the patient or very near the patient's skin. The dose near the cephalad margin of the field may be higher because of the smaller radius of the chest in this plane. This higher dose may, however, be balanced out by the increased SSD where the radius is smaller. If the dose is higher, the field can be shaped so that it is narrower where the radius is smaller. Thus the beam remains over any particular segment a shorter time. This particular aspect can be compared with photon rotation therapy (Chap. 6, Fig. 6.31).

Patients with parasternal tumors present a special problem because they are difficult to treat without also including a large volume of underlying lung tissue. When the parasternal mass is small, a direct electron field may be adequate. The electron cone should be placed perpendicular to the surface to minimize the air gap and thus improve dose uniformity at a specified depth. In patients with tumors that are large or contiguous with the breast tissue, it is necessary to treat both the parasternal mass and the breast in contiguous fields.

When an electron field is contemplated, the maximum depth of the tumor must be measured from the skin surface of each individual CT or MRI image and the appropriate electron beam energy is then determined (Fig. 11.39). In Fig. 11.39A, the maximum depth is measured in the direction of the beam and a composite of the tumor volumes in all levels is indicated to the right. In Fig. 11.39B, the composite tumor volume on the right is outlined with respect to the origin in the coordinate system. Here the tumor appears to be at a much greater depth and, in fact, a portion of the tumor lies outside the patient's skin surface contour indicated at the center of the tumor. The difference here is that when a tumor such as this

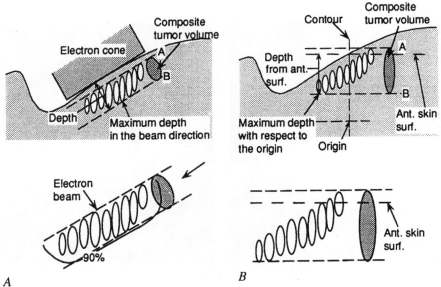

A   *B*

Figure 11.39   *A.* When an electron beam is used to treat a chest wall tumor, the greatest depth of the tumor should be determined in the beam's-eye view and not from a reconstruction of the tumor with respect to the coordinate system. *B.* The same tumor transposed to one level with respect to the origin in the coordinate system appears much larger.

is treated using electron beams, it is important to direct the beam in such a way that the tumor depth is minimal, while with photon beams, the beam orientation is unpredictable and therefore the tumor location must be known in three dimensions. For example, if the composite tumor was outlined as in Fig. 11.39A, it appears as if a very small field width would encompass the tumor. However, if a lateral or oblique field were used, a large portion of the tumor would be missed. This is also discussed in Chap. 7.

A boost to the site of the primary tumor is sometimes given using an electron beam. The location and beam orientation of the electron beam should be carefully determined. The scar may not always be a good indicator of the primary tumor site.[49] When the tumor bed is marked with metallic clips, these can be used as indicators for where to place the boost field (Fig. 11.40). Several CT images obtained through the tumor bed with reference marks on the skin sur-

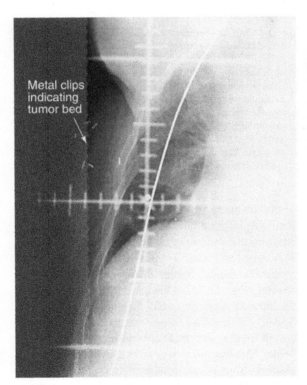

Figure 11.40 Metal clips indicating the tumor bed in a breast patient are useful both for setting the deep margin of the tangential fields and for the boost field.

face can also be helpful to localize the boost area.[50] The boost can also be delivered via an interstitial implant (Chap. 16).

TREATMENT SIMULATION

It would be impossible to describe simulation procedures for all of the treatment techniques used in breast treatment. This section is therefore limited to a description of the simulation of the treatment technique used at Duke University. That does not imply that this technique is superior, only that it is most familiar to the author.

An immobilization mold is made for all patients, either in the simulation or the CT room, depending on which procedure is first. When the treatment simulation is first, the Alpha Cradle with the patient is positioned so that the spinal column is parallel with the couch motion. This is ascertained by moving the couch along the longitudinal axis while watching the position of the beam's central axis with respect to the spinal column in fluoroscopy. When the position is satisfactory, the sagittal laser alignment line is marked on the chest and on the Alpha Cradle both superior to the head and between the knees (Fig. 11.19). When the internal mammary nodes are treated, a CT usually precedes the simulation to determine whether these lymph nodes can be included within the tangential fields without also including an excessive lung volume (Fig. 11.41). When the CT is obtained first, the sagittal laser line is marked as described above, with the patient in the position in which the CT was obtained. It is important to recognize that this line does not necessarily indicate the location of the isocenter, the midline, or a particular field, but that its sole purpose is to realign the patient on the couch for each procedure (Fig. 11.19). Occasionally, however, this line may coincide with the location of the isocenter or the central axis of a treatment field. Aligning two points separated by a long distance and using alignment lasers and immobilization devices improves the reproducibility of the setup from day to day.[5,25,51]

When a treatment-planning CT is obtained first to determine the field arrangement, the patient needs to be realigned in the simulator room with marks made during the CT procedure. Prior to the simulation

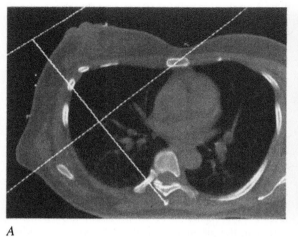

A

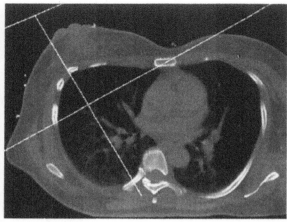

B

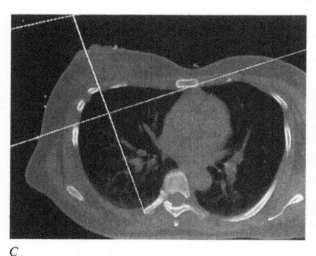

C

Figure 11.41 Often, CT images are obtained with the breast patient in treatment position to determine the possibility of including the internal mammary lymph nodes in the tangential fields. *A*. In an effort to cover the internal mammary lymph nodes with the tangential fields adequately without also including a large volume of the contralateral breast, too much lung tissue is included. *B*. When the medial margin is moved farther across the midline and the lateral margin is moved more anteriorly, the beams are including portions of the contralateral breast and the lung volume remains excessive. *C*. When the medial margin is moved farther across the midline and the lateral margin is moved more anteriorly, a larger volume of the contralateral breast is irradiated.

procedure, it is necessary to have all machine settings (gantry, collimator, and couch angles) set to 0°. Also, prior to beginning the simulation procedure, lead markers are placed on incisions, drain sites, or any other area that should be included in the fields.

When the internal mammary lymph nodes are treated in a separate field, it is usually 5 to 6 cm wide and extends 1 cm to the contralateral side of the midsternal line (Fig. 11.36). Traditionally, it extends from the match line superiorly to about 1 cm below the inframammary fold inferiorly. This field is treated with alternating a 6-MV photon beam (using an SSD technique) and a 10- to 12-MeV electron

beam. In many instances, it may be reasonable to omit the inferior portion of this field, thereby decreasing the volume of heart within the field.[52]

A thin lead wire is taped to the patient's chest where the medial border of the tangential fields is desired (Fig. 11.36). This can be the match line of the internal mammary field, the patient's midline, or across the midline when the internal mammary lymph nodes are included within the tangential fields. This lead wire is used as a guide when beam-shaping blocks are produced, as previously described. The length of the tangential fields is determined by setting the cephalad margin superior to the breast tissue and the inferior margin 1 cm inferior to the inframammary fold. The superior margin should be set so that the axilla, which is rarely irradiated when the patient has had an axillary dissection, is excluded from the beam. A lead shot is placed on the transverse laser line in the lateral aspect of the chest where the lateral tangential field should enter. After determining the separation between the two lead markers (medial and lateral), the isocenter is set approximately midway between the two lead markers and the central axis is centered on the lead wire. The gantry is turned, while viewing in fluoroscopy, until

the two lead markers are superimposed (Fig. 11.36B). This requires adjustments of the couch (vertical and left to right) and of the gantry angle. The central axis indicator of the simulator, the lead shot in the lateral chest, and the lead wire should be superimposed. The SSD is adjusted so that the isocenter is at the middepth between the two entrance points. The area anterior to the lead wire will be irradiated and the posterior area will be blocked (Fig. 11.36B). If the volume of lung tissue within the field is unsatisfactory, the lateral field margin is adjusted anteriorly if the lung volume is too large and posteriorly if it is too small. When there is no internal mammary field to match, the medial margin of the tangential fields can also be adjusted (Fig. 11.41).

The foot of the couch is turned away from the collimator an appropriate number of degrees, as described previously. The cephalad margin may have to be adjusted if the axilla lies within the tangential field. A radiograph is obtained and the field and laser lines are marked on the patient and the immobilization device. The gantry is then rotated 180° to the lateral tangential field and the couch angle is reversed. A radiograph is obtained and the field is marked.

The supraclavicular field is centered on the cephalad margin of the tangential fields and the caudal half overlying the tangential fields is blocked. The field is angled 15° to exclude the larynx, esophagus, and spinal cord and extends from the lateral aspect of the vertebral bodies medially to about 1 cm medial of the humeral head (Fig. 11.42). If the axillary lymph nodes also need to be irradiated, this field extends farther laterally and the axillary portion of the field is sometimes opposed to boost the dose to the axillary lymph nodes, which lie at a greater depth than the supraclavicular nodes (Fig. 11.43).

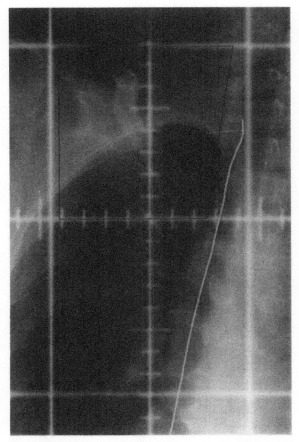

Figure 11.42 The supraclavicular lymph node field is usually angled 15° to avoid the spinal cord, esophagus, and trachea. The field usually extends from the lateral aspect of the vertebral bodies medially to about 1 cm medial of the humeral head.

TREATMENT

Special Situations. Because of the many variations in (1) the patient's size, (2) the presence or absence of the breast, (3) the breast size and shape, (4) the patient's ability to elevate the arm, (5) the size and location of an incision or drain site, and

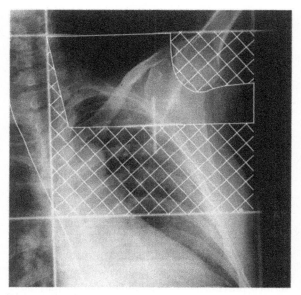

Figure 11.43   A simulation film of an anterior supraclavicular and axillary field.

(6) the thickness of the patient's chest wall, a technique developed for one patient may not be useful for treating another. Other factors that must be considered include, for example, whether the internal mammary or the axillary lymph nodes need treatment and whether the patient has had previous irradiation to the other breast or the lung or to the thoracic segment of the spinal cord. Breast treatment techniques that offer flexibility must be available in order to accommodate these situations.

In many patients, the sternum and spine are not aligned on a vertical plane (Fig. 11.44).[53] Alignment of the patient's body under fluoroscopy, using the spinal axis to determine when the patient is straight, is a good practice. However, setting the anterior internal mammary field with respect to the spinal axis can cause great errors because of the sternum-spine relationship previously mentioned.[53]

When the breast is situated high on the chest, allowing the tangential fields to include the breast tis-

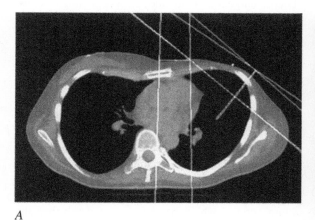

A

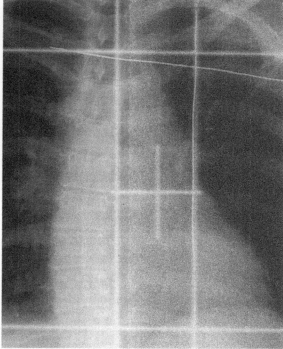

B

Figure 11.44   In many patients, the sternum and the spine are not aligned on a vertical plane. This internal mammary field, shown in a CT image *(A)* and a simulation radiograph *(B),* is centered on the ipsilateral internal mammary chain; it demonstrates the relationship between the sternum and the spine on a vertical plane. In most patients, the spinal column cannot be used to guide the position of an internal mammary field.

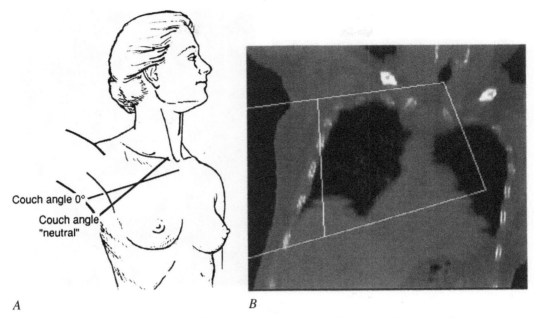

Figure 11.45   *A.* When the breast is very high on the chest wall, causing difficulties in excluding the arm and the axilla from the tangential fields, the couch can be turned so that the tangential fields cross the chest at an angle rather than transversely. *B.* The desired orientation of the tangential beams in the cephalad-caudal direction is adjusted by turning the couch.

sue while at the same time excluding the axilla, the cephalad margin of the tangential fields can be arranged so that they cross the patient's chest at an angle (Fig. 7.45). The desired orientation of the cephalad margin of the tangential fields (match line) is accomplished by turning the couch (Fig. 7.45*B*). The required couch angle, which is no longer 0°, is referred to as the "neutral" angle. The supraclavicular field, which is matched in the usual fashion, is treated with the couch in the neutral angle and the couch is then turned (from this position) the number of degrees needed to accomplish the match with the supraclavicular field. As an example, we can assume that the "usual" couch angle is 0° and the required couch angle to match the supraclavicular fields is + 5 and − 5°. If we turned the couch to + 10° (neutral angle) to accomplish the angled match line across the chest, the new couch angles to accomplish the match will be + 5 and + 15° (i.e., 5° in each direction figured from the + 10° neutral angle where we started). In this situation, the cephalad margins of

the tangential fields are not perpendicular to the sagittal axis of the patient as they were in the earlier description. In most patients, this angled match line is more cephalad in the medial aspect of the chest to include the breast and more caudal in the lateral aspect to exclude the axilla. When the angle of the supraclavicular-tangential field-match line is severe, the cephalad "deep" portion of the tangential fields may extend too far into the neck; however, frequently, this corner of the fields can safely be blocked (Fig. 11.46). The field match with the internal mammary field remains the same, since the matching field margin in the tangential fields, indicated by the lead wire, is defined by the customized blocks.

In other techniques, attempts of solving this problem have been made by the addition of an angled insert on top of the treatment couch which causes the patient's chest to be elevated, in the hope of lowering the breast by gravity. This technique is simple, but in patients who are also treated through a supra-

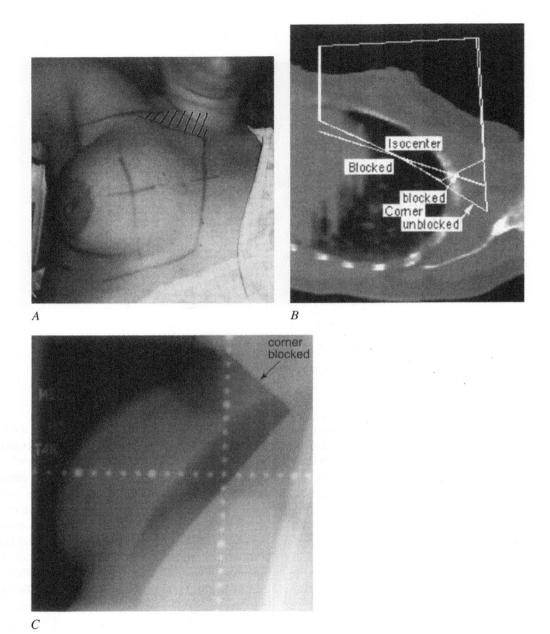

A

B

C

Figure 11.46 *A.* When the neutral couch angle is severe, the cephalad margin of the tangential fields may sometimes be too close to the neck. *B* and *C.* This deep cephalad corner can usually be blocked.

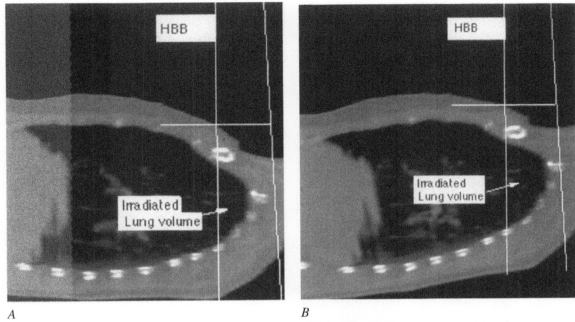

Figure 11.47 Elevating the patient's chest, in an effort to cause a gravitational shift of the breast caudally, causes more lung tissue to lie within the supraclavicular field. *A.* The patient's chest is horizontal. *B.* The chest is elevated 10°.

clavicular field, it will cause more lung volume to lie within this field (Fig. 11.47). The breast ring, described above, can be used to move the breast caudally.

Cardiac toxicity from breast irradiation can develop, particularly when the left breast is treated. To reduce the risk of this side effect, a modification can be made in the customized block of the tangential fields to protect the heart from irradiation.[52] In this technique, the tangential fields are designed to include only the cephalad portion of the internal mammary lymph nodes, while the caudal nodes are shielded by a heart block (Fig. 11.48*A*). The need for treating the internal mammary lymph nodes at all is uncertain, but irradiation of the cephalad lymph nodes may be more important than the caudal. The heart shield changes the location of where the beam intercepts the chest in the inferior half of the tangential fields (Fig. 11.48*B* and *C*). It is therefore important that the radiation oncologist actually verify vi-

sually that target tissues are not excluded due to the field modification. Sometimes a separate electron field can be used to treat superficial target tissues excluded by the heart block.

Including incisions and drain sites may not always be necessary, but when it is, this can cause a problem, particularly if they lie outside of typical treatment fields. A drain site, placed caudal to the conventional margin of the tangential fields, can be included by making the tangential fields slightly longer. Customized beam-shaping blocks can also be designed to include such a drain site. A lead marker should be placed on the site during the simulation procedure so that the blocks can be designed appropriately. If a drain site or scar lies outside either the medial or the lateral tangential fields, the customized beam-shaping blocks can be modified to include a slightly larger depth at this particular location (Fig. 11.49). Customized beam shaping provides the option of tailoring the treatment fields to the needs of

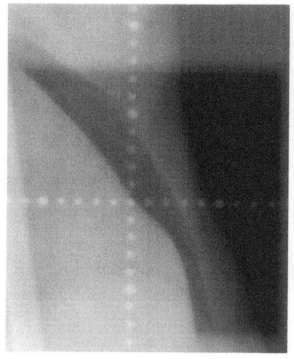

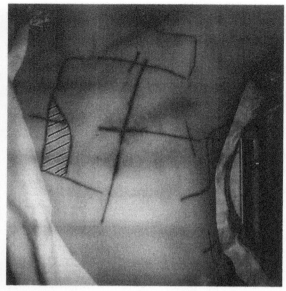

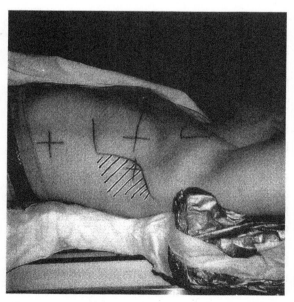

A

B

C

Figure 11.48   *A.* Left tangential fields can be shaped to include the internal mammary lymph nodes in the cephalad half of
the field while excluding the heart and the internal mammary
lymph nodes in the lower half. *B* and *C.* The field outline on the
skin surface is then changed and any target tissue that is excluded
may have to be treated via electron beams.

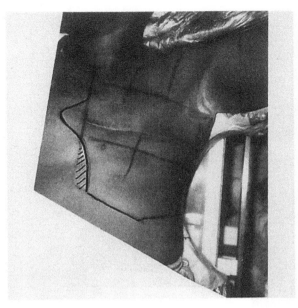

A

Figure 11.49   *A* and *B*. An incision that is very long and extends beyond the normal field boundaries may be included within the tangential fields by modifying the depth at just this location.

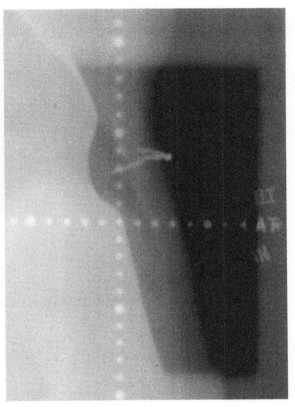

B

each patient. Figure 11.50 illustrates a patient presenting with a very difficult dilemma, which was solved by using customized beam shaping and non-opposed tangential fields.

In some cases, particularly with elderly or obese patients, the breast tends to fall laterally, thus making it difficult to include the entire breast without also including a large volume of lung tissue. Patients with large breasts are particularly difficult to treat, and there are often large dose heterogeneities within the breast tissue and the chest wall, giving rise to concerns related to the cosmetic outcome of the treatment.[54] Treatment of women with large or pendulous breasts is feasible only if there is sufficient expertise to ensure reproducibility of setup and the availability of 6- to 10-MV photon beams to obtain adequate

dose homogeneity. The breast ring described above, used to modify the breast position, can be useful in patients with large breasts and in those with small flaccid breasts. In some cases, when the breast is moved, the beam angles and entrance/exit points can be changed, resulting in reduced lung volume within the radiation fields.

Another difficult problem is posed by morbidly obese patients with large, pendulous breasts (Fig. 11.51). In this particular patient, a sitting position was found to be the most satisfactory though not ideal position. A Styrofoam block was strapped around the chest to elevate and support the breast and also to separate the breast tissue from the abdominal surface.

If no solution can be found and the entire target

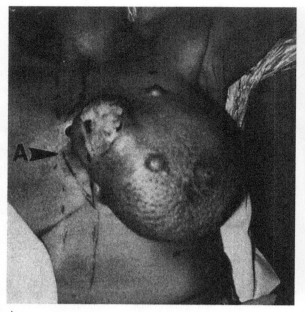

A

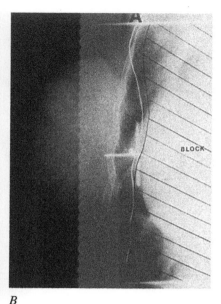

B

Figure 11.50 A patient with advanced disease in the breast creates very difficult geometric problems *(A)*, but the volume of irradiated lung can be minimized by using customized beam shaping *(B)*. This tumor extended across the patient's midline on the skin surface. A CT study *(C)* was used to determine beam angles and field shapes. The fields were not opposed but were instead angled, so that the large lymph node near the sternum could be included in both of the tangential fields without including more lung volume than absolutely necessary. A lead wire (A on the radiograph) was placed on the skin marks (A on the photograph) indicating palpable disease. The deep field margins, shaped by customized blocks, were extended to allow more margin around the breast.

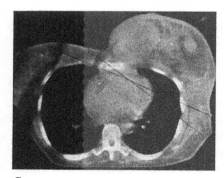

C

cannot be satisfactorily included in the tangential fields, the field borders may have to be compromised and the sections of the target beyond the tangential fields treated using electron fields. For example, breast tissues that lie too high on the chest for inclusion in the tangential fields can be treated using a separate electron field. If there is an adjoining supraclavicular field, alternating photon and electron beams can be used to reduce the dose to the underlying lung tissue.

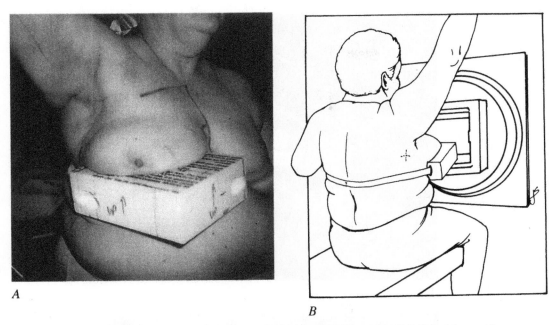

A

B

Figure 11.51 *A* and *B*. Very large patients with large breasts may have to be treated in a sitting position. This patient could be treated in a sitting position only with a Styrofoam block strapped to the chest to support the breast and to separate the breast from the abdomen.

Dose. Approximately 4600 cGy is given in fractions of 200 cGy to the breast. Higher doses or dose fraction sizes may compromise the cosmesis. A boost dose of 1500 to 2000 cGy is sometimes given using an electron beam or an interstitial implant to the site of the primary tumor. If the axillary lymph nodes are found to be positive, the supraclavicular and internal mammary lymph nodes may also be treated. It is generally agreed that the dissected axilla should not be irradiated unless there is strong suspicion of residual disease there. The dose to the regional nodes is approximately 4500 cGy in 4.5 to 5 weeks.

The beam energy usually used for breast treatment varies from a cobalt-60 to 8-MV photons. In the majority of patients, a 6-MV photon beam may be the most appropriate to achieve both adequate dose homogeneity and skin sparing. For large patients, even higher-energy beams may be needed to produce acceptable dose uniformity in the breast. Although some skin sparing is lost due to the beam being tan-gential with the breast tissue, when higher energies are used, a beam spoiler (Chap. 14) or bolus may be needed to assure adequate dose to shallower regions of the target. When the internal mammary lymph nodes are treated in a separate anterior field, a portion of the dose should be delivered via an electron beam to spare the underlying heart, lungs, and esophagus.

Delivering uniform dose to the entire breast is usually difficult due to the irregular shape of the breast tissues, causing varying degree of attenuation. Wedges are used in an attempt to improve the dose uniformity within the tangential fields (Fig. 11.52). Selection of the appropriate wedge angle can be difficult, but as a general rule, the following guidelines can be considered. In the patient who has had a mastectomy, the transverse chest wall contour often has a steep curvature; therefore, 45° wedges are usually needed to produce an acceptable dose distribution. In the patient with a moderately large breast, 30° wedges are often satisfactory. Generally, a patient

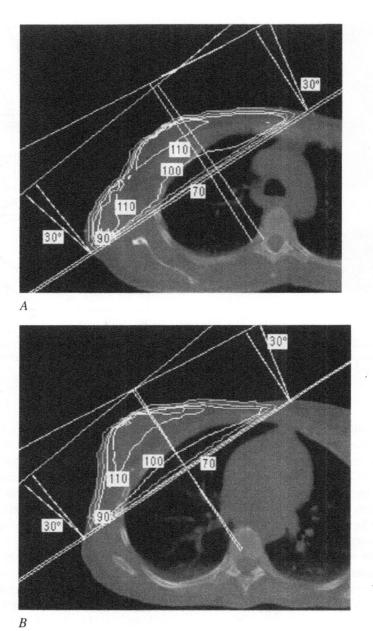

A

B

Figure 11.52 When the internal mammary lymph nodes are included within the tangential fields, the separation between the entrance points becomes larger. Wedges are used to compensate for the curvature of the chest and breast. The isodose distribution in a plane near the cephalad margin of the tangential fields *(A)*, through the central axis *(B)*, and near the caudal margin *(C)* illustrates relatively uniform dose within the fields. The same plan in the sagittal plane shows a small area of high dose near the apex of the breast *(D)*.

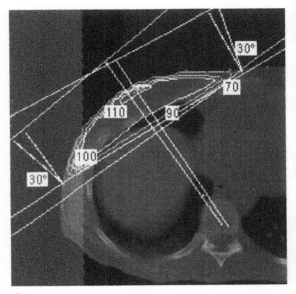

C

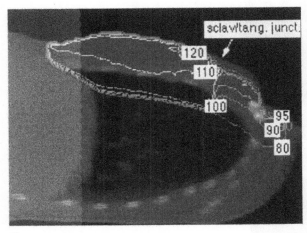

D

Figure 11.52 (*Continued*)

with a large breast requires less wedge angle; thus, in a patient with a very large breast, no wedge at all may result in the best dose uniformity.

Standard wedges affect the dose intensity only in the transverse direction and do not produce dose uniformity in the sagittal direction of tangential fields. In evaluating the dose distribution, dose variations within the tangential fields should also be considered

in the sagittal plane (Fig. 11.52*D*). A transverse contour through the central axes of the beams is useful in selecting the wedge angle that will give the most uniform dose distribution in that plane. Dose distributions calculated on transverse contours near the cephalad and caudal margins of the tangential fields, where the shape of the contour can be quite different, are needed to show whether the selected wedge angle

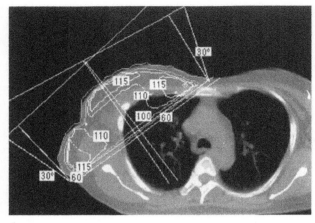

A

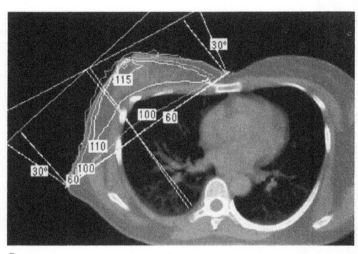

B

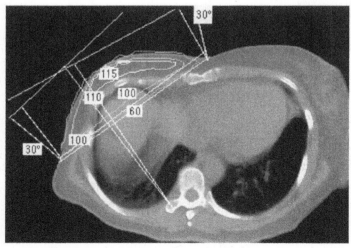

C

Figure 11.53 When the internal mammary lymph nodes are not treated, the medial field margin usually extends to the midline. Isodose distributions in a larger patient near the cephalad margin *(A)*, at the central axis plane *(B)*, and near the caudal margin *(C)* demonstrate relatively uniform dose.

is acceptable on these contours also. Figure 11.52 illustrates the isodose distribution in three transverse planes and one sagittal plane when the internal mammary lymph nodes are included in the tangential fields. A small area receives 120 percent, which is not apparent in either of the three transverse dose distributions.

Figure 11.53 illustrates the dose distribution in three transverse planes in a larger patient where the internal mammary lymph nodes are not treated. The highest dose (approximately 115 percent) in the cephalad plane is found at three locations; each entrance/exit region, where the separation is largest and the beam travels through a thin portion of the wedge, and at the apex of the breast. When a beam passes through a portion of a wedge that is thinner than at the central axis, the dose is increased. This dose increase with respect to the central axis dose is more pronounced with larger wedge angles. In the treatment technique using customized beam shaping, the beam passes through a thinner part of the wedge near the cephalad margin, where less than half of the beam width is blocked. This causes a progressively higher dose to occur as the width of the blocked area closer to the cephalad field margin becomes smaller and the beam passes through a decreasing thickness of the wedge (Fig. 11.50 and Chap. 6, Fig. 6.42). This problem is especially critical in large patients, where the slope is often more severe. It is therefore an advantage that the wedge angle usually needed in large patients is small.

Since standard wedges do not address dose heterogeneities in the sagittal direction and are limited in terms of the field size with which they can be used, a three-dimensional beam compensator would better address the issue of dose heterogeneities in breast treatment.[27] A quality-assurance program has also been described, in which routine in vivo dose determinations are made in breast patients to detect systematic errors in dose delivery and to identify inadequate treatment situations.[55]

Special Considerations. When tangential fields are treated, the dose to the unaffected breast should be considered.[56,57] Although the frequency is low, secondary cancer in the contralateral breast does occur.[58,59]

The effect of the radiation on the underlying lung is of great concern in breast irradiation. The volume of lung tissue included in the tangential fields should be kept to a minimum. However, to include the chest wall, some lung volume is unavoidable. It is estimated that when the distance from the deep margin of a tangential field to the inner part of the chest wall at the central axis of the field is 1.5 cm, approximately 6 percent of the ipsilateral lung volume is irradiated. When the same measurement is 2.5 cm, the lung volume is 16 percent; and when it is 3.5 cm, the lung volume is 26 percent.[60]

When isodose distributions are calculated in tangential breast treatments, corrections of lung inhomogeneity are not routinely included. The effect of the lung inhomogeneity has been studied by several authors.[61-63] The relative electron density of lung, using CT numbers, has been found to be approximately 0.25 for the entire lung volume but 0.17 in the anterior aspect of the lung.[64,65] This finding has been observed earlier and is thought to be due to larger accumulation of blood posteriorly when the patient is in the supine position. Inclusion of the lung density correction factor in the tangential fields may cause a reduction in the amount of wedge compensation needed.[39]

One problem sometimes encountered in breast irradiation is that of a surgically reconstructed breast where a prosthesis is implanted under the pectoralis major muscle. The concerns are related to the effect of the radiation on the prosthesis, the effect on the radiation by the prosthesis, and the cosmetic result of irradiating a reconstructed breast. The dosimetry of irradiation of the breasts with silicone implants appears to be satisfactory, as the prostheses are essentially tissue-equivalent.[66,67] The cosmetic results of irradiating augmented breasts is variable, and has been reported as being poor in some.[66,68,69] Doses of 4500 cGy in 5 weeks or the use of 6-MV photon beams is thought to produce less fibrosis and shrinkage of the breast. The cosmetic result also appears to be poorer when the irradiation is given immediately following the surgical reconstruction than if there was a time delay between the surgery and radiation therapy.[70]

MORBIDITY—BRONCHOPULMONARY AND BREAST

ESOPHAGUS

Acute radiation-induced esophagitis is usually experienced following approximately 2000 to 3000 cGy. Some chemotherapeutic agents, when used in combination with irradiation, may exacerbate the symptoms of esophagitis and cause them to occur at lower doses. Esophagitis is characterized by retrosternal discomfort and dysphagia (pain on swallowing). Patients with severe symptoms may resort to liquid intake only, and their nutritional status must be monitored. Some relief can be achieved by administering local analgesics, and the symptoms usually disappear a couple of weeks after the completion of radiation therapy. When large, infiltrating esophageal tumors are treated, a tracheoesophageal fistula may form as the tumor disappears, leaving an opening in the esophageal wall. This is a relatively rare occurrence but can arise if an accelerated treatment schedule is used. Long-term esophageal sequelae—such as stricture, perforation, and hemorrhaging—are rare but can occur.

LUNG

The incidence and severity of pneumonitis is thought to be related to the volume of lung tissue in the fields, dose, and fractionation schedule. The threshold for radiation-induced pneumonitis is approximately 2000 cGy. When chemotherapy is used in combination with irradiation, the symptoms of pneumonitis may develop earlier and be more severe. Patients with chronic obstructive pulmonary disease (COPD) appear to be at a higher risk of radiation-induced pulmonary symptoms. At Duke University, we have been using single photon emission computed tomography (SPECT) scans to better appreci-ate the three-dimensional distribution of functioning lung relative to the tumor. The information is then used to design beams that minimize incidental irradiation of functioning lung. This technique is unproven and appears to be potentially most useful in patients with small targets (providing flexibility in beam arrangement) and very poor pulmonary function.[71] Symptoms of pneumonitis are cough, dyspnea, congestion, and fever. Bed rest, oxygen, and steroids are used to treat the acute stages of pneumonitis. As the pneumonitis subsides, fibrosis is formed, which can later be seen on plain radiographs of the lungs.

HEART

Radiation-induced pericarditis is relatively rare but can occur following irradiation doses of approximately 2000 cGy. The incidence is also related to the volume of heart in the radiation fields and field size.

SPINAL CORD

Transverse myelitis is discussed in Chap. 10 and is therefore not considered here. It is obviously a serious sequela of thoracic irradiation, which can be prevented by careful treatment planning and meticulous setup of spinal cord–sparing boost fields.

MISCELLANEOUS

Rib fractures are rare but can occur with doses in excess of 5000 cGy. Approximately 1 percent of patients irradiated for breast cancer will experience rib fractures. Brachial plexus paralysis is also rare but may occur at doses in excess of 5500 cGy. Arm edema can occur if the axilla is irradiated following surgery.

PROBLEMS

11.1 The most commonly occurring cancer in the United States is
(*a*) Breast cancer

(*b*) Lung cancer

(*c*) Esophageal cancer

(*d*) Prostate cancer

11.2   When an immobilization device is needed, it is best to
(*a*) First build the device and then decide what the field orientation should be
(*b*) First determine the beam orientation and then build the device
(*c*) First determine what device to use and the patient's position
(*d*) First build the device and then decide what patient position is best

11.3   It is important to reproduce the patient's position
(*a*) During the first treatment only
(*b*) Only on the days when port films are taken
(*c*) As it was during the simulation procedure
(*d*) Perfectly straight even if he or she was not when the simulation procedure was performed

11.4   Opposed anterior and posterior fields in the chest
(*a*) Invariably causes a higher dose near the caudal margin than at the central axis
(*b*) Invariably causes a lower dose near the cephalad margin than at the central axis
(*c*) Invariably results in a uniform dose distribution
(*d*) Invariably causes a higher dose near the cephalad margin than at the central axis

11.5   A lung boost is often delivered via
(*a*) Opposed anterior and posterior fields with a midline block
(*b*) Opposed anterior and posterior fields off the spinal cord
(*c*) Opposed oblique fields
(*d*) Opposed lateral fields

11.6   Treatment fields in the chest should be designed
(*a*) With generous margins because these patients tend to move a lot
(*b*) With generous margins to allow for difficulty in appreciating the tumor volume on a chest radiograph
(*c*) With respiratory motion in mind
(*d*) With very small margins

11.7   Tumors in the lower two-thirds of the esophagus can be boosted via
(*a*) Opposed anterior and posterior fields off the spinal cord
(*b*) An anterior and two posterior oblique fields
(*c*) A posterior and two anterior oblique fields
(*d*) Opposed anterior and posterior fields and opposed lateral fields

11.8   Aligning two points separated by a long distance is
(*a*) Unreliable because the laser alignment lines are often not precise away from the isocenter
(*b*) Impossible to do because the laser alignment lines are very short
(*c*) A reliable method to reproduce the patient's position
(*d*) Less reliable than to align the patient with skin marks indicating the treatment field

11.9   In setting up opposed oblique boost fields to treat a lung tumor
(*a*) It is important to know the isocenter depth (SSD) in each field

(*b*) The isocenter must be midway between the two entrance points (same SSD)

(*c*) The location of the isocenter does not matter

(*d*) The location of the isocenter must always be in the center of the tumor

11.10 The number of U.S. women who will develop breast cancer is approximately

(*a*) 1/10

(*b*) 1/5

(*c*) 1/100

(*d*) 1/20

11.11 The regional lymph nodes in breast cancer are

(*a*) The internal mammary and axillary

(*b*) The internal mammary, hilar, and axillary

(*c*) The internal mammary and supraclavicular

(*d*) The internal mammary, supraclavicular, and axillary

11.12 In most breast treatment techniques, field matching is a problem between

(*a*) The supraclavicular and the internal mammary fields and between the tangential and an axillary field

(*b*) The internal mammary and tangential fields and between the tangential and supraclavicular fields

(*c*) The lateral tangential field and the supraclavicular field and between the internal mammary and medial tangential field

(*d*) The medial tangential field and the internal mammary field and between the axillary and supraclavicular field

11.13 The couch angle necessary to avoid beam divergence from the tangential fields into the supraclavicular field depends on the

(*a*) Length of the tangential field in the direction of the supraclavicular field and the distance

(*b*) Width of the tangential field and distance

(*c*) Length of the tangential field in the direction of the supraclavicular field and length of the supraclavicular field

(*d*) Width of the supraclavicular field and width of the tangential field

11.14 To avoid beam divergence from the tangential fields into the supraclavicular field,

(*a*) The foot of the couch is turned toward the collimator

(*b*) The direction of the couch rotation is irrelevant as long as the right number of degrees is used

(*c*) The head of the couch is turned away from the collimator

(*d*) The foot of the couch is turned away from the collimator

11.15 To avoid beam divergence into the lung by the tangential fields

(*a*) The central axes of the tangential fields can be separated by slightly more than 180° until the deep margins become parallel

(*b*) The central axes of the tangential fields can be separated by slightly less than 180°

(*c*) The couch can be turned 5° toward the collimator when the medial field is treated and 5° away from the collimator when the lateral field is treated

(*d*) The collimator can be rotated to follow the slope of the chest wall

11.16 Multiple adjacent electron fields to treat a chest wall recurrence
   (*a*) Can easily be carried out in any department
   (*b*) Should be considered only when proper dosimetry is available
   (*c*) Are easy to set up, since field junctions are of no concern because electron beams do not penetrate very deep
   (*d*) Pose no risk of overlap at a depth because the beams do not penetrate very deep

11.17 A boost is sometimes delivered to the tumor bed in breast cancer using
   (*a*) External photon beams or multiple electron beams
   (*b*) An electron beam or an interstitial implant
   (*c*) Opposed tangential fields supplemented by an electron beam
   (*d*) Opposed photon beams and an interstitial implant

11.18 The internal mammary lymph nodes are
   (*a*) Usually treated via a separate field using a 6-MV photon beam
   (*b*) Always included in the tangential fields
   (*c*) Usually not treated
   (*d*) Sometimes treated in a separate field using a photon and an electron beam or are included in the tangential fields

11.19 Cardiac toxicity from breast irradiation is
   (*a*) Sometimes a serious problem
   (*b*) Never heard of
   (*c*) Never occurs because the heart is outside the fields
   (*d*) Occurs following 1000 cGy

11.20 The most important considerations to avoid radiation-induced pneumonitis is
   (*a*) Total dose and also which portion of the lung was irradiated
   (*b*) Total dose, fractionation schedule, and volume of irradiated lung
   (*c*) Daily fractionation schedule and the patient's weight
   (*d*) The patient's smoking history and the total dose

REFERENCES

1. Wingo AP, Tong T, Bolden S: Cancer statistics 1995. *CA* 45:8, 1995.
2. Yang CS: Research in esophageal cancer in China: A review. *Cancer Res* 40:2633, 1980.
3. Corn BW, Coia LR, Chu JCH, et al: Significance of prone positioning in planning treatment for esophageal cancer. *Int J Radiat Oncol Biol Phys* 21:1303, 1991.
4. Vijayakumar S, Muller-Runkel R: Irradiation of the thoracic esophagus: Prone versus supine treatment position. *Acta Radiol Oncol* 25:187, 1986.
5. Bentel GC: Positioning and immobilization device for patients receiving radiation therapy for carcinoma of the breast. *Med Dosim* 15:3, 1990.
6. Bentel GC: Positioning and immobilization of patients undergoing radiation therapy for Hodgkin's disease. *Med Dosim* 16:111, 1991.
7. Marcus KC, Svensson G, Rhodes LP, Mauch PM: Mantle irradiation in the upright position: A technique to reduce the volume of lung irradiated in patients with bulky mediastinal Hodgkin's disease. *Int J Radiat Oncol Biol Phys* 23:443, 1992.
8. Hishikawa Y, Taniguchi M, Kamikonya N, et al: External beam radiotherapy alone or combined with high-dose-rate intracavitary irradiation in the treatment of cancer of the esophagus: Autopsy findings in 35 cases. *Radiother Oncol* 11:223, 1988.
9. Hishikawa Y, Kurisu K, Taniguchi M, et al: High-dose-rate intraluminal brachytherapy for esophageal cancer: 10 years experience in Hyogo College of Medicine. *Radiother Oncol* 21:107, 1991.
10. Petrovich Z, Langholz B, Formenti S, et al: The importance of brachytherapy in the treatment of unresectable carcinoma of esophagus. *Endocuriether Hyperther Oncol* 5:201, 1989.

11. Syed AMN, Puthawala AA, Severance SR, Zamost BJ: Intraluminal irradiation in the treatment of esophageal cancer. *Endocuriether Hyperther Oncol* 3:105, 1987.

12. Perez CA, Purdy J, Rezak A: Radiation therapy of carcinoma of the lung and esophagus, in Levitt SH, Tapley N (eds): *Technological Basis of Radiation Therapy: Practical Clinical Applications.* Philadelphia: Lea & Febiger, 1984.

13. Rosenberg JC, Schwade JG, Vaitkevicius VK: Cancer of the esophagus, in DeVita VT, Hellman S, Rosenberg SA (eds): *Cancer: Principles and Practice of Oncology.* Philadelphia: Lippincott, 1982.

14. Veronesi U, Saccozzi R, Del Vecchio M: Comparing radical mastectomy with quadrantectomy, axillary dissection, and radiotherapy in patients with small cancers of the breast. *N Engl J Med* 305:6, 1981.

15. Veronesi U, Zucali R, Luini A: Local control and survival in early breast cancer: The Milan trial. *Int J Radiat Oncol Biol Phys* 12:717, 1986.

16. Veronesi W, Salvadori B, Luini A: Conservative treatment of early breast cancer: Long-term results of 1232 cases treated with quadrantectomy, axillary dissection, and radiotherapy. *Ann Surg* 211:250, 1990.

17. Veronesi U, Banfi A, Salvadori B: Breast conservation is the treatment of choice in small breast cancer: Long-term results of a randomized trial. *Eur J Cancer* 26:668, 1990.

18. Ege GN: Internal mammary lymphoscintigraphy in breast carcinoma: A study of 1072 patients. *Int J Radiat Oncol Biol Phys* 2:755, 1977.

19. Rose CM, Kaplan WD, Marck A, et al: Parasternal lymphoscintigraphy: Implications for the treatment planning of internal mammary lymph nodes in breast cancer. *Int J Radiat Oncol Biol Phys* 5:1849, 1979.

20. Siddon RL, Chin LM, Zimmerman RE, et al: Utilization of parasternal lymphoscintigraphy in radiation therapy for breast carcinoma. *Int J Radiat Oncol Biol Phys* 8:1059, 1982.

21. Chu FCH, Huh SH, Nisce LZ, Simpson LD: Radiation therapy of choroid metastasis from breast cancer. *Int J Radiat Oncol Biol Phys* 2:273, 1977.

22. Merchant TE, McCormick B: Prone position breast irradiation. *Int J Radiat Oncol Biol Phys* 30:197, 1994.

23. Cross MA, Elson HR, Aron BS: Breast conservation radiation therapy technique for women with large breasts. *Int J Radiat Oncol Biol Phys* 17:199, 1989.

24. Gagliardi G, Lax I, Rutquist LE: Radiation therapy of stage I breast cancer: Analysis of treatment technique accuracy using three-dimensional treatment planning tools. *Radiother Oncol* 24:94, 1992.

25. Creutzberg AL, Althog VG, Huizenga H, Visser AG: Quality assurance using portal imaging: The accuracy of patient positioning in irradiation of breast cancer. *Int J Radiat Oncol Biol Phys* 25:529, 1993.

26. Redpath AT, Thwaites DI, Rodger A, et al: A multidisciplinary approach to improving the quality of tangential

27. Valdagni R, Ciocca M, Busana L, et al: Beam modifying devices in the treatment of early breast cancer: 3-D stepped compensating technique. *Radiother Oncol* 23:192, 1992.

28. Zierhut D, Flentje M, Frank C, et al: Conservative treatment of breast cancer: Modified irradiation technique for women with large breasts. *Radiother Oncol* 31:256, 1994.

29. Bentel GC, Marks LB: A simple device to position large/flaccid breasts during tangential breast irradiation. *Int J Radiat Oncol Biol Phys* 29:879, 1994.

30. Bentel GC: A reproducible field matching technique for treatment of breast carcinoma (abstr). *Int J Radiat Oncol Biol Phys* 10:177, 1984.

31. Klein EE, Taylor M, Michaletz-Lorenz M, et al: A mono isocentric technique for breast and regional nodal therapy using dual asymmetric jaws. *Int J Radiat Oncol Biol Phys* 28:753, 1994.

32. Lichter AS, Fraass BA, van De Geijn J, Padikal TN: A technique for field matching in primary breast irradiation. *Int J Radiat Oncol Biol Phys* 9:263, 1983.

33. Podgorsak EB, Pla M, Kim TH, Freeman CR: Center-blocked field technique for treatment of extensive chest wall disease. *Int J Radiat Oncol Biol Phys* 7:1465, 1981.

34. Podgorsak EB, Gosselin M, Kim TH, Freeman CR: A simple isocentric technique for irradiation of the breast, chest wall and peripheral lymphatics. *Br J Radiol* 57:57, 1984.

35. Siddon RL, Tonnesen GL, Svensson GK: Three-field technique for breast treatment using a rotatable half-beam block. *Int J Radiat Oncol Biol Phys* 7:1473, 1981.

36. Svensson GK, Bjärngard BE, Chen GTY, Weichselbaum RR: Superficial doses in treatment of breast with tangential fields using 4 MV x-rays. *Int J Radiat Oncol Biol Phys* 2:705, 1977.

37. Svensson GK, Bjärngard BE, Larsen RD, Levene MB: A modified three-field technique for breast treatment. *Int J Radiat Oncol Biol Phys* 6:689, 1980.

38. Siddon RL: Solution to treatment planning problems using coordinate transformation. *Med Phys* 8:766, 1981.

39. Cross P, Joseph DJ, Cant J, et al: Tangential breast irradiation: Simple improvements. *Int J Radiat Oncol Biol Phys* 23:433, 1992.

40. Rosenow UF, Valentine ES, Davis LW: A technique for treating local breast cancer using a single set-up point and asymmetric collimation. *Int J Radiat Oncol Biol Phys* 19:183, 1990.

41. Leavitt DD: Electron arc therapy, in *Varian Users Meeting.* San Diego, CA, 1978.

42. Leavitt DD, Peacock LM, Gibbs FA, Stewart JR: Electron arc therapy: Physical measurement and treatment planning techniques. *Int J Radiat Oncol Biol Phys* 11:987, 1985.

43. Leavitt DD, Stewart JR, Moeller JH, Earley L: Optimization of electron arc therapy doses by multivane collimator control. *Int J Radiat Oncol Biol Phys* 16:489, 1989.

44. Leavitt DD, Stewart JR, Lee WL, Takach GA: Electron arc therapy: Design, implementation, and evaluation of a dynamic multi-vane collimator system. *Int J Radiat Oncol Biol Phys* 17:1089, 1989.

45. Leavitt DD, Earley L, Stewart JR: Design and production of customized field shaping device for electron arc therapy. *Med Dosim* 15:25, 1990.

46. Leavitt DD, Stewart JR, Earley L: Improved dose homogeneity in electron arc therapy achieved by a multi-energy technique. *Int J Radiat Oncol Biol Phys* 19:159, 1990.

47. Leavitt DD, Stewart JR: Electron arc therapy of the postmastectomy prosthetic breast. *Int J Radiat Oncol Biol Phys* 28:297, 1993.

48. Swalec JJ, Leavitt DD, Moeller JH: Improved field edge definition in electron arc therapy with dynamic collimation techniques. *Int J Radiat Oncol Biol Phys* 30:205, 1994.

49. Machtay M, Lanciano R, Hoffman J, Hanks GE: Inaccuracies in using the lumpectomy scar for planning electron boosts in primary breast carcinoma. *Int J Radiat Oncol Biol Phys* 30:43, 1994.

50. Regine WF, Ayyanger KM, Komarnicky LT, et al: Computer-CT planning of the electron boost in definitive breast irradiation. *Int J Radiat Oncol Biol Phys* 20:121, 1991.

51. Bentel GC: Laser repositioning in radiation oncology. *Applied Radiol* 13:46, 1984.

52. Marks LB, Hebert ME, Bentel G, et al: To treat or not to treat the internal mammary nodes: A possible compromise. *Int J Radiat Oncol Biol Phys* 29:903, 1994.

53. Bentel GB, Marks LB, Torano AE, Prosnitz LR: Correlation of mid-sternum and mid-spine positions in 82 patients irradiated for breast cancer. *Radiother Oncol* 31:248, 1994.

54. Gray JR, McCormick B, Cox L, Yahalom J: Primary breast irradiation in large-breasted or heavy women: Analysis of cosmetic outcome. *Int J Radiat Oncol Biol Phys* 21:347, 1991.

55. Leunens G, VanDam J, Dutreix A, Van der Schueren E: Importance of *in vivo* dosimetry as part of a quality assurance program in tangential breast treatments. *Int J Radiat Oncol Biol Phys* 28:285,˙1993.

56. Fraass BA, Roberson PL, Lichter AS: Dose to the contralateral breast due to primary breast irradiation. *Int J Radiat Oncol Biol Phys* 11:485, 1985.

57. Tercilla O, Krasin F, Lawn-Tsao L: Comparison of contralateral breast doses from 1/2 beam block and isocentric treatment techniques for patients treated with primary breast irradiation with ⁶⁰Co. *Int J Radiat Oncol Biol Phys* 17:205, 1989.

58. Boice JD, Land CE, Shore RE, et al: Risk of breast cancer following low-dose radiation exposure. *Radiology* 131:589, 1979.

59. DeLaney TF, Pierce LJ: Cancer in the contralateral breast after radiotherapy for breast cancer. *N Engl J Med* 327:430, 1992.

60. Bornstein BA, Cheng CW, Rhodes LM, et al: Can simulation measurements be used to predict the irradiated lung volume in the tangential fields in patients treated for breast cancer. *Int J Radiat Oncol Biol Phys* 18:181, 1990.

61. Chin LM, Cheng CW, Siddon RL, et al: Three-dimensional photon dose distributions with and without lung corrections for tangential breast intact treatments. *Int J Radiat Oncol Biol Phys* 17:1327, 1989.

62. Fraass BA, Lichter AS, McShan DL, et al: The influence of lung density corrections on treatment planning for primary breast cancer. *Int J Radiat Oncol Biol Phys* 14:179, 1988.

63. Mijnheer BJ, Heukelom S, Lanson JH, et al: Should inhomogeneity corrections be applied during treatment planning of tangential breast irradiation? *Radiother Oncol* 11:239, 1991.

64. Mira JG, Fullerton GD, Ezekiel J, Potter JL: Evaluation of computed tomography numbers for treatment planning of lung cancer. *Int J Radiat Oncol Biol Phys* 8:1625, 1982.

65. Rotstein A, Lax I, Svane G: Influence of radiation therapy on the lung-tissue in breast cancer patients: CT assisted density changes and associated symptoms. *Int J Radiat Oncol Biol Phys* 18:173, 1990.

66. Krishnan L, Krishnan EC: Electron beam irradiation after reconstruction with silicone gel implant in breast cancer. *Am J Clin Oncol* 9:223, 1986.

67. Shedbalkar AR, Devata A, Padanilam T: A study of effects of radiation on silicone prosthesis. *Plast Reconstr Surg* 65:805, 1980.

68. Jacobson GM, Sause WT, Thompson JW, Plank HP: Breast irradiation following silicone gel implants. *Int J Radiat Oncol Biol Phys* 12:835, 1986.

69. Liskow A, Shank B: Breast irradiation for recurrence in a patient with silicone implant. *Oncology* 2:58, 1988.

70. Halpern J, McNeese MD, Kroll SS, Ellerbroek N: Irradiation of prosthetically augmented breasts: A retrospective study on toxicity and cosmetic results. *Int J Radiat Oncol Biol Phys* 18:189, 1990.

71. Marks LB, Spencer DP, Bentel GC, et al: The utility of SPECT lung perfusion scans in minimizing and assessing the physiologic consequences of thoracic irradiation. *Int J Radiat Oncol Biol Phys* 26:659, 1993.

12

Treatment Planning—Abdomen

The abdomen is defined as the portion of the body between the thorax and the pelvis that contains the peritoneal cavity. The abdomen is separated from the thoracic cavity by the diaphragm above and from the pelvic cavity by the plane of the pelvic inlet below.

Irradiation of the whole abdomen or portions of the abdominal cavity is necessary in the management of various diseases, including some gynecologic malignancies, gastric and hepatobiliary tumors, pancreatic cancer, colon cancer, lymphomas, Wilms' tumor, and neuroblastoma. Careful consideration of critical organs within the abdominal cavity, including kidneys, liver, and bowel, is necessary.

In many situations, the treatment is delivered through anterior and posterior opposed fields, although, with the utilization of three-dimensional treatment planning, other field arrangements resulting in superior sparing of normal tissues are sometimes possible.

PATIENT POSITIONING

The patient's position is generally supine, with supports under the knees to relax the back. When lateral or large anterior/posterior abdominal fields are treated, the arms may be elevated above the head or extended away from the torso to reduce the amount of scatter or direct radiation of the arms. A Plexiglas extension can be added to the width of the treatment couch to support the arms, as shown in Chap. 7, Fig. 7.50.

WHOLE ABDOMEN

Irradiation of the abdominal cavity and pelvis is usually referred to as whole-abdominal or abdominopelvic irradiation. This treatment is primarily used in the management of ovarian and endometrial malignancies, where it is intended to deliver therapeutic doses to the entire peritoneal cavity and the pelvis.

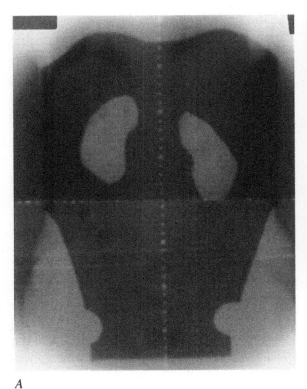

A

Figure 12.1   *A*. Port film of a posterior whole-abdominal field with 5-HVT kidney blocks in place. *B*. A typical anterior whole-abdominal field of another patient.

The dose that can safely be delivered to the whole abdomen is limited by the tolerance of the organs within the abdomen. For gynecologic tumors, the whole abdominal dose usually ranges from 125 to 150 cGy up to 3000 cGy. This is often followed by a boost to the pelvis or the pelvis and paraaortic lymph nodes, depending on the presence of gross disease. Radioactive chromic phosphate (^{32}P) or radioactive colloidal gold (^{198}Au) are sometimes administered intraperitoneally in an effort to treat tumor cells that may have spread into the peritoneal cavity. This is also discussed in Chap. 15. The combination of intraperitoneal ^{32}P with external beam treatment is associated with a relatively high incidence of bowel complications and therefore this combination should be used with caution.[1]

TARGET LOCALIZATION AND TREATMENT SIMULATION

Generally speaking, whole-abdominal irradiation involves the use of large anterior and posterior fields with shielding of dose-limiting organs at appropriate dose levels. The treatment distance must be sufficiently long to include the entire peritoneal cavity and pelvis from the pelvic floor to about 2 cm above the dome of the diaphragm in a single field (Fig. 12.1). Due to the constant motion of the diaphragm with respiration, the cephalad margin is best determined under fluoroscopy with the patient breathing quietly. The lateral field margins should include the peritoneal cavity. It is highly recommended that intravenous contrast (60 mL Isovue®*, organically bound iodine) be given during the simulation of these fields to assess the position and function of the kidneys and facilitate the design of kidney shields. The dose to the whole kidneys must be limited to 2000 cGy in adults and about 1500 cGy in children. When the patient is also receiving chemotherapy, these doses should be lower. It is important to recog-

* Squibb Diagnostics, New Brunswick, NJ.

nize that parts of the liver[2] and the kidneys can safely be irradiated to higher doses if other parts of the organ receive lower doses.

Since the kidneys are not midplane structures, their position with respect to the central axis of the beam will be different in the anterior and posterior fields. It is therefore necessary to obtain a simulation radiograph of each field for proper positioning of the kidney shields.

Preferably, both fields should be treated with the patient in the supine position. In some circumstances, however, the treatment couch cannot be elevated high enough to achieve the treatment distance required to produce the necessary field size for the posterior field, or the field may be too large to fit within the window in the couch. It is then usually necessary to reposition the patient in the prone position. If the required treatment distance for the posterior field can be achieved with the treatment machine but not with the simulator, one can treat both fields in the supine position, but special care must be taken in block design, since a proper simulation radiograph is not available. When this situation occurs in our practice, a CT scan of the upper abdomen is obtained with the patient in the treatment position. The kidneys are then outlined on each image using a three-dimensional treatment planning system (the Virtual Simulator™*). Kidney blocks are outlined in the beam's-eye view (Fig. 12.2) and templates are produced for block cutting. In the absence of this technology, the patient must be positioned prone when the posterior field is simulated and treated. The virtues of anterior versus posterior kidney shielding are discussed below.

TREATMENT TECHNIQUES

Whole-abdominal treatment fields should be shaped to minimize the volume of irradiated bone marrow, thus reducing the risks of myelosuppression (Fig. 12.1). Due to the domelike shape of the diaphragm in the anterior-posterior view, it is impossible to treat the entire abdominal cavity without also treating some volume of lung and heart (Fig. 12.3A and B;

* Sherouse Systems, Inc., Charleston, SC.

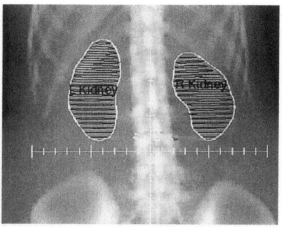

Figure 12.2   Digitally reconstructed radiograph of posterior kidney blocks outlined in the beam's-eye view in a three-dimensional treatment planning system.

see also Fig. 12.1). The beams must therefore be shaped to include the abdominal cavity while minimizing the amount of lung and heart in the radiation field (Fig. 12.1). Willett *et al.* have suggested gated irradiation, a technique in which the treatment is delivered during only one phase of the respiratory cycle.[3] The radiation is interrupted at short intervals while the patient is taking a new breath.

Kidney and liver doses can be kept below tolerance levels by partially shielding these organs during treatment of the whole abdomen. Kidney protection can be achieved by three methods: (1) fully blocking both kidneys once the tolerance dose is reached, (2) using shielding blocks that allow only partial transmission of the radiation beam during the entire treatment course, or (3) fully shielding from one field only. The dose distribution and biological effect will be different in these three methods because of the fractionation scheme in which the dose within the shielded area is delivered. The choice will depend on the prescribed dose to the abdominal fields and must be tailored to the specific situation.

In practically all of these patients, blocks used to shield kidneys will also shield possible tumor sites. Therefore, in patients where it is urgent to treat the entire abdomen, it might be advantageous to deliver the initial treatment without any shielding. When

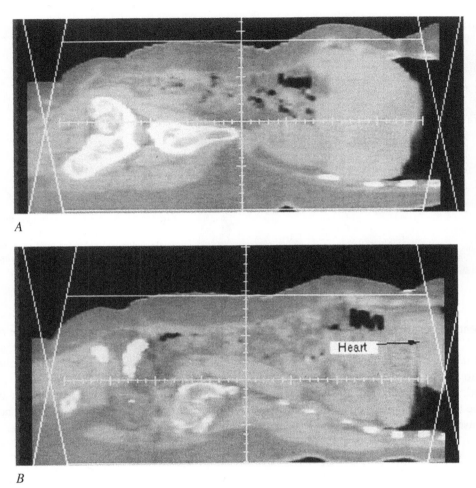

Figure 12.3 Computed tomography images reconstructed in the sagittal plane through the right *(A)* and left *(B)* abdomen. Anterior and posterior whole-abdominal fields extend above the diaphragm to include the abdominal cavity; therefore a portion of the lungs and the heart cannot be avoided.

tolerance doses have been reached, 5-HVT shielding can be added in both fields to prevent further irradiation of the kidneys and liver. This method of shielding may also be selected for the treatment of patients where it is uncertain whether the planned course of treatment can be completed because of the hematologic picture, the patient's general condition, or the level of patient compliance. Using 5-HVT blocks in both fields when kidney tolerance doses have been reached would deliver uniform dose throughout the organs (Fig. 12.4). Insertion of a 1-HVT block in both fields during the entire course of treatment would deliver approximately 50 percent of the dose in the shielded organs, and the dose distribution under these shields would be similar to that of using 5-HVT shields during a portion of the treatments only. Adding a 5-HVT shield in the posterior field only during a portion of the treatment course would cause most of the dose to the kidneys to be delivered through the anterior field, resulting in a

15 MV photons, 2000 cGy open + 1000 cGy 5 HVT A/P shield

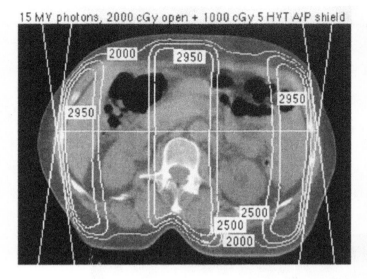

Figure 12.4 Isodose distribution through the kidneys resulting when open anterior and posterior whole-abdominal fields are used to deliver 2000 cGy followed by an additional 1000 cGy with 5-HVT kidney blocks inserted in both fields.

dose gradient in the anterior-posterior direction (Fig. 12.5).

When shielding of the kidneys is considered, it is important to recognize that even when the kidneys are blocked, a significant dose is deposited in the kidneys due to scattered radiation (10 to 15 percent) and by transmission in the 5-HVT shields (about 3 percent). The dose depends on the size of the irradiated area, the beam energy, and the size of the block. The dose can be significantly higher near the edge of the kidney shields (Fig. 12.6).

Rosenthal et al. studied the virtues of anterior versus posterior kidney shielding and concluded that although posterior shields block a larger portion of

15 MV photons, AP open, PA 5 HVT shield to 3000 cGy

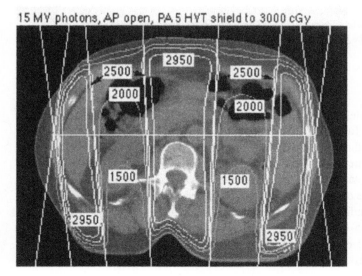

Figure 12.5 Isodose distribution through the kidneys resulting when 3000 cGy is delivered to the whole abdomen via anterior and posterior fields with 5-HVT kidney blocks in the posterior field only during the entire treatment course.

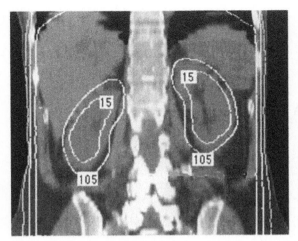

Figure 12.6 Isodose distribution in the coronal plane through the kidneys. A posterior whole-abdominal field is used, delivering 100 cGy at middepth using a 6-MV photon beam. The isodose line surrounding each kidney (105 percent) is higher than the middepth dose because the kidneys are located at a shallower depth from the posterior surface. The minimal dose in the kidneys at this depth was 11 cGy.

the anterior abdomen due to the divergence, these blocks are more effective because of the smaller depth of the kidneys from the posterior surface.[4]

The anterior portions of the peritoneal cavity can also be treated with lateral fields that exclude the kidneys. The best treatment technique for a particular patient depends on the disease, but it is important to recognize that in either of the options described here, a section of the abdominal cavity is unavoidably also shielded.

A strip technique for whole-abdominal irradiation has also been described,[5,6] wherein the whole abdomen is divided into strips that are 2.5 cm in the cephalad-caudal direction. On the first treatment, only one strip is treated via opposed anterior and posterior fields. On each subsequent treatment, one strip is added, until four strips are treated (10 cm). During each treatment that follows, one strip is excluded and a new one is added until the field has moved to the opposite extent of the abdomen, where the field-reduction process is reversed. The dose delivered to each segment of the field ranges from 2250 cGy in 10 fractions without shielding of the

liver to 2800 cGy in 8 fractions with shielding of the liver. The kidneys are also shielded, usually by 5-HVT blocks in the posterior field. While this technique was designed to reduce morbidity, a prospective comparison with open fields suggest a higher incidence of late toxicity.[7] This technique is rarely used at the present time, due to concerns of complexity, small bowel mobility, and the time lapse of several weeks before reaching the last strip. Other dissuasive factors are concerns that tumor cells that may be floating around in the peritoneal space escape radiation altogether or are irradiated with every treatment. Also, if a patient is unable to complete the course of treatment, portions of the abdomen would have received a full dose while other portions would have received some or no dose.

MORBIDITY

Because of the large volume of irradiated tissues, the acute tolerance of whole-abdominal irradiation is sometimes poor. Acute toxicity primarily takes the form of nausea, vomiting, diarrhea, fatigue, and loss of appetite. Late sequelae such as enteritis and small bowel obstruction are far less common. Late renal and hepatic injury is uncommon if appropriate shielding is used, as noted above. The toxicity of whole abdominal irradiation has been studied by several authors.[8–10]

SUBTOTAL ABDOMEN

Intraabdominal tumors include those arising in the stomach, duodenum, bowel, hepatobiliary tract, pancreas, colon, kidneys, and ureters. The delivery of cancerocidal doses of ionizing radiation in this region is limited by the tolerance of adjacent normal organs, primarily kidneys, liver, small intestine, stomach, and spinal cord. Both the target and the normal organs in the vicinity must therefore be carefully localized. A diagram illustrating the pertinent anatomy is shown in Fig. 12.7.

When the treatment involves only a portion of the abdomen, sparing of the small bowel may, in some patients, be accomplished by placing the patient in a

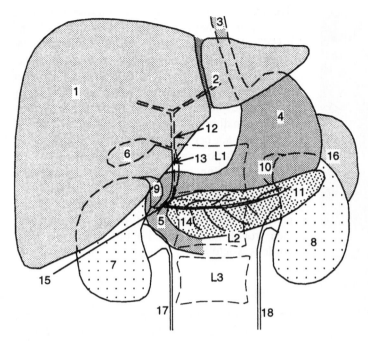

Figure 12.7 A diagram showing the location of some of the organs in the upper abdomen. 1 = R. lobe of liver; 2 = L. lobe of liver; 3 = esophagus; 4 = stomach; 5 = duodenum; 6 = gallbladder; 7 = R. kidney; 8 = L. kidney; 9 = R. adrenal gland; 10 = L. adrenal gland; 11 = pancreas; 12 = hepatic duct; 13 = common bile duct; 14 = pancreatic duct; 15 = ampulla of Vater; 16 = spleen; 17 = R. ureter; 18 = L. ureter.

decubitus position (Fig. 12.8*A*). It is difficult to reproduce this position; therefore an immobilization device should be made to support the patient (Fig. 12.8*B*).

TARGET LOCALIZATION AND TREATMENT SIMULATION

Intraabdominal tumors are localized with the help of various contrast studies. The administration of oral contrast (1 pt of barium sulfate) during the simulation procedure demonstrates the position of the stomach and the duodenum. A diagnostic study, referred to as the endoscopic retrograde cholangiopancreatography (ERCP), which demonstrates the position of the biliary tree and the pancreatic duct, is helpful to have available during the simulation procedure. Intravenous injection of contrast (60 mL Isovue) should be considered during the simulation to assess kidney position and function (Fig. 12.9). Placement of metallic clips in the tumor bed during a prior surgical procedure will increase the confidence with which the target is radiographically localized. When tumors in the colon are localized, bowel con-

trast may also be useful. Since barium contrast usually obscures surgical clips and renal contrast, an orthogonal set of radiographs should be taken prior to the administration of oral contrast. Magnetic resonance imaging (MRI) and computed tomography (CT) studies show the position of the kidneys, liver, and spinal cord with respect to the target.

TREATMENT TECHNIQUES—PANCREAS

The prognosis for most patients with pancreatic cancer is dismal, and the goal of radiation therapy is usually palliation. Anterior and posterior fields can be used until spinal cord tolerance has been reached (about 4500 cGy). If more aggressive therapy is warranted, additional treatments can be delivered through small lateral fields, thus minimizing the volume of liver within the fields.

The size and precise position of the fields depends on the tumor location. The most common location of pancreatic tumors is in the head of the pancreas. The target volume is the primary or residual tumor and nodal areas at risk. The nodal areas include the pancreaticoduodenal, porta hepatis, suprapancreatic, and

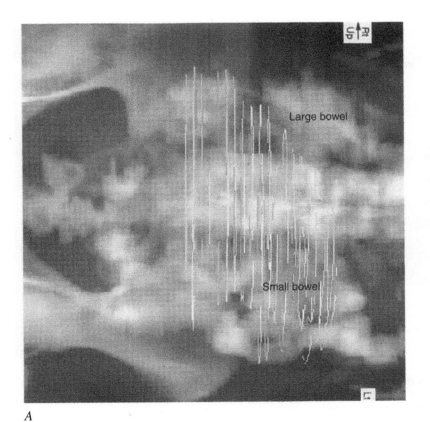

A

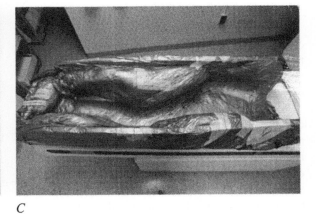

B   *C*

Figure 12.8 *A.* A decubitus position may, in some patients, cause a gravitational shift of the small bowel. *B* and *C*. An immobilization device is usually necessary for reproducibility of the position. This patient is being treated for a retroperitoneal liposarcoma.

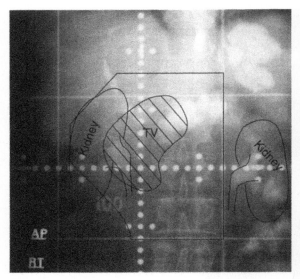

A

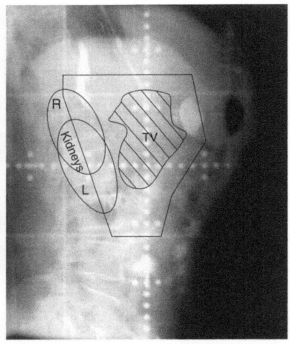

B

Figure 12.9 *A* and *B*. Typical simulation films of anterior and lateral pancreas fields. The tumor volume was outlined from CT images. Intravenous contrast was administered to demonstrate the function and location of the kidneys. In this patient, the right kidney (B) is higher than the left (A) which is unusual. Oral contrast shows the stomach and the duodenum. Anterior and a lateral films should be taken prior to administering oral barium, which otherwise would obscure metallic clips marking the tumor bed and kidney contrast.

celiac lymph nodes. Generous margins are sometimes used when these fields are designed due the uncertainty in target localization and the motion caused by respiration.

For treatment of tumors in the head of the pancreas, the target includes the previously mentioned nodal groups and the entire duodenum, since it is at risk. Anterior and posterior treatment fields usually extend from the mid- or upper T11 to include the L3 vertebra (Fig. 12.9A). When the primary tumor is in the body or tail of the pancreas, the splenic hilar lymph nodes are also at risk. The fields are slightly more cephalad and must usually extend farther to the left. As much of the kidneys as possible should be blocked in these fields (Fig. 12.9A). The lateral fields will have the same cephalad and caudal margins as the anterior and posterior fields. The lateral field anterior margin must be 1.5 to 2 cm anterior of gross disease and the

posterior margin must extend approximately 1.5 cm posterior to the anterior portion of the vertebral body to include the paraaortic lymph nodes, which are also at risk in patients with posterior tumor extension. The treatment fields are then shaped to minimize the kidney volume within the fields (Fig. 12.9B). In many patients, the lateral fields may still include a large portion of the kidneys, and in some patients the lateral fields may have to be angled slightly to avoid at least one kidney. It is important to recognize that the fields must be individualized to each patient's disease.

Achieving a uniform dose in the target while minimizing the dose in the kidneys, liver, and spinal cord when pancreatic tumors are treated presents a challenging proposition. The use of different wedge angles and variations in the weighting of the dose give the planner a wide variety of options. Since the pancreas is bordered by the liver (right), spinal cord (posteriorly), and kidneys (posteriorly bilaterally), multiple beams are generally used to ''spread out the

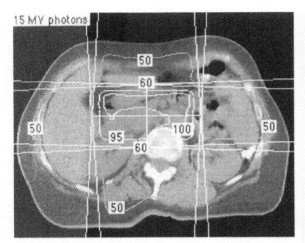

Figure 12.10 Isodose distribution resulting from using a four-field technique to treat a pancreatic tumor. The fields are weighted equally and a 15-MV photon beam is used. The dose in the liver is between 50 and 60 percent and the right kidney (outside this plane) is also high.

dose.'' The exact combination of wedges and weighting is determined and depends on the goal of therapy.

The field arrangement used for the treatment of pancreatic tumors is often opposed anterior and posterior fields and opposed lateral fields, as previously described. The dose distribution shown in Fig. 12.10 results when the fields are equally weighted. The dose in the spinal cord, right kidney, and a section of the liver is between 50 and 60 percent of the dose at the isocenter. The kidney tolerance may be exceeded when this plan is used; however, that may be of no consequence in patients with a functioning left kidney.

The dose in the right kidney can be lowered somewhat by omitting the posterior field, which delivers a higher dose to the kidney(s) and the spinal cord than to the anteriorly located pancreas. In a three-field technique, the kidney(s) and spinal cord receive exit dose from the anterior field only. Of course, in some patients, the anterior portion of the kidneys may lie within the lateral fields, thus receiving the same dose as the target. A typical dose distribution resulting from treating via an anterior and two lateral fields weighted equally is shown in Fig. 12.11A. The dose

in the right kidney is now lower, while the dose in the liver is higher. The dose is also higher in the anterior portion of the treatment volume, and the dose gradient is poor (105 to 90 percent). The addition of wedges and changing the weights, favoring the anterior field, will increase the dose in the right kidney, decrease the dose in the liver, and improve the dose gradient within the treatment volume (Fig. 12.11B). The choice of wedge angle and weighting must be determined for each situation. For example, the dose in the liver can be decreased by increasing the weight of the anterior and left lateral fields or by the addition of a posterior field. When it is important to spare the right kidney (as in patients where the left kidney function is poor), the weight can be increased on the lateral fields.

A treatment technique described by Dobelbower et al. uses opposed lateral fields with a 45-MV photon beam and an anterior field mixing a 45-MV photon beam (50 percent) and a 15- to 35-MeV electron beam (50 percent).[11] The electron energy is determined from the depth of the posterior extent of the target. For large patients, a three- or four-field technique with 45-MV photon beams is used.

The dose delivered via external beam irradiation is usually about 4000 to 6000 cGy at conventional fractionation (200 cGy per fraction), usually concurrently with chemotherapy. The total dose depends on the clinical situation. Shrinking-field techniques are used to limit the normal tissue volume exposed to high doses. Other methods to deliver a boost include intraoperative irradiation using an electron beam[12-14] and interstitial implants.[15]

TREATMENT—GALLBLADDER AND BILIARY DUCT TUMORS

Tumors in the gallbladder and biliary tree are not very common. They are usually treated through a field arrangement similar to that described for pancreatic tumors or through opposed anterior and posterior fields. Bile duct tumors frequently grow along the ducts but can also invade adjacent tissues (i.e., liver) and lymph nodes. Obstruction of biliary flow is common. The target includes the primary lesion, adjacent tissues, and sometimes the regional nodes (pancreaticoduodenal, porta hepatis, and the celiac).

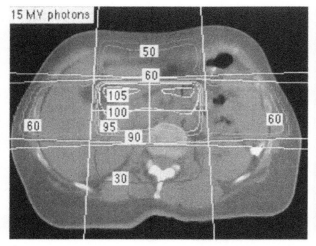

A

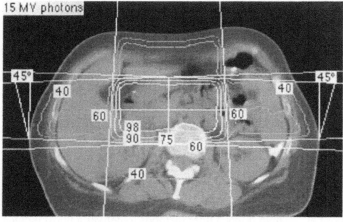

B

Figure 12.11   *A*. When a three-field technique consisting of equally weighted anterior and opposed lateral fields is used, the dose in the liver is high (> 60 percent) while the dose in the right kidney is lower than with the four-field technique. The dose gradient through the target is poor. *B*. The addition of wedges in the lateral fields and increasing the weighting in the anterior field (50 percent) reduces the dose in the liver and improves the dose gradient. The lateral fields are equally weighted (25 and 25 percent).

The treatment simulation procedure is basically the same as for the pancreas, possible with the additional aid of a diagnostic study using contrast in the transhepatic catheter to demonstrate the position of the bile duct (Figs. 12.7 and 12.12).

The dose that can safely be delivered in these tumors is limited by the volume of liver inevitably included in the fields. Higher doses are tolerated if the treated volume is small. A dose of 4000 to 4500 cGy is commonly delivered with the initial fields, followed by a boost of about 1500 cGy to a small volume. This boost can be delivered via a variety of beam arrangements, including anterior and lateral wedged fields or a three-field technique using wedges and weighting the beams unequally (Fig. 12.13*A*), or an arc with wedges—a technique described in Chap. 6 (Fig. 12.13*B*). Intraluminal insertion of an ^{192}Ir wire in the bile duct is also commonly used as a method of delivering high local dose in bile duct tumors (Chap. 16). The role of radiation therapy in the treatment of bile duct carcinoma has been described.[16,17]

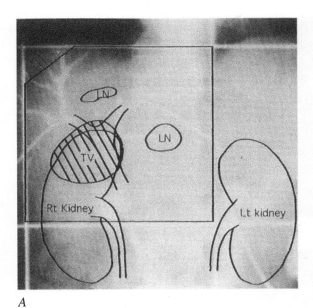

A

B

Figure 12.12 Typical anterior and lateral treatment fields for a bile duct tumor. Contrast in a transhepatic catheter is useful to localize the target volume.

TREATMENT—STOMACH

Radiation therapy in the treatment of gastric carcinoma is not very common. Target localization is usually with oral contrast given during the simulation procedure. The treatment technique usually consists of opposed anterior and posterior fields including the tumor and major nodal regions (Fig. 12.14). The lymph nodes at risk are the pancreaticoduodenal, porta hepatis, suprapancreatic, and splenic hilar lymph nodes. Also at risk are the lymphatic chains in the lesser and greater curvature of the stomach. The fields are, as in most other sites, customized to exclude adjacent normal tissues and include the appropriate areas in any particular patient, depending on the extent of the disease. Care must be taken to minimize cardiac volume within the fields, particularly when the fields must also include a portion of the esophagus. The treatment should also be delivered prior to a meal or the consumption of carbonated drinks, which might overextend the stomach.

TREATMENT—COLON

The field arrangement used in the treatment of colon cancer is usually opposed anterior and posterior fields including the tumor bed with adequate margins. The dose is usually approximately 4500 cGy at 180 to 200 cGy per fraction, frequently with chemotherapy. If the treatment fields are small and include very little or no small bowel, the dose may be slightly higher. Small bowel contrast should be given during the simulation procedure to determine the volume of small bowel within the fields. Placing the patient in the decubitus position may sometimes cause the small bowel to be displaced by gravity out of the treatment fields. Assessment of the function and location of the kidneys is necessary prior to initiation of the treatments. The volume of liver must also be considered when fields are designed and the dose is prescribed.

TREATMENT—KIDNEY AND URETERS

Radiation therapy in the management of renal cell carcinoma of the kidney has been tried for many years as a preoperative, postoperative, solitary, or as a palliative measure, and its role is still uncertain. Treatment fields generally include the renal bed and

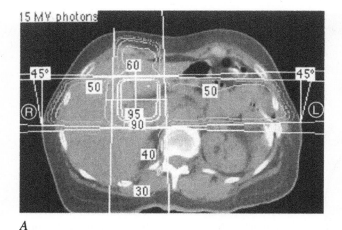

A

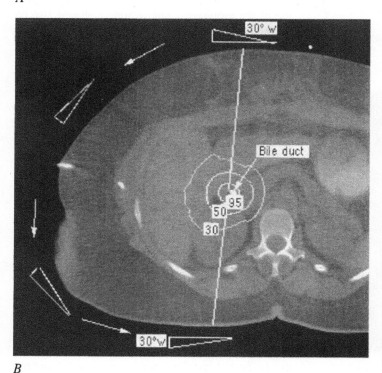

B

Figure 12.13 *A.* A boost dose can be delivered in bile duct tumors via a three-field arrangement, similar to that used in the pancreas. In this plan, the anterior field is weighted 50 percent, the right lateral 30 percent, and the left lateral 20 percent. The difference in the weighting of the lateral fields is due to the difference in the depth of the isocenter. A 15-MV photon beam is used and the wedges in the lateral fields are 45°. *B.* As an alternative, an arc with wedges that are reversed midway through the arc can also be used. In this plan, a 6-MV photon beam is used with 30° wedges. The arc is from 170° anterior to 350° posterior. In this plan, the dose in the surrounding liver, kidneys, and spinal cord is considerably lower than in the three-field plan. Moving-beam techniques are usually not appropriate for large tumors, when the target is irregularly shaped, or when the target volume lies at an angle relative to the axis of the rotation.

paraaortic lymph nodes while sparing as much liver as possible. The dose is on the order of 4500 to 5000 cGy.

The role of radiation therapy in the management of tumors in the renal pelvis and ureters is still unde-fined. Theoretically, preoperative radiation therapy may prevent dissemination of tumor cells during the surgical procedure and sterilize subclinical disease. Postoperative radiation therapy could possibly sterilize microscopic disease left behind at surgery. The

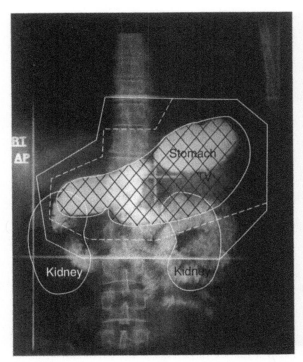

Figure 12.14   Typical treatment field for gastric carcinoma. The solid line indicates the original fields and the hatched line the boost field.

treatment fields should include the entire length of the involved ureter.

Wilms' tumor, occurring almost exclusively in children, is a highly malignant tumor of the kidney. Postoperative radiation therapy of the tumor bed, meaning the entire preoperative tumor extent, is sometimes given, depending on the stage and histologic subtype (Fig. 12.15). Opposed anterior and posterior fields are usually used. Margins are generally determined from an intravenous pyelogram (IVP), MRI or CT images, and the operative report. The lateral margin includes the abdominal wall and the medial margin includes the entire width of the vertebral bodies with enough contralateral extension to include the paraaortic lymph nodes while excluding the opposite kidney. Inclusion of the entire width

of the spine will uniformly affect the epiphyseal growth plates on both sides of the spinal column and reduce the incidence of subsequent scoliosis. The dose to these fields varies depending on the ability to limit normal tissues within the fields; they range from 1080 to 3000 cGy, depending on the age of the child, stage of disease, and histology. A boost may be given to sites of gross residual disease. The sequelae of irradiating the spine in a small child must be weighted against the benefits of irradiation in this disease. In patients with diffuse implants, massive intraabdominal disease, or rupture of the capsule, whole-abdominal irradiation is often considered. When Wilms' tumor metastasizes to the lungs, whole-lung irradiation is employed. The dose ranges from 1050 to 1500 cGy at 150 cGy per fraction, usually via anterior and posterior fields.

TREATMENT—NEUROBLASTOMA

Neuroblastoma is a tumor of the sympathetic nervous system that may arise in the abdomen, chest, or neck in children. Many young children with abdominal primary node-negative disease are cured by surgical excision. In some patients where gross residual tumor remains after surgery and in patients with positive lymph nodes, postoperative irradiation of the tumor bed with wide margins has been shown to be beneficial if chemotherapy does not produce a complete response. Treatment fields should be designed to include the tumor bed and regional lymph nodes (Fig. 12.16). When the field must include part of the spinal column, it is important to extend it across the entire width of the spine to reduce the severity of subsequent scoliosis. Treatment fields should be arranged and designed to minimize incidental irradiation of the kidneys and of the ovaries in female patients. Anterior and posterior fields are usually used. Oblique beam arrangements may be used in special situations. The dose varies depending on the stage of the tumor, size of the fields, and age of the child. Boost doses of irradiation to the primary tumor bed may precede high-dose chemotherapy or chemotherapy plus total body irradiation for stage IV neuroblastoma.

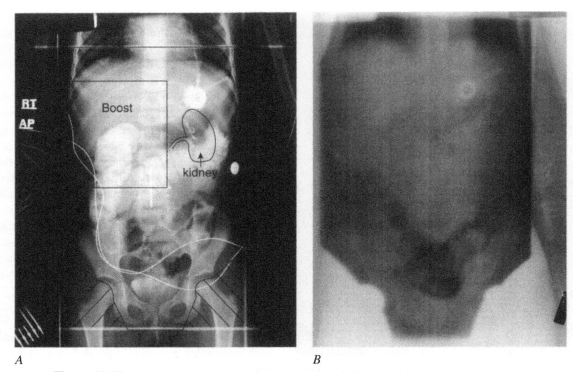

A   *B*

Figure 12.15   A simulation *(A)* and port film *(B)* of a whole-abdominal field used to treat a 4-year old child with stage III Wilms' tumor. The surgical margins were positive and tumor cells were found in the vein at the aortic bifurcation. The patient received 1050 cGy to the whole abdomen. A smaller field would typically be treated in a patient with Wilms' tumor delivering 1800 to 4000 cGy, depending on the age of the child and the stage of disease.

MORBIDITY

The ability to deliver high doses in the upper abdomen is compromised by the tolerance of organs in the vicinity. The right kidney is usually included when tumors in the gallbladder, head of the pancreas, bile duct, and distal stomach are treated, and the left kidney usually lies with the fields when tumors in the body or tail of the pancreas or in the proximal and mid-gastric area are treated. The function of the opposite kidney must be determined prior to irradiation, and at least two-thirds of this kidney must be excluded from the fields. Clinically significant renal dysfunction is uncommon if care is taken to shield some renal tissue. Subclinical renal injury, noted as a reduction in creatinine clearance following incidental kidney irradiation, appears to depend on the percentage of kidney volume irradiated.[18] The liver volume may be excessive when large fields are used. Shrinking-field techniques with reduction at 3000 to 3500 cGy are recommended when gallbladder or proximal bile duct lesions are treated, especially if the fields are large.

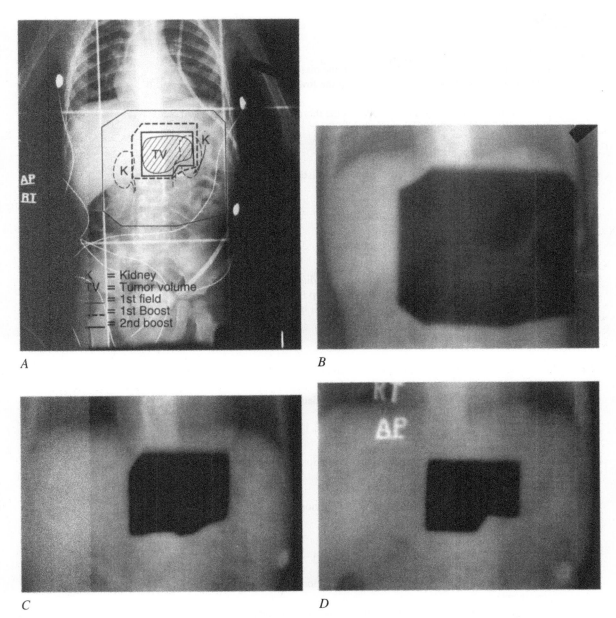

Figure 12.16   A simulation film *(A)* and three port films *(B, C,* and *D)* showing the field reduction for a neuroblastoma. The tissues within the large field *(B)* received 1440 cGy, the first field reduction *(C)* received 360 cGy, and the final boost field *(D)* received 600 cGy, for a total dose of 2400 cGy delivered in twice a day (bid) fractions of 120 cGy each (240 cGy per day).

PROBLEMS

12.1 The abdomen is defined as
   (*a*) The portion of the body that lies between the diaphragm and the iliac crests
   (*b*) The portion of the body that lies between the lowest aspect of the rib cage and the pelvic floor
   (*c*) The portion of the body that lies between the thorax and the pelvis and that contains the peritoneal cavity
   (*d*) The peritoneal cavity

12.2 The following radioisotopes are sometimes administered intraperitoneally in the treatment of gynecologic malignancies:
   (*a*) ^{137}Cs
   (*b*) ^{192}Ir
   (*c*) ^{131}I
   (*d*) ^{32}P

12.3 The cephalad field margin in whole-abdominal irradiation should be set
   (*a*) At the superior aspect of the diaphragm on deep inhalation
   (*b*) At the superior aspect of the diaphragm in quiet breathing
   (*c*) By palpating the 12th rib
   (*d*) At the xiphoid

12.4 Whole-abdominal treatment fields can be set so that
   (*a*) They include some lung and some heart tissue
   (*b*) They do not include any heart but a small segment of lung
   (*c*) They do not include any heart or lung
   (*d*) They include a small section of the heart but no lung tissue

12.5 Generally speaking, the kidney tolerance to irradiation in the adult is
   (*a*) 2000 cGy delivered in five fractions
   (*b*) 1500 cGy delivered in three fractions
   (*c*) 2000 cGy delivered at 180 to 200 cGy per fraction
   (*d*) 2500 cGy delivered in 200 cGy per fraction

12.6 Partial kidney shielding in a patient who is likely not to complete the course of treatment is best accomplished by means of
   (*a*) 5-HVT blocks in both the anterior and posterior fields, throughout the course of treatment
   (*b*) Partial shielding of the kidneys during the first week of treatment only
   (*c*) Partial shielding of the kidneys in the anterior and posterior fields until kidney tolerance is reached, followed by total removal of the blocks
   (*d*) No shielding of the kidneys until kidney tolerance dose has been reached and then insertion of 5-HVT blocks in both the anterior and posterior fields

12.7 The time/dose schedule in the kidney is the same regardless of which shielding method is used.
   (*a*) True
   (*b*) False

12.8   The dose under a 5-HVT kidney block is
  (*a*) None
  (*b*) Approximately 5 to 10 percent of the dose delivered at middepth on the central axis
  (*c*) Approximately 10 to 20 percent of the dose delivered at middepth on the central axis
  (*d*) Approximately 20 to 25 percent of the dose delivered at middepth on the central axis

12.9   The amount of dose under a 5-HVT kidney block
  (*a*) Depends on the beam energy, the size of the field, and the size of the kidney block
  (*b*) Depends on the size of the patient, the size of the field, and the distance from the central axis
  (*c*) Depends on the beam energy, the size of the patient, and the distance from the central axis
  (*d*) Can be disregarded because there is none

12.10   The most common site of pancreatic tumors is
  (*a*) The midsection of the pancreas
  (*b*) The tail of the pancreas
  (*c*) The head of the pancreas
  (*d*) Langerhans' islands

12.11   The organs in which normal tissue tolerance is of concerns when treating pancreatic tumors are
  (*a*) The kidneys, the liver, and the spinal cord
  (*b*) The liver and the spinal cord
  (*c*) The lungs, the heart, and the kidneys
  (*d*) The heart and the kidneys

12.12   When a three-field technique (anterior and opposed lateral fields) is used in the treatment of pancreatic tumors, the best dose distribution is achieved with
  (*a*) Open fields and equal weighting
  (*b*) Open fields and weighting the lateral fields more to avoid exit in the kidneys
  (*c*) Wedges in the lateral fields and more weighting on the anterior field
  (*d*) Open fields and more weighting on the anterior field

12.13   Wilms' tumor is a tumor originating in the
  (*a*) Hepatobiliary system
  (*b*) Kidneys
  (*c*) Sympathetic nervous system
  (*d*) Spinal cord

12.14   Neuroblastoma is a tumor most often originating in the
  (*a*) Kidneys
  (*b*) Hepatobiliary system
  (*c*) Sympathetic nervous system
  (*d*) Spinal cord

12.15   When children are treated for Wilms' tumor,
  (*a*) The medial field margin should be in the midline of the spinal cord
  (*b*) The medial field margin should include the width of the spine
  (*c*) The spine should not be irradiated at all
  (*d*) The medial margins should only include the spinous processes on the involved side

REFERENCES

1. Klaassen D, Stavreveld A, Shelly W, et al: External beam pelvic radiotherapy plus intraperitoneal radioactive chromic phosphate in early stage ovarian cancer: A toxic combination. *Int J Radiat Oncol Biol Phys* 11:1801, 1985.
2. Lawrence TS, TenHaken RK, Kessler ML, et al: The use of 3-D dose volume analysis to predict radiation hepatitis. *Int J Radiat Oncol Biol Phys* 23:781, 1992.
3. Willett CG, Linggood RM, Stracher MA, et al: The effect of the respiratory cycle on mediastinal and lung dimensions in Hodgkin's disease. *Cancer* 60:1232, 1987.
4. Rosenthal DI, Sailer SL, Varia M, et al: Optimizing peritoneal surface and renal dose distribution in whole abdominal radiation therapy (abstr). *Int J Radiat Oncol Biol Phys* 19(suppl 1): 256, 1990.
5. Delclos L, Quinlan EJ: Malignant tumors of the ovary managed with postoperative megavoltage irradiation. *Radiology* 93:659, 1969.
6. Dembo AJ, Van Dyk J, Japp B, et al: Whole abdominal irradiation by a moving strip technique for patients with ovarian cancer. *Int J Radiat Oncol Biol Phys* 5:1933, 1979.
7. Dembo AJ: Radiotherapeutic management of ovarian cancer. *Semin Oncol* 11:238, 1984.
8. Hacker NF, Berek JS, Burnison CM, et al: Whole abdominal radiation as salvage therapy for epithelial ovarian cancer. *Obstet Gynecol* 65:60, 1985.
9. Reddy S, Hartsell W, Graham J, et al: Whole-abdominal radiation therapy in ovarian carcinoma: Its role as a salvage therapeutic modality. *Gynecol Oncol* 35:307, 1989.
10. Schray MF, Martinez A, Howes AE: Toxicity of open-field whole abdominal irradiation as primary postoperative treatment in gynecologic malignancy. *Int J Radiat Oncol Biol Phys* 16:397, 1989.
11. Dobelbower RR, Borgelt BB, Strubler KA, et al: Precision radiotherapy for cancer of the pancreas: Technique and results. *Int J Radiat Oncol Biol Phys* 6:1127, 1980.
12. Abe M, Takahashi M: Intraoperative radiotherapy: The Japanese experience. *Int J Radiat Oncol Biol Phys* 7:863, 1981.
13. Goldson AL, Ashaveri E, Espinoza MC, et al: Single high dose intraoperative electrons for advanced stage pancreatic cancer: Phase I pilot study. *Int J Radiat Oncol Biol Phys* 7:869, 1981.
14. Wood CW, Shipley WU, Gunderson LL, et al: Intraoperative irradiation for unresectable pancreatic carcinoma. *Cancer* 49:1271, 1982.
15. Shipley WU, Nardi GL, Cohen AM: Iodine-125 implant and external beam irradiation in patients with localized pancreatic carcinoma: A comparative study to surgical resection. *Cancer* 45:709, 1980.
16. Fritz P, Brambs H-J, Schraube P, et al: Combined external beam radiotherapy and intraluminal high dose rate brachytherapy on bile duct carcinomas. *Int J Radiat Oncol Biol Phys* 29:855, 1994.
17. Veeze Kuijpers B, Meerwaldt JH, Lameris JS, et al: The role of radiotherapy in the treatment of bile duct carcinoma. *Int J Radiat Oncol Biol Phys* 18:63, 1990.
18. Willett CG, Tepper JE, Orlow EL, Shipley WU: Renal complications secondary to radiation treatment of upper abdominal malignancies. *Int J Radiat Oncol Biol Phys* 12:1601, 1986.

13

Treatment Planning—Pelvis

In this chapter, treatment planning concepts concerning some of the most common tumor sites in the pelvis are described.

PATIENT POSITIONING AND IMMOBILIZATION

As with any other treatment site, it is important to place the patient in a position that is comfortable and reproducible and at the same time allows the treatment to be delivered with optimal sparing of normal tissues.

Patients are most frequently treated in the supine position because it is usually considered easier and more comfortable, however, treatment of prostate patients in the prone position has been described.[1] A support under the patient's knees helps to relax the lower back which is especially important when lying on a rigid treatment couch (Chap. 7, Fig. 7.50). To help reproduce the position of the patient's feet, a support made from Styrofoam®* can be used (Chap. 7, Fig. 7.51). Changes in the foot position also change the relative position of bony reference points that are used to determine the accuracy of the setup —an important consideration when port films are reviewed.

In some patients, a prone position is preferred. It is generally thought that when a patient lies prone, gravitational displacement of the small bowel out of the pelvis may be promoted. Another reason for the prone position is the difficulty of repositioning the treatment fields on morbidly obese patients, where skin marks on the anterior pelvic skin can shift, maybe by several centimeters. Some very obese patients also have tissue folds in the lower abdomen, which can be the cause of undesirable skin reactions due to lack of skin sparing in the folds. The rubbing of two skin surfaces against each other causes irritation and inhibits healing of the reaction. This problem is less apparent with higher-energy radiation beams, where the maximum dose lies at a greater depth, but it must still be given proper consideration. Skin folds can be reduced in the prone patient by having the patient pull them up while getting into the prone position. In the supine patient, straps and tape can be used to eliminate the skin folds, or the patient can be asked to hold them during the treatment. These methods of eliminating skin creases are unsatisfactory because they may cause the patient's thickness to vary from treatment to treatment. Because of slippage or nonuniform taping, it can even vary during the treatment, thus resulting in uncertainty of the delivered dose. As in all other instances, it is important that the contour on which the dose calculations are made truly represent the size and shape that the patient maintains during the treatment. Many of the problems just described can be reduced by treating the patient in the prone position, particularly if sparing of the small bowel is not of paramount concern. In the prone position, the abdomen is flattened against the hard treatment couch and thus the patient's thickness is consistent; it is also reduced in

many patients. The patient's posterior skin surface is usually quite flat and less mobile, providing a more reliable surface on which to mark the treatment fields.

For most patients, the prone position is less comfortable and is therefore more difficult to maintain. It is important to make the patient as comfortable as possible. A prone patient may be more comfortable with a pillow under the ankles to allow the knees to be bent during the treatments. Some patients are more comfortable holding the arms above the head while in the prone position. The degree of arm elevation and the side to which the head is turned are important to daily reproducibility of the relationship between the skin marks and the underlying anatomy.

IMMOBILIZATION MOLDS

Half-body positioning molds, extending from the midchest to below the feet, are used in many radiation therapy departments to immobilize patients receiving prostate irradiation, particularly when small target margins are used.[2-4] Here, the reproducibility is extremely important, and vigorous immobilization is necessary in order to accurately reproduce the position during the CT, treatment simulation, and treatment. At Duke University, an Alpha Cradle®,* with built-in knee supports, providing a very tight positioning support for the patient's chest, pelvis, and legs, is used (Fig. 13.1). Setup marks are made on the cradle and the posterior and lateral fields are treated through the cradle, using 15-MV photons. Alignment marks are made on the right and left sides of the cradle and between the legs from the thighs down to between the feet. Additional marks are made on each leg just below the knees and on the cradle. The purpose of these marks is to make sure that the patient is returned to the mold correctly in the cephalad-caudal direction.

SMALL BOWEL SPARING

Injury to the small bowel as a result of radiation therapy is an important dose-limiting factor to con-

---

* Dow Chemical, Midland, MI.

* Smithers Medical Products, Inc., Akron, OH.

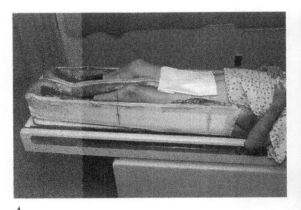

A

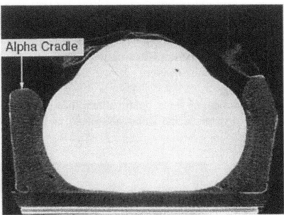

C

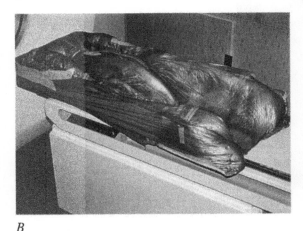

B

Figure 13.1   *A*. Immobilization device for prostate irradiation. Sagittal alignment marks are made between the legs, and marks across the legs below the knees are used to verify that the patient is returned to the Alpha Cradle correctly in the cephalad/caudal direction. *B* and *C*. The immobilization device fits tightly to the patient's body.

sider when radiation therapy of the pelvis or abdomen is contemplated. Letschert et al. found a 37 percent incidence of severe small bowel injury when large opposed anterior and posterior (AP-PA) pelvic fields were used to deliver 4500 to 5000 cGy in 5 weeks and only 6 percent when smaller fields were treated using a three-field technique.[5] The authors suggest that when the small bowel volume is increased by a factor of 2, the dose has to be reduced by 17 percent for the same incidence of small-bowel injury. The problem of small bowel injury following pelvic irradiation have been studied by several other authors.[6-11]

Several methods to reduce the volume of small bowel within pelvic fields have been described, including placement of the patient in the supine, prone, decubitus, or Trendelenburg position.[12-14] Other nonsurgical techniques, including custom molds providing an opening for unobstructed gravitational displacement of the bowel, external low pelvis compression, and bladder distention have been described.[14-17] Surgical techniques, consisting of placement of an absorbable mesh sling that elevates the small bowel out of the pelvis, have also been described.[18-22] After several weeks, the mesh is absorbed and the bowel returns to its normal position. Placement of a pelvic spacer,[23] a permanent silastic prosthesis creating a barrier for the small bowel,[24] and a temporary tissue expander that excludes the small bowel from the pelvis[25] have been tried. Devices placed surgically to displace the small bowel out of the pelvis are usually limited to patients where a surgical procedure is necessary, either during the staging procedure or as an adjunct to radiation therapy. In either event, the use of radiation therapy in the management of the disease must be anticipated before the device is inserted.

Belly Board.   A belly board, sometimes used in an effort to displace the small bowel out of pelvic fields,[17] is an insert that fits over the treatment couch and has an opening which eliminates the pressure of the hard treatment couch on the abdomen of the prone patient. The technique is tried in an effort to promote a gravitational displacement of the small bowel out of pelvic treatment fields. The addition of a compression roll, immediately caudal to the opening and positioning the patient such that the lower

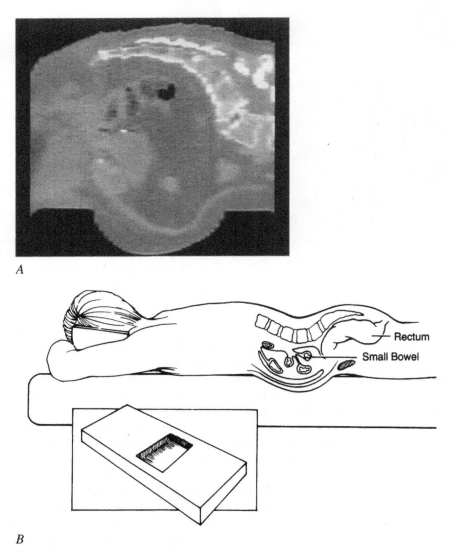

A

B

Figure 13.2   *A.* Sagittal view of the pelvis when the patient is on a belly board. *B.* A belly board with an opening, eliminating pressure on the abdomen and, instead, promoting gravitational displacement of the small bowel out of the pelvis.

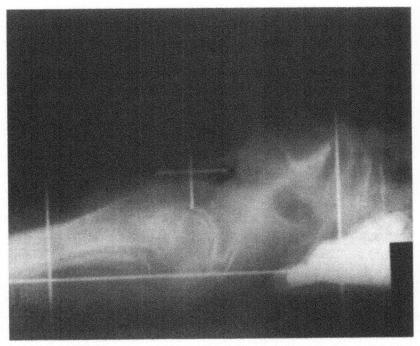

A

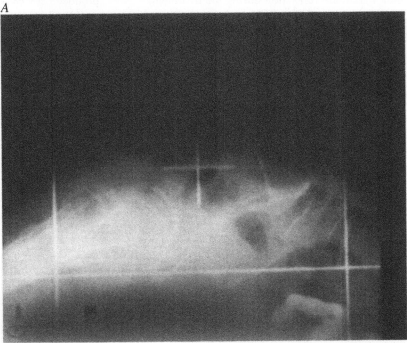

Figure 13.3 A prone patient without *(A)* and with *(B)* a compression roll. Some shift of the small bowel is noted in this very thin patient.

B

pelvis is on the compression roll, may also promote small-bowel displacement. The small bowel is confined inside the peritoneal cavity and is protected by the abdominal muscles. In patients with good abdominal muscle tone, the effect of gravity on the small bowel is thought to be less than in patients with poor tone. Thin patients benefit as much from the belly-board position as do obese patients. The absence of abdominal pressure from the tabletop is advantageous in practically all cases. In obese patients, the abdominal folds sometimes fall into the opening; it is a mistake to believe that it is the small bowel which falls anteriorly (Fig. 13.2A).

For many patients, especially those treated during the immediate postsurgical period, a prone position on a belly board rather than on the hard treatment couch may be more comfortable. The position of the patient on a belly board must be carefully reproduced, and the exact location of the compression is very important to the reproducibility (Fig. 13.2B). Adequate support must be provided to allow the patient maximum relaxation during the treatment.

The use of a belly board in very obese patients should be limited to patients being treated through a three-field technique consisting of posterior and opposed lateral fields. An anterior field should be omitted when possible, because when a large volume of abdominal tissue falls into the opening, an anterior field would pass through a very large thickness of normal tissue, and the dose here could be quite high. In a thin or moderately obese patient, either a three- or a four-field technique could be used while the patient is on a belly board.

Other Nonsurgical Methods.   In some patients, placement of a compression roll under the lower abdomen, with or without the help of a belly board, may promote small-bowel displacement out of the pelvis. Determination of which technique is most beneficial in each situation can only be made through comparison of lateral radiographs taken with the patient in each position 1 to 2 h after swallowing the barium contrast (Figs. 13.3, 13.4, and 13.5).

Sparing of the small bowel and bladder may also be achieved by treating the patient with a full bladder. The level of bladder fullness must then be reproduced for every treatment. Giving the patient a couple of glasses of water or a soft drink 1 h before the treatment may be necessary if the patient forgets or is unable to hold the urine.

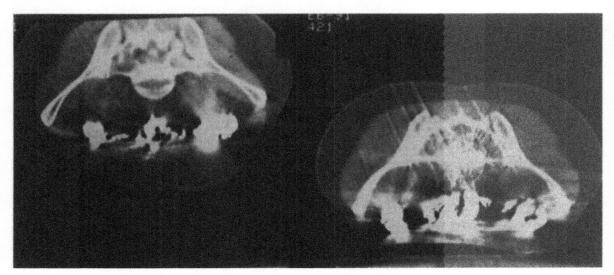

Figure 13.4   Computed tomography images with *(left)* and without *(right)* the belly board show a small displacement of the bowel in the patient in Fig. 13.3.

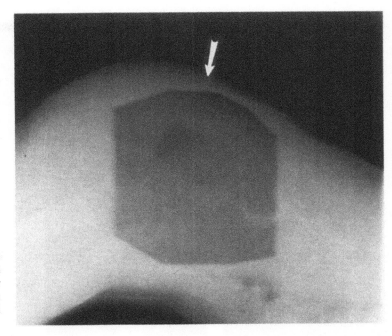

Figure 13.5   A compression roll under the patient changes the patient's position so that the anterior and posterior fields include a larger volume of the abdomen. By turning the couch 90° and then the gantry, the volume of normal tissue in the abdomen can be reduced.

Elderly, ill, and postsurgical patients are often limited as to the position they can tolerate. For these patients, compromises may have to be made in terms of positioning. For example, a patient who would be better treated in the prone position but is unable to tolerate it due to postsurgical discomfort may have to be treated in the supine or decubitus position. (See Chap. 12, Fig. 12.8, for a decubitus immobilization device.)

EFFECTIVENESS OF PATIENT IMMOBILIZATION

The effectiveness of an immobilization method is largely dependent on patient cooperation. A patient who understands the importance of the immobilization and is willing and able to cooperate is more likely to remain motionless during the therapy and is usually also willing to get into awkward positions. The effectiveness of an immobilization device is often determined by comparing simulation and portal films of the treatment fields. It is important to recognize, however, that many other factors play an important role in the accuracy of the patient-beam alignment observed on portal films. For example, the

fit of the immobilization device (clothing must be avoided), the precision with which the alignment system is calibrated, the amount of sag in the couch in the CT, simulation, and treatment rooms, and the patience and meticulousness of the treating technologists. The ability to reproduce the setup of pelvic fields is becoming very important as three-dimensional treatment-planning capabilities and the desire to spare normal tissues in the pelvis lead to smaller tumor margins.[2–4,26,27]

TREATMENT PLANNING—GYNECOLOGIC MALIGNANCIES

TARGET LOCALIZATION AND TREATMENT SIMULATION

The most common gynecologic malignancies treated with radiation therapy are carcinoma of the uterine cervix and endometrial carcinoma. The treatment fields used for these diseases are similar and are designed to include the primary tumor and the regional lymph nodes (Fig. 13.6). The treatment technique

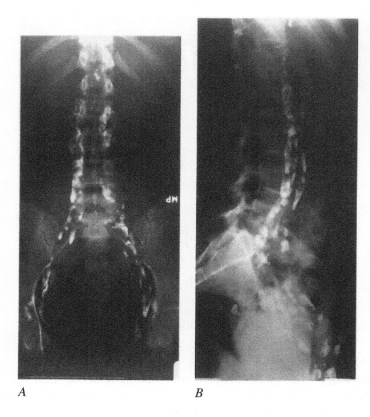

A   *B*

Figure 13.6   Anterior *(A)* and lateral *(B)* radiographs from a lymphangiogram demonstrating the location of paraaortic and pelvic lymph nodes.

usually consists of a four-field box technique, as described previously. The anterior treatment field usually extends cephalad from the L5-S1 interspace in early-stage disease and from the L4-L5 interspace in more advanced stages. The caudal margins should extend to the midobturator foramen if there is no known vaginal disease and, in patients with known vaginal involvement, the caudal margins are usually extended inferiorly to include the disease with at least a 1.5- to 2-cm margin. The lateral margins extend 1.5 to 2 cm beyond the widest section of the bony pelvis. The lateral fields should have the same cephalad and caudal extent as the anterior field. The anterior margin includes the symphysis pubis and the posterior margin extends to the S2-S3 interspace. Typical fields are shown in Fig. 13.7. The fields should be tailored to each patient's disease and the margins given here should be used only as a guide. For example, in patients with carcinoma of the uter-

ine cervix with known disease in the common iliac or paraaortic lymph nodes, the fields must extend cephalad to also include the paraaortic lymph nodes. In other patients, it may be necessary to treat the inguinal lymph nodes, and in patients with endometrial carcinoma, it may be necessary to treat the entire length of the vagina.

Approximately one hour prior to the simulation procedure, the patients are given oral barium sulfate* (one pint) contrast so that the location of small bowel with respect to the treatment fields can be visualized on the radiographs. When possible, the fields should be shaped to minimize small-bowel volume within the irradiated volume. The patient is placed in the anticipated treatment position and a contrast-enhanced vaginal cylinder is inserted in the vagina. A

---

* E-Z Paque barium sulfate for suspension, E-Z-EM, Inc., Westbury, NY.

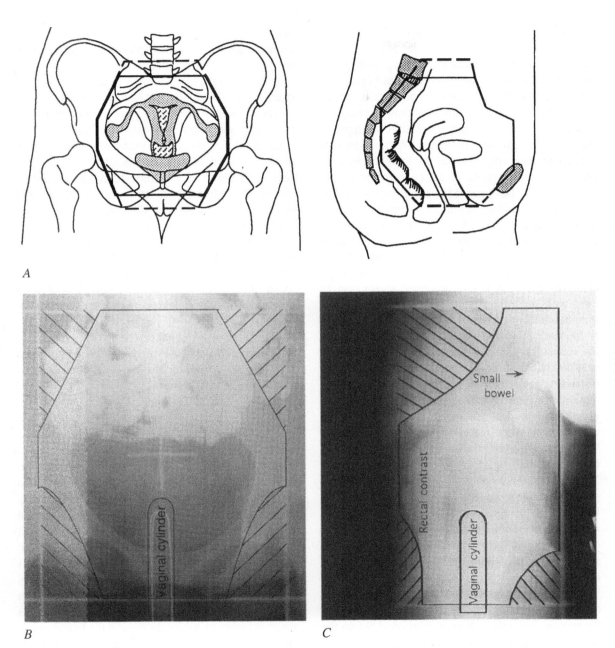

Figure 13.7 *A–C.* Typical treatment fields for treatment of carcinoma of the cervix. A vaginal cylinder is inserted to indicate the location of the vagina. Rectal contrast is used only in the lateral radiograph, as it would obscure the vaginal cylinder in the anterior radiograph. The volume of small bowel in these fields appears very large; however, most of the small bowel is spared by the lateral fields. The hatched lines in the diagram indicate typical fields used in patients with more advanced cervical disease or with endometrial carcinoma.

rectal tube is inserted in the rectum for later insertion of rectal contrast. It is a good practice to insert the rectal tube in advance so as to prevent patient movement once the simulation procedure has begun. The anterior field is then set while the position is viewed in fluoroscopy. An isocentric treatment technique is preferable, and the isocenter is therefore set approximately at the patient's middepth. Without moving the patient, the gantry is turned 90° to either side and, again, in fluoroscopy, the anterior and posterior margins are set by raising and lowering the couch. The cephalad and caudal margins must remain the same as in the anterior view. From these two orthogonal views, it is possible to appreciate the volume of small bowel that will be within the treatment fields. If it is considered excessive, the patient's position can be changed or a belly board, described above, can be used with or without compression in an effort to minimize the small-bowel volume within the fields. If the small-bowel volume is considered acceptable, the simulation procedure can continue.

If the height of the couch was changed considerably when the lateral field was viewed, the margins in the anterior field may need to be adjusted because, effectively, the distance and therefore the field size was changed when the couch height was adjusted. The radiograph, or simulation film, is exposed, and the field is marked on the patient's anterior pelvis. When two parallel opposed fields are used, a radiograph of only one field is necessary. However, it is important to recognize that the field margins with respect to reference structures will appear different on the two films. It may therefore be useful to have a simulation film of both fields when port films are reviewed.

Approximately 60 mL (60 cc) of barium contrast (the same as used for the small bowel) is inserted in the rectum. If the rectal barium is inserted before the anterior radiograph is taken, important anatomic references and the vaginal cylinder would be obscured. The gantry is again turned 90° to either side and the field margins are verified before the radiograph is exposed. The field is then marked on the skin surface or, alternatively, on the immobilization device. There are conflicting opinions as to how these fields should be marked. One philosophy is that these

marks represent the intended fields and that any subsequent adjustment is accomplished through changes in the customized shields and in the collimator setting. The central axis of these fields will thus not change and should be tattooed before the patient leaves the simulation room. Another philosophy is that these fields represent only the simulated treatment and should therefore be marked with temporary marks. Small discrepancies are often observed between the setup in the simulation and treatment rooms (laser alignment systems, couch surface, and so on), giving rise to small discrepancies in the first set of port films. It is therefore believed that subsequent field adjustments, required when the port film is examined, should be made by shifting the field; when port films are acceptable, the marks are tattooed. A contour, described in Chap. 7, should be obtained while the patient remains in treatment position.

In patients with vaginal extension of the disease, it is advisable to mark the inferior extent with a gold seed to ensure that the radiation field covers the disease with adequate margins.

TREATMENT TECHNIQUES—WHOLE PELVIS

The four-field arrangement described above is usually treated using high-energy photon beams (Fig. 13.8A). For comparison, the same treatment plan using 4-MV photon beams is also shown (Fig. 13.8B). Here we can see that using a 4-MV photon beam results in a fairly high dose in the lateral aspect of the pelvis. When the same plan is calculated using a 15-MV photon beam, the dose in these areas is considerably lower. In situations where high-energy beams are not available, the lower beam energy can be used and the anterior and posterior beams weighted more to reduce the dose in the lateral pelvis (Fig. 13.8C). Alternate field arrangements, eliminating anterior and posterior fields, may be necessary in patients with wound dehiscence (Fig. 13.9).

The use of anterior and posterior pelvic fields alone should be limited to palliative treatment of metastatic disease or to situations where the tumor extent is uncertain. This situation, although rare, could present itself in elderly patients in whom stag-

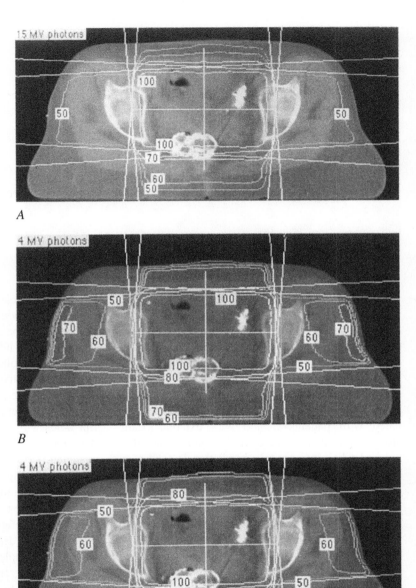

Figure 13.8 *A.* An isodose distribution from a four-field box technique using 15-MV photon beams and equally weighted. *B.* The same plan calculated using 4-MV photon beams results in higher dose in the lateral aspect of the pelvis. *C.* The same plan as in *B*, but with heavier weight on the anterior and posterior fields (1.5 to 1.0) reduces the dose in the lateral pelvis.

ing procedures are precluded due to the patient's physical condition. The addition of lateral fields in some patients would encompass the entire patient thickness. However, it is important to remember that although at some point the entire patient thickness is included in the lateral fields, some normal tissue sparing can be achieved by shaping these fields to the target in the beam's-eye view (Fig. 13.10). For example, segments of small bowel that lie within the anterior and posterior fields can often be spared by

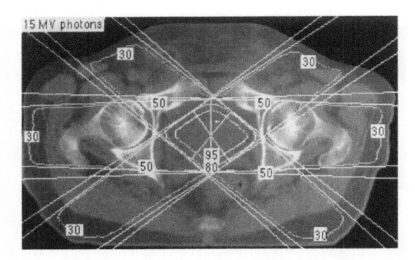

Figure 13.9 A six-field beam arrangement, omitting the anterior and posterior fields, may be needed in patients with wound dehiscence.

the lateral fields, thus reducing the dose within the segment (Fig. 13.7).

In practically all patients with carcinoma of the uterine cervix, the disease is managed by a combination of external beam irradiation and brachytherapy.[28,29] In patients where a portion of the treatment is delivered via intracavitary irradiation, the recurrence rates in all stages are decreased when compared with patients treated with external beam alone.[30] Furthermore, the complication rates are also reduced when intracavitary irradiation is used as a component of the treatment as compared with the use of external beam irradiation alone. In patients with carcinoma in situ or very early invasive carcinoma, a total abdominal hysterectomy is an acceptable treatment. An alternate treatment, often used in the management of medically inoperable patients and yielding similar results, is to deliver approximately 7000 cGy to point A via intracavitary insertions. A discussion of intracavitary insertions, including definition of point A, can be found in Chap. 16.

Patients with early-stage invasive disease, where the tumor is confined to the central part of the pelvis, may be treated by delivering 2000 cGy to the entire pelvis via anterior and posterior external beam fields, followed by one or two intracavitary placements to deliver 5500 to 6000 cGy to point A. The external beam treatment, generally used to treat more advanced disease, supplements the dose to regional lymph nodes situated too far from the intra-

cavitary application to receive adequate dose.

In patients with more advanced disease, a larger proportion of the dose is delivered via external beam therapy. Here, 4000 to 5000 cGy is delivered to the whole pelvis followed by one or two intracavitary applications delivering 3500 to 4500 cGy to point A. The dose in the parametria may have to be supplemented via external beam, using anterior and posterior fields with a midline shield to protect the bladder, rectum, and other normal tissues already irradiated to a very high dose via the intracavitary applications (Fig. 13.11). A typical isodose distribution from the external-beam treatment is shown in Fig. 13.12. The total dose and the sequencing of external beam therapy and intracavitary applications is individualized depending on the extent of the disease. For example, where the anatomy of the upper vagina and the cervix is distorted by disease, it may not be possible to achieve acceptable geometry with the intracavitary application. In anticipation of tumor regression, external beam irradiation is then delivered first, and, following a short rest period, an intracavitary application may be tried.

TREATMENT TECHNIQUES—PELVIS AND PARAAORTIC LYMPH NODES

The role and outcome of paraaortic lymph node irradiation in patients with cervical and uterine carcinoma has been studied by several authors.[31-41] The

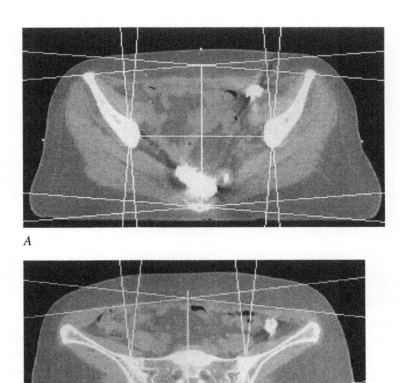

A

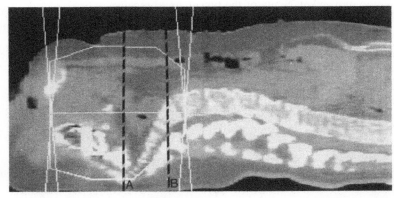

B

C

Figure 13.10   *A.* In a contour at the central axis, lateral pelvic fields may sometimes appear not to be of benefit because it would have to include the entire pelvis. *B.* Lateral fields may, however, be beneficial, because sparing of normal tissue at other levels is usually possible. *C.* A sagittal view showing the location of the two contours and sparing of normal tissue in the lateral fields.

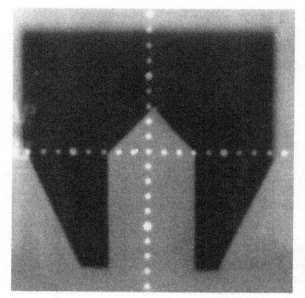

Figure 13.11 A midline block to spare the bladder, rectum, and other central pelvic normal tissues is used when the parametria are boosted following intracavitary implants.

both areas. Most authors propose treating both the pelvis and paraaortic lymph nodes in contiguous large fields. Some authors describe opposed anterior and posterior fields, while others suggest a four-field technique. Russell et al. report treating both the pelvis and paraaortic lymph nodes via a four-field technique, weighting the anterior and posterior fields 2 to 1 over the opposed lateral fields.[40] The lateral fields are carefully shaped to the target to minimize the risks of enteritis.

The paraaortic lymph node fields usually extend cephalad to the T12-L1 interspace and are wide enough to include the transverse processes (about 8 cm). During the simulation of these fields, it is highly recommended that intravenous contrast [60 mL (i.e., 60 cc) Isovue®, organically bound iodine]* be given to determine the function and position of the kidneys.

Treatment of the pelvis and paraaortic lymph nodes in one field is often complicated by the need for different dose fractionation schemes in the two sites. The fraction size to the pelvis is often 180 cGy, while that to the paraaortic lymph nodes is 150 cGy, so as to minimize the risks of small-bowel toxicity. A four-field technique can be used to treat both areas, but an attenuator that transmits about 83 percent (150/180) of the pelvic dose must be used in the segment of the fields that covers the paraaortic lymph nodes. As in all other off-axis dose calculations, the patient's thickness, the off-axis factor, and

technique, dose fractionation, and total dose vary among the authors. Some authors report treating the pelvis and paraaortic lymph nodes in separate fields.[33,34] This leads to concern with regard to field matching in an area where there is considerable peristaltic movement. Some of the bowel could receive very high doses, as peristaltic movements, at least theoretically, could cause some of the bowel to lie within the irradiated area during the treatment of

* Squibb Diagnostics, New Brunswick, NJ.

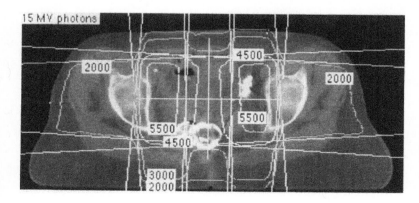

Figure 13.12 The dose distribution resulting from delivering 4500 cGy to the pelvis via a four-field box technique, followed by 1000 cGy to the parametria via anterior and posterior fields with a midline block.

the effect of field size and shape should be considered when the amount of beam attenuation is calculated. An alternative method is to deliver 150 cGy via all four fields and then reduce the size of the lateral fields to encompass only the pelvis and deliver another 30 cGy. This method requires longer setup time and is quite complicated to execute. A simpler method, although less sparing of normal tissue, is to deliver 150 cGy to the paraaortic lymph nodes through anterior and posterior opposed fields and then deliver the additional 30 cGy through lateral fields to the pelvis only. Isodose distributions in the transverse, coronal, and sagittal planes resulting from an equally weighted four-field technique are demonstrated in Fig. 13.13. The isodose distributions in Fig. 13.14 result from delivering 150 cGy

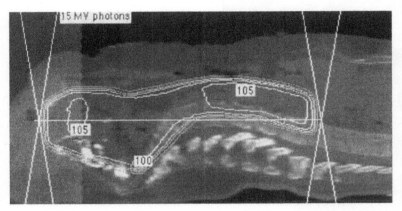

A

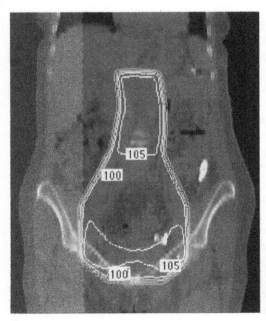

B

Figure 13.13 The isodose distribution in the sagittal *(A)* and coronal *(B)* planes, resulting from pelvic and paraaortic lymph node treatment through a four-field technique using equal weighting. The isodose distribution from the same plan in a transverse plane in the pelvis *(C)* and in the paraaortic region *(D).*

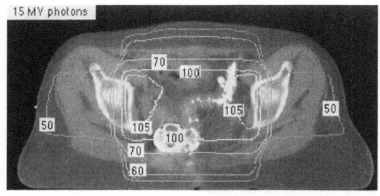

C

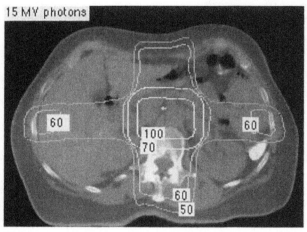

D

Figure 13.13 (*Continued*)

to the pelvic and paraaortic lymph nodes via anterior and posterior fields and then delivering an additional 30 cGy via lateral fields to the pelvis only.

TREATMENT TECHNIQUES—PELVIS AND INGUINAL LYMPH NODES

Primary tumors in the vulva, uterine cervix with involvement of the distal third of the vagina, urethra, penis, and anal canal can metastasize to the inguinal lymph nodes. Irradiation of both the primary disease in the pelvis and the inguinal lymph nodes can be quite difficult and requires careful planning.

In a study by the Gynecologic Oncology Group comparing inguinal lymph node dissection versus irradiation in patients with carcinoma of the vulva (with clinically negative or nonsuspicious regional lymph nodes following radical resection of the primary tumor), radiation therapy was found to be significantly inferior.[42] The protocol specified that a dose of 5000 cGy, calculated at 3-cm depth, be delivered in 25 fractions, and it was recommended that 50 percent of this dose be delivered with 12- to 13-MeV electrons to reduce the dose to the femoral head. It is possible that the radiation failure was due to the specified depth of dose calculation. The depth of the deep inguinal lymph nodes was studied by

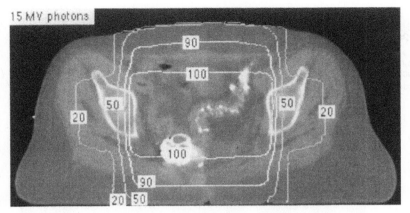

A

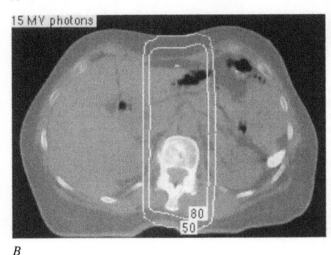

B

Figure 13.14   The isodose distribution in a transverse plane in the pelvis *(A)* and in the paraaortic region *(B),* resulting from pelvic and paraaortic lymph node treatment where 150 cGy is delivered via anterior and posterior fields to the entire volume followed by an additional 30 cGy via lateral fields to the pelvis only. In this plan, 180 cGy was delivered to the 95 percent isodose line; the 80 percent isodose line received about 150 cGy.

Koh et al.[43] They found that the mean average depth of the femoral lymph nodes in 50 patients was 6.1 cm; however, the range of depth varied from 2 to 18.5 cm. They also found a definite trend toward increased depth with increased patient obesity. This finding is significant, because the recommended depth for dose prescription is much shallower, possibly leading to underdosage of the inguinal lymph nodes.[43,44]

Treatment of the pelvis and inguinal lymph nodes is difficult when a four-field technique is used to treat the pelvis. It requires that large anterior and posterior fields be shaped to include the inguinal lymph nodes.[45] The lateral fields usually do not extend anterior enough to include the shallower inguinal lymph nodes. A separate electron field is therefore used to treat the inguinal lymph nodes, but it is critical that the risks of beam overlap be considered in three dimensions. The electron beam energy must therefore be selected so that there is no overlap with the lateral fields at depth, and it is highly recommended that the location of the field junctions on the skin surface be moved every 1000 cGy. This type of complex field matching must be carefully planned in advance. For example, the shape of the lateral photon fields must match that of the deep electron

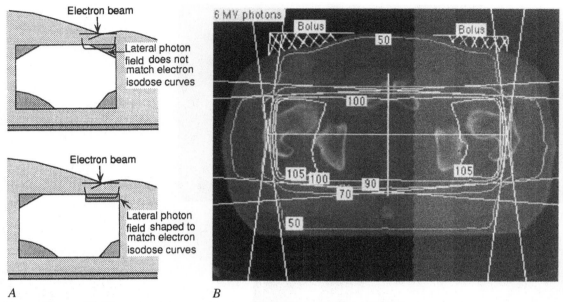

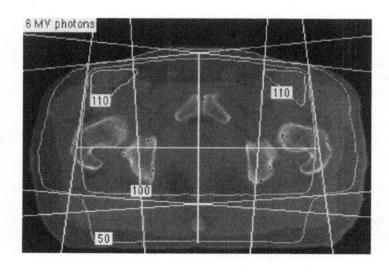

Figure 13.15 *A.* To avoid overlap at depth when anterior electron fields are used to treat the inguinal lymph nodes, the lateral photon fields must be shaped so they match the shape of the deep electron isodose curves. *B.* In the transverse direction, where shaping of the photon isodose curves is not possible, the anterior surface must be modified so that the electron isodose curves match the photon isodose curves.

isodose curves in the selected electron beam (Fig. 13.15*A*). In order for the electron isodose curves to also match the isodose distribution from the lateral fields in the transverse plane, compensating bolus material is usually needed over the inguinal lymph nodes (Fig. 13.15*B*). Alternatively, the lateral fields could also be shaped to include the inguinal nodes; however, the volume of bladder included in these fields may be excessive (Fig. 13.16).

Petereit et al. described a technique using only

Figure 13.16 If the lateral photon fields are extended anteriorly to include the inguinal lymph nodes, there is very little normal tissue sparing in the pelvis.

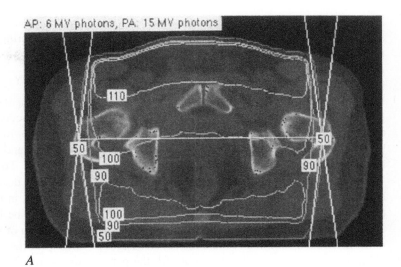

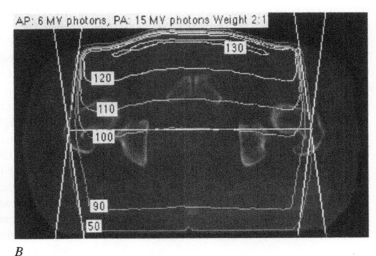

Figure 13.17   *A.* Isodose distribution resulting from treating the pelvis and inguinal lymph nodes using a 6-MV photon beam in the anterior and a 15-MV photon beam in the posterior field, equally weighted. *B.* The same treatment plan but weighted 2 to 1 favoring the anterior field.

A

B

anterior and posterior fields shaped to include the inguinal nodes.[46] They use a 2 : 1 weighting favoring the anterior field or a mixed-beam technique in which the anterior field was treated with 6-MV and the posterior with 10-MV photons. Figure 13.17*A* and *B* show two treatment plans in which an anterior field is treated using a 6-MV photon beam and a posterior field using a 15-MV photons beam. In Fig. 13.17*A*, the fields are equally weighted; in Fig. 13.17*B*, the fields are weighted 2 : 1 favoring the anterior.

Another technique, described by Kalend,[47] con-

sists of a large anterior field that encompasses the pelvis and the inguinal lymph nodes and a posterior field covering the pelvis only. The desired dose to the inguinal lymph nodes at a specified depth is delivered through the anterior field. A beam attenuator is used in the segment of the anterior field that is opposed by the posterior pelvic field. The amount of beam attenuation is calculated so that the midpoint of the pelvis receives the same dose from the anterior and the posterior fields. The anterior beam attenuator is fabricated with beveled edges that extend slightly out into the inguinal section of the field to compensate for the divergence of the posterior field. The width of the beveled section depends on the thickness of the patient; that is, the amount of divergence of the posterior field and the slope of the beveled edge depend on the penumbral width of the posterior beam. Figure 13.18 shows a port film with the pelvic compensator in place. A treatment plan simulating this technique is shown in Fig. 13.19A. (The additional dose delivered in the inguinal areas is here delivered through *separate* small inguinal fields.) When the compensator is used, both the inguinal areas and the pelvis are treated in a single field, causing the geometry to be slightly different from that in Fig. 13.19B. The dose is also somewhat less uniform in this illustration because the beveled edges of the compensator would compensate for the penumbra of the posterior field.

In the absence of a compensator, other, less sophisticated treatment techniques can be used. Figure 13.20 demonstrates isodose distributions using large opposed anterior and posterior fields with equal weight (A), a 2 to 1 weight favoring the anterior fields (B), and a large anterior pelvic and inguinal

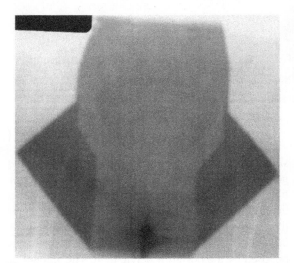

Figure 13.18   A port film of the anterior field including the pelvis and the inguinal lymph nodes. The pelvic portion of the field appears lighter because of the compensator present in the beam. This portion of the field is opposed by a posterior pelvic field.

field opposed by a smaller pelvic field and weighted 2 to 1 favoring the anterior (C).

MORBIDITY

The treatment results in patients with carcinoma of the uterine cervix are gradually improving and a high percentage of patients with early-stage disease (stages I and II) are cured with radiation therapy.[28,48–52] To achieve these encouraging results, very high doses of radiation are delivered to the pelvis and, in a relatively small number of patients, normal tissue injury occurs. The combined dose in the mucosa of the cervix and the distal vagina delivered via external beam and brachytherapy is often in excess of 10,000 cGy, while the dose in the paracervical triangle is often on the order of 7000 to 8000 cGy. The proximity of radiosensitive organs such as the bladder, rectum, and small bowel is of serious concern, and methods to reduce morbidity or complications while at the same time maintaining or improving cure rates must be pursued.

The most severe complication from radiation therapy, although not very common, is rectovaginal or vesicovaginal fistulas. Fistulas can be caused when a tumor in the vaginal wall is destroyed, leaving an opening between the rectum and the vagina or between the bladder and the vagina. It can also be caused by tissue necrosis resulting from excessive radiation dose. Other less severe but far from inconsequential complications include proctitis, cystitis, uretheral stricture, rectal ulcer, sigmoid stricture, small bowel obstruction, and pelvic abscess. Montana et al. reported a 6.3 percent incidence of cystitis — including six cases of vesicovaginal fistula and an 11 percent incidence of proctitis as well as seven cases of rectovaginal fistula — in a series of 527 patients. The mean bladder and rectal doses in the group with cystitis and proctitis was higher (6661 cGy and 6907 cGy, respectively) than in the patients without those side effects (6298 cGy and 6381 cGy, respectively).[53]

Among the factors associated with complications is the radiation dose to critical structures such as the bladder and rectum and the volume of these organs

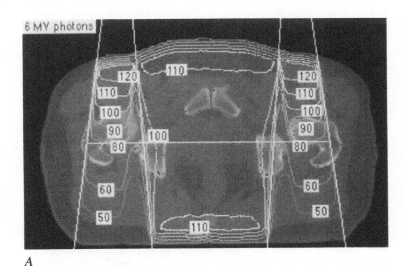

A

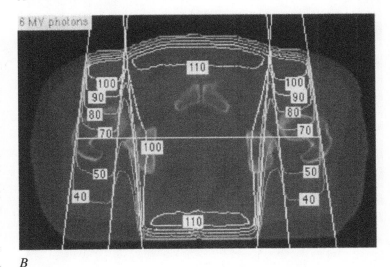

B

Figure 13.19 *A.* The dose distribution resulting from the anterior field in Fig. 13.18 with a compensator in the pelvic portion of the anterior field. The dose is calculated to deliver 100 percent at 6-cm depth in the inguinal lymph nodes. The compensator is of a thickness that reduces the dose in the pelvis to 50 percent at middepth. An additional 50 percent is then delivered only to the central pelvis via a smaller posterior field. *B.* The same plan, but here the dose is prescribed to be 100 percent at 3-cm depth in the inguinal lymph nodes. A thinner compensator is needed when the dose is prescribed at a shallower depth. In these two plans, the dose in the inguinal regions is delivered via separate inguinal fields rather than by using an attenuator in the pelvic portion of the anterior field.

included in the treatment fields. In general, the tolerance of an organ to the radiation is inversely proportional to the volume of the organ irradiated,[54] although this is not universally agreed upon.[55,56] Pourquier et al. reported a 7 percent incidence of urinary tract complications in patients where the total bladder dose was 7000 to 7500 cGy.[56] Esche et al. reported that frequency and severity of rectosigmoid complications increased with increased dose and volume treated.[54] The majority of rectosigmoid complications occurred with total doses in excess of 7000 cGy. Orton et al. also reported a correlation between dose and complication rates for both bladder and rectal injuries in a group of 410 patients.[57] Perez et al. reported that the frequency of genitourinary and rectosigmoid complications with bladder and rectal doses of 8000 cGy is 5 percent but that it rises steeply with higher doses.[58]

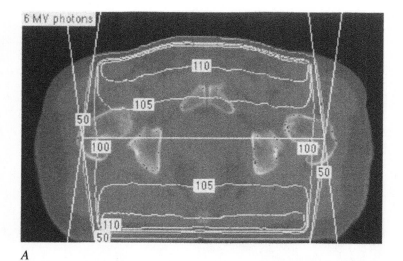

A

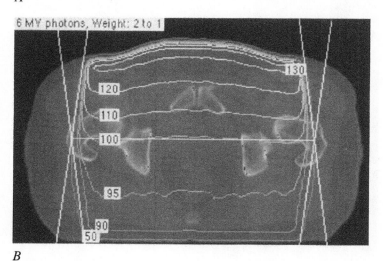

B

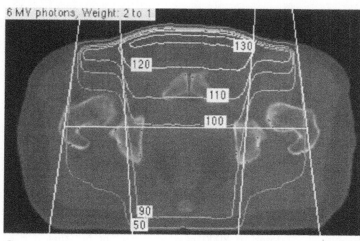

C

Figure 13.20 Isodose distributions resulting from using large opposed anterior and posterior fields with equal weight *(A)*, a 2-to-1 weight favoring the anterior fields *(B)*, and a large anterior pelvic and inguinal field opposed by a smaller pelvic field and weighted 2 to 1 favoring the anterior *(C)*.

TREATMENT PLANNING— PROSTATE CARCINOMA

The treatment philosophy of prostatic carcinoma is quite complex; with the introduction of the prostate specific antigen (PSA) test, the issue has become further compounded. Surgery, radiation therapy, and hormonal manipulation are the primary treatment modalities. The treatment depends largely on the patient's age, stage and differentiation of the tumor, PSA level, underlying medical problems, and patient preference. The reliability of clinical staging of prostate carcinoma is not very good, and a large percentage of patients are found at the time of prostatectomy to have extension into the seminal vesicles, capsular penetration, and/or histologically positive margins.[59] Staging lymphadenectomy is the preferred procedure to determine the presence of lymph node metastases.

When the tumor is confined to the prostate, the treatment usually consists of radiation therapy or a radical prostatectomy. If the tumor is felt to have penetrated the capsule or to involve the seminal vesicles, radiation therapy is the treatment of choice. Most patients with prostate carcinoma who have positive regional nodes are incurable and are not offered definitive radiotherapy. Those few patients who may benefit from radiotherapy are treated to the prostate, seminal vesicles, and periprostatic tissues only on the assumption that the majority of patients have undetected hematogenous metastasis at the time of the diagnosis[60] and that the potential gain from elective nodal irradiation is not worth the increased risk of complications from large-field radiation therapy. Furthermore, since a randomized study by the Radiation Therapy Oncology Group (RTOG) comparing results between large-field whole-pelvis versus limited-field treatment in early-stage prostate carcinoma showed equal results,[61] the trend is not to treat the whole pelvis.

In cases where whole-pelvis treatment is carried out, the seminal vesicles are unintentionally included; however, when smaller fields are used, it is important to know whether the seminal vesicles are at risk. Involvement of the seminal vesicles is difficult to detect on physical and radiographic examination but is important for designing the radiation ther-apy fields. Patients with well-differentiated T1 or T2 tumors appear to be at a low risk for occult seminal vesicle involvement; therefore the seminal vesicles can be excluded from the target volume, thus also reducing the volume of rectum and bladder in the irradiated fields.[62]

Radiation therapy of prostate carcinoma is usually delivered via external beam therapy alone, but in some institutions interstitial irradiation is employed either as primary therapy, usually in conjunction with a lymph node dissection, or to deliver a boost to the prostate gland[63–70] (Chap. 16). Locally advanced prostatic cancer is sometimes managed with a regimen consisting of external beam therapy followed by brachytherapy and interstitial hyperthermia[71] or with neoadjuvant androgen deprivation.

External beam radiation therapy of early-stage prostate carcinoma involves the treatment of the prostate gland, seminal vesicles, and periprostatic tissues to approximately 6000 cGy, followed by a boost to the prostate gland to 6800 to 7000 cGy. Higher doses are given in some trials where the margins around the target are very tight, the patients are aggressively immobilized (Fig. 13.1), and the planning is carried out on a three-dimensional treatment planning system.[1,72,73] The ability to visualize the three-dimensional geometry of the prostate and its position relative to the bladder and rectum and to shape the radiation beam so that it conforms to the shape of the target has led to increased confidence in designing treatment fields with smaller tumor margins (Fig. 13.21).[3,4,26,27,60,72,74–76] Studies with respect to changes in the size and location of the bladder and rectum and their effect on the location of the prostate gland and seminal vesicles has been prompted by the small margins often used in prostate treatments designed with the aid of a three-dimensional treatment planning system.[74,77–82]

In advanced-stage disease, palliative irradiation of the entire pelvis to approximately 5000 cGy followed by a boost to the prostate gland may be given.

TARGET LOCALIZATION AND TREATMENT SIMULATION

The four-field box technique described for treatment of gynecologic malignancies is often also used in the

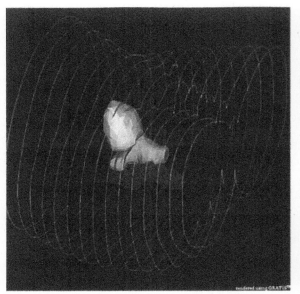

A

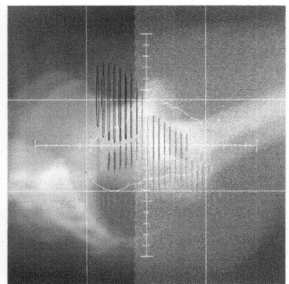

B

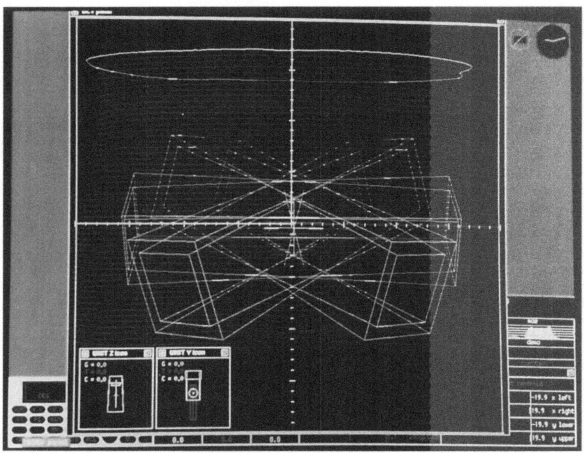

C

treatment of prostate cancer, and the treatment simulation procedure is therefore similar.

In the treatment of advanced disease, where the whole pelvis is treated, the inferior border encompasses the inferior border of the prostate with a 1.5- to 2-cm margin and is usually at the inferior aspect of the ischial tuberosities. The cephalad margin should include the common iliac lymph nodes (i.e., approximately the L4-L5 interspace), and the lateral borders should include the bony pelvis with a 1.5- to 2-cm margin. The lateral fields should have the same caudal and cephalad extent as the anterior and posterior fields. The anterior margins should include the pubis symphysis and the posterior margins should transect the rectum (Fig. 13.22). The fields should be shaped to avoid large volumes of small bowel, rectum, and bladder. Treatment of these fields is often followed by a boost dose to the prostate. Radical prostate irradiation is usually delivered via smaller fields that include the prostate gland, seminal vesicles, and the periprostatic tissues (Fig. 13.23). These fields must usually be at least 10×10 cm. Custom design of these fields must be seriously considered, since the size and location of the prostate and seminal vesicles varies among patients and from day to day, depending on the fullness of the bladder and rectum. The boost volume just described cannot be encompassed by 8×8 cm fields, as shown by several authors.[76,83-87] A boost is often delivered to the prostate gland only, using small margins (usually less than 1.5 cm).

In the absence of three-dimensional treatment-planning capabilities and aggressive immobilization methods, the target margins must be quite generous, because the precise target is difficult to localize. In some patients, it is possible to insert a metal clip to mark the palpable inferior and posterior aspects of the prostate gland prior to the simulation procedure. Some authors recommend a urethrogram to define the caudal margin of the treatment field.[88-92]

Contrast should be inserted into the bladder prior to taking an anterior simulation film. Ten mL (10 cc) of Renografin®* is inserted in the bulb of a Foley catheter, and 60 mL (60 cc) of Renografin diluted in saline (50/50) is inserted in the bladder. The catheter should be retracted until the balloon is at the uretheral orifice. Localization of the prostate gland, situated immediately below the bladder neck and surrounding the proximal urethra, is aided by visualization of the contrast in the uretheral segment of the catheter as it emerges from the bladder (Fig. 13.23). When large whole pelvis fields are simulated, small bowel contrast should also be given prior to the simulation procedure.

To include the prostate gland, the seminal vesicles and the periprostatic tissues, 10×10 cm to 12×12 cm fields may be necessary. The fields should be centered from left to right in the pelvis with the inferior margin usually at or slightly caudal of the ischial tuberosities (Fig. 13.23). After the anterior simulation film has been obtained and prior to taking the lateral radiograph, approximately 60 mL (60 cc) of E-Z Paque barium sulfate is inserted in the rectum. The lateral fields should have the same cephalad and caudal margins as the anterior and posterior fields and be centered, in the anterior-posterior direction, on the prostate and seminal vesicles (Fig. 13.23). The anterior margin should transect the pubic symphysis and the posterior collimator margin may include the entire circumference of the rectum. The

* Squibb Diagnostics, New Brunswick, NJ.

◀ **Figure 13.21** *A.* Surface-rendered illustration of the anatomy pertinent to prostate treatment planning. The prostate and seminal vesicles in red are immediately adjacent to the bladder in yellow and the rectum in green. *B.* A digitally reconstructed radiograph (DRR) with the prostate and seminal vesicles in red, the bladder in green, and the rectum in yellow with the conformal lateral field superimposed. *C.* With three-dimensional treatment-planning tools, treatment fields with small tumor margins and complex field orientations can be delivered with more confidence than with standard methods. (See color illustration 4, which appears between pages 532 and 533.) (The Virtual Simulator™, Sherouse Systems, Inc., Charleston, SC.)

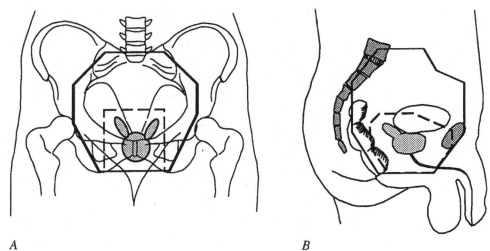

A   *B*

Figure 13.22   *A* and *B*. Diagram illustrating typical treatment fields for prostate treatment. The solid lines indicate the fields for whole-pelvic treatment while the hatched lines indicate the boost, which includes the prostate gland, seminal vesicles, and periprostatic tissues.

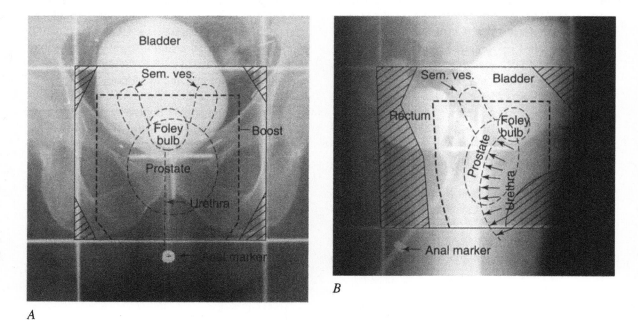

Figure 13.23   *A* and *B*. Typical prostate fields for radical prostate treatment. In the anterior simulation film, contrast is inserted into the bladder and the balloon of the Foley catheter. In the lateral radiograph, contrast has also been inserted in the rectum. The Foley catheter is retracted until the balloon is at the uretheral orifice. The course of the urethra can be followed as it exits the bladder and continues through the prostate. The prostate gland and the seminal vesicles are outlined on each film. The solid lines indicate the treatment fields for prostate, seminal vesicles, and periprostatic tissues, while the hatched lines indicate the boost to the prostate gland only.

fields should then be shaped to spare the posterior half of the rectum and as much as possible of the bladder volume without compromising the target volume. The normal prostate gland is situated anterior to the rectum, but it is important to recognize that the cancerous gland may extend farther posterior on either side of the rectum (Fig. 13.24).

For the final boost, treating the prostate gland only, the field size is reduced to approximately 9 × 9 cm or 10 × 10 cm, with the caudal margin remaining unchanged.

When CT-assisted treatment-planning technology is available, the field margins can be determined with greater confidence and the margins given here may be modified. The need for bladder and rectal contrast is usually obviated.[93]

TREATMENT TECHNIQUES

Many different techniques for the treatment of prostate cancer have been described, including arc and

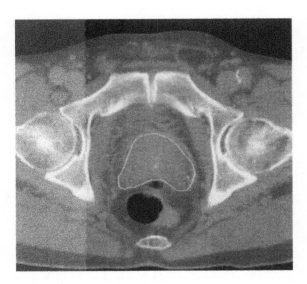

Figure 13.24 Although the prostate gland is located anterior to the rectum, it is not unusual to note that, in patients with prostate cancer, the prostate tissues may actually extend farther posterior on either side of the rectum. Rectal sparing in the lateral fields is therefore difficult, and at least the anterior half of the rectum must be included in the treatment fields during the first part of the treatment. The need for rectal sparing may indeed be more important than to risk missing a small portion of the prostate gland.

rotation techniques often used in combination with a four-field stationary field technique. With the availability of improved methods to localize the target (CT and MRI) and three-dimensional treatment-planning systems allowing more complex field arrangements, better sparing of adjacent normal tissues can be achieved.[94] A six-field technique using opposed lateral fields and two sets of opposed oblique fields angled ± 45° with respect to the lateral fields has been described by Ten Haken et al.[76] A noncoplanar multiple-field technique, which includes lateral fields and two anterior inferior oblique fields, has also been described (Fig. 13.21).[95]

In a treatment technique described by Bijhold et al. and Lebesque et al., the boost to the prostate gland is delivered simultaneously with the large-field treatment (i.e., during the same few minutes of the treatment).[26,96,97] A partial transmission block is used in the portions of the large field that are to receive a lower dose, while the segment that is to receive a higher dose remains unobstructed, i.e., without an attenuating device.

The favored treatment technique in external-beam radiation therapy of prostate carcinoma remains a four-field box technique, primarily because of the ease in setup and in review of portal films. High-energy (> 6-MV) photon beams should be used to keep the dose in the femoral head and neck low. The dose distribution resulting from a four-field technique using 15-MV photons and treating the entire pelvis is shown in Fig. 13.25. When high-energy beams are not available, heavier weighting on the anterior and posterior fields is necessary in order to keep the dose in the entrance/exit regions of all four fields fairly uniform (Fig. 13.8). This should not be done without due consideration of the inability to protect the bladder and rectum in the anterior and posterior fields. A compromise between the high dose in the bladder, rectum, and femoral head and necks may be necessary; however, a large patient may be better treated in a clinic with access to higher beam energy.

Isodose distributions using a four-field technique with 15-MV photons to treat the prostate gland, seminal vesicles, and periprostatic tissues are shown in Fig. 13.26*A*. A treatment plan for the boost to the prostate gland alone is shown in Fig. 13.26*B*. The anterior and posterior fields include the entire blad-

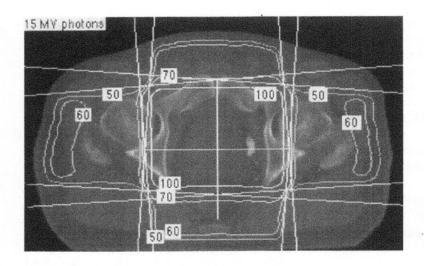

Figure 13.25   The isodose distribution resulting from a four-field whole-pelvis treatment using 15-MV photon beams with equal weighting.

der and rectum but exclude the femoral head and neck. The lateral fields, on the other hand, include the femoral head and neck but exclude large sections of the bladder and rectum (Fig. 13.27). The combined dose distribution of delivering 5000 cGy to the larger fields and 2000 cGy to the prostate boost fields is shown in Fig. 13.26C.

Alternate field arrangements are sometimes necessary when a patient presents with a metal hip prosthesis. Oblique fields to avoid the prosthesis on the proximal side of the target are then used to prevent dose reduction caused by the higher-density prosthesis.[98–102] No adverse effect on the prosthesis of the exiting radiation beam has been reported. Sometimes, alternate field arrangements may also be necessary in patients with wound dehiscence or inguinal hernia.

In a study of dose-volume histograms comparing different treatment techniques using 15-MV photons, it was found that in terms of bladder and rectum sparing, the lateral fields were superior, followed by a six-field conformal technique.[76] Other techniques studied were bilateral arcs, a four-field open-box technique, and a four-field conformational technique. Ten Haken et al. describe a treatment policy applying to all prostate boost treatments delivered via a conformational six-field technique, where half of the dose is delivered through lateral fields.[76]

Treatment of lateral fields, shaped to conform to the target, provides the highest degree of sparing of rectum and bladder, as shown in the Ten Haken et al. study. The dose in the acetabulum, on the other hand, is very high; therefore these fields cannot be used alone. It is important to recognize that this higher weighting on the lateral fields is used only for the boost treatment. Another study comparing the three-dimensional dose distributions among three-, four-, and six-field treatment plans using 24-MV photon beams in the treatment of the prostate has also been published.[103]

MORBIDITY

Minimizing the volume of rectal and bladder tissues in the fields is crucial when the doses are high. With the advent of CT-based three-dimensional treatment-planning capabilities, considerable progress has been made in the accuracy with which we can now localize the target volume and reduce the volume of bladder and rectal tissue within the high-dose isodose contours. Hopefully, this will minimize the morbidity of the irradiation.

Acute toxicities include but are not limited to diarrhea, tenesmus, rectal bleeding, abdominal pain, urinary frequency, dysuria, and hematuria. Late sequelae of radiation therapy include persistent procti-

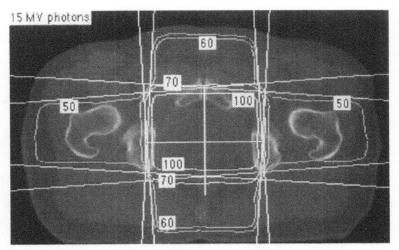

A

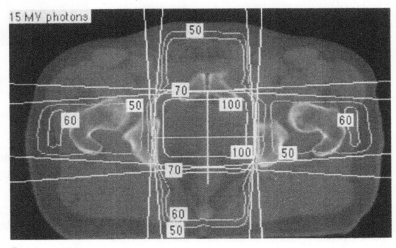

B

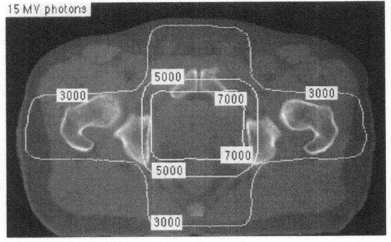

C

Figure 13.26 *A.* Isodose distribution resulting from a four-field plan to treat the prostate gland, seminal vesicles, and periprostatic tissues. *B.* Isodose distribution resulting from the same treatment plan but including only the prostate gland with small margins. *C.* A composite dose distribution from delivering 5000 cGy using the fields in *A* and 2000 cGy using the fields in *B.*

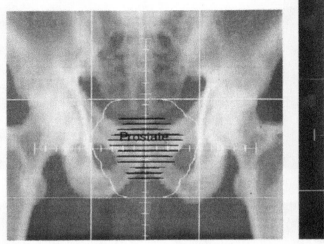
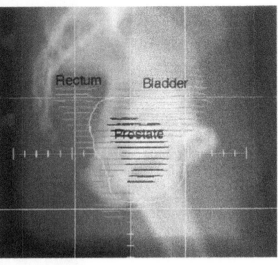

A   *B*

Figure 13.27 Digitally reconstructed radiographs (DRR) demonstrating the treatment fields for prostate boost treatment designed in a three-dimensional treatment planning system (The Virtual Simulator, Sherouse Systems, Inc.).

tis or proctosigmoiditis, fistula or perforation, bowel or bladder obstruction, chronic cystitis, and impotence. A comparison of the frequency and severity of acute toxicities between CT-based, manual, and beam's-eye-view based treatment techniques has been studied.[104] Some studies have shown a reduction in acute toxicities when conformal radiation therapy techniques are used.[73,75,105] Late toxicity as a consequence of radiation therapy is also well documented.[61,106–112]

TREATMENT PLANNING— BLADDER CARCINOMA

In the United States, most muscle-invading bladder tumors are treated with total cystectomy; radiation therapy is limited to patients with diffuse, multicentric lesions, medically or surgically inoperative patients, or patients who prefer organ preservation. Preoperative radiation therapy delivering 5000 cGy in 5 weeks, 1600 cGy in 4 fractions, or 2000 cGy in 1 week has been used.[113–115] Primary radiation therapy is more commonly used in Europe than in the United

States. The role of chemotherapy for organ preservation is currently being studied.

TARGET LOCALIZATION AND TREATMENT SIMULATION

Radiation therapy usually consists of a three-field technique using anterior and opposed lateral fields. In some very large patients, the addition of a posterior field with low weighting may be necessary. The simulation procedure is similar to that described for gynecologic tumors; however, bladder contrast is necessary in order to determine the size and position of the bladder. It is often beneficial to treat the patients with an empty bladder, thus reducing bladder size.

If the whole pelvis is to be treated, the anterior field usually extends inferiorly to the lower aspect of the obturator foramen and the cephalad margin to include the common iliac lymph nodes or to the L4-L5 interspace. This margin is often brought down to the L5-S1 interspace if the patient is also receiving chemotherapy. The lateral margins should extend approximately 1.5 to 2 cm beyond the widest aspect

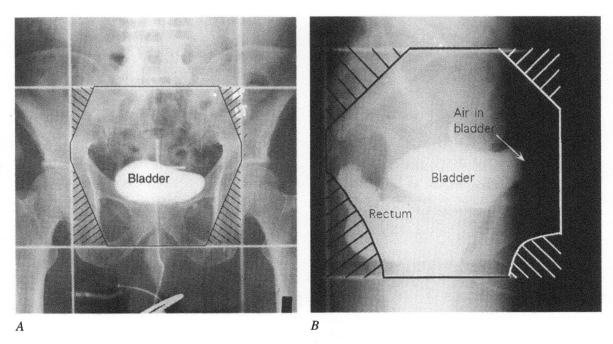

A   *B*

Figure 13.28 *A* and *B*. Typical treatment fields for treatment of bladder cancer. Contrast is inserted only in the bladder for the anterior simulation film. Rectal contrast is also inserted for the lateral film and, in female patients, a contrast-enhanced vaginal cylinder should also be used. A small volume of air in the bladder indicates the anterior extent of the bladder and is helpful when the lateral treatment fields are designed.

of the bony pelvis (Fig. 13.28). The lateral fields should have the same caudal and cephalad margins. The anterior margin should include the bladder, with at least a 1.5-cm margin, and the posterior margins should transect the rectum (Fig. 13.28).

Ten mL (10 cc) of Renografin is inserted in the bulb of the Foley catheter and 60 mL (60 cc) of Renografin diluted (50/50) in saline is inserted into the bladder along with about 10 mL (10 cc) of air. The purpose of the air, which will rise to the top, is to define the anterior extension of the bladder. A contrast-enhanced vaginal cylinder should be inserted to identify the location of the vagina in female patients. If large fields are contemplated, oral small-bowel contrast should also be given so that the treatment fields can be shaped to minimize the small-bowel volume within the fields. Following simulation and radiographic exposure of the anterior field, rectal contrast is added and the lateral simulation film is exposed.

Custom shaping of the fields is done in an attempt to minimize morbidity. The anterior field should not include the femoral head and necks and the upper corners can be shielded to reduce small bowel volume. The lateral fields can also be shaped to exclude small bowel and a large volume of the rectum. Approximately 5000 cGy is delivered to these large fields and a boost dose of approximately 1500 cGy is then delivered to the tumor-bearing portion of the bladder if this can be accurately identified. It is important to have the urologist provide a diagram of the findings at cystoscopy to facilitate boost treatment if the entire bladder is not to be included in the boost fields. The fields should be reduced to include the bladder contrast with a 2-cm margin. It is important to recognize that the bladder contrast only demonstrates the cavity of the organ and allowance must be made for the bladder wall, variations in the fullness in the bladder, and small discrepancies in setup reproducibility (Fig. 13.29).

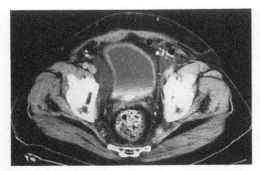

Figure 13.29 When treatment fields are designed, it is important to recognize that the contrast seen on radiographs represents only the cavity of an organ and that margins for the wall should be considered.

TREATMENT TECHNIQUES

The anteriorly situated bladder can be treated using an anterior field and two opposed lateral fields with wedges (Fig. 13.30). The purpose of the wedges is to cause the combined dose from the opposed fields to increase in a posterior direction at the same rate as the anterior field dose decreases in the same direction. A high-energy beam is necessary in order to minimize the dose in the adjacent normal tissues. A higher dose must be delivered via the anterior field to avoid excessive doses in the lateral aspect of the

pelvis near the thin edge of the wedges. The difficulties with hot spots under the thin portion of a wedge is also demonstrated in Chaps. 6 and 11. The wedges are necessary to compensate for the gradual fall-off of dose from the anterior field and for the curvature of the patient's contour. A balance must be found between the weighting and wedge angle to achieve desired dose distribution. A higher weighting on the anterior field causes a higher dose in the rectum and would also require a steeper wedge angle in the lateral fields. A steeper wedge angle increases the hot spot under the thin edge of the wedges. Higher weighting on the lateral fields also increases the dose in the lateral pelvis and femoral head and necks. In a large patient, it is sometimes necessary to add a posterior field, weighted lightly, to eliminate hot spots in the lateral aspect near the thin edge of the wedges (Fig. 13.31).

MORBIDITY

Acute morbidity consists primarily of cystitis. Diarrhea and mild proctitis may occur if the rectal wall is included in the high-dose area. Late sequelae consist of teleangiectasia in the bladder mucosa, which can lead to hematuria. Rectal bleeding may also occur. Contraction of the bladder wall can occur as a result of radiation fibrosis, leading to reduced bladder capacity.

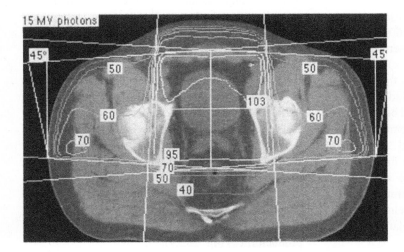

Figure 13.30 Bladder cancer is usually treated via anterior and opposed lateral wedged fields. The precise combination of weighting and wedge angles depends on the beam energy and the patient's size and shape. In this treatment plan, the anterior field is weighted 0.5 and the lateral fields with 45° wedges are weighted 0.25 each. The dose in the lateral pelvis under the thin portion of the wedges is relatively high in this particular plane but, depending on the field shape, it could be even higher in other planes.

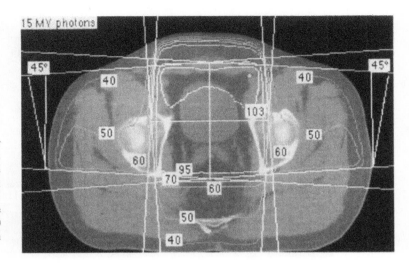

Figure 13.31   In this plan, a posterior field has been added to reduce the hot spots under the thin portions of the wedges. The anterior field is weighted 0.50, the lateral fields 0.20 each, and the posterior field 0.10. The hot spots under the thin portions of the wedges have been reduced from about 70 percent to about 55 percent, while the dose in the rectum is increased slightly.

TREATMENT PLANNING— COLORECTAL CARCINOMA

Colorectal cancer is often treated with surgery alone or with a combination of surgical resection and radiation therapy. As an adjuvant to surgery, the radiation therapy is delivered preoperatively or postoperatively and in some situations both pre- and postoperatively often in conjunction with concurrent chemotherapy. In locally advanced tumors, high-dose preoperative irradiation is the preferred treatment.[116] The intent of preoperative irradiation is to reduce the risk of tumor seeding at the time of surgery and to take advantage of the increased radiosensitivity due to better oxygenation. Preoperative irradiation is sometimes given in anticipation of reducing the extent of the surgical procedure.

TARGET LOCALIZATION AND TREATMENT SIMULATION

Radiation therapy in the treatment of colorectal cancer involves irradiation of the entire pelvis, sometimes with the addition of a boost to the site of the original tumor. When the boost is planned, it is helpful if the target is marked by surgical clips. In the absence of surgical clips, a barium enema study may be helpful to localize the target volume.

The treatment technique frequently consists of posterior and opposed lateral fields. The preferred patient position is prone to allow visualization of the sacrum on the lateral radiograph and to promote a gravitational shift of small bowel out of the pelvis. More aggressive techniques to displace small bowel have been described.[6,16,17] The prone position also reduces the risk of excessive skin reaction in and between the gluteal folds. The lateral fields are usually flashing over the posterior skin surface; therefore, when the patient is treated in the supine position, they also include the couch top, causing scatter off the couch. The skin sparing is further reduced when the patient is in the supine position because the gluteal folds are squeezed together, and when the beam is parallel with the skin surface, the skin-sparing effect of high-energy beams is decreased. The resulting reaction can be very uncomfortable and painful, and the injury is often exacerbated because the two skin surfaces constantly rub against each other. As a result, the healing process is often protracted and the patient can be incapacitated for a long time. Placing the patient in the prone position would spread the buttocks apart, thus improving the skin sparing in the crease. The treatment fields would no longer include the treatment couch, so the problem of scattering from the couch is eliminated (Fig. 13.32).

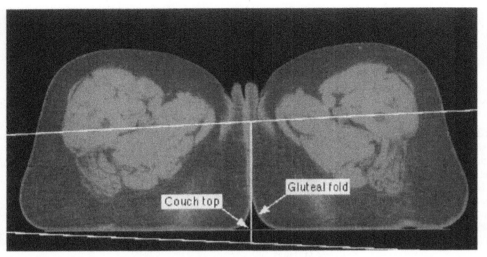

Figure 13.32   When lateral fields flash over the posterior skin surface of a supine patient, the skin reaction in the gluteal fold can be severe. Secondary scatter off the treatment couch can cause high skin dose and the skin sparing is lost from the lateral fields in this region.

The simulation procedure is similar to that described for gynecologic disease. Approximately 1 h prior to the simulation procedure, the patients are given oral barium sulfate (1 pt) contrast so that the location of small bowel with respect to the treatment fields can be visualized on the radiographs. In patients with an intact rectum (inoperative and preoperative patients), rectal contrast consisting of approximately 60 mL (60 cc) of barium contrast (same as used for small bowel) is inserted in the rectum before the simulation procedure begins. In postoperative patients, the rectal contrast should not be inserted until after anterior and lateral radiographs have been obtained to ascertain the position of surgical clips, which are sometimes left to mark the tumor bed. The rectal contrast would obscure these small metal clips. Ten mL (10 cc) of Renografin is inserted in the bulb of a Foley catheter and 60 mL (60 cc) of Renografin diluted in saline (50/50) and about 10 mL (10 cc) of air is inserted in the bladder. The catheter should be retracted until the balloon is at the uretheral orifice. The purpose of the air, which will rise to the top, is to define the posterior extension of the bladder and aid in the design of the lateral fields in the prone patient. The patients should be treated with a full bladder in an effort to reduce the volume of bladder mucosa within the treatment fields. It is also hoped that the bladder will displace small bowel out of the treatment fields. In a small group of patients with tumor adherence to or invasion of the dome of the bladder, bladder distention could displace not only the small bowel but also the necessary tumor volume outside the treatment fields. The location of the anus can be indicated by a short lead wire, formed into a circle and inserted into the rectum with the two ends of the wire extending along the external surface of the perineum (Fig. 13.33). In the postoperative setting, the incision is marked by a lead wire. In female patients, it is advantageous to indicate the vagina by the insertion of a contrast-enhanced vaginal cylinder.

The lateral field margins should extend approximately 1.5 to 2 cm beyond the widest point of the bony pelvis, and the cephalad margin should be at the L4-L5 interspace. The caudal margin varies depending on the surgical procedure but should include the obturator foramina. After an abdominoperineal resection, the inferior margin should include the perineum and the incision. The lateral fields should have the same cephalad and caudal margins as the

TREATMENT TECHNIQUES

There are differences of opinion regarding the sequencing of radiation therapy and surgical resection. The major advantage of postoperative radiation therapy is the ability to treat patients at high risk for recurrence on the basis of operative findings and to exclude those patients who were found at surgery to have metastatic disease. It also makes it possible to identify the patients who are at low risk for recurrence and therefore do not need postoperative irradiation. Preoperative radiation therapy is delivered in the hope of making unresectable tumors resectable and reducing the risk of spread during the surgical procedure. A "sandwich" technique in which both pre- and postoperative irradiation is given has also been tried. Approaches to preoperative radiation therapy have varied widely, ranging from 500 cGy in one fraction to 2000 to 2500 cGy in 2 to 2.5 weeks or 4500 to 4700 cGy followed by a boost of approximately 400 cGy to the tumor site.[116] Postoperative doses are usually on the order of 4500 to 5000 cGy in 4.5 to 5 weeks, followed by a boost to the site of the original tumor.

Patients with colorectal carcinoma are usually treated in the prone position, using a posterior and opposed lateral wedged fields (Fig. 13.35). In large patients, it might be necessary to add an anterior field with low weight to reduce the dose in the lateral aspect of the pelvis (Fig. 13.36). High-energy photon beams should be used for improved dose uniformity.

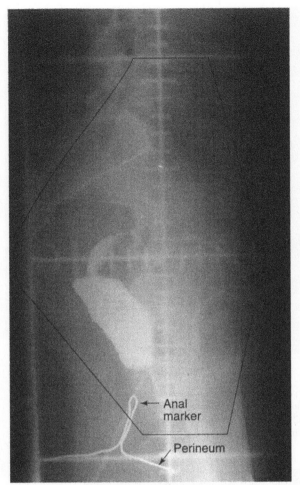

Figure 13.33   A lead wire, formed into a circle, can be inserted in the anal sphincter with the two ends extending out along the perineum. This prevents the anal marker from slipping out or otherwise being displaced during the simulation procedure.

posterior fields. The posterior margin should be approximately 1.5 cm posterior to the anterior aspect of the sacrum to provide adequate coverage of the presacral space. The anterior margins should be set to cover the site of the original tumor with a 2-cm margin. Typical treatment fields are shown in Fig. 13.34. If there is invasion of structures that drain into the external iliac nodes (i.e., bladder, uterus, or prostate), the anterior field margin may have to be placed anterior to the pubic symphysis in order to include these lymph nodes adequately.

TREATMENT PLANNING— TESTICULAR TUMORS

Testicular seminoma, the most common malignancy in the testicles, is a relatively radiosensitive tumor. Following orchiectomy, the involved or potentially involved regional lymph nodes are irradiated. In early stages, the fields include the paraaortic, ipsilateral renal hilar, and ipsilateral iliac lymph nodes. An intravenous pyelogram is recommended in order to evaluate the position and function of the kidneys prior to or during the treatment simulation.

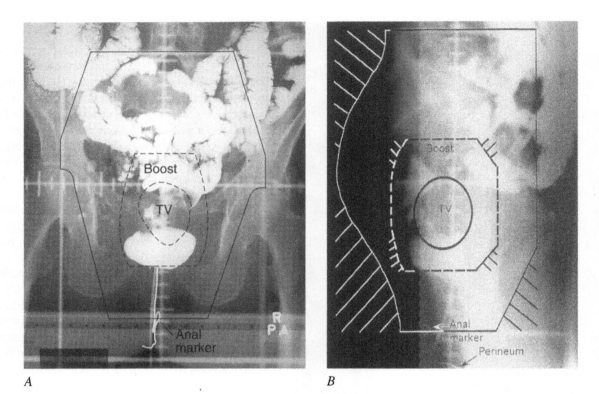

A   *B*

Figure 13.34   *A* and *B*. Typical treatment fields for preoperative irradiation of rectal cancer. Small bowel contrast given prior to the simulation procedure is helpful for field shaping. Rectal contrast is inserted prior to simulation of the lateral fields. If a boost is given, a small volume of air can be inserted in the bladder. The air will rise and indicate the posterior aspect of the bladder in the prone patient, which is helpful when the lateral fields are designed.

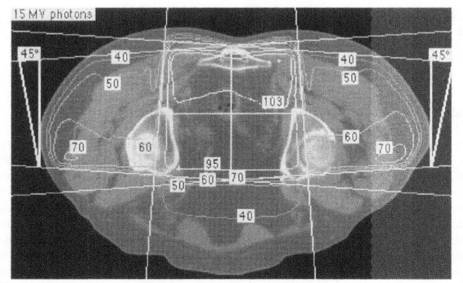

Figure 13.35   Isodose distribution for a rectal cancer using a posterior field weighted 0.5 and opposed lateral fields with 45° wedges and weighted 0.25 each. As in the bladder tumor, hot spots are present under the thin portion of the wedges.

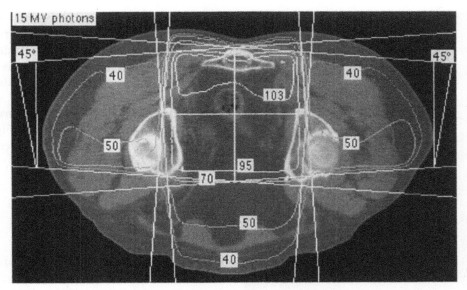

Figure 13.36 The addition of an anterior field reduces the hot spots in the lateral aspect of the pelvis. The posterior field is weighted 0.5, the lateral fields 0.2 each, and the anterior 0.1.

TREATMENT TECHNIQUE

The treatment of seminoma is usually through opposed anterior and posterior fields extending cephalad to approximately the T11 vertebra and caudal to the pubic symphysis. The lateral margins include the ipsilateral renal hilum and the contralateral paraaortic and ipsilateral iliac lymph nodes (Fig. 13.37). These fields should be shaped to conform to the lymph nodal areas just described. In some patients, a modification of these fields may be necessary, depending on their particular situation.

Previous surgery, such as a herniorraphy or orchiopexy, may cause the lymphatic drainage to be altered. Therefore, in these situations, the inferior region of the field should be extended to also include the contralateral pelvic lymph nodes. The dose depends on the histology of the tumor, but for seminoma it is usually about 2400 cGy in the absence of gross tumor and 3000 to 3500 cGy when gross tumor is present. The dose is delivered with conventional fractionation using a 6- to 10-MV photon beam.

SCROTAL SHIELD

A small amount of dose to the testicles is unavoidable when pelvic fields are treated in male patients. Temporary aspermia in the postirradiation period may follow.[117-119]

Primarily, the dose is caused by internal scatter, which is very difficult to prevent. Methods to minimize this dose have been explored by several authors. A device that retracts the penis and the remaining testicle out of the treatment field has been described.[120] The scrotal dose was reduced by approximately 40 percent when this device was used. When an 11-mm-thick shield was added, the dose was further reduced by 50 percent. With a gonadal shield, forming a cup around the testes only, the dose to the testes was reduced 3- to 10-fold.[121] The amount of dose reduction was primarily related to the distance from the proximal edge of the field to the gonads.

A shielding technique described by Kubo et al. lowered the dose to the contralateral testicle to 0.1 percent of the treatment dose.[122] The technique uti-

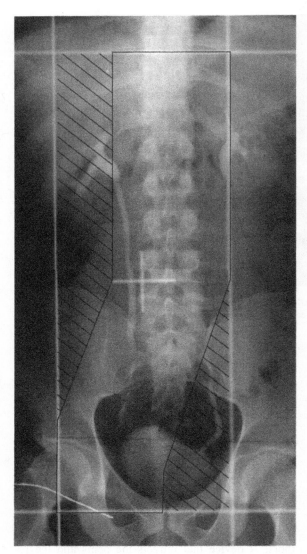

Figure 13.37 A typical treatment field for seminoma, including the paraaortic and ipsilateral pelvic lymph nodes. Intravenous kidney contrast was administered during the simulation procedure to identify the function and location of the kidneys.

lizes three additional shielding blocks as follows: a 10-cm-thick lead block is placed immediately above the contralateral testicle, the field-shaping block is extended caudal for an additional 5 cm below the inferior border of the collimated field, and a gonadal shield is used to prevent internal scatter from reaching the remaining testicle.

The primary purpose of a testicular shield is to reduce the amount of internal scatter arriving at the testes (Fig. 13.38). It is important that the shield be small to allow more room for thick walls of the lead shield. Shielding of the penis does not affect gonadal function and would only increase the size of the shield. Therefore, the most effective gonadal shields are those that shield only the testes. Figure 13.39 illustrates the components of two different shields.

TREATMENT—OTHER PELVIC SITES

ANAL CANAL

Carcinoma of the anus is usually treated by irradiation with or without chemotherapy. Radiation therapy consists of delivering 4500 to 5000 cGy via anterior and posterior external beam fields including the entire pelvis, inguinal lymph nodes, and the perineum. A boost of 1500 to 2000 cGy to the primary tumor can be delivered via reduced external beam fields or an interstitial implant. The anal verge should be marked during the simulation to assure adequate coverage.

VAGINA

Carcinoma of the vagina is usually treated via external beam irradiation to the entire pelvis to 4500 to 5000 cGy. For lesions in the middle or lower third of the vagina, the inguinal and femoral lymph nodes also need to be treated. This treatment is followed by intracavitary or interstitial therapy delivering an additional 2000 to 3000 cGy (Chap. 16).

VULVA

Carcinoma of the vulva is usually treated with surgical resection with or without adjuvant radiation therapy. Patients are treated via external beam irradiation using anterior and posterior fields including the inguinal, femoral, and deep pelvic lymph nodes, the vulva, and the entire pelvis (Fig. 13.40). Doses vary according to the clinical situation. A boost of 1000 to 2000 cGy to the vulva is then delivered via an elec-

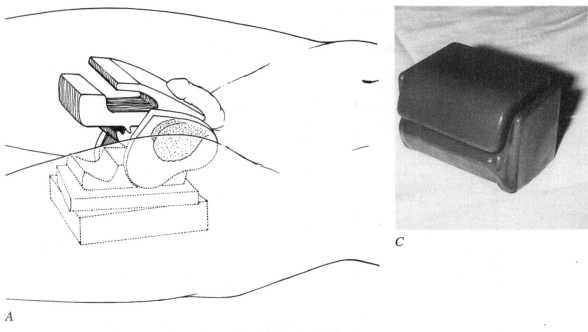

C

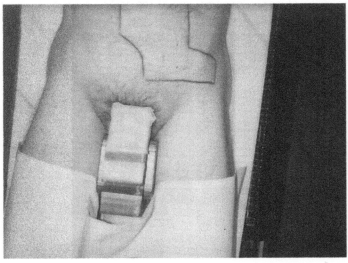

A

B

Figure 13.38 *A* and *B*. A diagram and a photograph illustrating the placement of a testicular shield. The proper placement of testicular shields can have an impact on the testicular dose. The shield may have to be supported by Styrofoam blocks of varying height and angle. *C*. Another testicular shield made from several sheets of lead to minimize the needed thickness. The shield is coated by liquid vinyl (less durable paraffin can also be used) to remove secondary scatter. The shield is mounted on an arm, which allows variable height and angle. (Courtesy of Thomas Mitchell, University of Florida.)

tron beam or an implant. In patients with known lymph node involvement, these should be treated also.

Preoperative irradiation is sometimes used to promote resectability in patients with extensive disease. Postoperative irradiation to 4500 to 5000 cGy is often given where the resection margins are inade-

quate. In patients with known gross residual tumor, the postoperative dose should be about 6000 to 7000 cGy.

PENIS

In carcinoma of the penis, the primary disease is most often treated by penectomy. The regional

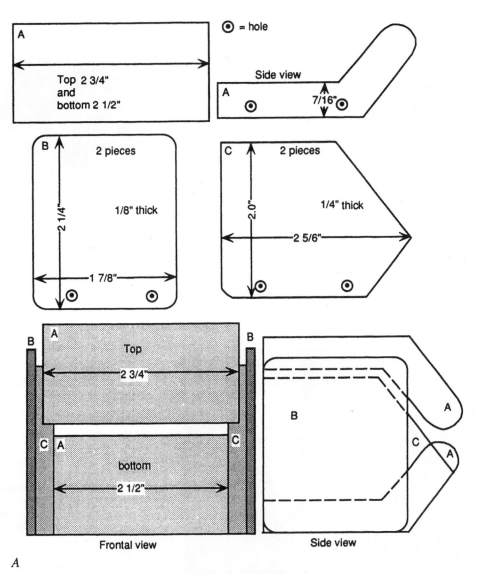

A

Figure 13.39 *A.* A diagram of the different sections of the shield shown in Fig. 13.38*C. B.* The components of the shield shown in Fig. 13.38*A* and *B.* (Courtesy of Thomas Mitchell, University of Florida.)

lymph nodes (inguinal and iliac lymph nodes) are usually treated by lymphadenectomy; however, this procedure is sometimes complicated by wound infection, necrosis, dehiscence, and lymphedema. In patients who prefer organ preservation, a brachytherapy surface mold, formed to the penis and de-

livering 6000 to 7000 cGy, can be used to treat the primary lesion. External beam irradiation can also be used to treat both the penis and regional lymph nodes to approximately 6000 cGy. A boost of 500 to 1000 cGy is then delivered to the primary lesion. Bolus material would be needed over the penis and

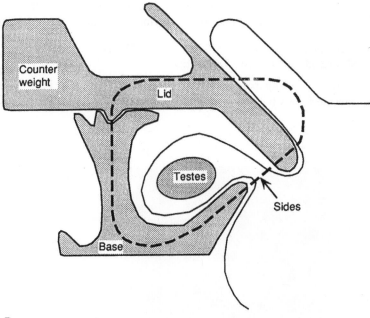

Figure 13.39 *(Continued)* *B*

also, in thin patients, over the inguinal lymph nodes.

URETHRA

Malignancies in the male urethra are relatively rare. The majority of patients present with locally advanced disease, which is difficult to manage with either radiation therapy or surgery. Radiation therapy of tumors in the distal urethra is similar to that of penal carcinoma, while tumors presenting in the middle urethra are treated with opposed anterior and posterior fields including the urethra and the inguinal and iliac lymph nodes. Tumors presenting in the prostatic urethra are treated using the same technique as that used for prostatic carcinoma.

Small meatal tumors in the female urethra are usually treated with an implant delivering 6000 to 7000 cGy.[123,124] Larger lesions, extending into adjacent organs such as the labia, vagina, or bladder, require surgical excision or external irradiation delivering 4000 to 5000 cGy through anterior and posterior fields. An interstitial implant, delivering an additional 2000 to 3000 cGy, should follow either

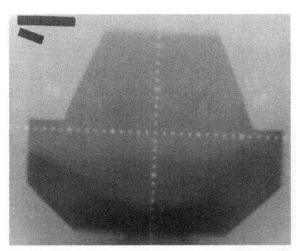

Figure 13.40 Typical treatment field for carcinoma of the vulva, including the inguinal lymph nodes.

procedure. Total doses may be dictated by the patient's age, general condition, and perineal reaction.

GENERAL CONSIDERATIONS WHEN PELVIC MALIGNANCIES ARE TREATED

In the following paragraphs, some of the general considerations for pelvic treatment are given.

In low pelvic tumors—such as in the uterine cervix, vagina, and prostate gland—the inferior extent should be marked with a gold seed or other radiopaque seed so that the inclusion of the lower margin of the tumor can be verified on simulation films. This is particularly important when the field size is reduced for a boost.

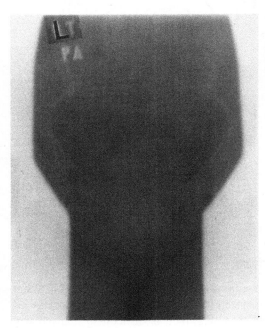

A

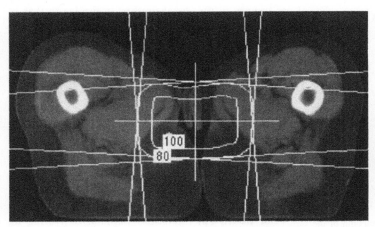

B

Figure 13.41 *A.* Treatment fields extending inferiorly to include the perineum may cause skin reaction in the perineum because the beam is more or less parallel with the skin and the thickness of attenuating tissue becomes smaller. *B.* When a four-field treatment plan is used and the beams extend inferior to include the perineum, skin sparing in the medial aspects of the thighs and in the perineum from the lateral fields is lost, since these beams travel through the thighs before reaching the perineum.

If it is necessary to include the perineal surface in the treatment fields, consideration must be given to the decreased skin sparing when the radiation beam travels parallel with the skin surface (Chap. 6). Lateral fields, which include the perineal surface, provide no skin sparing at all, since the beams will travel through one of the thighs before reaching the perineum (Fig. 13.41). The most caudal part of the perineum will often receive a higher dose than intended because the thickness decreases as the perineum slopes posteriorly and caudally. Consideration should also be given to the dose and lack of skin sparing in the male genitalia, which, of necessity, sometimes are partly included in the anterior and posterior fields. To reduce some of the problems just described, the couch can be turned 90° with respect to its normal 0° position and then the gantry can be turned to avoid or minimize radiation to the male genitalia. An electron field can be added to treat the perineal incision when needed.

When extremely obese patients are treated, an isocentric technique may not be possible because the clearance between the patient's skin surface and the collimator of the machine is insufficient. Electron contamination, mainly due to secondary electron scatter off the collimator, reduces the skin-sparing effect when the distance between the collimator and the patient's skin surface is too short. A distance of 15 to 20 cm is recommended to keep the surface dose within acceptable levels in most high-energy radiation beams.[125-127] The risk of a collision with the patient or the treatment couch is also increased when the clearance is decreased (Chap. 2, Fig. 2.11).[128,129]

The factors to consider in deciding whether to use an isocentric technique or SSD technique are as follows: (1) the importance of reproducibility in the particular patient, (2) the amount of dose delivered through the field, and (3) the actual distance between the collimator and the patient's skin surface. The first depends on how generous the margins around the target are and how well the patient cooperates.

PROBLEMS

13-1   When pelvic irradiation is delivered in an obese patient, the advantage of a prone position is that

    (a) The patient is more comfortable

    (b) Skin marks are more reliable to set up the fields

    (c) Sparing of the small bowel is improved

    (d) The abdomen is flattened against the couch, causing the small bowel to move anteriorly

13-2   When pelvic irradiation is delivered in an obese patient in the supine position, the concern is that

    (a) The small bowel would be in different positions each day

    (b) There would be difficulties in reproducing the patient's position each day

    (c) Uncertainty of dose due to variations in patient thickness would be caused when attempts were made to eliminate skin folds

    (d) The patient's hands might be in the treatment field when they were pulling up the skin folds

13-3   To reduce the volume of small bowel within a pelvic field,

    (a) The patient should be supine with the knees bent

    (b) The patient should be in the prone position with a compression roll under the upper abdomen

    (c) The patient's position should be prone on a belly board

    (d) The patient should be prone with the arms above the head

13-4   Methods to reduce the volume of small bowel in the pelvis include
   (*a*) Surgically implanted expander, placement of a mesh sling, and a prone position
   (*b*) Surgically implanted expander, a compression roll under the upper abdomen, and alternating the patient's position each day
   (*c*) Surgically implanted prosthesis, bladder distention, and a compression roll under the upper abdomen
   (*d*) Decubitus position, arms above the head, and a surgically placed prosthesis

13-5   When a pelvic four-field treatment plan used for treatment of carcinoma of the cervix is simulated, which of the following should be used?
   (*a*) A gold seed in the rectum, a contrast-enhanced vaginal cylinder, and small bowel contrast
   (*b*) A contrast-enhanced vaginal cylinder, small bowel contrast, bladder contrast, and a gold seed in the rectum
   (*c*) Small bowel contrast, gold seed in the inferior aspect of the palpable or visible tumor, rectal contrast, and a barium swallow
   (*d*) Small bowel contrast, gold seed in the inferior aspect of the palpable or visible tumor, a contrast-enhanced vaginal cylinder, and rectal contrast

13-6   A patient has a large pelvic tumor that involves the bladder and prostate and there is a presacral mass. Therefore
   (*a*) The treatment should be given through opposed anterior and posterior fields only because lateral fields would have to cover the entire pelvis and shielding of normal tissues would not be possible in the lateral fields
   (*b*) The treatment should be given through opposed anterior and posterior fields only and lateral fields should be used only in very sick patients
   (*c*) The treatment should be given through a four-field box technique because it is possible to shield normal tissues within the cephalad portion of the lateral fields
   (*d*) The treatment should be given through lateral fields alone because a larger volume of normal tissues can be shielded in these fields

13-7   Patients with carcinoma of the cervix are treated with a combination of external beam and intracavitary irradiation. However,
   (*a*) In patients with more advanced disease, a larger proportion of the dose is delivered using intracavitary irradiation
   (*b*) In patients with more advanced disease, a larger proportion of the dose is delivered using external beam irradiation
   (*c*) In patients with early-stage disease, a larger proportion of the dose is delivered using external beam irradiation
   (*d*) In patients with early-stage disease, a larger proportion of the dose is delivered using intracavitary irradiation

13-8   A central pelvic shield is sometimes used in the treatment of opposed anterior and posterior fields following intracavitary irradiation
   (*a*) To protect the bladder, rectum, and tissues irradiated to a high dose via the intracavitary implant
   (*b*) To protect the external iliac lymph nodes
   (*c*) Because no additional dose is needed in the vaginal apex
   (*d*) To protect the small bowel already irradiated to a high dose

13-9   Treating the pelvis and paraaortic lymph nodes in separate fields
    (*a*) Is preferred because it is easier to deliver different size dose fractions in the two areas
    (*b*) Is preferred because it is easier to set up
    (*c*) Is not preferred because of concerns regarding field matching
    (*d*) Is not preferred because the size of the dose fraction is always the same in the two areas

13-10   Treating the whole pelvis and inguinal nodes can be done using one of the following techniques:
    (*a*) Delivering 100 percent of the prescribed inguinal dose via an anterior pelvic and inguinal field with a pelvic beam attenuator, made to a thickness that allows 50 percent of the midpelvic dose to be delivered via this field while 50 percent of the pelvic dose is delivered via a posterior field covering the pelvis only
    (*b*) Delivering 50 percent of the prescribed pelvic and inguinal dose via an anterior pelvic and inguinal field with a beam attenuator, made to a thickness that allows 25 percent of the inguinal dose to be delivered via this field while 50 percent of the pelvic dose is delivered via a posterior field covering the pelvis only
    (*c*) Delivering 100 percent of the prescribed pelvic dose via an anterior pelvic and inguinal field with an inguinal beam attenuator, made to a thickness that allows 50 percent of the inguinal dose to be delivered via this field while 50 percent of the pelvic dose is delivered via a posterior field covering the pelvis only
    (*d*) Delivering 50 percent of the prescribed inguinal dose via an anterior pelvic and inguinal field with a pelvic beam attenuator, made to a thickness that allows 50 percent of the midpelvic dose to be delivered via this field while 25 percent of the pelvic dose is delivered via a posterior field covering the pelvis only

13-11   In a four-field box technique, used to treat a prostate tumor, the best rectal and bladder protection is achieved
    (*a*) Through conformal anterior and posterior fields
    (*b*) When all four fields are treated each day
    (*c*) When a larger proportion of the dose is delivered via the anterior and posterior fields
    (*d*) Through conformal lateral fields

13-12   When bladder tumors are treated, the field arrangement is usually
    (*a*) A posterior and opposed lateral open fields
    (*b*) A four-field box technique
    (*c*) An anterior and opposed lateral fields with wedges
    (*d*) An anterior and opposed lateral unwedged fields

13-13   When a posterior and opposed lateral fields with wedges are used to treat a rectal tumor, to reduce the hot spot under the thin portion of the wedges, we can
    (*a*) Increase the weight of the lateral fields and decrease the wedge angle
    (*b*) Decrease the weight of the posterior field and add an anterior field
    (*c*) Add an anterior field and decrease the weight on the lateral fields
    (*d*) Increase the weight on the lateral fields and add an anterior field

13-14   When a patient treated for rectal carcinoma is treated in the prone position as opposed to a supine position
    (*a*) The scatter off the couch is increased
    (*b*) The skin reaction between the buttocks is reduced

(c) The skin sparing is lost

(d) The skin reaction on the anterior surface is increased

13-15 The primary purpose of a testicular shield is to

(a) Shield the testes from the primary beam

(b) Shield the testes and the penis from scattered dose off the collimator

(c) Shield the testes from scatter off the treatment couch

(d) Reduce the amount of internal scattered dose in the testes

13-16 To assure inclusion of the inferior aspect of a vaginal lesion in the treatment fields

(a) A radiopaque gold seed should be inserted in the inferior aspect of the tumor prior to the simulation

(b) A contrast-enhanced cylinder should be inserted into the vagina during the simulation

(c) Barium should be smeared on the lesion prior to the simulation

(d) A lead wire should be inserted to the inferior aspect of the lesion during the simulation

13-17 When a large patient is treated for a pelvic tumor using a four-field box technique

(a) Secondary scatter off the collimator and block trays is irrelevant

(b) Secondary scatter off the collimator and block trays may be a problem

(c) Secondary scatter off the collimator and block trays is worse when the distance is longer

(d) Secondary scatter off the collimator and block trays is increased when a smaller patient is treated

13-18 Of gynecologic tumors treated with radiation therapy, the most common type is

(a) Benign ovarian cyst

(b) Adenocarcinoma of the endometrium

(c) Squamous cell carcinoma of the cervix

(d) Squamous cell carcinoma of the vagina

13-19 For small bowel contrast during simulation of a four-field pelvic plan, the patient should drink the barium

(a) 1 to 1.5 h prior to the simulation

(b) 30 min prior to the simulation

(c) 15 min prior to the simulation

(d) On the way into the simulator room

13-20 The depth of the deep inguinal lymph nodes

(a) Can vary from 5 to 10 cm and does not vary with the patient's size

(b) Is always 4 cm and does not vary with the patient's size

(c) Can vary from 2 to 18 cm depending on the patient's size

(d) Is always one-third of the patient's anterior-posterior diameter

REFERENCES

1. Leibel SA, Heimann R, Kutcher GJ, et al: Three-dimensional conformal radiation therapy in locally advanced carcinoma of the prostate: Preliminary results of a phase I dose-escalation study. *Int J Radiat Oncol Biol Phys* 28:55, 1994.

2. Bentel GC, Marks LB, Sherouse GW, et al: The effectiveness of immobilization during prostate irradiation. *Int J Radiat Oncol Biol Phys* 31:143, 1995.

3. Rosenthal SA, Roach M III, Goldsmith BJ, et al: Immobilization improves the reproducibility of patient positioning during six-field conformal radiation therapy for prostate carcinoma. *Int J Radiat Oncol Biol Phys* 27:921, 1993.

4. Soffen EM, Hanks GE, Hwang CC, Chu JCH: Conformal static field therapy for low volume low grade prostate cancer with rigid immobilization. *Int J Radiat Oncol Biol Phys* 20:141, 1991.

5. Letschert JGJ, Lebesque JV, deBoer RW, et al: Dose-volume correlation in radiation-related late small-bowel complications: A clinical study. *Radiother Oncol* 18:307, 1990.

6. Gallagher MJ, Brereton HD, Rostock RA, et al: A prospective study of treatment techniques to minimize the volume of pelvic small bowel with reduction of acute and late effects associated with pelvic irradiation. *Int J Radiat Oncol Biol Phys* 12:1565, 1986.

7. Kinsella TJ, Bloomer WD: Tolerance of the intestine to radiation therapy. *Surg Gynecol Obstet* 151:273, 1980.

8. Palmer JA, Bush RS: Radiation injuries to the bowel associated with the treatment of carcinoma of the cervix. *Surgery* 80:458, 1976.

9. Potish RA, Jones TK, Levitt SH: Factors predisposing to radiation-related small-bowel damage. *Radiology* 132:479, 1979.

10. van Nagell JR, Maruyama Y, Parker JC, Dalton WL: Small bowel injury following radiation therapy for cervical cancer. *Am J Obstet Gynecol* 118:163, 1974.

11. Yoonessi M, Romney S, Dayem H: Gastrointestinal tract complications following radiotherapy of uterine cervical cancer: Past and present. *J Surg Oncol* 18:135, 1981.

12. Caspers RJL, Hop WCJ: Irradiation of true pelvis for bladder and prostatic carcinoma in supine, prone, or Trendelenburg position. *Int J Radiat Oncol Biol Phys* 9:589, 1983.

13. Green N, Iba G, Smith WR: Measures to minimize small intestine injury in the irradiated pelvis. *Cancer* 35:1633, 1975.

14. Green N: The avoidance of small intestine injury in gynecologic cancer. *Int J Radiat Oncol Biol Phys* 9:1385, 1983.

15. Gunderson LL, Russell AH, Llewellyn HJ, et al: Treatment planning for colorectal cancer: Radiation and surgical techniques and value of small-bowel films. *Int J Radiat Oncol Biol Phys* 11:1379, 1985.

16. Mak AC, Rich TA, Schultheiss TE, et al: Late complications of postoperative radiation therapy for cancer of the rectum and rectosigmoid. *Int J Radiat Oncol Biol Phys* 28:597, 1994.

17. Shanahan TG, Mehta MP, Bertelrud KL, et al: Minimization of small bowel volume within treatment fields utilizing customized "belly boards." *Int J Radiat Oncol Biol Phys* 19:469, 1990.

18. Devereux DF, Chandler JJ, Eisenstat T, Zinkin L: Efficacy of an absorbable mesh in keeping the small bowel out of the human pelvis following surgery. *Dis Colon Rectum* 31:17, 1988.

19. Feldman MI, Kavanah MT, Devereux DF, Choe S: New surgical method to prevent pelvic radiation enteropathy. *Am J Clin Oncol* 11:25, 1988.

20. Kavanah MT, Feldman MI, Devereux DF, Kondi ES: New surgical approach to minimize radiation-associated small bowel injury in patients with pelvic malignancies requiring surgery and high-dose irradiation. *Cancer* 56:1300, 1985.

21. Rodier JF, Janser JC, Rodier D, et al: Prevention of radiation enteritis by an absorbable polyglycolic acid mesh sling. *Cancer* 68:2545, 1991.

22. Soper JT, Clarke-Pearson DL, Creasman WT: Absorbable synthetic mesh (910-Polyglactin) intestinal sling to reduce radiation-induced small bowel injury in patients with pelvic malignancies. *Gynecol Oncol* 29:283, 1988.

23. Durig M, Steenblock U, Heberer M, Harder F: Prevention of radiation injuries to the small intestine. *Surg Gynecol Obstet* 159:162, 1984.

24. Sugarbaker PH: Intrapelvic prosthesis to prevent injury of the small intestine with high dose pelvic irradiation. *Surg Gynecol Obstet* 157:269, 1983.

25. Herbert SH, Solin LJ, Hoffman JP, et al: Volumetric analysis of small bowel displacement from radiation portals with the use of a pelvic tissue expander. *Int J Radiat Oncol Biol Phys* 25:885, 1993.

26. Bijhold J, Lebesque JV, Hart AAM, Vijbrief RE: Maximizing setup accuracy using portal images as applied to a conformal boost technique for prostatic cancer. *Radiother Oncol* 24:261, 1992.

27. Dunscombe P, Loose S, Leszczynski K: Sizes and sources of field placement error in routine irradiation for prostate cancer. *Radiother Oncol* 26:174, 1993.

28. Fletcher GH: *Textbook of Radiotherapy,* 3d ed. Philadelphia: Lea & Febiger, 1980.

29. Perez CA, Brady LW: *Principles and Practice of Radiation Oncology,* 2d ed. Philadelphia: Lippincott, 1992.

30. Hanks GE, Herring DF, Kramer S: Patterns of care outcome studies—results of the National Practice in Cancer of the Cervix. *Cancer* 51:959, 1983.

31. Brookland RK, Rubin S, Danoff BF: Extended field irradiation in the treatment of patients with cervical carci-

noma involving biopsy proven para-aortic nodes. *Int J Radiat Oncol Biol Phys* 10:1875, 1984.

32. Cheung AY: Extended field irradiation for invasive carcinoma of the cervix. *Obstet Gynecol* 9:280, 1980.

33. Corn BW, Lanciano RM, Greven KM, et al: Endometrial cancer with para-aortic adenopathy: Patterns of failure and opportunities for cure. *Int J Radiat Oncol Biol Phys* 24:223, 1992.

34. Feuer GA, Calanog A: Endometrial carcinoma: Treatment of positive para-aortic nodes. *Gynecol Oncol* 27:104, 1987.

35. Fletcher GH, Rutledge FN: Extended field technique in the management of the cancers of the uterine cervix. *Am J Roentgenol* 114:116, 1972.

36. Nori D, Valentine E, Hilaris BS: The role of paraaortic node irradiation in the treatment of cancer of the cervix. *Int J Radiat Oncol Biol Phys* 11:1469, 1985.

37. Piver MS, Barlow JJ: High dose irradiation to biopsy confirmed aortic node metastases from carcinoma of the uterine cervix. *Cancer* 39:1243, 1977.

38. Potish RA, Twiggs LB, Adcock LL, et al: Paraaortic lymph node radiotherapy in cancer of the uterine corpus. *Obstet Gynecol* 65:251, 1985.

39. Rose PG, Cha SD, Tak WK, et al: Radiation therapy for surgically proven para-aortic node metastasis in endometrial carcinoma. *Int J Radiat Oncol Biol Phys* 24:229, 1992.

40. Russell AH, Jones DC, Russell KJ, et al: High dose para-aortic lymph node irradiation for gynecologic cancer: Technique, toxicity, and results. *Int J Radiat Oncol Biol Phys* 13:267, 1987.

41. Silverstein AB, Aron BS, Alexander LL: Para-aortic lymph node irradiation in cervical carcinoma. *Radiology* 95:181, 1970.

42. Stehman FB, Bundy BN, Thomas G, et al: Groin dissection vs. groin radiation in carcinoma of the vulva: A gynecologic oncology group study. *Int J Radiat Oncol Biol Phys* 24:389, 1992.

43. Koh WJ, Chiu M, Stelzer KJ, et al: Femoral vessel depth and the implications for groin node radiation. *Int J Radiat Oncol Biol Phys* 27:969, 1993.

44. Lanciano RM, Corn BW: Groin node irradiation for vulvar cancer: Treatment planning must do more than scratch the surface (editorial). *Int J Radiat Oncol Biol Phys* 27:987, 1993.

45. Henderson RH, Parsons JT, Morgan L, Million RR: Elective ilioinguinal lymph node irradiation. *Int J Radiat Oncol Biol Phys* 10:811, 1984.

46. Petereit DG, Metha MP, Buchhler DA, Kinsella TJ: A retrospective review of nodal treatment for vulvar cancer. *Am J Clin Oncol* 16:38, 1993.

47. Kalend AM, Park TL, Kalnicki S, et al: Clinical use of a wing field with transmission block for the treatment of the pelvis including the inguinal nodes. *Int J Radiat Oncol Biol Phys* 19:153, 1990.

48. Hanks GE, Herring DF, Kramer S: Patterns of care outcome studies: Results of the National Practice in Cancer of the Cervix. *Cancer* 51:959, 1983.

49. Kapp DS, Fisher D, Guttierrez E, et al: Pretreatment prognostic factors in carcinoma of the uterine cervix: A multivariate analysis of the effects of age, stage, histology, and blood counts and survival. *Int J Radiat Oncol Biol Phys* 9:445, 1983.

50. Montana GS, Fowler WCJ, Varia MA, et al: Analysis of results of radiation therapy for stage II carcinoma of the cervix. *Cancer* 56:956, 1985.

51. Montana GS, Fowler WCJ, Varia MA, et al: Analysis of results of radiation therapy for stage IB carcinoma of the cervix. *Cancer* 60:2195, 1987.

52. Perez CA, Camel HM, Kuske RR, et al: Radiation therapy alone in the treatment of carcinoma of the uterine cervix: A 20-year experience. *Gynecol Oncol* 23:127, 1986.

53. Montana GS, Fowler WC: Carcinoma of the cervix: Analysis of bladder and rectal dose and complications. *Int J Radiat Oncol Biol Phys* 16:95, 1989.

54. Esche BA, Crook MJ, Horiot JC: Dosimetric methods in the optimization of radiotherapy for carcinoma of the uterine cervix. *Int J Radiat Oncol Biol Phys* 13:1183, 1987.

55. Pourquier H, Dubois JB, Delard R: Cancer of the uterine cervix: Dosimetric guidelines for prevention of late rectal and rectosigmoid complications as a result of radiotherapeutic treatments. *Int J Radiat Oncol Biol Phys* 8:1887, 1982.

56. Pourquier H, Delard R, Achille E, et al: A quantified approach to the analysis and prevention of urinary complications in radiotherapeutic treatment of cancer of the cervix. *Int J Radiat Oncol Biol Phys* 13:1025, 1987.

57. Orton CG, Wolf-Rosenblum S: Dose dependence of complication rates in cervix cancer radiotherapy. *Int J Radiat Oncol Biol Phys* 12:37, 1986.

58. Perez CA, Breaux S, Bedwinek JM, et al: Radiation therapy alone in the treatment of carcinoma of the uterine cervix: II. Analysis of complications. *Cancer* 54:235, 1984.

59. Anscher MS, Prosnitz LR: Postoperative radiotherapy for patients with carcinoma of the prostate undergoing radical prostatectomy with positive margins, seminal vesicle involvement and/or penetration through the capsule. *J Urol* 138:1407, 1987.

60. Leibel SA, Fuks Z, Zelefsky MJ, Whitmore WF: The effects of local and regional treatment on the metastatic outcome in prostatic carcinoma with pelvic lymph node involvement. *Int J Radiat Oncol Biol Phys* 28:7, 1994.

61. Asbell SO, Krall JM, Pilepich MV, et al: Elective pelvic

irradiation in stage A2, B carcinoma of the prostate: Analysis of RTOG 77-06. *Int J Radiat Oncol Biol Phys* 15:1307, 1988.

62. Marks LM, Anscher MS: Radiotherapy for prostate cancer: Should the seminal vesicles be considered target? *Int J Radiat Oncol Biol Phys* 24:435, 1992.

63. Brindle JS, Benson RC, Martinez A, et al: Acute toxicity and preliminary results of pelvic lymphadenectomy combined with transperineal interstitial implantation of 192-iridium and external beam radiotherapy for locally advanced prostatic cancer. *Urology* 25:233, 1985.

64. Giles GM, Brady LW: [125]Iodine implantation after lymphadenectomy in early carcinoma of the prostate. *Int J Radiat Oncol Biol Phys* 12:2117, 1986.

65. Hilaris BS: *Handbook of Interstitial Brachytherapy.* Boston: Publishing Science Group, 1975.

66. Kumar PP, Good RR, Rainbolt C, et al: Low morbidity following transperineal percutaneous template technique for permanent iodine-125 endocurie therapy of prostate cancer. *Endocuriether Hyperther Oncol* 2:119, 1986.

67. Porter AT, Scrimger JW, Pocha JS: Remote interstitial afterloading in cancer of the prostate: Preliminary experience with the Microselectron. *Int J Radiat Oncol Biol Phys* 14:751, 1988.

68. Puthawala AA, Syed AM, Tansey LA, et al: Temporary iridium-192 implant in the management of carcinoma of the prostate. *Endocuriether Hyperther Oncol* 1:25, 1985.

69. Shipley WU, Kopelson G, Novack DJ, et al: Preoperative irradiation, lymphadenectomy, and I-125 implant for selected patients with localized prostatic carcinoma: A correlation of implant dosimetry with clinical results. *J Urol* 24:639, 1981.

70. Whitmore WF, Hilaris BS, Grabstald H: Retropubic implantation of I-125 in the treatment of prostatic cancer. *J Urol* 108:918, 1972.

71. Proinas SD, Kapp DS, Goffinet DR, et al: Thermometry of interstitial hyperthermia given as an adjuvant to brachytherapy for the treatment of carcinoma of the prostate. *Int J Radiat Oncol Biol Phys* 28:151, 1993.

72. Sandler HM, McShan DL, Lichter AS: Potential improvement in the results of irradiation for prostate carcinoma using improved dose distribution. *Int J Radiat Oncol Biol Phys* 22:361, 1991.

73. Sandler HM, Perez-Tamayo C, TenHaken RK, Lichter AS: Dose escalation for Stage C (T3) prostate cancer: Minimal rectal toxicity observed using conformal therapy. *Radiother Oncol* 23:53, 1992.

74. Roach M III, Pickett B, Rosenthal SA, et al: Defining treatment margins for six field conformal irradiation of localized prostate cancer. *Int J Radiat Oncol Biol Phys* 28:267, 1993.

75. Soffen EM, Hanks GE, Hunt MA, Epstein BE: Conformal static field radiation therapy of early prostate cancer versus non-conformal techniques. *Int J Radiat Oncol Biol Phys* 24:485, 1992.

76. TenHaken RK, Perez-Tamayo C, Tesser RJ, et al: Boost treatment of the prostate using shaped, fixed fields. *Int J Radiat Oncol Biol Phys* 16:193, 1989.

77. Balter J, Sandler HM, Lam K, et al: Measurement of prostate motion over the course of radiotherapy. *Int J Radiat Oncol Biol Phys* 27(suppl 1):227, 1993.

78. Beard CJ, Bussiere MR, Plunkett ME, et al: Analysis of prostate and seminal vesicle motion. *Int J Radiat Oncol Biol Phys* 27(suppl 1):136, 1993.

79. Forman JD, Mesina CF, He T, et al: Evaluation of changes in the location and shape of the prostate and rectum during a seven week course of conformal radiotherapy. *Int J Radiat Oncol Biol Phys* 27(suppl 1):222, 1993.

80. Melian E, Kutcher G, Leibel S, et al: Variation of prostate position: Quantification and implications for three-dimensional conformal radiation therapy. *Int J Radiat Oncol Biol Phys* 27(suppl 1):137, 1993.

81. Pickett B, Roach M, Rosenthal S, et al: Defining "ideal margins" for six field conformal irradiation of localized prostate cancer. *Int J Radiat Oncol Biol Phys* 27(suppl 1):223, 1993.

82. TenHaken RK, Forman JD, Heimburger DK, et al: Treatment planning issues related to prostate movement in response to differential filling of the rectum and bladder. *Int J Radiat Oncol Biol Phys* 20:1317, 1991.

83. Asbell SO, Schlager BA, Baker AS: Revision of treatment planning for carcinoma of the prostate. *Int J Radiat Oncol Biol Phys* 6:861, 1980.

84. Lee DJ, Leibel S, Shiels R, et al: The value of ultrasonic imaging and CT scanning in planning the radiotherapy for prostatic carcinoma. *Cancer* 45:724, 1980.

85. Pilepich MV, Perez CA, Prasad S: Computed tomography in definite radiotherapy of prostatic carcinoma. *Int J Radiat Oncol Biol Phys* 6:923, 1980.

86. Pilepich MV, Prasad SC, Perez CA: Computed tomography in definitive radiotherapy of prostatic carcinoma, part 2: definition of target volume. *Int J Radiat Oncol Biol Phys* 8:235, 1982.

87. ShankarGiri PG, Walsh JW, Hazra TA, et al: Role of computed tomography in the evaluation and management of carcinoma of the prostate. *Int J Radiat Oncol Biol Phys* 8:283, 1982.

88. Hafermann MD, Gibbons RP, Murphy GP: Quality control of radiation therapy in multi-institutional randomized clinical trials for localized prostate cancer. *Urology* 31:119, 1988.

89. Murphy DJ, Porter AT: Prostate localization for the treatment planning of prostate cancer: A comparison of two techniques. *Med Dosim* 13:11, 1988.

90. Porter AT, Daly H: Retrograde urographic technique in the radiotherapy treatment planning of prostate cancer. *Med Dosim* 12:29, 1987.

91. Roach M, Pickett B, Holland J, et al: The role of the urethrogram during simulation for localized prostate cancer. *Int J Radiat Oncol Biol Phys* 25:299, 1993.

92. Schild SE, Buskirk SJ, Robinow JS: Prostate cancer: Retrograde urethrography to improve treatment planning for radiation therapy. *Radiology* 181:885, 1991.

93. Kuruvilla AM, Olch A, Kagan AR, et al: Radiotherapy planning for simulation of prostate cancer: Computerized tomographic scanning vs. conventional radiographic localization. *Med Dosim* 14:277, 1989.

94. Low NN, Vijyakumar S, Rosenberg I, et al: Beam's eye view based prostate treatment planning: Is it useful? *Int J Radiat Oncol Biol Phys* 19:759, 1990.

95. Marsh LH, TenHaken RK, Sandler HM: A customized non-axial external beam technique for treatment of prostate carcinoma. *Med Dosim* 17:123, 1992.

96. Heukelom S, Lanson JH, Mijnheer BJ: Quality assurance of the simultaneous boost technique for prostatic cancer: Dosimetric aspects. *Radiother Oncol* 30:74, 1994.

97. Lebesque JV, Keus R: The simultaneous boost technique: The concept of relative normalized dose. *Radiother Oncol* 22:45, 1991.

98. Biggs PJ, Russell MD: Effect of a femoral head prosthesis on megavoltage beam radiotherapy. *Int J Radiat Oncol Biol Phys* 14:581, 1988.

99. Erlanson M, Franzén L, Henriksson R, et al: Planning of radiotherapy for patients with hip prosthesis. *Int J Radiat Oncol Biol Phys* 20:1093, 1991.

100. Hazuka MB, Ibbott GS, Kinzie JJ: Hip prosthesis during pelvic irradiation: Effects and corrections. *Int J Radiat Oncol Biol Phys* 14:1311, 1988.

101. Hazuka MB, Stroud DN, Adams J, et al: Prostatic thermoluminiscent dosimeter analysis in a patient treated with 18 MV X-rays through a prosthetic hip. *Int J Radiat Oncol Biol Phys* 25:339, 1993.

102. Sibata CH, Mota HC, Higgins PD, et al: Influence of hip prostheses on high energy photon dose distributions. *Int J Radiat Oncol Biol Phys* 18:455, 1990.

103. Haraf DJ, Kuchnir FT, Watson-Bullock S, et al: A dosimetric study comparing three-, four-, and six-field plans for treatment of carcinoma of the prostate. *Med Dosim* 17:191, 1992.

104. Vijayakumar S, Awan A, Karrison T, et al: Acute toxicity during external-beam radiotherapy for localized prostate cancer: Comparison of different techniques. *Int J Radiat Oncol Biol Phys* 25:359, 1993.

105. Emami B, Purdy JA, Manolis JM, et al: 3-D static conformal radiotherapy: Preliminary results of a prospective clinical trail (abstr). *Int J Radiat Oncol Biol Phys* 21(suppl 1):147, 1991.

106. Lai PP, Perez CA, Shapiro SJ, Lockett MA: Carcinoma of the prostate Stage B and C: Lack of influence of duration of radiotherapy on tumor control and morbidity. *Int J Radiat Oncol Biol Phys* 19:561, 1990.

107. Leibel SA, Hanks GE, Kramer S: Patterns of care outcome studies: Results of the National Practice in Adenocarcinoma of the Prostate. *Int J Radiat Oncol Biol Phys* 10:401, 1984.

108. Mameghan H, Fisher R, Mameghan J, et al: Bowel complications after radiotherapy for carcinoma of the prostate: The volume effect. *Int J Radiat Oncol Biol Phys* 18:315, 1990.

109. Pilepich MV, Krall J, George FW: Treatment-related morbidity in phase III RTOG studies of extended-field irradiation for carcinoma of the prostate. *Int J Radiat Oncol Biol Phys* 10:1861, 1984.

110. Pilepich MV, Asbell SO, Krall JM, et al: Correlation of radiotherapeutic parameters and treatment related morbidity—Analysis of RTOG study 77-06. *Int J Radiat Oncol Biol Phys* 13:1007, 1987.

111. Pilepich MV, Krall JM, Sause WT, et al: Correlation of radiotherapeutic parameters and treatment related morbidity in carcinoma of the prostate—Analysis of RTOG study 75-06. *Int J Radiat Oncol Biol Phys* 13:351, 1987.

112. Smith WGJM, Helle PA, Van Putten WLJ, et al: Late radiation damage in prostate cancer patients treated by high dose external radiotherapy in relation to rectal dose. *Int J Radiat Oncol Biol Phys* 18:23, 1990.

113. Miller LS: Bladder cancer: Superiority of preoperative irradiation and cystectomy in clinical stages B2 and C. *Cancer* 39:973, 1977.

114. Skinner DJ, Tift JP, Kaufman JJ: High-dose short-course preoperative radiation therapy and immediate single stage radical cystectomy with pelvic node dissection in the management of bladder cancer. *J Urol* 127:1274, 1982.

115. Whitmore WF, Batata MA, Hilaris BS, et al: A comparative study of pre-operative radiation regimens with cystectomy for bladder cancer. *Cancer* 40:1077, 1977.

116. Minsky BD, Cohen AM, Enker WE, Sigurdson E: Phase I/II trial of pre-operative radiation therapy and coloanal anastomosis in distal invasive resectable rectal cancer. *Int J Radiat Oncol Biol Phys* 23:387, 1992.

117. Hahn EW, Feingold SM, Simpson L, Batata M: Recovery from aspermia induced by low-dose radiation in seminoma patients. *Cancer* 50:337, 1982.

118. Pedrick TJ, Hoppe RT: Recovery of spermatogenesis following pelvic irradiation for Hodgkin's disease. *Int J Radiat Oncol Biol Phys* 12:117, 1986.

119. Speiser B, Rubin P, Casarett G: Aspermia following lower truncal irradiation in Hodgkin's disease. *Cancer* 32:692, 1973.

120. Harter DJ, Hussey DH, Delclos L, et al: Device to position and shield the testicle during irradiation. *Int J Radiat Oncol Biol Phys* 1:361, 1976.

121. Fraass BA, Kinsella TJ, Harrington FS, Glatstein E: Peripheral dose to the testes: The design and clinical use of a practical and effective gonadal shield. *Int J Radiat Oncol Biol Phys* 11:609, 1985.

122. Kubo HD, Shipley WU: Reduction of the scatter dose to the testicle outside the radiation treatment field. *Int J Radiat Oncol Biol Phys* 8:1741, 1982.

123. Pierquin B, Chassagne D, Cox JD: Toward consistent local control of certain malignant tumors: Endoradiotherapy with iridium 192. *Radiology* 99:661, 1971.

124. Taggart CG, Castro JR, Rutledge FN: Carcinoma of the female urethra. *Am J Roentgenol* 114:145, 1972.

125. Johns HE, Epp ER, Cormack DV, Fedoruck SO: Depth dose data and diaphragm design for the Saskatchewan 1000 curie cobalt unit. *Br J Radiol* 25:302, 1952.

126. Khan FM, Moore VC, Levitt SH: Effect of various atomic number absorbers on skin dose for 10 MeV x-rays. *Radiology* 109:209, 1973.

127. Richardson JE, Kerman HD, Brucer M: Skin dose from cobalt 60 teletherapy unit. *Radiology* 63:25, 1954.

128. Bentel GC: Collimator and treatment couch design in radiation therapy equipment. *Radiat Ther J Radiat Oncol Sci* 1:250, 1992.

129. Humm JL: Collision avoidance in computer optimized treatment planning. *Med Phys* 21:1053, 1994.

CHAPTER

14

Treatment Planning—Miscellaneous Treatments

Treatment techniques that involve more than one anatomic region or require complex equipment or setup techniques are described in this one chapter rather than in several smaller chapters.

TREATMENT PLANNING—HODGKIN'S DISEASE

Hodgkin's disease is a curable disease that strikes approximately 7400 young Americans annually, the majority of them less than 35 years old. This disease, which earlier was considered fatal, is now consid-

ered curable in the majority of previously untreated patients. The mortality rate decreased by more than 60 percent between 1950 and mid-1980, and the 10-year survival for patients with all stages of Hodgkin's disease is now approximately 80 percent. The improved prognosis for patients with this disease represents one of the major accomplishments of cancer therapy in recent years. Its success can be attributed to improved radiation therapy techniques as well as the development of many new chemotherapeutic regimes.

Improvements in radiation techniques include the

ability to treat the major lymph node groups in two or three large adjacent fields rather than several small fields, thus minimizing the risks associated with field matching. Also, the ability to utilize custom-designed shielding blocks to tailor the treatment fields to suit each particular patient's disease has contributed to the accuracy of treatment delivery. The accuracy with which the target can be delineated has also been improved by the use of modern imaging tools. Linear accelerators allow large fields to be treated at normal distances and without changing the patient's position. This facilitates the treatment of both the anterior and the posterior mantle fields and the anterior and posterior paraaortic fields with the patient in the same position. The dose uniformity within the fields is thus improved and the risks of over- or underdosage in the match region between these areas is also minimized. Last, positioning and immobilization devices, along with laser alignment systems, greatly improve the ability to reproduce the treatment setup from treatment to treatment.[1]

TREATMENT

Appropriate treatment decisions in the management of cancer are always important for successful outcome but, in the management of Hodgkin's disease, they are especially critical. The prognosis for patients with Hodgkin's disease is largely determined by the stage at diagnosis and initial management. Failure to control the disease on the first attempt often constitutes a life-threatening situation for the patient. Future radiation therapy, which may be necessary to treat recurrent disease, is limited by the tolerance of the adjacent normal tissue and will increase the risks of long-term adverse consequences. Serious attention must therefore be given to precision in the delivery of the initial, often complex radiation treatments in these relatively young and curable patients.

The extent of radiation therapy in Hodgkin's disease depends on the stage of disease, but it often involves total lymphoid irradiation (TLI) or subtotal lymphoid irradiation (STLI). The lymph nodal groups above the diaphragm consists of the cervical, supraclavicular, infraclavicular, axillary, medias-

tinal, and hilar lymph nodes. These are treated through large opposed anterior and posterior fields, usually referred to as *mantle fields*.

The lymph nodal groups below the diaphragm, the paraaortic, pelvic, and inguinal lymph nodes, are often treated after mantle-field irradiation but following a rest period. The splenic pedicle (or spleen, if it is *in situ*) is also usually treated, depending on the findings during a staging laparotomy.

The radiation dose prescription for Hodgkin's disease is currently controversial. A balance must be struck between two conflicting endpoints: the use of doses high enough to eradicate the tumor and low enough to cause little or no injury to normal tissue. The precise dose varies depending on the technique used by the individual radiation oncologist, the ability to shield normal tissues, and whether chemotherapy is used. The dose prescription varies from 3500 to 4000 cGy at 150 to 180 cGy/fraction in the absence of chemotherapy and 2000 to 2500 cGy with chemotherapy. These doses may be lower in children.

POSITIONING AND IMMOBILIZATION

The ability to reproduce the treatment fields precisely on a daily basis is crucial and may have a role in the final outcome of the treatment, both to limit the risk of toxicity and reduce the risk of "geographic miss." When confidence in treatment reproducibility is increased, the tumor margins may be reduced, minimizing the volume of normal tissue being irradiated.[2-6] Aggressive immobilization should therefore be utilized to offer these patients the best possible chances of cure.

The patient's position is usually supine, with the arms raised above the head and the chin extended. Optimally, the same position is maintained during the treatment of all fields, both above and below the diaphragm, to minimize changes in the relationship between skin marks and the spinal cord near the field junctions. Extension of the chin allows the submental, submandibular, and cervical lymph nodes to be treated while keeping the oral cavity out of the treatment field. The arms are elevated in an effort to move the axillary lymph nodes out and away from

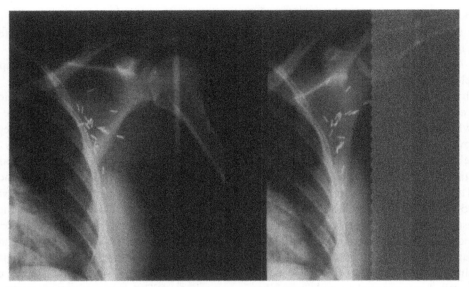

Figure 14.1 Elevating the patient's arm pulls axillary lymph nodes out away from the chest wall, allowing larger margins around the lymph nodes while sparing the lung parenchyma. (Reprinted from Bentel GC: Positioning and immobilization of patients undergoing radiation therapy for Hodgkin's disease, in *Medical Dosimetry,* vol 16, p 111, copyright © 1991, with kind permission from Elsevier Science Ltd., The Boulevard, Langford Lane, Kidlington OX5 1GB, UK.)

the lung parenchyma (Fig. 14.1). This allows shielding of lung tissue while maintaining adequate margins around the axillary lymph nodes.

In some patients with large mediastinal disease, it may be impossible to protect a sufficient volume of lung and heart in the mantle field. In these situations, an upright position can shift the configuration of the mass, allowing a larger volume of normal tissue to be shielded.[7] The disadvantages are the poor reproducibility of the position, potential for tumor misses, and difficulties with field matching when the paraaortic/splenic fields are treated. It is therefore recommended that this technique be used only during the initial 1500 to 2000 cGy, in the hope that the size of the mass will decrease, allowing adequate lung shielding when the patient lies down.

It is fundamental to successful immobilization that the patient be comfortable and provided with supports that will make the position as comfortable as possible. Maintaining an uncomfortable position for a long period of time is difficult, and the patient may involuntarily move slightly. In addition to providing support for the patient, an immobilization device should also be used to aid in reproducing the position from day to day. Customized foam molds, referred to as Alpha Cradles®* and used at Duke University since the 1970s, satisfy both needs (Fig. 14.2). The mold consists of a Styrofoam®† form that extends from above the patient's head and elevated arms to just below the knees. It provides indentations for the elevated arms (45°) and offers a barrier for the foam around the patient's head, thorax, pelvis, and thighs. This form is placed inside a large polyvinyl bag. The foam is mixed and poured inside the polyvinyl bag; then the patient lies down on the bag. The foam expands inside the bag and fills the space between the Styrofoam and the patient, forming a mold within which the patient can be positioned for each treatment. Two handles that the patient can grasp during the treatment are also added to help the patient maintain the elevated-arm position without straining.[1]

* Smithers Medical Products, Inc., Akron, OH.
† Dow Chemical, Midland, MI.

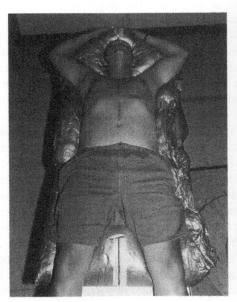
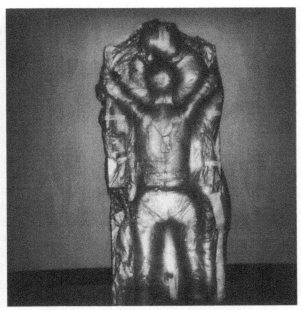

Figure 14.2   Patients are positioned supine in a customized mold, with the arms raised above the head and the chin extended. Sagittal alignment marks are made on the Alpha Cradle above the head and between the knees *(left)*. These marks are used to align the patient correctly on the treatment couch for each treatment. (Shorts are not worn for paraaortic and pelvic lymph node treatment.) The mold fits the patient's body tightly *(right)*.

Reproducing the arm elevation precisely each day eliminates the problems associated with skin marks moving with respect to deeper internal tissues.

To produce a tight-fitting mold, it is important that the patient wear no or minimal clothing during the fabrication of the immobilization device. Differences in clothing worn by the patient can give rise to variations in the fit of the mold and thus compromise the ability to reposition the patient correctly.

The Alpha Cradle used for the treatment of patients with Hodgkin's disease is approximately 5 ft long and offers reproducibility of the patient's position while all the major lymph node regions are treated. It also allows several positioning marks to be made on the device.

TREATMENT SIMULATION

The patient is positioned in the immobilization device and a chin strap, which helps to maintain the desired chin extension, is attached. The large perimeter of the mantle and subdiaphragmatic fields are very sensitive to small errors in misalignment between the radiation beam and the patient's anatomy. An alignment error, which can occur even if the central axis of the beam is correct, becomes more severe as the distance from the central axis increases, as shown in Fig. 14.3. Therefore, since the treatment fields used in the treatment of Hodgkin's disease often are large, the patient-beam alignment is very important when these fields are treated. It is also important that the position of the patient on the treatment couch be reproduced, not only from treatment to treatment but also from treatment course to treatment course.

The immobilization mold with the patient in it is first positioned straight on the couch. This can be accomplished by palpating the sternum and pubic symphysis or by viewing the spinal column in fluoroscopy. The sagittal laser alignment line is then

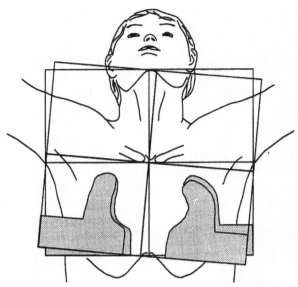

Figure 14.3 If a patient is not aligned with the sagittal laser alignment line, a misalignment occurs between the planned and the treated field, even when the central axis of the field is set correctly. The misalignment becomes larger farther away from the central axis.

marked on the foam mold both between the patient's knees and above the head. Laser alignment lines are usually arranged so that they coincide at the axis of rotation or the isocenter, but because they are projected over long distances, the plane they represent may be slightly tilted. This tilt may be different from one system to another, and it therefore becomes necessary to move the couch so that the point where the mark is made is near the isocenter. This requires that the couch be moved out from the gantry to make the mark above the head and moved in toward the gantry to make the mark between the knees. When the patient returns for treatment of the subdiaphragmatic areas, the position is resumed in the same foam mold and the marks, indicating the sagittal laser line, are again aligned with the alignment system. Failure to realign the patient with the sagittal alignment line will have the same effect as having turned the couch. It is therefore crucial that all machine settings (i.e., the couch, collimator, and gantry angles) be set to 0° prior to the simulation procedure. In patients where CT imaging is used to outline the target, the align-

ment in the simulation and treatment rooms must mimic that in the CT room.

When radiation alone is used, the mantle fields extend cephalad to include the submandibular nodes, caudal to the level of the diaphragm or T-10 vertebra, and lateral to include the axillary nodes. When radiation therapy is used in conjunction with chemotherapy, the mantle field is often modified to treat only the lymph nodes involved with disease at presentation. In patients who have palpable lymph nodes, it is helpful to mark them with lead wire or lead shot during the simulation procedure, when the treatment fields are designed. It is also good practice to palpate these lymph nodes during the first setup to ensure that they are actually included in the treatment field with acceptable margins.

Efforts should be made to treat both the anterior and posterior fields with the patient supine to minimize the risks of under- or overdosage at the junction between the mantle and subsequent paraaortic fields. The mantle fields are, however, often very large and

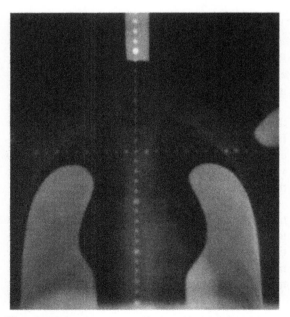

Figure 14.4 A typical mantle field with 5-HVT shields over the lungs, humeral heads, larynx, and the left ventricle of the heart. The larynx and left ventricle blocks are inserted after approximately 2000 cGy.

may require that the treatment be delivered at an extended distance with the patient in supine and prone positions. The entire field can rarely be included on a single radiograph and may require that several films be taken and then be taped together appropriately for block making. Simulation radiographs of both the anterior and the posterior fields should be obtained, since the areas to be shielded are not midplane structures and therefore will be projected differently with respect to the central axis in the two radiographs. The transverse and lateral (horizontal) alignment lines should be marked on the immobilization device and can also be marked on the patient's skin. The marks on the foam mold are more reliable in terms of patient realignment and are not subject to fading or

migration during remarking each day. By repositioning the patient properly in the mold and aligning the marks made on the foam mold with the laser alignment system, the position can be reproduced for each treatment without making marks on the patient's skin. The caudal extent of the mantle field is tattooed on the patient's skin on the anterior chest to aid in setting the gap between the mantle and the paraaortic fields when the patient returns for subsequent treatment.

The shape of the mantle fields is complex and require customized beam shaping. A typical mantle field is demonstrated in Fig. 14.4. The lung parenchyma, humeral heads, oral cavity, and posterior fossa are usually shielded during the entire treat-

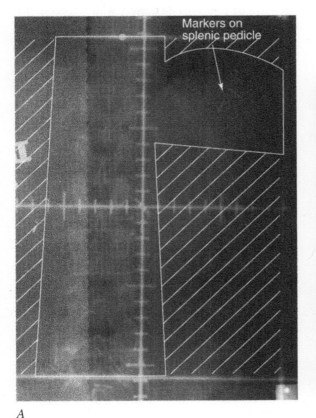

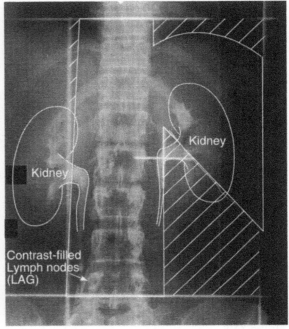

A   *B*

Figure 14.5   Metallic clips marking the position of the splenic pedicle *(A)*. When the spleen is *in situ,* the field must be larger *(B)*. Intravenous contrast was administered to identify the location of the kidneys. Contrast in the paraaortic lymph nodes remains after lymphangiography.

ment. A shield is often introduced over the left ventricle of the heart and the larynx after 2000 cGy.

The paraaortic lymph nodes and splenic pedicle are also treated through parallel opposed anterior and posterior fields. The fields extend from the inferior margin of the mantle field, allowing a sufficient gap between the fields, to the L4-L5 interspace. The right lateral margin should extend approximately 4 cm across the patient's midline, and the left margin should include the abdominal wall with a 1.5-cm margin. Marking the splenic pedicle with metallic clips during the removal of the spleen will facilitate the design of the paraaortic/splenic pedicle treatment fields (Fig. 14.5). In patients without metallic clips, other means of localizing the splenic pedicle, such as ultrasound or CT, can be used. Caution should be used when the fields are designed on the basis of marks made in ultrasound (Fig. 14.6). Due to the divergence of the beam, the spleen could be missed.

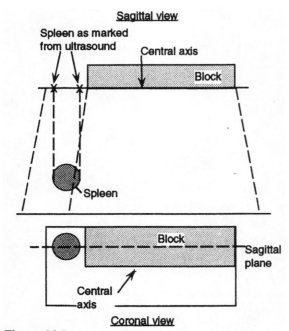

Figure 14.6   When the spleen or splenic pedicle is localized with ultrasound, marks are usually made on the anterior abdomen. When the fields are designed using these marks, the spleen could be missed by the diverging beam since the central axis typically is at some distance from the spleen.

A gap is calculated between the mantle and the paraaortic fields. During the simulation of the paraaortic fields, a lead marker is placed on the tattoo indicating the caudal margin of the anterior mantle field. If the gap is set correctly, the cephalad margin of the posterior paraaortic field should traverse the spinal column at the same level as the caudal margin of the anterior mantle field and vice versa (Fig. 14.7; also see Chap. 6, Fig. 6.54). It is highly recommended that intravenous contrast (60 cc Isovue®,* organically bound iodine) be given during the simulation of the paraaortic/splenic fields so that the position and function of the kidneys can be determined and appropriate shielding provided. Alternatively, the kidneys can be localized by using three-dimensional treatment planning (Fig. 14.8A). Since the organs to be shielded are not midplane structures, they will be projected differently with respect to the central axis of the beam in the anterior and the posterior radiographs. It is therefore necessary to obtain a simulation radiograph of each field for the design of shielding blocks. In some patients, the paraaortic lymph nodes may be enlarged and could be missed if a routine paraaortic field or an inadequate immobilization is used (Fig. 14.8B).

When the simulation films have been obtained, the transverse or axial laser alignment line indicating the position of the central axis in the cephalad-caudal direction is marked on the positioning mold. Since the central axis of these fields usually is moved to the patient's left side, the sagittal laser line, which is parallel with but to the left of the previous line, is marked on the foam mold. The paraaortic field is also tattooed on the patient's abdomen and, in the case of subsequent pelvic/inguinal node irradiation, the gap is similarly determined and marked.

The fields are then shaped to include the spleen or splenic pedicle, which, at the time of the staging laparotomy, should be marked with surgical clips. The fields are also designed to shield as much as possible of the left kidney (Fig. 14.5). In an adult, the paraaortic segment of the field should be approximately 8 cm wide so as to include the paraaortic lymph nodes with adequate margins. It is important

---

* Squibb Diagnostics, New Brunswick, NJ.

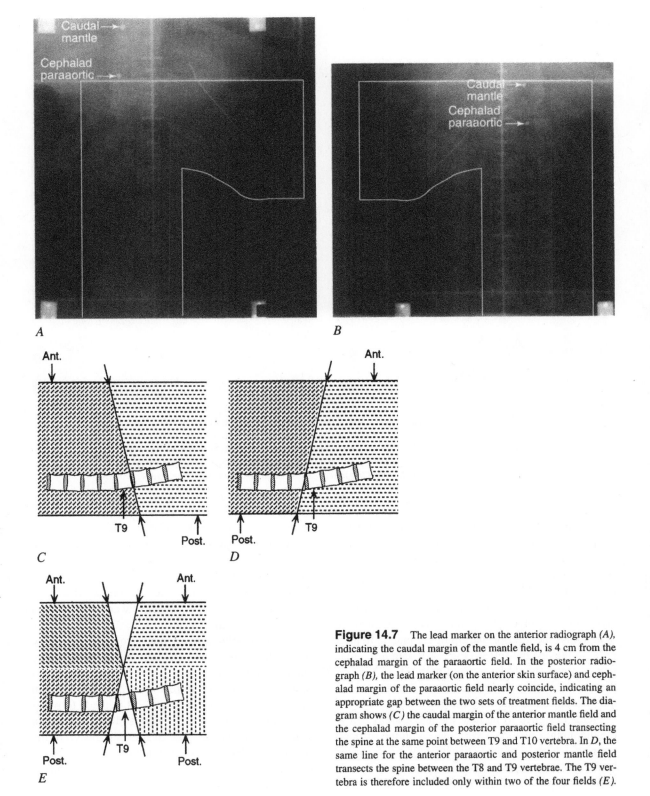

Figure 14.7 The lead marker on the anterior radiograph *(A)*, indicating the caudal margin of the mantle field, is 4 cm from the cephalad margin of the paraaortic field. In the posterior radiograph *(B)*, the lead marker (on the anterior skin surface) and cephalad margin of the paraaortic field nearly coincide, indicating an appropriate gap between the two sets of treatment fields. The diagram shows *(C)* the caudal margin of the anterior mantle field and the cephalad margin of the posterior paraaortic field transecting the spine at the same point between T9 and T10 vertebra. In *D*, the same line for the anterior paraaortic and posterior mantle field transects the spine between the T8 and T9 vertebrae. The T9 vertebra is therefore included only within two of the four fields *(E)*.

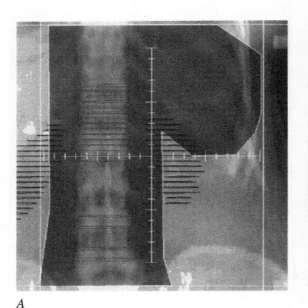

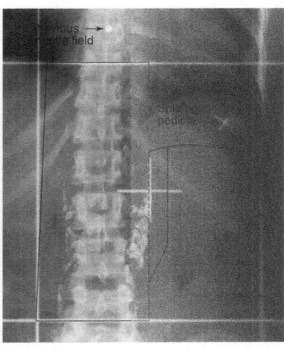

A   *B*

Figure 14.8 A typical paraaortic and spleen field (shaded area) designed using three-dimensional treatment planning tools *(left)*. The spleen, kidneys, and positive lymph nodes were outlined on sequential CT images. The lower part of the field is flared as the lymph node chains begin to bifurcate. Lymphangiography demonstrates the location of the paraaortic lymph nodes *(right)*. In this patient, the margins would be inadequate had a routine paraaortic field *(hatched line)* been used. A modification was therefore made *(solid lines)*.

to recognize that the spleen is a posteriorly situated organ; therefore the posterior field must be larger than the anterior to cover the spleen adequately (Fig. 14.9). Similarly, the kidney shield must be larger in the posterior field than in the anterior.

In some situations, it is necessary to extend the cephalad margin of the paraaortic/splenic pedicle field across the inferior margin of the mantle field in order to include the spleen (Fig. 14.10). In this situation, the gap should be marked with a lead wire on the patient's skin to indicate where a shielding block must be placed to facilitate the gap.

Fields designed to include the nodal areas below the diaphragm include a very large volume of bone marrow, which, if treated concurrently, often causes hematopoietic depression. The paraaortic lymph nodes and splenic pedicle are therefore often treated

in a separate treatment course and then, following a rest period, the pelvic and inguinal nodes are treated. Depending on the stage of the disease, the pelvic and inguinal lymph nodes may not need to be treated. This eliminates the difficulties associated with treating a large volume of bone marrow and also reduces the exposure to the gonads.

When the pelvic and inguinal lymph nodes need to be treated, the fields are custom-designed, using shielding blocks to protect bone marrow, bowel, and bladder (Fig. 14.11). In patients where preservation of fertility is of concern, an effort is made to minimize the exposure of the ovaries and the testicles. In young female patients, the ovaries are moved to the midline or laterally to the pelvic brim (oophoropexy) during staging laparotomy and the position is marked with surgical clips. The pelvic midline block,

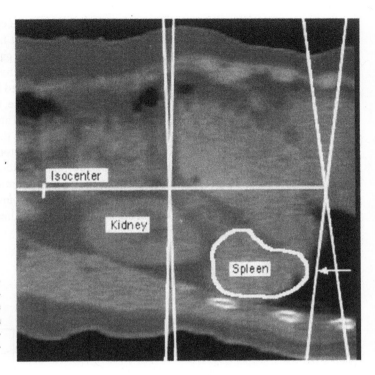

Figure 14.9   When both the anterior and posterior spleen fields are designed on an anterior simulation film, the posteriorly located spleen could be missed in the posterior field due to the difference in beam divergence. The arrow points at the small distance between the spleen and the posterior field margin.

intended to shield the bladder and rectum, may then be designed to also shield the ovaries without compromising the coverage of pelvic and inguinal lymph nodes. The dose in the ovaries consists of transmission through the block (approximately 3 percent) and scattered dose from the adjacent irradiated tissues. Although the testicles lie outside the pelvic/inguinal node fields, they receive scattered radiation from the adjacent irradiated tissues. This scattered radiation can be reduced by the use of an effective testicular shield (Chap. 13). Male patients who desire preservation of fertility should also be offered sperm banking.

In some patients it is necessary also to treat Waldeyer's ring, which includes the lymphoid tissues formed by the lingual, pharyngeal, and faucial tonsils. This area is usually treated through parallel opposed lateral fields that must be matched by the cephalad margin of the mantle fields. This creates a very difficult problem because the anterior and posterior mantle fields diverge in opposite directions.

This divergence is also quite severe due to the size of the mantle fields. Since the oral cavity and posterior fossa are usually shielded in the mantle fields, the potential for dose heterogeneity is greatest in the lateral tissues. Every effort should be made to avoid an overlap in organs such as the salivary glands and the auditory canals.

Another problem encountered when the Waldeyer's ring fields are treated is the patient's position. The raised arms would be in the path of the lateral fields and must therefore be moved when the lateral fields are treated.

As described above, the lymph nodal areas are often treated sequentially in two or three adjacent areas through opposed fields, leading to difficulties in matching field borders without causing overdosage at the field junctions. To reduce the risks of overdosage, a small block may be placed over the spinal cord when the paraaortic field is treated. This block should be quite narrow so as to avoid inadvertent shielding of the paraaortic lymph nodes. It can be used in the posterior field only, be used during some treatments only, or be of only 1 half-value thickness (HVT).[8] Other techniques to reduce the risks of under- or overdosage near the junction of these adjacent fields includes the use of a penumbra generator to make the dose less sensitive to small variations in the setup.[9-12] A similar effect will result if the gap between the fields is shifted several times during the treatment.[13-15] This technique requires very careful documentation of the direction and size of the shift as well as of the dose level at which the shift took place.[16] The use of the immobilization device described here reduces misalignment errors and

also reduces the risks of inadvertent mismatch of the adjacent field margins.

The gap between the mantle and paraaortic/splenic fields must be very carefully calculated and measured because the slope of the patient's chest can give rise to a significant error in the field separation.[17] Tattoos made on the patient's skin surface to indicate the margins of previously treated fields must not be totally relied on, because changes such as weight loss or gain, swelling, and growth (in the case of children) can alter the relationship between tattoos and the underlying anatomy.

An alternate treatment technique for Hodgkin's

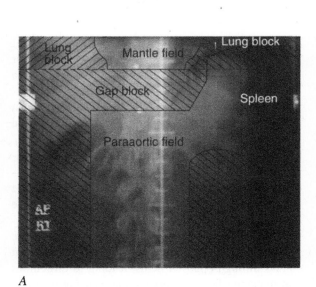

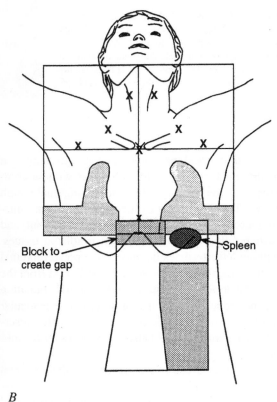

A   *B*

Figure 14.10   *A.* In patients where the spleen lies more cephalad than the caudal margin of the mantle field, the paraaortic/spleen field must extend into the mantle field in order to include the spleen. Since the lung block in the mantle field also shields the spleen, there is usually no problem with overlap here; however, there is an overlap in the mediastinum and spine. The necessary gap between the fields at this point must then be marked with a radiopaque marker so that a custom block can be produced to shield the overlap. The usual dose calculation points, representing the major lymph nodal groups, are indicated by an X in the diagram *(B).*

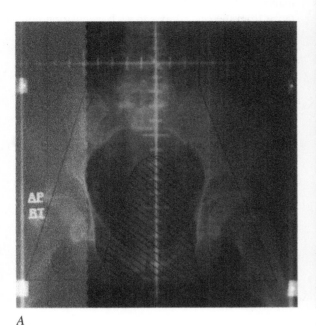

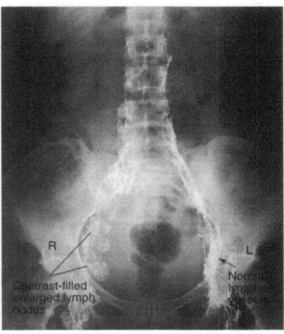

A   *B*

Figure 14.11   *A.* Typical treatment field including pelvic and inguinal lymph nodes. In this particular patient, the paraaortic lymph nodes and spleen were treated in the same opposed field. The bladder, rectum, small bowel, and bone marrow are shielded by a pelvic midline block. A scrotal shield is in place. *B.* A lymphangiogram from another patient, demonstrating large, contrast-filled lymph nodes in the right pelvis.

disease has been described.[18] In this technique, the lymph node areas are divided into three segments, which are irradiated sequentially. Following a rest period, the patient returns for additional treatment, during which the same area is divided into only two segments. In this "three and two" technique, the gap between the areas is thus shifted, reducing the risks of over- or underdosage at the junctions. The technique was designed in an attempt to improve the dose distribution and tolerance.

DOSE CALCULATION

Mantle fields are usually treated using a photon beam energy of 4 to 6 MV, since the cervical and supraclavicular lymph nodes can be situated at a shallow depth. With these relatively low beam energies, the dose within the rather large mantle fields

can vary 10 to 20 percent due to the often substantial difference in patient thickness (Fig. 14.12). In the cervical spine, for example, the patient's thickness is often about 14 to 15 cm, while in the inferior mediastinum, it could very well be 20 to 25 cm. The overflattening of the beam (off-axis ratio) frequently observed in large fields also causes the dose to be increased in the periphery of the field. Due to the differences in dose often observed in these fields, it is necessary to carry the dose at various points during the treatment course (Fig. 14.10). The use of compensators may be necessary in cases where the dose variations are excessive.[19-23]

Calculation of dose at an off-axis point requires knowledge of the SADs, SSDs, the patient's thickness, and the distance from the central axis of the beam to the calculation point, as described in Chap. 5. When the patient is treated supine and in a posi-

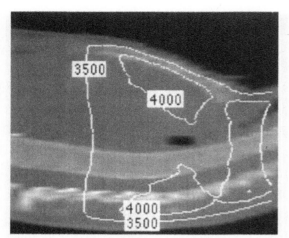

Figure 14.12 The dose distribution in the chest from anterior and posterior mantle fields. The dose at the patient's midplane on the central axis is 3500 cGy, while large areas in the thinner part of the chest and anteriorly and posteriorly receive 4000 cGy. In the neck, where the patient's diameter is smaller than at the central axis, the dose is often higher.

tioning device, obtaining some of these measurements can be difficult. The anterior SSD and the distance from the central axis to each calculation point can first be obtained with the patient in the immobilization device. The patient is then removed from the immobilization device and, by using calipers, the thickness is measured with the patient in treatment position (i.e., with the arms raised and a support of similar height under the head). In this method it is assumed that the patient's thickness is the same whether he is in an immobilization mold or not.

Another method is to first find the distance from the source to the top of the couch, which usually is also the back of the immobilization device (Fig. 14.13). The couch is then navigated horizontally, such that each calculation point is at the central axis of the beam, the SSD is determined, and the sagittal and transverse laser alignment lines are marked on the immobilization device. With the patient removed, the couch with the immobilization device is

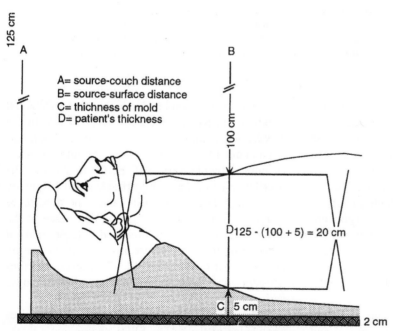

A= source-couch distance
B= source-surface distance
C= thichness of mold
D= patient's thickness

To set the posterior Source-Surface Distance at 100 cm, the source-couch distance should be 93 cm [100 cm minus 5 cm (immobilization device) minus 2 cm (couch thickness)]

Figure 14.13 Diagram of the various distances and measurements of the patient needed for dose calculation.

again navigated such that each of the calculation points are at the central axis of the beam. The thickness of the mold is determined at each point by pushing a pin through the material. To find the patient's thickness at each calculation point, the SSD and thickness of the immobilization device are subtracted from the source-to-couch distance (Fig. 14.13). In this method, the SSDs in the posterior field can be found by adding the thickness of the couch and mold at each point to the distance at the undersurface of the couch (Fig. 14.13).

A third method is to place lead shots on the calculation points on the anterior and posterior surfaces before the patient lies down in the immobilization device and then take a lateral radiograph. When two points lie close to one another, it is sometimes difficult to distinguish one from the other; unique markers should therefore be used. The separation between the anterior and posterior marks are then measured and demagnified in the same fashion as described previously (Chap. 7). The SSDs at each point are found by measuring and demagnifying the distances between a horizontal line drawn where the central axis of each beam intersects the skin surface and the mark indicating the calculation point.

Figures 14.14 and 14.15 illustrate yet another method by which the measurements can be deduced when an SAD or SSD technique is used. This assumes that the patient's thickness at the different off-axis points has been measured using calipers, as previously explained.

In the SAD technique, the isocenter is set to be 100 cm at the midplane of the patient (point A in Fig. 14.14A). In this example, the patient's thickness at the central axis is 20 cm, therefore the SSD is 90 cm and the depth of the calculation point is 10 cm. When the gantry is rotated 180°, the distance to point A is also 100 cm and the depth of the calculation point is 10 cm. Therefore, the distance between the two source positions (anterior and posterior) is 200 cm. As a matter of fact, the combined dimension between these two source positions is 200 cm everywhere within these fields.

In an SAD technique, it is not necessary to know the SSD when the dose is calculated, but we need to know the SAD and the depth of the calculation point.

When parallel opposed fields are treated, it is often assumed that the dose is essentially the same throughout the patient in the anterior-posterior direction. Therefore, the dose is generally calculated at middepth at the off-axis point, assuming that the calculation point is on the same plane as the isocenter, which it often is not (Fig. 14.16). There are, however, two other options: (1) to calculate the dose at middepth and using the distance to this point (it could be more or less than 100 cm) or (2) to calculate the dose at the plane of the isocenter, but that point may not be at middepth. The latter, demonstrated in Fig. 14.14B, also requires knowledge of the anterior SSD.

At the central axis point, the SAD is set so that it is 100 cm at the middepth in the patient and the dose calculation is straightforward. Calculating the dose at point B is more complicated because the plane of the isocenter may not be at the middepth in the neck. In Fig. 14.14B, we can determine the depth from the anterior surface by subtracting the SSD (93 cm) from the SAD (100 cm) and find that the depth is 7 cm. Since the thickness at this point is 12 cm, the depth from the posterior field is 5 cm (12 cm minus 7 cm). If we would like to find the posterior SSD at point B, we subtract the depth (5 cm) from the SAD (100 cm) and find that it is 95 cm.

In an SSD treatment technique, where %DD often is used, we must know the SSD and the depth of each calculation point. From Fig. 14.15, it is clear that the posterior SSD and the thickness of the couch top and the immobilization device are unknown. First, we must find the thickness of the couch top and the immobilization device at the central axis, so that the posterior SSD can be set to 100 cm (or an extended distance if it is needed in order to accomplish the desired field size). The thickness of the couch top can be measured using a ruler, and the thickness of the immobilization device can be determined by pushing a needle through it as described earlier. To set the posterior SSD to 100 cm, we must know what the distance to the undersurface of the couch should be. This distance should be 100 cm minus the combined thickness of the couch and immobilization device (4 cm in Fig. 14.15A). Therefore, the distance to the undersurface of the couch should be set to 96 cm.

As in the SAD example above, we can now find the total distance between the two source positions (anterior and posterior) at the central axis by adding the anterior SSD (100 cm), the patient's thickness (20 cm), the posterior couch distance (96 cm), and the thickness of the couch and the immobilization device (4 cm). In this case it is 220 cm (i.e., 100 cm SSD in both fields plus the patient's thickness). The

total distance is 20 cm longer than in the SAD technique, as we should have expected, since, in effect, the isocenter was moved to the patient's surface in both fields.

To find the thickness of the couch and the immobilization device at point B in Fig. 14.15A, we subtract the anterior SSD (103 cm), the distance to the couch (96 cm), and the patient's thickness at this

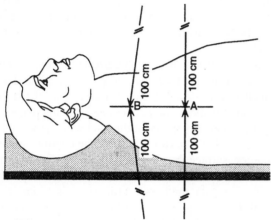

Point A: 100 cm SAD (ant) + 100 cm SAD (post) = 200 cm
Point B: 100 cm SAD (ant) + 100 cm SAD (post) = 200 cm

A

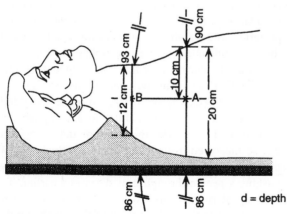

Point A (ant): 90 cm SSD + 10 cm (d) = 100 cm
Point A (post): x cm SSD + 10 cm (d) = 100 cm (x = 100 - 10 = 90 cm)
Point B (ant): 93 cm SSD + x cm (d) = 100 cm (x = 100 - 93 = 7 cm
Point B (post): x cm SSD + 6 cm (d) = 100 cm (x= 100 - 5 cm = 95 cm)

B

Figure 14.14 *A* and *B*. Diagrams of the various distances measured for central axis and off-axis calculation points when an SAD treatment technique is used.

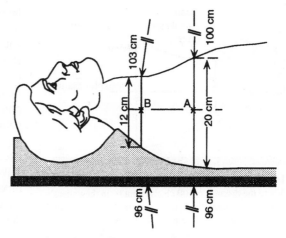

Point A: 100 cm SSD (ant) + 96 cm to couch (post) +
   4 cm (couch & immob.) + 20 cm thickn. = 220 cm
Point B: 103 cm SSD (ant) + 96 cm to couch (post) +
   x cm (couch & immob.) +12 cm thickn. = 220 cm
   x = 220 cm - (103 + 96 + 12) = 9 cm

A

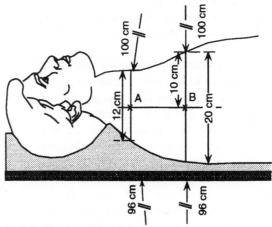

Point A (ant): 100 cm SSD
   10 cm depth (half of 20 cm)
Point A (post): 100 cm SSD (96 cm to couch + 4 cm couch & immob.)
   10 cm depth (half of 20 cm)
Point B (ant): 103 cm SSD
   6 cm depth (half of 12 cm)
Point B (post): x cm SSD (x = 220 - (103 + 12) = 105 cm)
   6 cm depth (half of 12 cm)

Figure 14.15   *A* and *B*. Diagrams of the various distances measured for central-axis and off-axis calculation points when an SSD treatment technique is used.

B

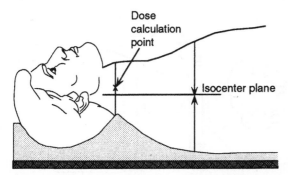

Figure 14.16   Due to the surface topography, the plane of the isocenter where the distance is 100 cm may not be in the patient's midplane within the entire field. In this example, the isocenter plane is posterior of the midplane point in the neck.

point (12 cm) from the total separation between the two source positions (220 cm) and find that it is 9 cm. To find the posterior SSD at point B (Fig. 14.15*B*) we subtract the anterior SSD (103 cm) and the patient's thickness at this point (12 cm) from the total separation between the two source positions (220 cm). Thus, we find that the posterior SSD is 105 cm.

These dimensions can also be obtained by using the same principle as in the SAD example, i.e., for the purpose of determining the distances and the patient's dimensions, we can set the isocenter at mid-depth and then find the dimensions as just described.

Determination of the dimensions described above is necessary for any off-axis calculation point. It has been discussed in detail here because the mantle field is probably the most common field where off-axis dose calculations are necessary and where patients invariably are positioned in an immobilization device.

In situations where the dose calculation is performed on a computer, where the shape of the treatment field must be digitized, a simulation film with lead shots marking the calculation points can be obtained.

One difficulty encountered when the two opposing mantle fields must be treated with the patient in supine and prone position is that the calculation points in the upper thorax and neck may be closer to

he source than the central axis dose calculation point in both positions, causing the dose to be higher than anticipated (Fig. 14.17). For example, in an SAD technique where the central axis is at 100 cm, a point in the midneck may also be at 100 cm when the patient is supine. When the patient is prone, the same point should be at 100 cm distance, but because the patient's head often is raised to allow free breathing, the distance may be 95 cm, causing the dose to be excessive.

When typical mantle fields are treated, 5-HVT blocks are commonly used to shield the lung parenchyma. The dose in the lungs can still be significant due to transmission and scatter (Fig. 14.18).

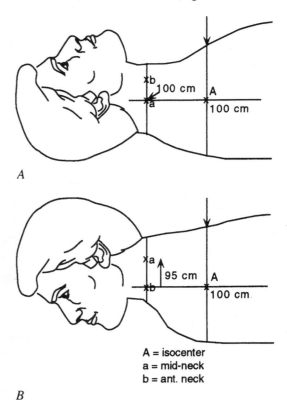

A = isocenter
a = mid-neck
b = ant. neck

B

Figure 14.17   When the patient's position is changed for the posterior field, the off-axis dose-calculation point may be at a distance that is less than 100 cm in both the anterior and the posterior fields, causing unexpectedly high dose. In this example, when the patient is in the supine position *(A)*, the midneck point is at 100 cm; but when the patient is in the prone position *(B)*, the same point is at a shorter distance (95 cm).

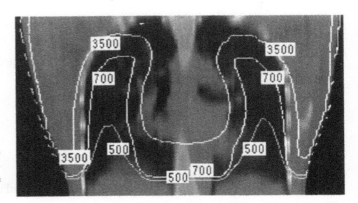

Figure 14.18   The dose in the lungs can be significant when mantle fields are treated. The prescribed central-axis dose in this patient was 3500 cGy, and a large volume of lung receives 700 cGy, or about 20 percent.

When only beams with energies higher than 6-MV photons are available or when it is necessary to take advantage of the superior dose uniformity of higher beam energies, some of the superficial lymph nodes in the mantle field may be in the buildup region of the beam and therefore receive a lower dose. To reduce the depth of the maximum dose while maintaining some skin sparing, a sheet of Lucite can be placed in the beam at a short distance from the skin surface.[24,25] The thickness of this "beam spoiler" and the distance at which it should be placed depend on the beam energy and the distance by which the location of D_{max} need to be shifted[26,27] (Chap. 6). The subdiaphragmatic fields are usually treated using a higher beam energy, since the target volume lies at a greater depth. Placing some bolus over the inguinal nodes may be necessary if the beam energy is higher than 10-MV photons. The dose calculation in the subdiaphragmatic region is straightforward because the patient's thickness varies less in this region. The dose should be carried at some off-axis points where, due to the irregular shape of the fields, the dose may be quite different from that calculated at the central axis.

MORBIDITY

The morbidity is directly related to the area treated.[28] When the mantle fields are treated, the acute symptoms are occipital epilation, dysphagia, sore throat, and sometimes nausea, vomiting, fatigue, and myelosuppression. If the salivary glands are included in the fields, dry mouth (xerostomia) and changes in taste can be experienced. When the paraaortic/splenic pedicle fields are treated, the patient may also experience nausea, vomiting, diarrhea, and myelosuppression.

Late sequelae of mantle irradiation consist of thyroid dysfunction, pneumonitis, carditis, myelitis, and development of secondary malignancies.[29–33] Thyroid dysfunction is observed in approximately 40 percent of patients who have received mantle irradiation. Patients with elevated TSH levels should receive thyroid supplementation. Pneumonitis is seen in about 15 percent of patients with large mediastinal disease. Radiation pneumonitis, in severe cases, can be fatal. The risk of radiation-induced carditis depends on the volume of heart irradiated (subject to the location of the disease) as well as the use of cardiotoxic chemotherapy and modern radiation therapy techniques. The most severe complications are myelitis and the development of second malignancies.

TREATMENT PLANNING—EXTREMITIES

Malignancies frequently occurring in the extremities that require radiation therapy include soft tissue sarcomas, Ewing's sarcoma, osteosarcoma, and metastatic disease. The most commonly occurring soft tissue sarcomas are malignant fibrous histiocytoma (MFH), fibrosarcoma, leiomyosarcoma, and synovial cell sarcoma. These tumors can occur anywhere but are most frequently found in extremities,

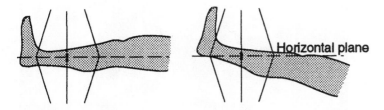

Figure 14.19 To achieve superior dose uniformity, the axis of the extremity should be perpendicular to the beam.

the most common site being the thigh. Soft tissue sarcomas usually spread locally along muscle planes, tendinous attachments, and the tissue compartments from which they originate. Bone, interosseous membranes, and major fascial planes can provide a barrier for spread outside the compartment. True sarcomas are not encapsulated and tumor contamination can be assumed to occur several centimeters from the primary site. Radiation therapy fields should therefore

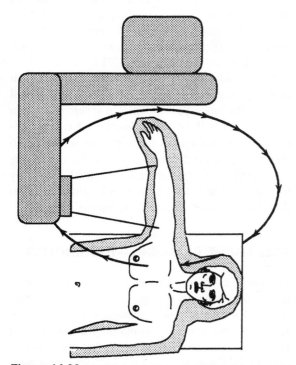

Figure 14.20 When the couch is turned 90° with respect to its normal position, the gantry can be turned to practically any angle around the arm.

extend well beyond the tumor mass. The grade of the tumor is of great importance for the prognosis and treatment approach, while histologic subgroup is less important.

POSITIONING AND IMMOBILIZATION

In contrast to many other tumor sites, the field arrangement in soft tissue sarcomas is heavily dependent on many variables, so the treatment approach must be highly individualized. This text is therefore aimed at outlining some basic principles that may aid in the treatment of extremities.

In an effort to produce a uniform dose distribution, the extremity must be positioned so that the long axis is perpendicular to the direction of the beam (Fig. 14.19). When an arm is treated, it is important to extend the afflicted arm away from the trunk so as to minimize scattered dose to the body and allow the needed beam angles while clearing the trunk. An arm, for example, may be best treated while it is extended out 90° and with the couch turned 90°, allowing the gantry to be turned to any angle without a collision or interception of the beam by portions of the couch (Fig. 14.20). Treatment of the lower extremities is more complicated because it is often difficult to move the unaffected leg out of the way. In soft tissue sarcomas occurring in the thigh, it is often necessary to extend the field cephalad so that part of the hip and pelvis is included. In these patients, the beam angles are limited by the presence of many radiosensitive organs (rectum, bladder, ovaries, testicles, vulva), which should be excluded from the beams when possible (Fig. 14.21).

Positions and Beam Directions for Various Sites

Thigh. The muscles in the thigh consist of three basic groups: the anterior, anteromedial, and posterior. Tumors in the anterior group can usually be treated by opposed oblique anteromedial to posterolateral beams with the patient supine. Tumors in the anteromedial group can often be treated using opposed anterior and posterior fields or with a small gantry angle with the patient in the supine position. When tumors originating in the posterior group are treated, the patient should be in the decubitus position and opposed vertical fields can be used.

Leg and Foot. The muscles in the leg also consist of three major groups. These are the anterior, posterior, and a small lateral group. Tumors in the anterior group can generally be treated via opposed anteromedial and posterolateral fields, while tumors in the posterior group can be treated with the patient in decubitus position via opposed lateral fields (i.e.,

the beam pointing vertically). Tumors in the lateral compartment can be treated with anterior-posterior fields with the patient in the supine position. Soft tissue sarcomas in the foot are rare; however, while treating some tumors in the leg, it may be necessary to extend the field to also include a portion of the foot. Treatment of soft tissue sarcomas in the foot has been described by several authors.[34-38] Every effort should be made to avoid treating joints, the heel, and the sole of the foot. The sole of the foot is exposed to harsh treatment from standing, walking, and supporting the body weight. High-dose irradiation of the sole of the foot should therefore be avoided.

Arm. The major muscle groups in the arm are the anterior and posterior compartments. These can usually be treated via opposed vertical fields with the arm extended 90° from the trunk, as shown in Fig. 14.20. Tumors in the forearm and hand can be treated with opposed fields at some oblique angle with the arm extended, as previously described (Fig.

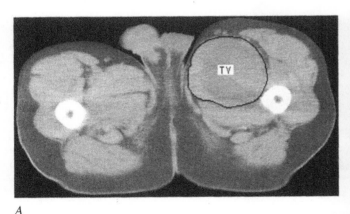

A

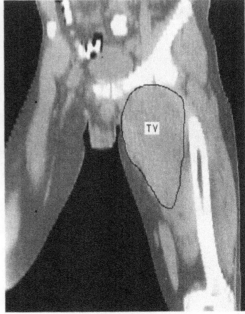

B

Figure 14.21 *A* and *B*. Soft tissue sarcomas situated medially in the upper portion of the thigh are very difficult to treat without also including some pelvic organs. In this patient, the tumor is very close to the genitals. Beam angles to avoid the genitals can best be determined using three-dimensional planning tools.

14.20). Treatment of soft tissue sarcoma in the hand, which is relatively rare, has been described by several authors.[34-38] The tumor margins are generally smaller and an effort should be made to spare a strip of tissue on the lateral or medial side of the hand. The treatment fields must be customized to individual needs and as much as possible of the joints should be spared. The dose in the skin surface where the beam exits can be very high, since the hand is thin and there is no skin sparing in the exit. In this situation, it is beneficial to use opposed beams, so that some skin sparing is achieved in both the dorsal and palmar surfaces.

The suggested patient positions and beam directions also apply to other less frequently occurring tumors in the extremities.

The position of the patients is often complicated by efforts to avoid unnecessarily irradiating volumes of normal tissue. When one lower extremity is treated, for example, it is crucial to move the opposite lower extremity out of the path of the beam. Treating very long and often large target volumes in an extremity of relatively small diameter can be difficult. Furthermore, efforts to spare a strip of soft tissue and as much bone marrow as possible in the final boost leads to very small tumor margins. Meticulous immobilization is therefore crucial to reproducibility of the patient's position.

In patients requiring treatment of an extremity, it is critical that the treatment-planning team know the anticipated beam arrangement prior to immobilizing the patient. The patient's position plays an important

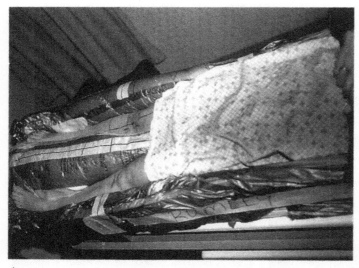

A

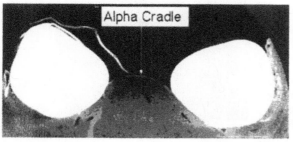

B

Figure 14.22 *A.* Immobilization devices for patients treated for malignancies in the lower extremities extend from the waist to below the feet. Sagittal alignment marks are made on the Alpha Cradle so the patient can be repositioned correctly with respect to the beam for each treatment.   *B.* The Alpha Cradle is a tight-fitting mold that assures reproducibility of the patient's position.

role in the ability to select the appropriate gantry angle. The foam molds, previously described, are also used for patients treated for tumors in an extremity. Some muscle compartments move when the position of the patient's foot changes or when the leg changes position relative to the hip. It is therefore important that the pelvis and the entire limb be immobilized. At Duke University, immobilization foam molds are built to extend from the waist to below the feet when the lower extremity is treated (Fig. 14.22). When one upper extremity is treated, the entire chest and arm are included in the mold, with particular emphasis on the position of the hand. As with all immobilization devices, it is important that the expanding foam be allowed to form itself around the patient so that the patient can fit in it in only one way. The bag containing the foam must therefore be pulled up between the fingers, the legs,

and between the arms and the trunk of the body so that the foam has room to expand. The foam will expand in the direction of least resistance and should therefore be guided up around the patient's body. Setup marks should be made on the immobilization device so that the mold carrying the patient can be repositioned on the treatment couch in the same position each day.

TREATMENT SIMULATION

Tumor localization is most reliably carried out with computed tomography (CT) or magnetic resonance imaging (MRI) (Fig. 14.23) with the patient in treatment position. In most situations, due to the often very elongated treatment fields, parallel opposed fields (AP-PA or oblique) are preferred. The separation between the two fields is also quite small in the

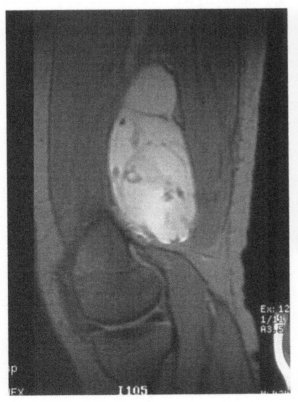

A

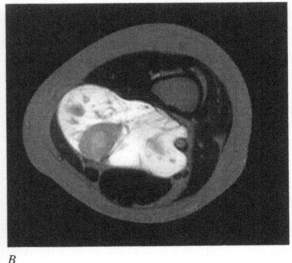

B

Figure 14.23 An oblique *(A)* and a transverse *(B)* MRI clearly demonstrating a tumor (soft tissue sarcoma) above the knee.

extremities, eliminating concerns for high doses in the entrance/exit regions of parallel opposed fields. The beam angles must be selected so that it is possible to include the entire target volume while still sparing a strip of soft tissue along the entire extremity. In these patients it is extremely important that the radiation oncologist and the treatment-planning team communicate clearly with regard to the approach prior to immobilizing the patient. The position and length of the target will influence how the patient is positioned to facilitate the needed beam angles.

During the simulation procedure, the immobilization device carrying the patient should be repositioned on the couch with the guidance of the alignment marks made during CT or other target localization procedure. Due to the design of the simulator and therapy machine, patients treated for malignancies in the lower extremity must usually be reversed on the couch, i.e., the feet toward the gantry. This can lead to difficulties in interpreting the beam angles, particularly the gantry angle. In these situations, it is crucial that the patient's position on the couch and the beam angles be very clearly indicated in the chart, preferably by using diagrams. It is also very important that the diagram and treatment plan be labeled clearly, indicating whether it is the right or left leg, right or left side of the leg, whether the fields are medial or lateral, anterior or posterior, and whether the patient's position is supine, prone, or decubitus.

Lead wires should be placed on incisions and around a palpable tumor. A note of caution: lead wires placed on the skin surface around a palpable mass during the simulation procedure can easily be misinterpreted when seen on an oblique simulation film (Fig. 14.24). The wire represents only the skin surface and yields no information about the tumor depth.

The setup (anterior and lateral) and treatment marks (often oblique) are made both on the patient and on the immobilization device. Simulation radiographs should be obtained of both opposed fields, since the projection of reference anatomy will appear different on the two films. The fields are then shaped by customized blocks to minimize irradiation to bone marrow and normal soft tissues (Fig. 14.25).

TREATMENT—SOFT TISSUE SARCOMAS

For many years surgery has been the primary modality in the management of soft tissue sarcomas. The surgical procedure consisted of radical resection, often leaving unacceptable functional and cosmetic sequelae, or amputation. During the last several decades limb-preserving alternatives—including radiation therapy, chemotherapy, and hyperthermia[39]—have been successfully employed. Radiation therapy has been given either preoperatively[40] or postoperatively.[41] In one study, it was found that the preoperative volume could be smaller than the postoperative volume.[42] Although not proven, the authors speculated that the complication rate may therefore be lower if the treatment is given preoperatively.

The basic principle of combining radiation therapy and surgery is the use of conservative resection of gross tumor without undue mutilation and radiation therapy to eradicate microscopic extension of tumor within the muscle compartment. In some locations—i.e., near major neurovascular or bony structures—the surgeon may not be able to remove all gross tumor or obtain adequate margins; however, these areas can usually be included in the irradiation field without any problems.

In situations where wide surgical margins are not possible or where gross tumor was removed with small margins for other reasons, radiation therapy to a larger area may follow the surgical resection. When gross tumor is resected with wide surgical margins, the tumor bed is considered ''contaminated'' and should therefore be irradiated. A dose of 6000 to 6500 cGy is considered adequate to eradicate microscopic disease. In patients where radical surgery is precluded—either because of location, patient preference, or functional and cosmetic outcome—less radical surgery combined with radiation therapy can give results similar to those of radical surgery alone.

Amputation should be reserved for special situations where limb-preserving therapy is not possible.

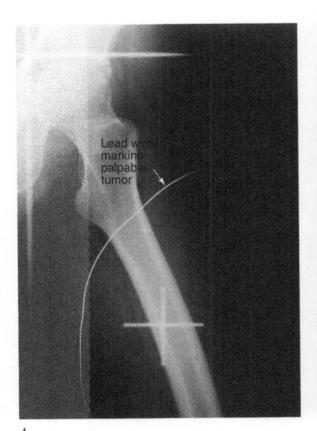

A

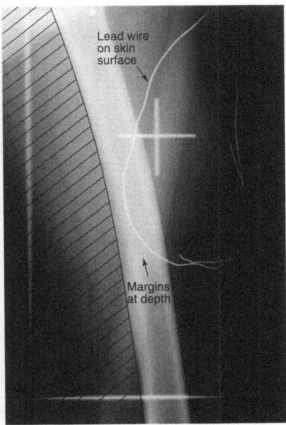

B

Figure 14.24   A lead wire outlining an incision that must be treated is useful when treatment fields are designed. A lead wire around a palpable tumor will only indicate the skin surface overlying a tumor and does not give information about the depth *(radiograph, A)*. When the beam is set to include the lead wire and is then angled, the tumor could be missed at depth *(radiograph, B)*. Also, see the diagram *(C)*.

C

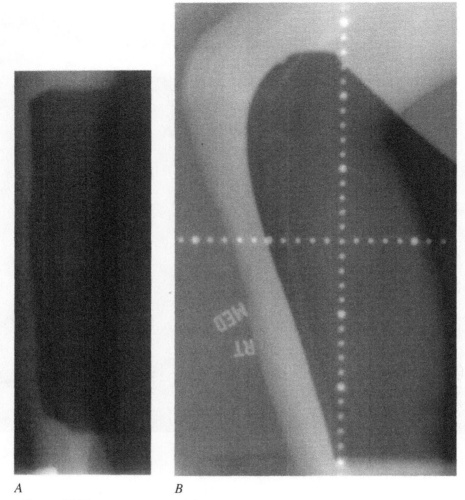

A   *B*

Figure 14.25   A port film of a soft tissue sarcoma *(A)* in the right arm of a preteen child where sparing of epiphyseal plates was essential. A port film of a soft tissue sarcoma *(B)* in the calf of the leg, where sparing of the knee joint was important.

Less aggressive surgery in combination with radiation therapy leaves good functional and cosmetic results. Reliable patient immobilization[43] and choice of radiation therapy technique is important to the outcome. Target and nontarget structures must be defined. Dose constraints by adjacent tissues should be determined and fields reduced at appropriate dose levels. Three-dimensional treatment-planning tools are very useful in the selection of appropriate beam directions and the design of the field margins. The

beam directions and field shapes used in Fig. 14.26 were determined using three-dimensional treatment-planning tools. Large volumes of interstitial infiltrates of contaminated blood spread during surgery would have been missed if the beam directions had been chosen on the basis of tumor location alone.

The tumor margins are generally quite generous when soft tissue sarcomas in the extremities are treated. This is because the tumor tends to grow along the muscle planes. Following compartment re-

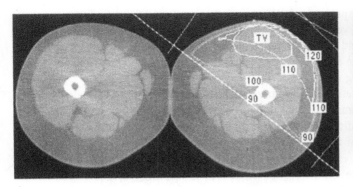

A

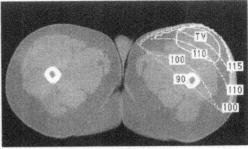

B

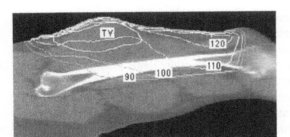

C

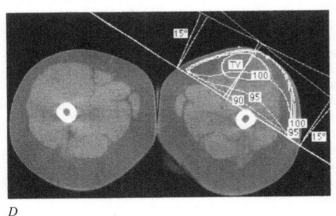

D

Figure 14.26 The dose distribution in the central axis plane *(A)* and near the cephalad margin near the testicles *(B)* (the testicles were moved to the right during treatment) in a patient where large volumes of tissue potentially had been ''contaminated'' by tumor cells during surgery. The length of these fields exceeded the maximum field length for which wedges were available. *C.* The dose distribution is also demonstrated in an oblique plane along the thigh. There were large areas that received about 20 percent higher dose, but much of these areas were not included in the boost fields. *D.* The boost field was shorter and 15° wedges were used to improve the dose uniformity.

section, the entire compartment from the origin to the insertion of the muscle is considered the target. The margins in the long axis of the extremity should be generous, but the exact dimensions must be determined for each situation.[44] High-grade tumors require larger margins than low-grade tumors; however, size and location of the tumor also play a role in the determination of margins. Margins may have to

be compromised when soft tissue sarcomas in sites other than an extremity are treated. It is also not necessary to extend the margins beyond the muscle compartment from which the tumor originates. Concessions may have to be made in both volume and dose due to the normal tissue tolerance.

At the site of the tumor mass, the entire circumference of the muscle compartment must be included in the radiation field. Care should be taken to spare joints whenever possible. When the target lies very close to a joint, at least a part of the joint should be shielded. To preserve long-term function of the extremity, a strip of tissue should be spared along the entire extremity. Delivering high doses of irradiation to the entire circumference of an extremity causes obstruction of lymphatic return, resulting in distal swelling (edema), which can be devastating for the patient.

The recommended minimum tumor dose is 5000 cGy in 5 to 5 1/2 weeks to tissues suspected of tumor involvement. This volume is reduced one or two times and a total dose of 6500 cGy is given to the tumor bed when surgery and radiation therapy are used together. When radiation therapy is given preoperatively, 5000 cGy to a large volume, covering the entire circumference of the muscle compartment where the gross tumor is and with generous margins in the long axis of the extremity, is recommended. This is followed, after approximately a 2-week rest, by conservative resection. A boost of 1000 cGy is then given to a smaller volume encompassing the tumor bed with some margins and an additional 500 cGy to the tumor bed only. It is important that the tumor bed be marked with surgical clips so that the treatment fields can be designed appropriately. The boost can also be given via an interstitial implant or intraoperatively using an electron beam. Postoperative radiation therapy is given approximately 2 to 3 weeks after surgery. The initial volume, receiving 5000 cGy, must include the entire surgical area, including the incision and any drain site. A shrinking-field technique is then used to a total dose of 6500 cGy. If gross tumor remains, the dose may have to be 7000 to 7500 cGy to small fields, using appropriate field reductions. The radiation dose should be lower if chemotherapy is also given.

Small tumors of low grade may be treated with wide radical surgical resection alone. Depending on the location, less radical surgery along with radiation therapy may result in a superior functional and cosmetic result. Where surgery is technically or medically not possible, radiation therapy alone to 6500 cGy may be successful if the treatment technique is carefully chosen and the margins are gradually reduced. Conservative surgery and carefully delivered radiation therapy to sarcomas of the hands and feet can give acceptable functional and cosmetic results.[38,45]

Other treatment modalities used in the treatment of soft tissue sarcomas include heavy-particle irradiation (i.e., protons and neutrons),[46-49] hyperthermia,[39] and brachytherapy.[50,51]

TREATMENT TECHNIQUES—SOFT TISSUE SARCOMAS

Isocentric treatment techniques should be used, since the reproducibility is superior to that of source-surface distance (SSD) techniques. In some instances, however, the length of the target volume may not be encompassed in a single field. Rather than treat at an extended SSD, the volume can be treated in two adjacent areas or the patient may be referred to a center with more sophisticated equipment. When the volume is treated in two adjacent areas, the gap between the two sets of fields should be placed away from the tumor mass and the junction should be shifted at approximately every 1000 cGy.

It is important to calculate isodose distributions in multiple levels within these often long fields to determine the variation of dose and the need for compensators. Compensators or wedges may also be necessary in some cases to compensate for the transverse curvature of the extremity. Since most commercial wedges do not cover the entire length of the maximum field, wedges may have to be customized. Compensators may also be needed to make up for variations in the thickness of the extremity in the long axis as well. A crude method of making the dose distribution more uniform is to gradually reduce the field off areas with higher dose.

INTRAOPERATIVE IRRADIATION

Intraoperative radiation therapy (IORT) is used mostly in the treatment of locally advanced unresectable tumors in the upper abdomen, primarily pancreatic carcinoma, but has also been used in the treatment of pelvic tumors. The advantages of IORT are that (1) the radiation dose can be delivered directly to the tumor without the beam having to pass through normal tissues before it reaches the tumor; (2) the radiation beam, usually electrons, can be directed to the tumor mass with great precision; and (3) normal tissues in the vicinity can be moved out of the way, allowing very high doses of radiation to be delivered.

Some radiation therapy departments have a therapy unit dedicated to IORT, which is located in the operating room suite. Alternatively, an operating room may be available within the radiation therapy department with easy access to a radiation therapy machine. Depending on the number of cases, these two alternatives might not be economically feasible. In another alternative, used in most IORT facilities, the patient, still under anesthesia, is transported from the operating room to the radiation therapy department with the surgical incision temporarily closed and with sterile drapes in place. Following the treatment, if no further surgery is necessary, the abdomen is closed in the radiation therapy department.

The IORT is delivered using a specially designed cone. The cone, made of clear plastic to permit direct visualization of the tumor during placement, is also of great value in trying to keep normal tissues out of the way of the radiation beam. A hole on the side of the cone is desirable to allow instruments to be inserted into the tumor while the cone is being placed. Following placement of the cone, the head of the linear accelerator is docked to the cone. The accurate placement of the field is then confirmed by visualizing the tumor through a periscope inserted into the side of the head of the machine. Because the tumor is directly visible, it is not necessary to allow margins for patient motion or inaccuracies in field placement. It is very important to select the electron-beam energy in such a way that the fall-off of dose at a depth occurs immediately beyond the tumor, so as to protect tissues at greater depth. The tumor thickness must therefore be carefully determined.

There must be no gap between the cone and the tumor because the cone acts as a normal tissue retractor as well as a radiation beam collimator. If the cone is not placed firmly against the tumor, normal tissues, such as a loop of small bowel, can slide into the radiation beam. In areas where the tumor has a sloping surface, a cone with beveled edges can be used to provide a better fit with the tumor.

Field sizes are usually limited by the presence of normal organs in the upper abdomen and by the size of the incision. Circular cones with an inner diameter of 5 to 10 cm are commonly used. A single dose of intraoperative irradiation consisting of 1000 to 2000 cGy is usually given following external beam irradiation and at the time of surgical resection.

TOTAL-BODY IRRADIATION

TREATMENT

Only 12 years after Roentgen's discovery of x-rays, total body irradiation (TBI) was described by Dessauer.[52] In its early days, TBI was used for the purpose of eradicating tumor cells in patients with disseminated disease. More recently, low-dose TBI has been employed in the treatment of chronic lymphocytic leukemia (CLL)[53,54] and high-dose TBI in the preparation of patients for bone marrow transplant (BMT) in the treatment of various malignant diseases, including leukemia. The doses in low-dose TBI range from 5 to 10 cGy three to five times per week to a total dose of 100 to 400 cGy.[53]

High-dose TBI has been used routinely since 1969 to condition patients undergoing BMT in the treatment of leukemia. More recently, the use of TBI and BMT has been expanded to the treatment of several other diseases, including lymphomas, neuroblastomas, sarcomas, brain tumors, and breast cancer. The primary function of TBI is immunosuppression to prevent organ rejection, elimination of malignant cells, and ablation of the bone marrow. Chemotherapy, primarily cyclophosphamide, is also used in conditioning the patient prior to the transplant.

There are three types of BMT:

1. *Autologous,* in which marrow is removed from the patient, generally during remission, and is reinfused following the conditioning regimen described above
2. *Allogeneic,* in which the marrow is removed from a sibling who is immunologically compatible with the patient

3. *Syngeneic,* in which the marrow is removed from an identical twin, significantly limiting the problems of graft-versus-host disease

Originally, a single dose of 1000 cGy was given.[55,56] Because such a single-fraction dose produced significant toxicity, multiple-fraction treatments were initiated in an effort to improve normal tissue tolerance and thus reduce late effects of TBI. The dose is often delivered in fractions of 120 to 200 cGy bid (twice a day) to a total dose of 900 to 1200 cGy. The dose rate is thought to have some effect on the tolerance of the treatment and is therefore kept at approximately 5 to 10 cGy per min. The central nervous system and testis appear to be sanctuaries for leukemia cells, and a boost is therefore often delivered to these areas (Fig. 14.27).

MORBIDITY

The toxicity of low-dose TBI is primarily thrombocytopenia, which usually occurs after doses of 100 to 150 cGy. The acute toxicity from the combination of high-dose chemotherapy and high-dose TBI can be

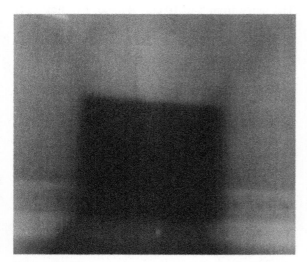

Figure 14.27 A port film of a testicular field treated in preparation for a bone marrow transplant. The patient is positioned in the lithotomy position and the beam is angled from the cephalad direction to avoid irradiating the pelvis and thighs. The penis is taped to the abdomen out of the radiation field.

quite severe, with nausea, vomiting, diarrhea, fever, chills, decreased saliva and tear production, skin erythema, oral mucositis, and alopecia. The most serious late effect is interstitial pneumonitis, which can be fatal.[56-63] Other less severe late sequelae are development of cataracts, growth retardation in children, and endocrine dysfunction. Parotitis, recognized by sudden painless swelling of the parotid gland, sometimes occur after the first treatment of TBI and usually subsides without intervention within a couple of days.

TREATMENT TECHNIQUES

The techniques and dosimetry of large-field irradiation have been studied by several authors.[64-70] The technical difficulties in delivering TBI are different from those of most other radiation therapy treatments.

In most radiation therapy departments, TBI is delivered using a conventional cobalt machine or linear accelerator; however, in some departments where TBI is delivered routinely, a special treatment room is designed for large-field irradiation. In some techniques, the treatment is delivered from two or more sources simultaneously, while in others, a beam "sweeps" over the patient or, alternatively, the patient is moved under a fixed beam (Fig. 14.28). In one treatment technique, the patient is placed in a reclining position with the knees bent and the treatment is delivered via opposed lateral fields.[66,68,70,71] In another technique, patients are treated through anterior and posterior fields (Fig. 14.28).[64,65,71,72] In some treatments, a combination of these two techniques is used.[71] Consideration must be given to the penumbra of the beam and to the shape of the effective radiation field of a linear accelerator when the patient is positioned within the field. As shown in Chap. 8 (Fig. 8.1), even though the field light appears square, the radiation field frequently does not extend to the corners.

Field Size and Treatment Distance. The field size must be large enough to cover the patient's entire body. To achieve this, treatment distances, which are often limited by the size of the treatment room, are usually 3 to 4 m. A treatment field that is 40 ×

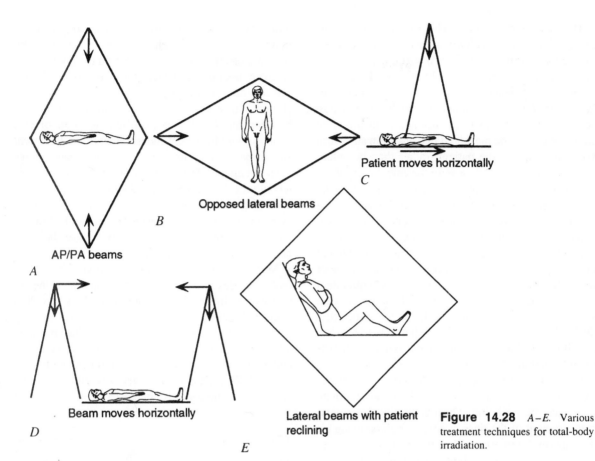

Opposed lateral beams

B

AP/PA beams

A

Patient moves horizontally

C

Beam moves horizontally

D

Lateral beams with patient reclining

E

Figure 14.28 *A–E.* Various treatment techniques for total-body irradiation.

40 cm at 1 m would be 120×120 cm at 3 m. Even its diagonal diameter of 167 cm would be too small to cover the entire body of the average adult lying on a stretcher or standing erect. Patients are therefore usually treated in a sitting or reclining position.

Dose Distribution. Variations in the patient's thickness and the presence of inhomogeneous tissues, particularly the lungs, make it difficult to achieve a uniform dose within the whole body. Compensators are therefore needed to reduce the dose in the lungs and areas where the patient's thickness is smaller—for example, the head, neck, lower legs, and feet.[66,68,71,73] When lateral fields are used, the patient's arms can be placed along the sides to reduce the dose in the lungs. When anterior and posterior fields are used, other means of reducing the

dose to the lungs must be used. Full-thickness blocks can be placed over the lungs, and then the tissues between the skin surface and the lungs are treated with an electron beam.[64] Partial transmission blocks or full-thickness blocks on some treatments will also reduce the dose in the lungs.

Beam Energy. In a survey of several clinics, the most commonly reported beam energy for TBI ranged from cobalt-60 to 10-MV photons, although the use of 16- and 18-MV photons was also reported.[74,75] The advantage of higher-energy beams is the improved dose uniformity across the patient's body; however, bolus material[65] or a beam spoiler, described in this chapter in the discussion of Hodgkin's disease, may be needed to increase the dose in the superficial tissues.

Dose Determination. The extreme conditions under which TBI is delivered create a unique set of problems in terms of determining the dose. The inverse square law may not hold at these long treatment distances because of the changed geometric relationship with the collimators, which gives rise to scattered radiation at shorter distances. The dose rate should therefore be measured in a phantom similar in size and shape to the patient, rather than be calculated. Percentage depth dose in the calculation of the treatment time or monitor unit setting should not be used. Instead, tissue-air ratio (TAR) or tissue-maximum ratio (TMR), which are independent of distance, should be used.[67] At these extreme distances, even these factors may show distance-dependent changes; they should therefore be measured under treatment conditions. Estimation of the equivalent square for the purpose of dose calculation is also very difficult and depends on the patient's position during the treatment. With the patient placed close to a wall or the floor in the treatment room, scatter off the wall and the floor can give rise to inaccuracies in "in air" measurements.[67,69,70] A barrier placed between the patient and the wall or floor can eliminate this scattered radiation. During the first treatment, measurement of the dose at several points, using either thermoluminescent dosimeters (TLDs) or an ionization chamber, is highly recommended.

TOTAL-SKIN ELECTRON IRRADIATION

Total-skin treatment using x-rays was first described in 1939.[76] During the 1950s, a technique using an electron beam was developed at Stanford University. This total-skin electron irradiation (TSEI) technique has undergone some modifications and is now used at many other institutions. It is used in the treatment of cutaneous diseases such as mycosis fungoides and Kaposi's sarcoma, where a high dose is needed in the first centimeter of tissue over the entire body while the underlying tissues are spared.

TREATMENT TECHNIQUES

Techniques to deliver a uniform dose to the entire skin surface are very complex. The treatment re-quires large fields; therefore the treatment distances must be long. Larger fields can be accomplished by omitting electron cones that are used in conventional electron treatments. Under these extreme circumstances, dose uniformity and dose rates are severely altered. Since there can be significant differences between measured dose distributions in air or in a phantom and in patient measurements, no treatment should be initiated until patient measurements have been obtained.[77] The dose uniformity is poor in most techniques due to the forward peaked dose near the central axis of the beam and also due to the irregular skin surface and the presence of skin folds. For example, it is almost impossible to expose the perineum to the electron beam.

Many different techniques of delivering TSEI have been described.[78–91] In most techniques, the patient is standing with arms raised and legs spread to avoid self-shielding (Fig. 14.29). The arm and leg surfaces are exposed to the electron beam. In many techniques, the patient is turned so that six fields, equally spread around the circumference, are treated (Fig. 14.30A). Due to the lower dose away from the central axis, the beam is angled 15 to 30° above and

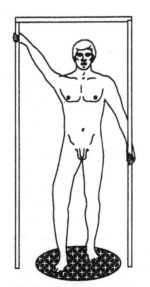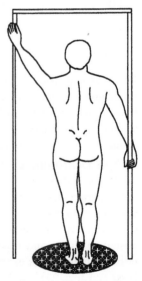

Figure 14.29 In most techniques for total-skin electron irradiation, the patient stands with the legs separated and the arms raised to expose as much of the skin as possible. The position is changed six times during the treatment.

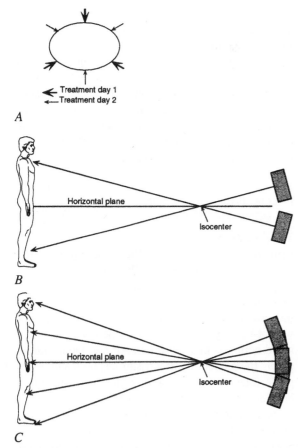

Figure 14.30 Diagram showing the six angles for TSEI *(A)*. Each position is treated every other day. The treatment consists of 12 fields; 6 in the upper and 6 in the lower half of the body *(B)*. Only 3 in the upper and 3 in the lower are treated in one day, and on alternate days the other 6 fields are treated. Diagram of a pendulum-arc technique *(C)*.

below the horizontal plane (Fig. 14.30*B*). Six fields are therefore used to treat the upper half of the body and another six fields to treat the lower half; thus twelve fields are used. Given the time required to deliver the dose at these long distances, only six fields per day are treated and the remaining six fields are treated on alternate days (Fig. 14.30*A*).

As an alternative to the patient turning and changing position several times during the treatment, the patient could stand on a slowly turning platform during the treatment, exposing the skin surfaces to the electron beam.[81,89] In another technique, a pen-

dulum-arc is used (Fig. 14.30*C*). This technique consists of six arc fields symmetrically spread around the circumference of the patient while the beam is arcing in the direction of the patient's longitudinal axis.[88]

DOSE

The dose often prescribed for the treatment of mycosis fungoides is 3600 cGy, and the electron beam energy used is 4 to 6 MeV. Bremsstrahlung, which is present in all electron beams, penetrates much deeper than electrons and increases with higher-beam energies. It is therefore important to deliver TSEI using low electron beam energies. When six and possibly twelve fields overlap at a depth, the x-ray dose can be significant.

Due to the irregular shape of the skin surface and the difference in the sizes and shapes of patients, significant dose heterogeneity often occurs. Since it is impossible to predict what the effect of these variations and the overlap from different fields will be, careful measurements must be made. Higher doses are generally found in the head, particularly the nose and the ears, while the hands, soles of the feet, scalp, areas between the thighs, underarms and breasts, and perineum are severely underdosed. The dose in these areas and areas with extensive disease can be boosted via separate fields.

It is important to recognize that in TSEI, as opposed to photon treatment, the prescribed dose must be delivered from each field. In photon treatments, all beams are contributing dose to the target; therefore, only some of the prescribed dose is delivered from each field. Here, each field is effectively treating only a portion of the target, although there is an overlap among several fields. For example, when a right anterior oblique (RAO) field is treated, skin surfaces that are irradiated via the neighboring fields will unavoidably also be irradiated, but to a lower dose. As a result of this overlap, the dose from a given field must be adjusted so that the combined dose from all fields meets the prescription. A lower dose may also be delivered from the RAO field in the left anterior oblique field (LAO). The dose given via the anterior and LAO fields must therefore be lower, depending on the amount of dose contributed by other fields. On the other hand, when the anterior and LAO fields are treated, the skin surface treated via the RAO field will also receive some dose. Obviously, the dose determination in this type of treatment can be very complicated.

MORBIDITY

In general, TSEI is well tolerated; however, some adverse effects are unavoidable. The acute toxicities include erythema, hyperpigmentation, dry desquamation, conjunctivitis, some extremity edema, decreased lacrimation, and epilation of eyebrows and eyelashes as well as partial epilation of the scalp. Wax-coated internal eye shields can be used to protect the cornea. If the eyelids do not have to be treated, external wax-coated shields protecting the cornea, conjunctiva, and eyelashes should be used. The relationship between acute toxicity and dose measured at different anatomic sites has been studied.[92]

TREATMENT OF METASTATIC DISEASE

Radiation therapy in the management of metastatic disease is almost always palliative. The goal of palliative irradiation is to improve quality of life by achieving pain relief, the cessation of hemorrhaging, improved breathing or swallowing, and/or improved mental status. Palliative irradiation should be delivered in a fashion that will not result in side effects worse than the symptoms the treatments are supposed to alleviate. Treatment decisions should include consideration of the patient's overall prognosis, length of the treatment course, transportation and travel time to and from the treatment center, the possibility of hospitalization for treatment of possible complications, and the cost versus benefit of the treatments as well as the duration of the benefits. For example, a patient with brain metastasis and a prognosis of a couple of months should not be subjected to a long treatment course requiring that most of his or her remaining life is spent coming to the hospital for treatment.

Many patients return on several occasions for treatment of various areas. Meticulous record keeping is critical in avoiding overlap or overdosage. Adjacent fields are often treated and small areas of overlap may be necessary. This is acceptable if the combined dose is low. However, when tolerance doses have been reached, it is necessary to carry the combined dose in the overlap region, particularly in the spine, and to reduce the fields off previously treated areas at the appropriate dose level.

PALLIATIVE IRRADIATION OF BONE METASTASIS

The goal of irradiating bony metastases is to relieve pain and prevent fractures. The most common sites for bony metastases are the ribs, spine, sacrum, and long bones in extremities. Metastases in the bones of extremities often threaten mechanical stability and increase the risk of fractures, particularly in the weight-bearing bones. If half of the combined measured cortex is missing on an AP and lateral radiograph, the probability of a fracture is high and orthopedic intervention to stabilize the bone should be considered.[93] Lytic lesions, appearing on a radiograph as a less dense area in the bone, are most frequently multiple myeloma or metastasis from malignant disease in breasts, kidneys, or the thyroid gland, while osteoblastic lesions, appearing denser than bone on a radiograph, can be from breasts, prostate gland, or Hodgkin's disease.

Treatment fields used in the irradiation of metastases in the pelvic bones should be designed to maximize sparing of the small bowel, rectum, and bladder. The volume of bone marrow is often quite large when the pelvic bones are treated; the patient's blood counts should therefore be closely monitored, particularly if the patient has also received chemotherapy.

Opposed tangential photon fields can be used to spare underlying lung tissue when rib metastases are irradiated. Electron beams can also be used; however, consideration should be given to the increased attenuation of the electron beam by bone.

When bone metastases in extremities are treated, it is important to spare a strip of soft tissue along the entire length of the extremity to allow lymphatic return from the distal portion of the limb. The same consideration should be given to patients irradiated for other conditions in an extremity (soft tissue sarcomas, Ewing's sarcoma, and osteosarcoma).

Simultaneously appearing metastases in several sites can be treated in multiple fields but should be carefully set up so that no overlap occurs at a depth. It is also important to document what areas have been irradiated, because many of these patients return for additional radiation therapy. If an excessive volume of bone marrow would be included, it is advisable to treat the areas causing the most severe symptoms first. Other areas can be treated subsequently when the symptoms become more severe and the myelodepression has subsided.

The total dose is determined by the histology of the tumor and the size of the field. The volume of bone marrow and normal tissues within the irradiated field may limit the dose that can safely be delivered. In patients with poor prognosis, a short course of irradiation (2000 cGy in 1 week) to relieve pain may be beneficial, while a patient with longer expected survival time may benefit from a more protracted course, resulting in longer-lasting pain relief. In patients who respond to initial irradiation of painful bone metastases, a similar response can be expected when they are reirradiated for a relapse.[94]

HALF-BODY IRRADIATION

In severe cases of widespread bone metastases, single-dose or fractionated hemibody irradiation may be tried.[95,96] In this type of treatment, where large fields and long treatment distances are necessary, the same considerations must be given to the dose calculation as described for TBI. Most of these patients are too weak to stand up for the treatment and are therefore often placed on the floor to achieve the needed treatment conditions. When it is difficult to obtain the needed field size to include half of the body, the beam can be angled slightly (Fig. 14.31). If this angle is equal to the angle of the diverging beam edge, matching of the field edges of subsequent fields will be easier. Another method of achieving better coverage of the body is to turn the collimator 45° to take advantage of the larger diagonal field

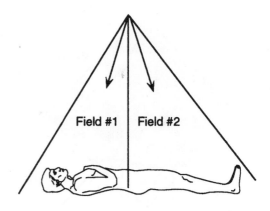

Or divide into 3 segments

Figure 14.31   To achieve a larger field in half-body treatments, the gantry can be angled a few degrees. The angles of each field should be away from the junction to prevent an overlap. Alternatively, the volume can be divided into three rather than two segments.

dimension (Fig. 14.32). In situations where neither method is adequate, treating in three rather than two treatment regions may be considered. The area that includes most of the metastases can be treated initially and, following bone marrow recovery, the remaining two segments can be treated.

The dose delivered in a single fraction is usually on the order of 600 cGy to the upper and 800 cGy to the lower half of the body. When the upper half of the body is irradiated, the toxicity is more severe and requires premedication, including hydration, antiemetics, and corticosteroids. Hospitalization may also be required. The toxicity of upper-half body irradiation is usually nausea and vomiting and occasionally pneumonitis, while diarrhea more frequently occurs following lower-half body irradiation. Myelosuppression frequently occurs, primarily in patients who have received prior chemotherapy. High-dose half-body irradiation should therefore be reserved for patients whose bone marrow reserve has not been compromised by prior chemotherapy.

Single-fraction high-dose hemibody irradiation can be as effective as conventional fractionated radiation therapy in achieving pain relief in patients with metastatic disease; it therefore represents an accept-

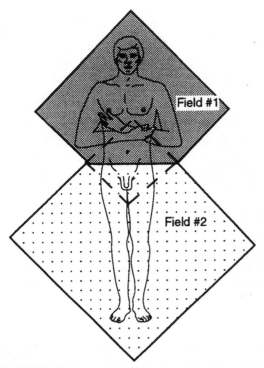

Figure 14.32 When the collimator is turned 45°, the longer diagonal direction can be used to achieve a larger treatment field along the patient's torso. The corner near the junction must be blocked so that the match line is straight across the torso.

able alternative in the management of patients with disseminated tumors involving multiple sites and whose survival is limited.[97,98]

SPINAL-CORD COMPRESSION

Spinal-cord compression caused by metastatic disease can be disastrous for the patient. Epidural compression of the spinal cord, usually caused by vertebral metastasis extending into the epidural space, causes motor and sensory dysfunction below the level of the compression. If the patient presents with early symptoms of compression with minimal neurological compromise, radiation therapy, along with steroids, is effective in the reversal of neurological symptoms and prevention of tumor progression in more than half of these patients. In patients with rapid progression of neurological dysfunction

presenting with paraplegia, immediate surgical decompression is usually necessary. Chances of reversing the symptoms decrease as the time interval between loss of function and decompression increases. Total resection is often impossible and postoperative radiation therapy is therefore recommended. Spinal-cord compression can occur simultaneously at more than one level. A more caudad compression can be masked by sensory and motor loss caused by the compression more cephalad in the spine. A myelogram from above and below or an MRI is useful to rule out the presence of a second compression site and in demonstrating the level of the compressions.

The treatment is often delivered through a single posterior photon field. It is the custom in many centers to treat these patients in the prone position. This gives rise to many difficulties associated with field matching, particularly if the patient has received previous treatments in an adjacent area while in the supine position. Tattoos on the anterior chest, indicating previous treatment fields, cannot be visualized when the patient is prone and will also move relative to the spine. It is also conceivable that the patient might return later for further treatment and is then unable to lie in the prone position. Thus the same field-matching problem is present, but in the opposite direction—i.e., tattoos made on the posterior surface cannot be visualized when the patient is in the supine position. Most modern radiation therapy couches allow unobstructed irradiation of posterior fields through a window in the couch. This improvement should be taken advantage of by treating posterior spine fields with the patient in the supine position. For optimal field matching, the patient's position should be repeated from one treatment course to the next, even if these treatments are separated by several years. If the entire spinal axis must be treated, the fields are often too long to pass through the window in the couch. However, since the entire spinal canal is treated, there is no field-matching problem and the patient may be positioned prone. Matching of adjacent fields is also discussed in Chap. 6.

The depth of the spinal canal from the posterior skin surface varies from 4 to 6 cm in the thoracic spine to 8 to 10 cm in the lumbar spine, with the anterior aspect of the vertebral body at about 2 to 2.5 cm greater depth. These dimensions are smaller in children and also vary with the size of the adult patient. The depth of the dose prescription should be decided with consideration given to the location of the tumor. Since tumors causing the cord compression often originate in the vertebral body, the depth of the dose prescription, particularly in the lumbar spine, may necessitate an opposing anterior field to prevent excessive doses in the subcutaneous tissues. The width of the treatment field should be about 7 to 8 cm and the length should extend approximately two vertebral bodies beyond demonstrable disease. In a few instances, a spinal-cord compression can be caused by invasion of paraspinous tumors such as lymphomas, sarcomas, and neuroblastomas. In these cases, the width of the field must be modified to include the entire tumor.

Total dose and fractionation schemes are determined based on the urgency of the relief of symptoms and the tumor histology. The total dose is limited by the tolerance of the spinal cord and previous irradiation. If the compression is acute and cannot be relieved by surgery, a high dose (400 cGy) is often given in the first one or two fractions, followed by 250 to 300 cGy per fraction to a total dose of 3000 to 4000 cGy. This dose may be modified depending on the histology of the tumor and the length of spinal cord treated. In patients with less acute onset, 3000 to 4000 cGy in 2 to 4 weeks can be considered. Previous irradiation of the same segment of spinal cord should be considered when the prescription is written, and clear documentation of overlap areas should be made. Field reduction off previously treated spinal cord must be made at appropriate doses.

BRAIN METASTASIS

The primary treatment of brain metastasis is radiation therapy, particularly when multiple metastases are present. If a solitary metastasis is present, surgical resection may be possible; however, most patients with brain metastasis present with multiple lesions, and whole-brain irradiation is given. The dose is usually 2000 cGy in 1 week or 3000 cGy in 2 weeks.[99] No significant difference in duration of improvement or survival has been found in studies comparing several fractionation schemas.[100] Treatment techniques are discussed in Chap. 10.

LIVER METASTASIS

The role of radiation therapy in the palliative treatment of liver metastasis is uncertain. The survival of patients with liver metastasis is usually short (months), and the goal of therapy is to relieve pain. A dose of 2000 to 2500 cGy in 2 to 3 weeks to the whole liver is generally well tolerated and may be effective in reducing the size of the liver and thus relieving pain.

SUPERIOR VENA CAVA OBSTRUCTION

Obstruction of the superior vena cava is usually caused by pulmonary tumors. Patients usually present with shortness of breath, swelling, and discoloration of the skin in the head, arms, and chest above the site of obstruction. Due to the hazards of obtaining a biopsy in patients with this condition, radiation therapy may be initiated without a tissue diagnosis. The patients are usually unable to lie down and must be treated sitting in a chair (Chap. 7, Fig. 7.53) or in the bed. Initially, daily high doses are given to relieve the obstruction. The patient's condition usually improves within a few days and a tissue diagnosis can then be obtained. When the patient is able to lie down, appropriate treatment fields can be designed and the treatment continued via anterior and posterior fields.

PALLIATIVE RADIATION THERAPY FOR OTHER CONDITIONS

Palliative irradiation is sometimes required in situations where tumors are causing obstructive symptoms, as in the trachea, esophagus, bile duct, ureters, or urethra. In other situations, irradiation may be necessary to stop hemorrhage caused by extensive tumors in the bladder, uterus, cervix, rectum, or stomach. Prompt irradiation to a localized area to relieve obstruction or bleeding is usually necessary.

Following a few fractions of high-dose irradiation, a larger field including the entire tumor can be treated using smaller dose fractions. In this treatment schedule, the boost, which usually follows large-field irradiation, is given first in order to relieve the obstructive symptoms quickly.

Orbital metastasis causing severe proptosis may occasionally require radiation therapy. Field matching is impossible if the patient has received previous whole-brain irradiation and a small overlap may be necessary, thus limiting the total dose which can safely be delivered.

PROBLEMS

14.1 The 10-year survival for patients with all stages of Hodgkin's disease is approximately
   (a) 30 percent
   (b) 50 percent
   (c) 80 percent
   (d) 90 percent

14.2 The patient position for treatment of a mantle field in Hodgkin's disease is usually
   (a) Supine with the chin extended and the arms by the sides
   (b) Supine with the chin extended and the arms raised above the head
   (c) Supine with the chin in neutral position and the arms by the sides
   (d) Prone with the chin extended and the arms by the sides

14.3 Patients with Hodgkin's disease being treated with parallel opposed anterior and posterior fields to mantle and paraaortic and spleen fields are best positioned
   (a) In the supine position when all fields are treated
   (b) In the supine position when the anterior mantle field and the two paraaortic fields are treated
   (c) In the supine position for the two anterior fields and prone position for the two posterior fields
   (d) The position is not important

14.4 It is always important to align the patient with the sagittal laser alignment line every day because
   (a) When large fields are treated, it is sufficient to make sure the central axis of the beam is in the right position
   (b) If it is not, the field is rotated with respect to the patient's body
   (c) The central axis will be in the right position and the blocks will shield the appropriate areas
   (d) Otherwise the central axis may not be in the right position

14.5 To assure inclusion of palpable lymph nodes within the radiation field,
   (a) The lymph nodes should be outlined on a diagnostic radiograph and then transposed to the simulation film before blocks are drawn
   (b) The lymph nodes should be palpated by the technologist during the simulation procedure to make sure they are within the fields
   (c) The lymph nodes should be ignored as long as they are small
   (d) The lymph nodes should be indicated by radiopaque marker during the simulation procedure

14.6 The gap between mantle and paraaortic fields, assuming the same field length and SAD, is calculated and set correctly if the patient is in the same position and
   (a) The cephalad margin of the posterior paraaortic field is 1.5 cm from the marker indicating the caudal margin of the anterior mantle field
   (b) The cephalad margin of the posterior paraaortic field coincides with the marker indicating the caudal margin of the anterior mantle field
   (c) The cephalad margin of the anterior paraaortic field coincides with the marker indicating the caudal margin of the anterior mantle field
   (d) The cephalad margin of the anterior paraaortic field is about 1.5 cm from the marker indicating the caudal margin of the anterior mantle field

14.7 Tattoos made on the patient's skin indicating irradiated areas
   (a) Can always be trusted
   (b) Can shift due to growth and weight changes
   (c) Can be misleading because they may have been made in error
   (d) Can be trusted only if there also is a photograph showing the field

14.8 If the SAD at the central axis in two opposed mantle fields is 100 cm and the patient's thickness is 20 cm, we can find the thickness of the tabletop and the immobilization device under the patient by
   (a) Determining the SSD on the anterior skin surface and subtracting this distance from 100 cm
   (b) Rotating the gantry 180° and determining the SSD to the bottom of the couch then subtracting this distance from 110 cm
   (c) Push a pin through the immobilization device at the thickest point and measure the thickness of the couch top with a ruler
   (d) Rotating the gantry 180° and determining the SSD to the bottom of the couch, then subtracting this distance from 100 cm

14.9 In an isocentric treatment technique using a machine with 100-cm SAD, the total distance between the two sources positions in parallel opposed fields
   (a) Is found by determining the SSD on the anterior and posterior surfaces of the patient and adding them together
   (b) Is found by determining the anterior SSD and adding the patient's thickness, then multiplying by 2
   (c) Is found by determining the SSD on the anterior and the posterior surfaces of the patient and subtracting the patient's thickness
   (d) Is always 200 cm

14.10 In an SSD technique using a machine with 100-cm SAD, the total distance between the two source positions in parallel opposed fields can be determined by
   (a) Adding the SSD for the anterior field and the patient's thickness and multiplying by 2
   (b) Adding the patient's thickness to the anterior and posterior SSDs
   (c) Subtracting the patient's thickness from the sum of the two SSDs
   (d) Adding the anterior and the posterior SSDs and then subtracting half of the patient's thickness

14.11 When a soft tissue sarcoma in an extremity is treated, it is important to
   (a) Use very generous tumor margins and include at least one joint and the entire circumference of the extremity within the fields

(b) Use generous tumor margins and spare a small strip of the muscle compartment

(c) Use small tumor margins and spare a small strip of the muscle compartment

(d) Use generous tumor margins including the entire circumference of the muscle compartment and spare a small strip of tissue along the extremity

14.12 When a lower extremity is treated, it is almost necessary to

(a) Treat the patient in the prone position with the feet toward the gantry

(b) Reverse the patient's position on the couch with the feet toward the gantry

(c) Treat the patient in the supine position with the head toward the gantry

(d) Reverse the patient's position on the couch and treating the prone position

14.13 The advantage of intraoperative radiation therapy is

(a) That it provides superior normal-tissue sparing and improved precision

(b) That because electrons are used, more normal tissues are spared

(c) That the treatment is always delivered immediately following surgery when tissues are more radiosensitive

(d) That higher doses can be delivered

14.14 High- and low-dose total body irradiation is used in the

(a) Preparation of the patient for high-dose chemotherapy treatment for chronic lymphocytic leukemia

(b) Preparation of the patient for high-dose chemotherapy to minimize myelosuppression

(c) Management of patients undergoing a bone marrow transplant to minimize the effects of high-dose chemotherapy

(d) Preparation of patients for a bone marrow transplant and in the treatment of chronic lymphocytic leukemia

14.15 An allogenic bone marrow transplant is one in which

(a) The bone marrow is removed from the patient when the tumor appears most aggressive, the marrow is treated with high-dose irradiation, and is then reinfused into the patient

(b) The bone marrow is removed from the patient when the disease is in remission and is then reinfused following conditioning

(c) The patient receives bone marrow from a sibling who is immunologically compatible with the patient

(d) The bone marrow is removed from an identical twin and is infused into the patient following conditioning

14.16 The most serious late consequence of high-dose total-body irradiation is

(a) Hair loss

(b) Loss of vision

(c) Chronic liver disease

(d) Radiation pneumonitis

14.17 The most common position for patients receiving total-skin electron irradiation is

(a) Standing with legs spread and arms raised

(b) Resting in the reclining position

(c) Lying supine on the treatment couch

(d) Standing with the legs together and arms along the side and turning to six different positions

14.18 The main goal of radiation therapy in patients with bone metastasis is to
(*a*) Eradicate the tumor
(*b*) Prevent fractures and reduce nausea
(*c*) Prevent fractures and reduce pain
(*d*) Prevent the tumor from spreading further

14.19 When a patient requires half-body treatment but the necessary distance cannot be achieved, one can
(*a*) Turn the collimator 45° taking advantage of the diagonal direction of the field or angle the gantry a few degrees
(*b*) Turn the gantry 45° or rotate the collimator a few degrees to take advantage of the larger direction
(*c*) Have the patient sit in a chair with the knees bent for lower half-body irradiation and with the neck flexed for the upper half of the body
(*d*) Have the patient stand against the wall of the room, where the longest distance can be achieved

14.20 In patients treated for a spinal-cord compression, the treatment field should
(*a*) Include a very short segment of the vertebral bodies on each side beyond demonstrable disease
(*b*) Include at least a 10-cm margin along the spinal cord beyond demonstrable disease
(*c*) Include approximately two vertebral bodies in each direction beyond demonstrable disease
(*d*) Include only the area of the spinal cord that hurts

REFERENCES

1. Bentel GC: Positioning and immobilization of patients undergoing radiation therapy for Hodgkin's disease. *Med Dosim* 16:111, 1991.
2. Creutzberg CL, Visser AG, DePorre PMZR, et al: Accuracy of patient positioning in mantle field irradiation. *Radiother Oncol* 23:257, 1992.
3. Hulshof M, Vanuytsel L, van den Bogaert W, van der Schueren E: Localization errors in mantle-field irradiation for Hodgkin's disease. *Int J Radiat Oncol Biol Phys* 17:679, 1989.
4. Kinzie JJ, Hanks GE, MacLean CJ, Kramer S: Patterns of Care Study: Hodgkin's disease relapse rates and adequacy of portals. *Cancer* 52:2223, 1983.
5. Marks JE, Haus AG, Sutton HG, Griem ML: Localization error in the radiotherapy of Hodgkin's disease and malignant lymphoma with extended mantle fields. *Cancer* 34:83, 1974.
6. Taylor BW, Mendenhall NP, Million RR: Reproducibility of mantle irradiation with daily imaging. *Int J Radiat Oncol Biol Phys* 19:149, 1990.
7. Marcus KC, Svensson G, Rhodes LP, Mauch PM: Mantle irradiation in the upright position: A technique to reduce the volume of lung irradiated in patients with bulky mediastinal Hodgkin's disease. *Int J Radiat Oncol Biol Phys* 23:443, 1992.
8. Lutz WR, Larsen RD: Technique to match mantle and para-aortoic fields. *Int J Radiat Oncol Biol Phys* 9:1753, 1983.
9. Armstrong DI, Tait J: The matching of adjacent fields in radiotherapy. *Radiology* 108:419, 1973.
10. Fraass BA, Tepper JE, Glatstein E, van de Geijn J: Clinical use of a match-line wedge for adjacent megavoltage radiation field matching. *Int J Radiat Oncol Biol Phys* 9:209, 1983.
11. Griffin TW, Schumacher D, Berry HC: A technique for cranial-spinal irradiation. *Br J Radiol* 49:887, 1976.
12. Hale J, Davis LW, Block P: Portal separation for pairs of parallel opposed portals at 2 MV and 6 MV. *Am J Roentgenol* 114:172, 1972.
13. Bukovitz AG, Deutsch M, Slayton R: Orthogonal fields: Variations in dose vs. gap size for treatment of the central nervous system. *Radiology* 126:795, 1978.
14. Haie C, Schlienger M, Constans JP, et al: Results of radiation treatment of medulloblastoma in adults. *Int J Radiat Oncol Biol Phys* 11:2051, 1985.
15. Johnson PM, Kepka AG: A double-junction technique for total central nervous system irradiation with a 4-MV accelerator. *Radiology* 145:467, 1982.

16. Bentel GC, Halperin EC: High dose areas are unintentionally created as a result of gap shifts when the prescribed doses in the two adjacent areas are different. *Med Dosim* 15:179, 1990.

17. Keys R, Grigsby PW: Gapping fields on sloping surfaces. *Int J Radiat Oncol Biol Phys* 18:1183, 1990.

18. Nisce LZ, D'Angio GJ: A new technique for the irradiation of large fields in patients with lymphoma. *Radiology* 106:641, 1973.

19. Faw FL, Johnson RE, Warren CA, Glenn DW: A standard set of "individualized" compensating filters for mantle field radiotherapy of Hodgkin's disease. *Am J Roentgenol* 111:376, 1971.

20. Gray L, Prosnitz LR: Dosimetry of Hodgkin's disease therapy using a 4 MV linear accelerator. *Radiology* 116:423, 1975.

21. Page V, Gardner A, Karzmark CJ: Physical and dosimetric aspects of the radiotherapy of malignant lymphomas: I. The mantle technique. *Radiology* 96:609, 1970.

22. Svahn-Tapper G: Dosimetric studies of mantle fields in cobalt-60 therapy of malignant lymphomas. *Acta Radiol Ther* 9:190, 1970.

23. Svahn-Tapper G, Landberg T: Mantle treatment of Hodgkin's disease with cobalt-60. Technique and dosimetry. *Acta Radiol Ther* 10:33, 1971.

24. Doppke KP, Novack D, Wang CC: Physical considerations in the treatment of advanced carcinomas of the larynx and pyriform sinuses using 10 MV x-rays. *Int J Radiat Oncol Biol Phys* 6:1251, 1980.

25. Wang CC: *Clinical Radiation Oncology*. Littleton, MA: PSG Publishing, 1988.

26. Kubo H, Russel M, Wang CC: Use of 10 MV spoiled x ray beam for the treatment of head and neck tumors. *Int J Radiat Oncol Biol Phys* 8:1795, 1982.

27. Lee PC, Thomason C, Glasgow GP: Characteristics of a spoiled 6-MV beam from a dual-energy linear accelerator. *Med Phys* 20:717, 1993.

28. Kinsella TJ, Fraass BA, Glatstein E: Late effects of radiation therapy of Hodgkin's disease. *Cancer Treat Rep* 66:991, 1982.

29. Boivin JF, Hutchison GB: Coronary heart disease mortality after irradiation for Hodgkin's disease. *Cancer* 49:2470, 1982.

30. Brosius FC, Waller BF, Roberts WC: Radiation and heart disease: Analysis of 16 young (aged 15–33 years) necropsy patients who received over 3500 rads to the heart. *Am J Med* 70:519, 1981.

31. Mefferd JM, Donaldson SS, Link MP: Pediatric Hodgkin's disease: Pulmonary, cardiac, and thyroid function combined modality. *Int J Radiat Oncol Biol Phys* 16:679, 1989.

32. Morgan GW, Freeman AP, McLean RG, et al: Late cardiac, thyroid, and pulmonary sequelae of mantle radiotherapy for Hodgkin's disease. *Int J Radiat Oncol Biol Phys* 11:1925, 1985.

33. Tarbell NJ, Thompson L, Mauch P: Thoracic irradiation in Hodgkin's disease: Disease control and long-term complications. *Int J Radiat Oncol Biol Phys* 18:275, 1990.

34. Johnstone PA, Wexler LH, Venzon DJ, et al: Sarcomas of the hand and foot: Analysis of local control and functional result with combined modality therapy in extremity preservation. *Int J Radiat Oncol Biol Phys* 29:735, 1994.

35. Kinsella TJ, Loeffler JS, Fraass BA, Tepper J: Extremity preservation by combined modality therapy in sarcomas of the hand and foot: An analysis of local control, disease-free survival and functional results. *Int J Radiat Oncol Biol Phys* 9:1115, 1983.

36. Kinsella TJ: Limited surgery and radiation therapy for sarcomas of the hand and foot (editorial). *Int J Radiat Oncol Biol Phys* 12:2045, 1986.

37. Okunieff P, Suit HD, Proppe KH: Extremity preservation by combined modality treatment of sarcomas of the hand and wrist. *Int J Radiat Oncol Biol Phys* 12:1923, 1986.

38. Talbert ML, Zagars GK, Sherman NE, Romsdahl MM: Conservative surgery and radiation therapy for soft tissue sarcoma of the wrist, hand, ankle, and foot. *Cancer* 66:2482, 1990.

39. Leopold KA, Harrelson J, Prosnitz L, et al: Preoperative hyperthermia and radiation for soft tissue sarcomas: Advantage of two vs. one hyperthermia treatment per week. *Int J Radiat Oncol Biol Phys* 16:107, 1989.

40. Suit HD, Proppe KH, Mankin HJ, Wood W: Preoperative radiation therapy for sarcoma of soft tissue. *Cancer* 47:2269, 1981.

41. Eilber FR, Morton DL, Eckerdt J, et al: Limb salvage for skeletal and soft tissue sarcomas: Multidisciplinary preoperative therapy. *Cancer* 53:2579, 1984.

42. Nielsen OS, Cummings MB, O'Sullivan MB, et al: Preoperative and postoperative irradiation of soft tissue sarcomas: Effect on radiation field size. *Int J Radiat Oncol Biol Phys* 21:1595, 1991.

43. Niewald M, Berberich W, Schnabel K, Lehmann W: Ein einfache Methode zur Lagerung und Fixierung der Extreitatem bei der Strahlentherapie von Weichteilsarkomen. *Strahlenth Onkol* 166:295, 1990.

44. Tepper KJ, Rosenberg SA, Glatstein E: Radiation therapy technique in soft tissue sarcoma of the extremity — policies of treatment at the National Cancer Institute. *Int J Radiat Oncol Biol Phys* 8:263, 1982.

45. Selch MT, Kopald KH, Ferreiro GA, et al: Limb salvage therapy for soft tissue sarcomas of the foot. *Int J Radiat Oncol Biol Phys* 19:41, 1990.

46. Franke HD, Schmidt R: Clinical results after therapy with fast neutrons (DT, 14 MeV) since 1976 in Hamburg-Eppendorf, in Karcher KH (ed): *Progress in Radio-Oncology III: Proceedings of the Third Meeting on Progress of Radio-Oncology*. Vienna: International Club for Radio-Oncologists, 1987.

47. Griffin TW, Wambersie A, Laramore G, Castro J: High LET; Heavy particle trials. *Int J Radiat Oncol Biol Phys* 14:S83, 1988.

48. Pickering DG, Stewart JS, Rampling R, et al: Fast neutron therapy for soft tissue sarcoma. *Int J Radiat Oncol Biol Phys* 13:1489, 1987.

49. Schmitt G, Furst G, von Essen CF: Neutron and neutron boost irradiation of soft tissue sarcoma, in Karcher KH (ed): *Progress in Radio-Oncology III: Proceedings of the Third Meeting on Progress in Radio-Oncology.* Vienna: International Club for Radio-Oncologists, 1987.

50. Curran WJ, Littman P, Raney RB: Interstitial radiation therapy in the treatment of childhood soft tissue sarcomas. *Int J Radiat Oncol Biol Phys* 14:169, 1988.

51. Shiu MH, Turnbull AD, Nori D, et al: Control of locally advanced extremity soft tissue sarcomas by function-saving resection and brachytherapy. *Cancer* 53:1385, 1984.

52. Dessauer F: A new design for radiotherapy. *Arch Phys Med Med Tech* 2:218, 1907.

53. Johnson RE: Total body irradiation of chronic lymphocytic leukemia: Relationship between therapeutic response and prognosis. *Cancer* 37:2691, 1976.

54. Johnson RE: Role of radiation therapy in management of adult leukemia. *Cancer* 39(suppl 2):852, 1977.

55. Thomas ED: The role of marrow transplantation in the eradication of malignant disease. *Cancer* 49:1963, 1982.

56. Thomas ED, Clift RA, Hersman J, et al: Marrow transplantation for acute non-lymphoblastic leukemia in first remission using fractionated or single-dose irradiation. *Int J Radiat Oncol Biol Phys* 8:817, 1982.

57. Gluckman E, Devergie A, Dutreix A, et al: Total body irradiation in bone marrow transplantation: Hôspital Saint-Louis results. *Pathol Biol* 27:349, 1979.

58. Keane TJ, Van Dyk J, Rider WD: Idiopathic interstitial pneumonia following bone marrow transplantation: The relationship with total body irradiation. *Int J Radiat Oncol Biol Phys* 7:1365, 1981.

59. Kim TH, Rybka WB, Lehnert S, et al: Interstitial pneumonitis following total body irradiation for bone marrow transplantation using two different dose rates. *Int J Radiat Oncol Biol Phys* 11:1285, 1985.

60. Latini P, Aristei C, Aversa F, et al: Interstitial pneumonitis after hyperfractionated total body irradiation in HLA-matched T-depleted bone marrow transplantation. *Int J Radiat Oncol Biol Phys* 23:401, 1992.

61. Neiman PE, Thomas ED, Reeves WC, et al: Opportunistic infection and interstitial pneumonitis following marrow transplantation for aplastic anemia and hematologic malignancy. *Transpl Proc* 7:663, 1976.

62. Pino y Torres JL, Bross DS, Lam WL, et al: Risk factors in interstitial pneumonitis following allogeneic bone marrow transplantation. *Int J Radiat Oncol Biol Phys* 8:1301, 1981.

63. Thomas ED, Buckner CD, Clift RA, et al: Marrow trans-

plantation for acute nonlymphoblastic leukemia in first remission. *N Engl J Med* 301:579, 1979.

64. Breneman JC, Elson HR, Little R, et al: A technique for delivery of total body irradiation for bone marrow transplantation in adults and adolescents. *Int J Radiat Oncol Biol Phys* 18:1233, 1990.

65. Findley DO, Skov DD, Blume KG: Total body irradiation with a 10 MV linear accelerator in conjunction with bone marrow transplantation. *Int J Radiat Oncol Biol Phys* 6:695, 1980.

66. Galvin JM, D'Angio GJ, Walsh G: Use of tissue compensators to improve the dose uniformity for total body irradiation. *Int J Radiat Oncol Biol Phys* 6:767, 1980.

67. Galvin JM: Calculation and prescription of dose for total body irradiation. *Int J Radiat Oncol Biol Phys* 9:1919, 1983.

68. Khan FM, Williamson JF, Sewchand W, Kim TH: Basic data for dosage calculation and compensation. *Int J Radiat Oncol Biol Phys* 6:745, 1980.

69. Lam LW, Order SE, Thomas ED: Uniformity and standardization of single and opposing cobalt-60 sources for total body irradiation. *Int J Radiat Oncol Biol Phys* 6:245, 1980.

70. Van Dam J, Rijnders A, Vanuytsel L, Zhang HZ: Practical implications of backscatter from outside the patient on the dose distribution during total body irradiation. *Radiother Oncol* 13:193, 1988.

71. Shank B: Techniques of magna-field irradiation. *Int J Radiat Oncol Biol Phys* 9:1925, 1983.

72. Lam WC, Lindskoug BA, Order SE, Grant DG: The dosimetry of Co-60 total body irradiation. *Int J Radiat Oncol Biol Phys* 5:905, 1979.

73. Van Dyk J: Magna-field irradiation: Physical considerations. *Int J Radiat Oncol Biol Phys* 9:1913, 1983.

74. Engler MJ: A practical approach to uniform total body photon irradiation. *Int J Radiat Oncol Biol Phys* 12:2033, 1986.

75. Niroomand-Rad A: Physical aspects of total body irradiation of bone marrow transplant patients using 18 MV X rays. *Int J Radiat Oncol Biol Phys* 20:605, 1991.

76. Sommerville J: Mycosis fungoides treated with general x-ray "bath." *Br J Dermatol* 51:323, 1939.

77. Fraass BA, Roberson PL, Glatstein E: Whole-skin electron treatment: Patient skin dose distribution. *Radiology* 146:811, 1983.

78. Almond PR: Total skin/electron irradiation technique and dosimetry, in Kereikas JG, Elson HR, Born CG (eds): *Radiation Oncology Physics—1986.* New York: American Institute of Physics, 1987.

79. Bjärngard BE, Chen GTY, Piontek RN, Svensson GK: Analysis of dose distributions in whole body superficial electron therapy. *Int J Radiat Oncol Biol Phys* 2:319, 1977.

80. Edelstein GR, Clark T, Holt JG: Dosimetry for total-body

electron-beam therapy in the treatment of mycosis fungoides. *Radiology* 108:691, 1973.

81. Freeman CR, Suissa S, Shenouda G, et al: Clinical experience with a single field rotational skin electron irradiation technique for cutaneous T-cell lymphoma. *Radiother Oncol* 24:155, 1992.

82. Gerbi BJ, Khan FM, Deibel C, Kim TH: Total skin electron arc irradiation using a reclined patient position. *Int J Radiat Oncol Biol Phys* 17:397, 1989.

83. Holt JG, Perry DJ: Some physical considerations in whole skin electron beam therapy. *Med Phys* 9:769, 1982.

84. Karzmark CJ, Loevinger R, Steel RE: A technique for large-field, superficial electron therapy. *Radiology* 74:633, 1960.

85. Karzmark CJ: Large-field superficial electron therapy with linear accelerators. *Am J Radiol* 37:302, 1964.

86. Karzmark CJ: Physical aspects of whole-body superficial therapy with electrons. *Frontiers Radiat Ther Oncol* 2:36, 1968.

87. Page V, Gardener A, Karzmark CJ: Patient dosimetry in the electron treatment of large superficial lesions. *Radiology* 94:635, 1970.

88. Sewchand W, Khan FM, Williamson J: Total body superficial electron-beam therapy using a multiple-field pendulum-arc technique. *Radiology* 130:493, 1979.

89. Tetenes PJ, Goodwin PN: Comparative study of whole-body radiotherapeutic techniques using a 4-MeV nonangulated electron beam. *Radiology* 122:219, 1977.

90. Van Der Merwe DG: Total skin electron therapy: A technique which can be implemented on a conventional electron linear accelerator. *Int J Radiat Oncol Biol Phys* 27:391, 1993.

91. Williams PC, Hunter RD, Jackson SM: Whole body electron therapy in mycosis fungoides—Successful translational technique achieved by modification of an established linear accelerator. *Radiology* 52:302, 1979.

92. Desai KR, Pezner RD, Lipsett JA, et al: Total skin electron irradiation for mycosis fungoides: Relationship between acute toxicities and measured dose at different anatomic sites. *Int J Radiat Oncol Biol Phys* 15:641, 1988.

93. Ryan JR, Rowe DE, Salciccioli GG: Prophylactic internal fixation of the femur for neoplastic lesions. *J Bone Joint Surg* 58:1071, 1976.

94. Mithal NP, Needham PR, Hoskin PJ: Retreatment with radiotherapy for painful bone metastasis. *Int J Radiat Oncol Biol Phys* 29:1011, 1994.

95. Rider WD: Half-body radiotherapy: An update. *Int J Radiat Oncol Biol Phys* 4(suppl 2):69, 1978.

96. Salazar OM, Rubin P, Hendrickson FR, et al: Single-dose half-body irradiation for the palliation of multiple bone metastasis from solid tumors: A preliminary report. *Int J Radiat Oncol Biol Phys* 7:773, 1981.

97. Fitzpatrick PJ, Rider WD: Half body radiotherapy. *Int J Radiat Oncol Biol Phys* 1:197, 1976.

98. Salazar OM, Rubin P, Hendrickson FR, et al: Single-dose half-body irradiation for palliation of multiple bone metastases from solid tumors: Final Radiation Therapy Oncology Group report. *Cancer* 58:29, 1986.

99. Sheline GE, Brady LW: Radiation therapy for brain metastases. *J Neurooncol* 4:219, 1987.

100. Borgelt B, Gelber R, Kramer S, et al: The palliation of brain metastases: Final results of the first two studies by the Radiation Therapy Oncology Group. *Int J Radiat Oncol Biol Phys* 6:1, 1980.

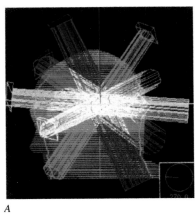

A

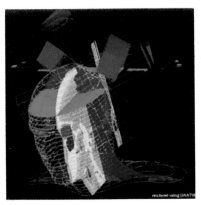

B

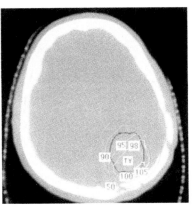

C

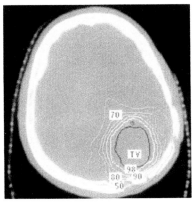

D

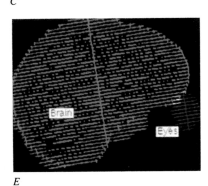

E

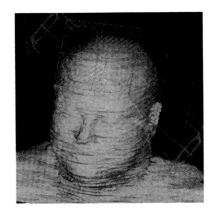

F

3. *(This illustration appears in Chapter 10 as Figure 10.24)* Retreatment of small brain tumors can also be delivered through a large number of conformal beams, none of which are opposed, to limit the dose in the entrance/exit regions. *A.* A "bouquet" of beams aimed at a small brain tumor with wedges oriented in an unconventional fashion to deliver a uniform dose in the tumor. *B.* A color display of the CT images in sagittal, coronal, and transverse planes and the location of the tumor *(red)* and the eyes *(green)*. Beam and wedge orientations are also shown in green. The resulting isodose distribution without wedges *(C)* and with wedges *(D)*. The maximum dose with wedges is 100.4 percent

and the target is covered by the 98 percent isodose line. *E.* The wire outline of the brain *(blue)* and the eyes *(red)* shows that the posterior superior portions of the eye and the brain are superimposed in the lateral beam's-eye view. *F.* A color wash of a patient with two small lesions treated through opposed fields angled such that the lesions are superimposed in the beam's-eye view. A third right anterior field was designed such that it included only the lesions with small margins, and the area between the tumors was blocked. Neither of these plans could be carried out without three-dimensional treatment planning tools. (The Virtual Simulator™, Sherouse Systems, Inc.)

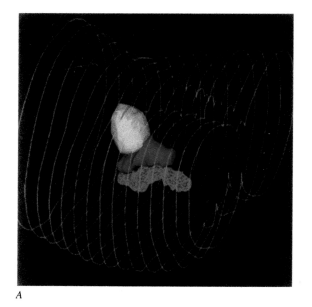

A

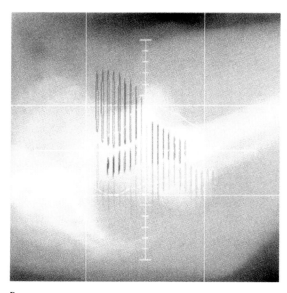

B

C

4. *(This illustration appears in Chapter 13 as Figure 13.21)* A. Surface-rendered illustration of the anatomy pertinent to prostate treatment planning. The prostate and seminal vesicles in red are immediately adjacent to the bladder in yellow and the rectum in green. ·B. A digitally reconstructed radiograph (DRR) with the prostate and seminal vesicles in red, the bladder in green, and the rectum in yellow with the conformal lateral field superimposed. C. With three-dimensional treatment-planning tools, treatment fields with small tumor margins and complex field orientations can be delivered with more confidence than with standard methods. (The Virtual Simulator™, Sherouse Systems, Inc.)

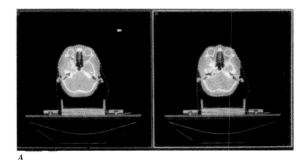
A

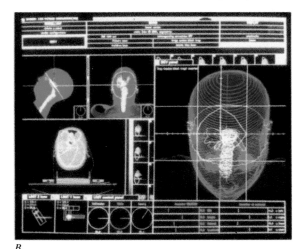
B

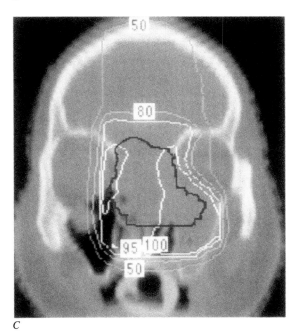
C

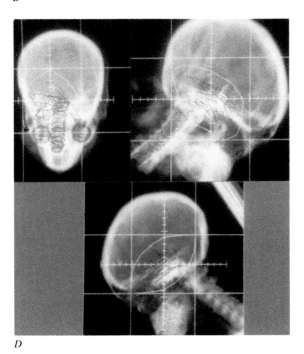
D

1. *(This illustration appears in Chapter 7 as Figure 7.46)* A. The target and pertinent anatomy are outlined in all CT images. B. The three-dimensional image of the patient is built. In the left lower corner are the icons showing the motions of the couch, gantry, and collimator as the beam directions are determined. In the lower right corner are dials for setting the field size and isocenter. Above is a three-dimensional rendering of the structures drawn on the CT images and the two perpendicular views of the patient. In the lower left of the screen is a CT image of the patient with outlined anatomy; while the planning takes place, the beams can be visualized on the image. Any CT image can be viewed in this window. At the top of the screen are the dials for choosing beam energy, wedges, trays, and other accessories along with options for outlining the treatment field in the beam's-eye view. An autocontour option allows the user to set the desired margin around the target; the program will then automatically draw the field around the target. C. Dose calculations in three dimensions are viewed on the screen or plotted on paper. D. Digitally reconstructed radiographs are calculated from the CT date for each field.

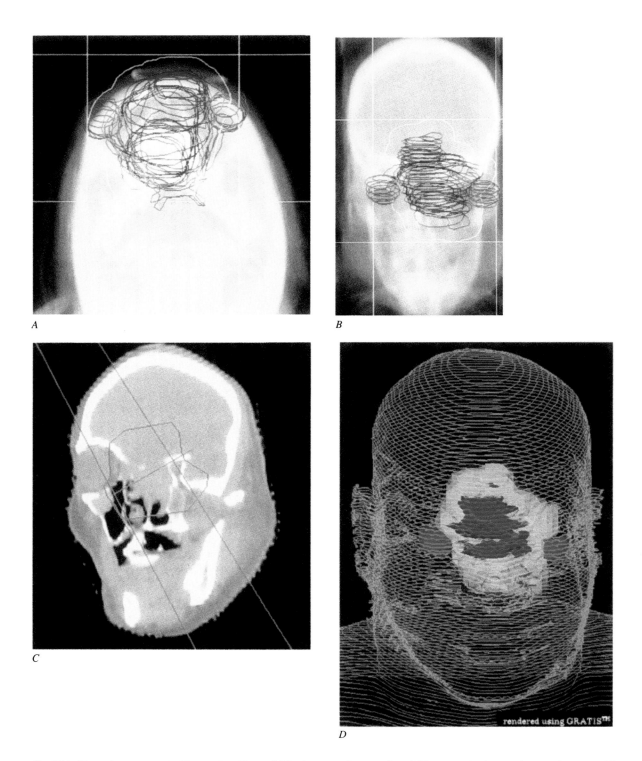

A

B

C

D

rendered using GRATIS™

2. *(This illustration appears in Chapter 9 as Figure 9.39)* An oblique vertex *(A)* and a frontal field *(B)* displayed on digitally reconstructed radiographs (DRR) used in treating an extensive carcinoma of the nasal cavity. *C.* The two treatment fields displayed on an oblique CT image. *D.* Surface-rendered tumor volume *(red)* and 98 percent isodose surface *(yellow).* The 98 percent isodose line does not totally enclose the tumor, which is seen outside the isodose surface. (The Virtual Simulator™, Sherouse Systems, Inc.)

15

Dose Calculations in Brachytherapy

Almost immediately following the discovery of radium by Marie and Pierre Curie in 1898, it was used to treat cancer by being placed in direct contact with the tumor. The placement of sealed radioactive sources into or immediately adjacent to tumors is referred to as *brachytherapy. Brachy,* meaning "short," is used here in the context of therapy at a short distance.

Isotopes used in brachytherapy can be embedded in surface applicators placed directly on the tumor, or they can be inserted into a specially designed apparatus that is placed into body cavities (intracavitary), various tubular organs (intraluminal), or directly through the tumor (interstitial). In each of these methods, the radioactive material is sealed inside a shell that prevents the escape of radioactivity into the tissues. One advantage of brachytherapy is that high doses can be delivered in a relatively short time (high dose rate, minutes; low dose rate, hours) locally to tumors that are accessible for insertion of the radioactive material, while the dose to surrounding tissues is minimal. The technical aspects of such brachytherapy applications are described in Chap. 16.

EMITTED RADIATION

Various types of radiation are produced by radioactive isotopes, including alpha, beta, and gamma rays. Emitted alpha particles are ineffective in the treatment of malignant disease because they lack penetrating power. Beta particles, which are somewhat more penetrating (the range is typically a few millimeters), may be useful for the treatment of very superficial lesions, especially those of the eye. Gamma rays have more penetrating power and are commonly used in the treatment of larger tumors.

Filters, consisting of platinum or a platinum/iridium alloy, are often built into the walls surrounding an isotope to prevent useless low-energy radiation from penetrating. The size and shape of a radioactive source depends on how it is to be used; it can be in the shape of a needle, seed, tube, or plaque, or it may be in solution.

ACTIVITY

Much of the early work with radioactivity and dose determination was carried out using radium. The very slow decay of radium makes it an excellent standard from which to determine the radioactivity of artificially produced isotopes.

The activity of an isotope is defined as the *number of disintegrations per time unit,* such as seconds, minutes, or hours. Because it is such an important concept, a special SI* unit for activity, the becquerel (Bq), has been defined. One becquerel equals one

* Système Internationale (International System).

disintegration per second. Another unit of activity, which has been used for many years, is the curie (Ci). Early experiments with radium indicated that 1 g of radium underwent 3.7×10^{10} disintegration per second, and this disintegration rate (or activity) was later chosen as the unit for the activity of all nuclides. A sample decaying at this rate of 3.7×10^{10} disintegration per second was said to have an activity defined as 1 Ci. Thus, a 1 g of radium has an activity of 1 Ci, and 1 mg of radium has an activity of 1/1000th curie, or 1 mCi. The becquerel and the curie are both named after famous physicists who did much of the early work on radiactivity and radium (Chap. 1).

DECAY

Radium decays to form daughter substances that are themselves unstable. Decay of successive daughters eventually results in a stable substance that does not decay any further. The rate at which this decay occurs is characteristic of the internal nuclear structures of the various daughters. The time required for a radioactive isotope to lose half of its original activity is the half-life, or $T_{1/2}$. The rate of decay of radium is very slow, and the half-life is about 1600 years. The half-lives of some of the radioactive isotopes frequently used in radiation oncology are listed in Table 15.1. Isotopes decay with half-lives ranging

Table 15.1 Physical Characteristics of Some Isotopes Used in Radiation Oncology

Isotope	Exposure Rate Constant, R/h/mCi at 1 cm	Half-Life	Energy of Gamma Ray, MeV	Half-Value Thickness, cmPb
Radium 226	8.25	1600 years	Avg. 1.2	1.3
Cesium 137	3.1	30 years	0.66	0.65
Cobalt 60	12.9	5.26 years	1.2	1.2
Strontium 90	—	28 years	Beta emitter	—
Iridium 192	4.61	74.3 days	Avg. 0.380	0.3
Gold 198	2.34	2.7 days	0.412–1.09	0.33
Iodine 125	1.66	59.6 days	0.035	0.003
Iodine 131	2.3	8 days	Many	0.31
Phosphorus 32	—	14.3 days	Beta emitter	—

from microseconds to millions of years. When the half-life and the present activity are known, it is possible to calculate the activity of a given isotopic sample at any future or past time.

Figure 15.1 shows the decay of a number of commonly used isotopes in radiation oncology. A straight line is drawn on semilogarithmic paper from the point, on day 0, when the activity is 100 percent, through a point one half-life later, when the activity is 50 percent, or half of its original value. Intermediate values can then easily be determined. Similar graphs are useful in a clinic where many isotopes are used and where it is frequently necessary to find the current activity of a given isotope quickly.

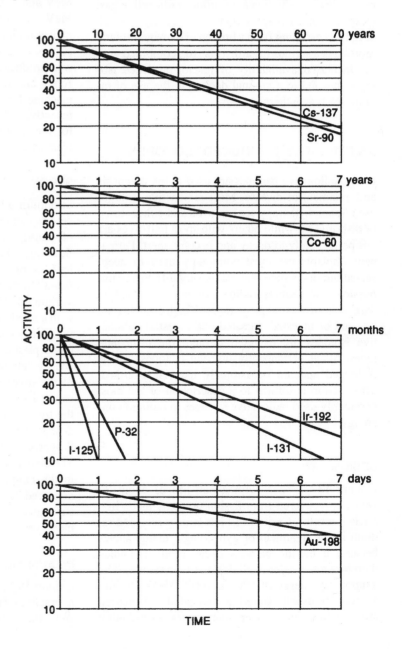

Figure 15.1 Decay of some commonly used isotopes plotted on semilogarithmic paper.

RADIUM

Radium 226, the earliest and once the most commonly used isotope in brachytherapy, has largely been replaced by artificially produced isotopes. This change is in part due to the hazards associated with radium. Radium disintegrates very slowly to form radon (^{222}Rn), which is a hazardous radioactive gas. Despite double encapsulation of the activity, the risk of radium escaping from a broken or damaged source represents a serious hazard. This risk, combined with the increased availability of reactor-produced isotopes, has led to a gradual decline in the use of radium for brachytherapy.

ARTIFICIALLY PRODUCED ISOTOPES

Many radioactive isotopes are used in the diagnosis and treatment of disease. Most radioactive isotopes used in brachytherapy are removed and either stored or disposed of, while others with short half-lives are left permanently to decay and become inert. Permanent implants are most commonly used in deep-seated tumors, where removal is very difficult or impossible. Sometimes radioactive isotopes used in diagnosis or treatment of thyroid malignancies are injected or ingested. Injected and ingested radioactive isotopes are excreted through the urine and feces. Some permanently inserted isotopes can be dislodged and are occasionally likewise excreted. This section is limited to a description of the most commonly used radioactive isotopes in radiation oncology.

CESIUM 137

Cesium 137 (^{137}Cs), with a half-life of about 30 years, is recovered from fission products made in a nuclear reactor. Cesium 137 has largely replaced radium in the treatment of gynecologic malignancies because it has no gaseous decay products and is therefore much safer in clinical use than radium. The gamma-ray energy of ^{137}Cs is 0.662 MeV. Cesium sources are usually stored in a shielded and secured area and are reused over many years. In radiation oncology, the most commonly used form of cesium is tubes.

COBALT 60

Cobalt 60 (^{60}Co) has a half-life of 5.26 years and in each disintegration produces two gamma-rays (1.17 MeV and 1.33 MeV) with an average energy of 1.2 MeV. The relatively high penetrating power of ^{60}Co makes it an excellent isotope for use in teletherapy (Chap. 2). The first source of ^{60}Co for medical use was produced in 1951 in Canada and was used by Johns and coworkers in the first ^{60}Co teletherapy machine for external beam therapy in 1952.[1] More recently, ^{60}Co has been used in ophthalmic plaques for the treatment of ocular melanomas. These eye plaques are stored and reused over several years.

STRONTIUM 90

Strontium 90 (^{90}Sr) became available in 1952 as a beta-ray applicator frequently used for the treatment of pterygium, a benign condition of the cornea. Strontium 90, a pure beta emitter, decays with a half-life of 28 years. The maximum beta-ray energy from ^{90}Sr is 0.54 MeV, while the daughter product, yttrium 90 (^{90}Y), produces a penetrating beta particle with a maximum energy of 2.27 MeV. The strontium 90, foil-bonded in silver, is covered with a polythene plastic of about 0.5-mm thickness. The low-energy beta particles from the strontium are stopped by the silver and are thus prevented from exiting the source itself. The beta particles from ^{90}Y are ideal for the treatment of superficial lesions of the eye. The dose falls very rapidly away from the applicator and is approximately 20 percent at 2-mm depth in tissue. The dose rate on the surface of such an applicator is in the range of 100 cGy/s; thus each treatment is delivered in seconds. Since the half-life is quite long, strontium 90 applicators are stored and used over many years.

IRIDIUM 192

Iridium 192 (^{192}Ir) is becoming increasingly popular in brachytherapy. Iridium has a half-life of 74.3 days and emits beta particles with a maximum energy of

0.670 MeV, which are largely eliminated by the stainless steel capsule, as well as 11 gamma rays with energies ranging from 0.136 to 0.613 MeV. The effective gammma energy is approximately 0.380 MeV and the half-value thickness (HVT) is approximately 3 mm lead (Pb). Iridium 192, a reactor-produced isotope, is usually manufactured in the shape of seeds approximately 3 mm long and 0.5 mm in diameter. Nylon ribbons containing iridium seeds can be purchased to specification as to seed spacing, ribbon length, and seed activity. The ribbons are placed inside hollow plastic tubing, which is first inserted into the tumor (Chap. 16). Following removal, seeds of iridium 192 are usually returned to the supplier and are not reused.

GOLD 198

Gold (^{198}Au) has a half-life of 64.7 h and emits primarily gamma rays, most of which have an energy of 0.412 MeV. In the form of seeds or grains, the material is suitable for permanent implants because of its relatively short half-life. After complete decay, the small inert masses cause no adverse effects and can remain in the tissues permanently. Gold seeds have largely replaced radon-222 seeds for permanent implantation. Because gold emits only three gamma rays (maximum energy is 0.412 MeV), in contrast to the complex penetrating spectrum of radium, protection problems are much more easily solved and exposure to personnel is minimal. Another advantage of gold over radon is that, although the major gamma activity of both isotopes disappears after about 1 month, some minor gamma activity from radon daughters persists for many years.

IODINE 125

Iodine 125 (^{125}I), which is also available in seed form (commonly 4.5 mm long and 0.8 mm in diameter), is used in permanent implants but can also be used in removable implants. Iodine 125 has a half-life of 59.6 days and, in addition to some very nonpenetrating radiations that are absorbed by the 0.05-mm titanium wall of the seed, emits 0.274- and 0.355-MeV photons. Some ^{125}I seeds are made with two to five resin spheres containing absorbed ^{125}I and an x-ray marker. The titanium end welds, sometimes seen on radiographs, will cause an asymmetrical dose distribution around the seed. This anisotropy should be taken into account in the dose calculation.[2-6] Another type of ^{125}I seed is made with a silver rod, serving both as an x-ray marker and as a carrier for the isotope (Fig. 15.2). The distribution of the activity within this type of seed may be sufficiently nonuniform to cause significant dose variations along the seed. A newly designed ^{125}I seed model contains radioactive iodine absorbed on a tungsten wire that is encapsulated by double walls of titanium. This model is easier to observe on radiographic implant documentation because the radiographic marker consists of tungsten. The dose distribution produced by this seed is more isotropic than from the seeds just described, because the iodine is distributed both on the circular surface around the seed and also on the ends of the wire.[7]

PHOSPHORUS 32 AND IODINE 131

Phosphorus 32 (^{32}P) and iodine 131 (^{131}I) are other artificially produced isotopes used for therapeutic purposes. Phosphorus 32 decays by beta-minus

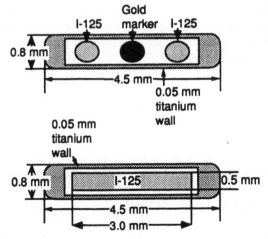

Figure 15.2 Two types of ^{125}I seeds; two resin spheres with ^{125}I and a gold x-ray marker in the center *(upper);* a silver rod with ^{125}I *(lower).*

emission with a maximum energy of 1.71 MeV and a half-life of 14.3 days.

Iodine 131, which has a half-life of 8 days, decays by beta and gamma emission. The maximum gamma energy is 0.723 MeV. Caution must be used due to the undesired gamma radiation from ^{131}I.

THE EXPOSURE RATE CONSTANT

The rate at which radiation arrives at a point near a radioactive source is related to the activity and to the energy and number of photons emitted in each decay. A quantity called the *exposure rate constant* and designated as Γ is used for this purpose. The exposure rate constant is defined as the *exposure rate in R/h at a point 1 cm from a 1-mCi point source.* Since the exposure rate at 1 cm from a 1-mg point source of radium 226 filtered by 0.5 mm of platinum (Pt) is 8.25 R/h, we can say that the exposure rate constant for radium is 8.25. This important value has been obtained experimentally rather than by calculation and forms the basis for all radium dosimetry. The source strength for radium is specified in terms of milligrams rather than millicuries.

From the inverse square law it is possible to calculate the exposure (X) at any distance (r), and by multiplying the exposure rate by the activity (A) in number of millicuries, it is possible to calculate the exposure rate at any distance and for any number of millicuries. By multiplying the exposure rate by the number of hours (t), the exposure for any length of time can also be found:

$$X = \frac{\Gamma \times A}{(r)^2} \times t \qquad (15.1)$$

The following example will illustrate calculation of the exposure at 70 cm from a 10-mg radium source filtered by 0.5 mmPt left unshielded for 8 h:

$$\frac{8.25 \text{ R cm}^2 \text{ h}}{\text{h mCi}} \times \frac{10 \text{ mCi}}{(70 \text{ cm})^2} \times 8 \text{ h} = 0.135 \text{ R}$$

A roentgen-to-centigray in tissue factor (f_{tis}) must be applied to convert exposure in air to absorbed dose in muscle. The recommended value is 0.963 f_{tis}.[8] All tables in this chapter have been converted to centigray.

The exposure rate at 1 cm away from a 1-mCi point source is called the *exposure rate constant* for that source material. The values for some commonly used sources in radiation oncology are given in Table 15.1. If we know the constant and the number of millicuries of the isotope in question, we can easily calculate the exposure at any distance, bearing in mind that the rate falls off as the inverse square of the distance. Thus, at 3 cm from a 1.5-mCi ^{192}Ir seed, the exposure rate is

$$\frac{1.5 \times 4.61}{(3)^2} = 0.7683 \text{ R/h}$$

It is often convenient to express the activity of other isotopes in terms of milligram radium equivalent (mg Ra eq). When the activity of another isotope is expressed in these terms, we mean that it produces the same exposure rate at a specified distance as a radium source of a specified activity. A ^{137}Cs source containing 1 mg Ra eq thus delivers the same dose rate at the treatment distance as 1 mg of ^{226}Ra filtered by 0.5 mmPt.

The exposure rate constant for ^{192}Ir, from Table 15.1, is 4.61. If we wanted to deliver 8.25 R/h at 1 cm (the same as 1 mCi of ^{226}Ra), it would be necessary to use

$$\frac{8.25}{4.61} = 1.79 \text{ mCi } ^{192}\text{Ir}$$

Thus, 1 mg Ra eq of ^{192}Ir contains 1.79 mCi of iridium.

In the rare event that we would need to find the number of milligrams of ^{226}Ra needed to deliver the same dose as 1 mCi of another isotope, the equation is inverted. To deliver 4.61 R/h (the exposure rate of 1 mCi of ^{192}Ir), the amount of ^{226}Ra is as follows:

$$\frac{4.61}{8.25} = 0.56 \text{ mg Ra}$$

One mCi of ^{192}Ir is thus equivalent to 0.56 mg of radium.

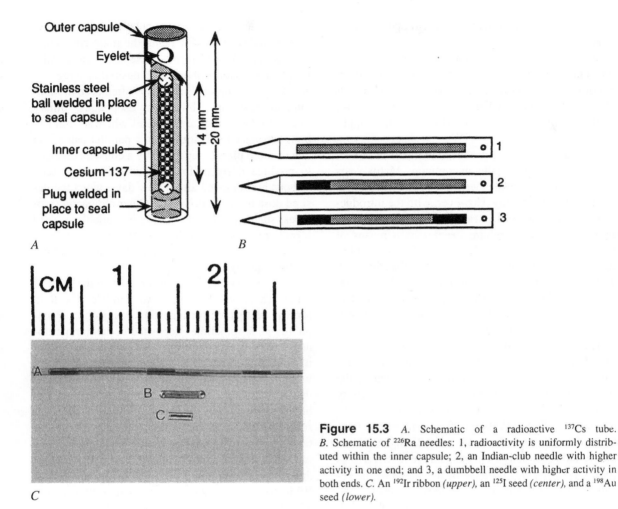

Figure 15.3 *A.* Schematic of a radioactive ^{137}Cs tube. *B.* Schematic of ^{226}Ra needles: 1, radioactivity is uniformly distributed within the inner capsule; 2, an Indian-club needle with higher activity in one end; and 3, a dumbbell needle with higher activity in both ends. *C.* An ^{192}Ir ribbon *(upper),* an ^{125}I seed *(center),* and a ^{198}Au seed *(lower).*

SPECIFICATION OF SOURCES

Radioactive sources are specified by their physical length, active length, activity or strength, and filtration. The active length is obviously always smaller than the physical length because of the encapsulating material that surrounds the radioactivity. The walls of each source consist of a platinum alloy and, in some sources, also of ordinary iridium (nonradioactive), which strengthens the walls. A 0.5-mm thick sheath of platinum surrounding the radium is sufficient to filter out all alpha and most beta particles emitted by the radium and its daughter products. Only the gamma rays (average energy 1.2 MeV)

escape. The encapsulating material also prevents escape of radioactive material into body tissues and fluids.

THE PHYSICAL FORM OF BRACHYTHERAPY SOURCES

Cesium 137 is most commonly available in the form of tubes that are 20 mm long and 3 mm in diameter, with an eyelet near one end to allow suturing the tube in tissues or to some apparatus (Fig. 15.3A). The active length of these tubes is usually about 14 mm and the activity of each tube usually ranges from 5 to

25 mg Ra eq. Other radioactive isotopes such as ^{226}Ra and ^{60}Co are also occasionally found in the form of tubes. The outer dimensions of these tubes are standardized to allow insertion into standard applicators used in intracavitary gynecologic implants (Chap. 16). Some smaller "microsources" are also available for specially designed intracavitary applicators.

Radioactive isotopes produced in the form of needles are becoming quite uncommon. Many years ago, radium-226 needles were the only means of interstitial brachytherapy. However, with the introduction of safer and less hazardous afterloading techniques, the use of radium needles as a means of interstitial treatment has fallen out of favor. Radioactive needles are usually longer than tubes, but with a smaller diameter and a sharp point to allow easier insertion (Fig. 15.3B). They also have an eyelet to allow suturing the needle to the tissue to prevent it from moving or falling out.

The activity of radium sources is always specified in milligrams of radium. This activity is usually uniformly distributed within the active segment of the tube or needle. Needles with uniform linear activity may be "full-strength" or "half-strength." A full-strength needle has 0.66 mg of radium per centimeter, and a half-strength needle has 0.33 mg/cm. Needles with higher activity in one end are referred to as *Indian club needles* because of the shape of the resulting dose distribution. A needle with higher activity in both ends is similarly referred to as a *dumbbell needle* (Fig. 15.3B). The significance of the differential in activity is explained in the Paterson-Parker dosage system.

The radioactive material in tubes and needles is usually double-encapsulated to minimize the risks of developing a leak. Leakage can also result if a tube or needle becomes bent during use. Prior to each use, each source should be tested for leaks by wiping a wad of cotton or gauze around the source and then, with a sensitive detector, testing if there is any activity on the cotton or gauze. If a leaking source is detected, it must not be used but should be returned to the supplier for repair.

Radioactive sources in the form of seeds (Fig. 15.3C) are one of the most popular forms of brachytherapy today, with ^{192}Ir being the most commonly used isotope in seed form. These seeds are usually supplied in nylon ribbons with desired spacing and activity. A ribbon of ^{192}Ir seeds is often used in intraluminal insertions (bronchus, esophagus, biliary tree, etc.). Other uses are implants where several ribbons are placed interstitially in a parallel pattern on one or more planes, separated by a constant distance to produce fairly uniform dose. Iridium-192 seed ribbons are removed after a few days, when the desired dose has been delivered. Other radioactive isotopes, such as ^{125}I and ^{198}Au, are available in seed form but not usually in ribbons. These isotopes have a shorter half-life and are often left in place permanently to decay.

Some radioactive isotopes are used in the form of fluids. These are ^{131}I, ^{32}P, ^{198}Au, and ^{90}Y. The fluid form is best suited for ingestion or injection. Phosphorus 32 is sometimes deposited in the intraperitoneal cavity in an attempt to treat peritoneal seeding in ovarian or endometrial carcinoma when peritoneal washings are positive for tumor cells. The effect of this is uncertain, since gravitational effects are believed to cause increased concentration in the lower segments of the cavity, which change with the patient's position. The risk of late bowel complications is increased if the addition of external beam radiation therapy is also required. The use of intraperitoneal ^{32}P is, for these reasons, on the decline. Phosphorus 32 is also sometimes deposited in the pleural space in patients with malignant pleural effusion in an effort to treat microscopic disease. Radioactive substances deposited in the intraperitoneal or intrapleural space cannot be removed; therefore isotopes with short half-lives must be used.

Injection of ^{90}Y[9,10] and ^{32}P[11] into cystic craniopharyngiomas has been tried, primarily in Europe and Japan. Strontium 90 in saline solution has also been tried in the treatment of extensive bone metastasis. Iodine 131 in doses of ≥ 100 mCi given orally is sometimes used in the treatment of thyroid malignancies, while lower doses (1 to 3 mCi) are used for diagnostic purposes. Many other radionuclides are used in fluid form for diagnostic purposes.

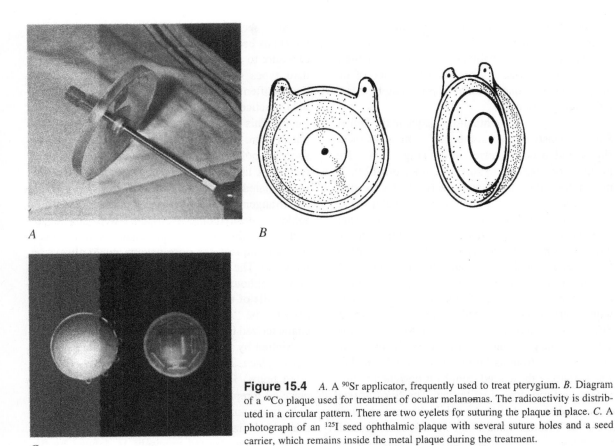

A

B

C

Figure 15.4 *A.* A ^{90}Sr applicator, frequently used to treat pterygium. *B.* Diagram of a ^{60}Co plaque used for treatment of ocular melanomas. The radioactivity is distributed in a circular pattern. There are two eyelets for suturing the plaque in place. *C.* A photograph of an ^{125}I seed ophthalmic plaque with several suture holes and a seed carrier, which remains inside the metal plaque during the treatment.

Many radionuclides are used in an experimental treatment modality called biologically targeted radiotherapy (BTR). This is a method in which the radiation is delivered to the tumor by tumor-seeking molecules such as monoclonal antibodies.

Radioactive isotopes in the form of ophthalmic applicators have been used for many years. An applicator using a ^{90}Sr source is often used in the treatment of pterygium, a benign condition of the conjunctiva. The daughter product, ^{90}Y, produces beta particles used in these treatments. The applicator has a circular shape with a concave surface, which fits directly on the surface of the cornea. The dose rate on the surface is about 100 cGy/s. The penetration of the beta particles is poor, making this a suitable treatment for very shallow lesions. The depth dose percentage at 1 mm is only about 50 percent of the surface dose; at 4 mm, it is only 5 percent. A ^{90}Sr ophthalmic applicator is shown in Fig. 15.4.

Other applicators in the form of plaques are used for the treatment of ocular melanomas (Fig. 15.4). The plaques are usually circular and have a concave surface to provide a snug fit over the curved surface of the eye. Several eyelets are provided for suturing the plaques onto the sclera, where they are usually left in place several days. Cobalt 60 plaques with diameters of 10 to 15 mm are available commercially, but other isotopes with shorter half-lives and less penetration such as ^{125}I or ^{192}Ir can be used in customized plaques. In ^{60}Co plaques, the radioactivity, which is not removable, is distributed in a circular pattern over the inner (concave) surface of the plaque. Each plaque contains approximately 2 to 3 mCi (not mg Ra eq).

The most popular ophthalmic plaque in the United States consists of two components: an outer metal shield and a seed carrier insert (Fig. 15.4). The plaques are available in sizes varying from 12 to 20 mm in diameter. The plaque size is selected to cover the tumor with a 2- to 3-mm margin. A metal shield, which consists of a gold alloy, is a spherical shell segment with a ''lip'' that is at right angles to the back of the plaque. The height of the lip depends on the thickness of the insert and the diameter of the plaque; it is designed to bring the lip to the outer scleral surface. Attached to the lip are several tabs with suture holes. The seed carrier insert, made of Silastic, is designed to fit snugly into the concave surface of the gold shield. Molded into the outer surface are seed ''troughs'' into which ^{125}I seeds will fit. The pattern of these seed troughs is designed to provide a uniform dose distribution. The Silastic seed carrier is discarded after use, while the gold plaque is reusable. These plaques hold 13 to 24 seeds, depending on the size, and the seed activity is usually about 1 to 3 mCi/seed but varies with prescription point, dose, and plaque size. The plaques usually remain in place for 4 to 6 days, delivering about 10,000 cGy at the apex of the tumor.

DOSE CALCULATION

Dose determination from radium, made by the pioneers in the early 1900s, is fundamental to all dose calculations in brachytherapy and can be applied to artificially produced isotopes. In dose calculations from radioactive implants, it is necessary to know the number of milligrams or millicuries in the implant and also the location of each source with respect to the dose calculation point. It is also necessary to know which isotope is being used, the filtration of the encapsulation, and the distribution of the activity within the capsule (seed, tube, etc.). In previous sections, the exposure rate (roentgens per hour) has been described, as well as how to convert exposure to absorbed dose. However, in many standard types of implants, such as the tandem and ovoids often used in gynecologic implants, it is common practice to express the dose in milligram hours (mgh). This practice stems from an era when computers were not available to calculate the dose to specified points. During the early years of the use of radium, a large volume of clinical experience was accumulated. From this experience, rules regarding the arrangement of the sources and their strength to achieve a desired clinical response were developed. If the rules for the source placement were followed for each implant, the dose pattern would always be the same. The dose distribution was not necessarily known, although it could be calculated provided that the details of the source strength and position were known. The ''dose'' delivered in such implants was characterized by the product of milligrams of radium multiplied by the number of hours the implant was left in place. This quantity was expressed in milligram hours. For example, a 20-mg source left in place 48 h represents 960 mgh.

In many implants, the patient's anatomy or the shape and size of the tumor may not permit the sources to be inserted precisely as defined by the rules. The difficulty with expressing a treatment in terms of milligram hours in such situations is the uncertainty of the dose distribution. For example, a 10-mg-Ra-eq source left in place for 1 h (10 mgh) delivers 79.5 cGy ($10 \times 8.25 \times 0.963$) at 1 cm from the source. However, 10 mg Ra eq in four sources arranged in a linear fashion and left in place for 1 h also represents 10 mgh, but the dose at 1 cm from the center of each source (19.86 cGy) cannot be added because this dose is delivered at four different points. The combined dose at 1 cm from either source is therefore less than 79.5 cGy. In most implants, several sources are used, and they are often arranged to produce a dose distribution that conforms to the target. It is therefore very unlikely that the sources are arranged so that all of them are at the same distance from a common dose calculation point. Ovoids of various diameters with a central canal for the source are often used in gynecologic implants. Here, the

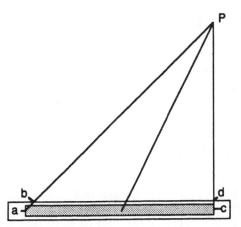

Figure 15.5 Illustration of the geometric relationships used in calculating the exposure at point P, from a linear source.

dose rate on the ovoid surface will vary depending on the diameter of the ovoid if the milligram hours remain unchanged. In this situation, the milligram hours must be increased in order to maintain the same dose rate on the ovoid surface (mucosa) as the ovoid diameter increases. The use of milligram hours to prescribe a treatment has given way in recent years as computers, capable of calculating the dose distribution around any implant, have been developed.

SIEVERT INTEGRAL

As shown in previous sections, the exposure rate applies only to point sources, while in most of brachytherapy, linear sources are used. Some smaller linear sources may be considered as point sources when the dose is calculated at long distances; however, in brachytherapy, the dose is commonly calculated at short distances. For example, in calculating dose from a ^{137}Cs tube in a tandem, the dose is often calculated at only 2 cm from the source. In this situation, a very complex calculation process must be carried out in which the contribution of dose from small segments of the activity and the variation of filtration that the radiation passes through at various angles is considered. This calculation process, too complicated to do by hand, is called the Sievert integral.[8,12,13]

The dose from a linear source can be found by considering the source to be divided into many small segments and applying an inverse square law calculation and a filtration correction factor to each segment. Adding together or "integrating" the doses contributed at the calculation point by each segment gives the dose rate from the entire source. Figure 15.5, for example, illustrates that the distance from segment a to the dose calculation point (P) is longer than from segment c to P. Furthermore, the thickness of filtration which the radiation from segment a traverses (a to b) is greater than that which the radiation from segment c traverses (c to d). The dose contributed at P by segment a is thus lower than that contributed by segment c because of the longer distance and also because of the increased attenuation by the greater thickness of filtration through which it travels. When a very large number of segments are considered, the mathematical expression used to add all of the segment doses together is called the *Sievert integral.*

Dose rates are similarly calculated around a source, and, by joining points of equal dose, dose-rate distributions are displayed. These calculations are very tedious to do by hand, but computer methods are routinely applied in clinical brachytherapy.

Figure 15.6 illustrates a computer-calculated dose-rate distribution around a 13.3-mg-radium source. The dose rate along the axis of the tube is lower than it is at right angles to the tube because of the increased effect of oblique filtration. Maximum oblique filtration occurs at the corners of the tube, while along the exact axis of the source, part of the attenuating encapsulation is replaced by the less attenuating radioactive material itself. As a result, there is a small cone of more intense radiation at the axis of the source.

For linear sources, the dose rate is lower than that calculated by the inverse square law, particularly at points close to the source. This is expected, since the photons traveling from the extremes of the source have a longer distance and also must traverse oblique filtration. As the distance from the source increases, the effect diminishes and the dose rates approach that of point sources (Fig. 15.7).

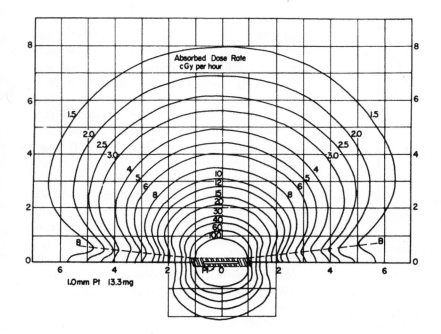

Figure 15.6   Dose-rate distribution around a 13.3-mg-radium tube filtered by 1.0-mm platinum. Note the small cone of more intense dose at 0 cm away from the source, that is, at the axis of the source. (From Johns HE, Cunningham JR: *The Physics of Radiology,* 4th ed., 1983. Courtesy of Charles C Thomas, Publisher, Springfield, Illinois.)

DOSAGE SYSTEMS

Several systems of dosimetric planning for brachytherapy have been devised over the past 50 years. The Paris system,[14-16] the Paterson-Parker, or Manchester, system,[17,18] and the Quimby system[19,20] are the most widely used. The three systems differ in the rules of implantation, definition of dose uniformity, and method used in reference-dose specification.[21] While the Paterson-Parker system was designed to distribute the radium in a nonuniform fashion to achieve a reasonably uniform dose distribution, the Paris and Quimby systems were designed to distribute the radium itself in a uniform fashion that provides a nonuniform dose distribution with substantially higher dose in the center than in the periphery. Figure 15.8 shows a comparison of dose-rate distributions from typical Manchester and Quimby systems.

Both the Manchester and Quimby systems provide tables giving the milligram hours necessary to deliver 1000 cGy for implants of various sizes and shapes. The original tables have been converted from roentgens to centigrays but have not been corrected for the attenuation and scattering of radiation in the surrounding tissue, which are assumed to compen-

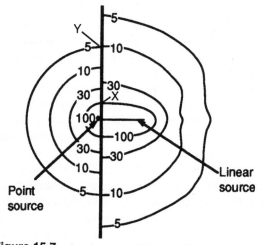

Figure 15.7   A point source *(left)* and a linear source *(right)* delivering the same dose (100 cGy/h) at a given distance from the source (X). However, at a longer distance, the linear source delivers a higher dose (Y). The inverse square law does not apply to linear sources.

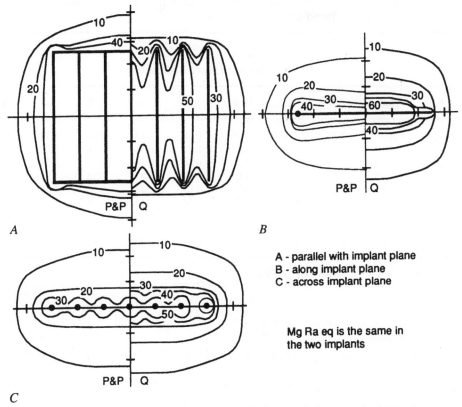

A - parallel with implant plane
B - along implant plane
C - across implant plane

Mg Ra eq is the same in
the two implants

Figure 15.8   Comparison of a Paterson-Parker-type and a Quimby-type implant. Only half of each implant *(Paterson-Parker, left, and Quimby, right)* is shown side by side.

Table 15.2   Centigrays per Milligram Hour Delivered to Locations *along* and *away* by Linear Radium Source (1.5-cm Active Length) Filtered by 0.5 mmPt (Ir)[a]

Distance away from Source, cm	Distance *along* Source, cm										
	0	0.5	1.0	1.5	2.0	2.5	3.0	3.5	4.0	4.5	5.0
0.5	20.4	16.9	8.06	3.25	1.62	0.90	0.56	0.37	0.24	0.15	0.10
0.75	10.9	9.30	5.64	2.92	1.62	0.99	0.66	0.44	0.32	0.24	0.17
1.0	6.69	5.95	4.11	2.48	1.54	0.99	0.68	0.48	0.35	0.26	0.21
1.5	3.27	3.03	2.41	1.75	1.23	0.88	0.64	0.48	0.36	0.29	0.23
2.0	1.89	1.79	1.56	1.25	0.97	0.74	0.57	0.45	0.36	0.28	0.23
2.5	1.23	1.18	1.07	0.92	0.75	0.62	0.50	0.40	0.33	0.27	0.23
3.0	0.86	0.84	0.77	0.70	0.60	0.51	0.42	0.36	0.29	0.25	0.22
4.0	0.49	0.48	0.46	0.43	0.39	0.35	0.31	0.28	0.24	0.21	0.19
5.0	0.31	0.31	0.30	0.29	0.27	0.25	0.22	0.21	0.19	0.17	0.15

[a] Modified from data of Greenfield et al.[23] With permission from RSNA.
Source: Reproduced with permission from Hendee WR: *Radiation Therapy Physics.* Chicago: Year Book Medical Publishers, Inc., 1981.[22]

Table 15.3   Centigrays per Milligram Hour Delivered to Locations *along* and *away* by Linear Radium Source (1.5-cm Active Length) Filtered by 1.0 mm Pt (Ir)[a]

Distance away from Source, cm	Distance *along* Source, cm										
	0	0.5	1.0	1.5	2.0	2.5	3.0	3.5	4.0	4.5	5.0
0.5	18.0	14.9	7.28	2.49	1.10	0.58	0.32	0.20	0.11	0.08	0.05
0.75	9.68	8.24	4.86	2.41	1.24	0.70	0.43	0.28	0.21	0.13	0.09
1.0	6.02	5.28	3.56	2.11	1.24	0.76	0.50	0.33	0.24	0.17	0.13
1.5	2.93	2.69	2.12	1.54	1.03	0.74	0.52	0.38	0.28	0.21	0.16
2.0	1.70	1.61	1.38	1.09	0.84	0.64	0.48	0.38	0.28	0.23	0.17
2.5	1.11	1.06	0.95	0.81	0.67	0.54	0.43	0.34	0.27	0.23	0.18
3.0	0.77	0.75	0.70	0.62	0.53	0.44	0.37	0.31	0.25	0.22	0.18
4.0	0.44	0.43	0.41	0.39	0.35	0.31	0.27	0.24	0.21	0.18	0.16
5.0	0.28	0.28	0.27	0.26	0.24	0.23	0.20	0.19	0.17	0.15	0.13

[a] Modified from data of Greenfield et al.[23] With permission from RSNA.
Source: Reproduced with permission from Hendee WR: *Radiation Therapy Physics.* Chicago: Year Book Medical Publishers, Inc., 1981.[22]

sate for each other. This approximation is valid to within a few percentage points.

The Quimby System.   Quimby calculated and tabulated dose distributions for linear radium sources with different active lengths and wall thicknesses. The tabulated data give the centigrays per hour at locations "along" as well as "away" from the axis of a 1-mg-radium source. Tables 15.2 and 15.3[22] take account of the f factor (roentgen-to-centigray conversion factor) and the oblique filtration through the radium salt and the source capsule.[23]

The example below illustrates the calculation of dose at a point using Quimby's tables for linear sources in a typical gynecologic implant consisting of a tandem containing three sources and a pair of ovoids, each containing one source (Fig. 15.9).

Calculating the dose at X from sources A, B, C, D, and E using Table 15.2:

Source A (2 cm away, 3 cm along):

$$0.57 \text{ cGy/mgh} \times 15 \text{ mg} = 8.55 \text{ cGy/h}$$

Source B (2 cm away, 1 cm along):

$$1.56 \text{ cGy/mgh} \times 10 \text{ mg} = 15.6 \text{ cGy/h}$$

Source C (2 cm away, 1 cm along):

$$1.56 \text{ cGy/mgh} \times 10 \text{ mg} = 15.6 \text{ cGy/h}$$

Source D (4.5 cm away, 0 cm along):

$$.4 \text{ cGy/mgh} \times 15 \text{ mg} = 6.0 \text{ cGy/h}$$

Source E (2 cm away, 0 cm along):

$$1.89 \text{ cGy/mgh} \times 15 \text{ mg} = 28.35 \text{ cGy/h}$$

Total dose in cGy/h at X = 74.1.

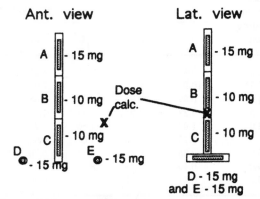

Figure 15.9   Diagram illustrating point calculation from linear sources.

Table 15.4 Milligram Hours Required for Absorbed Dose of 1000 cGy at Locations along a Line Perpendicular to Center of Applicator or Implant Plane[a,b]

Distance, cm	Circular Applicators (Diameter in Centimeters)					
	1	2	3	4	5	6
0.5	47	80	110	181	234	319
1.0	145	187	234	319	394	482
1.5	301	345	426	506	598	725
2.0	528	577	646	745	846	977
2.5	782	846	920	1016	1229	1346
3.0	1160	1224	1298	1404	1522	1665

Distance, cm	Square Applicators (Length of Side in Centimeters)					
	1	2	3	4	5	6
0.5	49	85	122	210	266	372
1.0	150	200	253	348	431	544
1.5	314	367	442	544	638	782
2.0	532	606	686	795	910	1064
2.5	777	846	952	1075	1213	1458
3.0	1160	1224	1351	1479	1617	1777

Distance, cm	Rectangular Applicators (Length of Side in Centimeters)					
	1 × 1.5	2 × 3	3 × 4	4 × 6	6 × 9	8 × 12
0.5	54	110	152	305	606	1016
1.0	157	228	291	453	772	1181
1.5	317	394	496	664	1005	1442
2.0	538	628	761	930	1319	1777
2.5	767	894	1053	1213	1617	2128
3.0	1181	1266	1420	1617	2054	2660

[a] The radium sources are distributed uniformly across the plane and filtered by 0.5 mmPt (Ir).
[b] Modified from data of Quimby.[24] With permission from RSNA.
Source: Reproduced with permission from Hendee WR: *Radiation Therapy Physics.* Chicago: Year Book Medical Publishers, Inc., 1981.[22]

Quimby's system of uniform distribution of radioactivity within one- or multiple-plane implants give a nonuniform dose distribution within the implanted volume. The center of the volume receives substantially higher dose than the periphery (Fig. 15.8).

The following example of dose calculation illustrates the use of Quimby's tables giving the milligram hours necessary to deliver 1000 cGy at differ-

ent distances from a surface applicator. Using Quimby's approach, a surface mold is to be constructed to treat a 4 × 6 cm lesion. A dose of 3000 cGy is to be delivered in 48 h at the center of the lesion, which is 1 cm below the plane of the radium sources (filtration 0.5 mmPt [Ir]).

Here we use Table 15.4, modified from Quimby's data,[24] providing the product of the amount of radium and exposure time in hours, that is, the milligram hours required to deliver 1000 cGy at various distances along a line perpendicular to the center of the implant plane. From Table 15.4, 453 mgh are required for 1000 cGy. The number of milligram hours required for 3000 cGy is

$$\frac{453 \text{ mgh} \times 3000 \text{ cGy}}{1000 \text{ cGy}} = 1359 \text{ mgh}$$

To deliver the treatment in 48 h, the required milligrams of radium is

$$\frac{1359 \text{ mgh}}{48 \text{ h}} = 28.3 \text{ mg}$$

The radioactivity must be uniformly distributed over the mold.

In small surface applicators, the radioactive sources must be placed closer to the tumor than in larger applicators (Fig. 15.10). In Fig. 15.10A, the source is placed 0.5 cm from the surface and the dose rate is 40 cGy/h at 0.5 cm depth in tissue. In Fig. 15.10B, six sources are placed 1.0 cm from the surface. The dose rate at 0.5-cm depth in tissue is also 40 cGy/h; however, the surface dose is approximately 63 cGy/h in *(B)* and 100 cGy/h in *(A)*. (See

inverse square law for point sources versus linear sources, Fig. 15.7.)

If all dimensions (length, width, and height) of an implant are approximately the same, tables for volume implants must be used. As an example, a cylindrical volume 3 cm in diameter and 4 cm long is implanted and 3000 cGy is desired in 72 h. (See the Manchester system for a similar case.)

Here we use Table 15.5, which is modified from Quimby's data,[24] providing the milligram hours required to deliver 1000 cGy in a volume implant designed according to the Quimby system. We find that for a volume of 28 cm³, 554 mgh (interpolated value) is required to deliver 1000 cGy.

The number of milligram hours required to deliver 3000 cGy is

$$\frac{554 \text{ mgh} \times 3000 \text{ cGy}}{1000 \text{ cGy}} = 1662 \text{ mgh}$$

To obtain 1662 mgh in 72 h, we need

$$\frac{1662 \text{ mgh}}{72 \text{ h}} = 23 \text{ mg Ra}$$

Caution must be used when tables of dose rates or

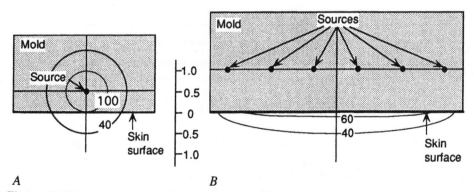

A   *B*

Figure 15.10 A very small surface mold *(A)* with a radioactive source embedded 0.5 cm above the surface delivers 40 cGy/h at 0.5-cm depth in tissue. A larger surface mold *(B)* with several radioactive sources embedded 1.0 cm above the surface also delivers 40 cGy/h at 0.5-cm depth in tissue. The maximum tissue dose in *A* is 100 cGy, while in *B* it is 63 cGy/h; there is a considerable improvement in %DD in *B*.

Table 15.5 Milligram Hours Required for Minimum Absorbed Dose of 1000 cGy in Volume Implant[a]

Volume, cm³	Mgh for 1000 cGy	Diameter of Sphere	Mgh for 1000 cGy
5	213	1.0	43
10	340	1.5	106
15	415	2.0	192
20	468	2.5	298
30	575	3.0	415
40	660	3.5	505
60	798	4.0	612
80	926	4.5	718
100	1064	5.0	841
125	1192	6.0	1138
150	1330	7.0	1490
175	1479		
200	1596		
250	1788		
300	1915		

[a] Modified from data of Quimby.[24] With permission from RSNA. The radium sources are distributed uniformly and filtered by 0.5 mmPt (Ir). *Source:* Reproduced with permission from Hendee WR: *Radiation Therapy Physics.* Chicago: Year Book, 1981, based on data from Goodwin et al.[24]

milligram hours are consulted. For example, using Quimby's tables with a Paterson-Parker system implant would be erroneous, and vice versa.

The Paterson-Parker System. The Paterson-Parker system was devised to deliver a reasonably uniform dose to a plane or volume. Elaborate rules for distribution of the radioactivity within the volume were developed along with tables, which give the milligram hours necessary to deliver 1000 cGy at various treatment distances from the implant. In Quimby's approach, the number of milligram hours required to deliver 1000 cGy is higher than in the Manchester system, because with Quimby's approach, the *minimum* dose is 1000 cGy, while in the Manchester system the absorbed dose is approximately 1000 cGy *throughout the volume.*

An exposure rate constant correction from 8.4 R/h at 1 cm from 1 mg of radium to the current value of 8.25 must be made when using older Paterson-Parker tables. A roentgen-to-cGy in tissue factor (f_{tis}) of 0.963 should be applied to convert exposure in air to absorbed dose in muscle.

The distribution rules for surface applicators and planar implants are as follows:

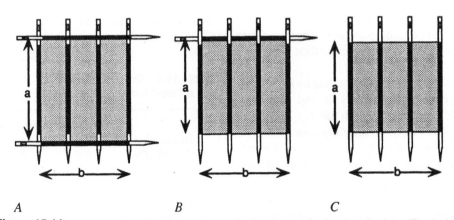

A   *B*   *C*

Figure 15.11 Diagrams of different arrangements of radioactive needles for planar implants. The shaded areas indicate the sizes of the areas used for calculating the dose. To calculate the number of cubic centimeters (cm³) of the treated slice of tissue, one would use a × b × 2 h, where h is the treatment distance in the third dimension and 2 h is the thickness of the slice of tissue treated. If the treatment distance (h) is 0.5 cm, the slice thickness (2 h) is 1 cm.

1. On a single plane, a fraction of the radium should be arranged uniformly around the periphery, while the remainder should be spread as evenly as possible over the area itself. The fraction of the radium used in the periphery should be as follows:

Area	< 25 cm²	25–100 cm²	> 100 cm²
Peripheral fraction	2/3	1/2	1/3

2. A common arrangement is a row of parallel needles with active ends crossed by means of needles at right angles to the first part of the implant (Fig. 15.11). In many anatomic situations, it is impossible to cross one or both ends of the implant. When only one end is crossed, the area that is treated should be considered as 90 percent of the length of the implant; when neither end is crossed the treated area should be considered as 80 percent—that is, for each uncrossed end, the treated area should be taken as 10 percent less than the nominal area. Use of Indian club needles, previously described, eliminates the need for a crossing needle at the end of uniformly implanted needles. Dumbbell needles, also previously described, have greater activity at both ends and do not require crossing needles at either end.

3. Needles arranged as such a series of parallel lines should not be more than 1 cm from each other or from the crossing ends. Similarly, when seeds are used, they should not be spaced more than 1 cm from each other.

4. In two-plane implants, the radium on each plane should be arranged as in rules 1, 2, and 3, and the planes should be parallel to each other.

5. If two planes differ in area, the area to be used for table-reading purposes is the average of the two, and the total amount of radium is prorated to each plane.

When the radium is distributed on two planes, the number of milligram hours found from the table has to be increased by a factor depending on the distance between the planes, except for planes separated by 1 cm. These factors are

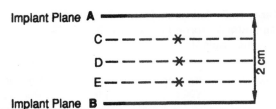

Figure 15.12   Two implant planes separated by 2 cm. The dose at X on plane D is the same from both implant planes, while the dose at X on planes C and E is higher. Point X on plane C receives a higher dose from implant plane A than from B.

Separation, cm	1.5	2.0	2.5
Factor	1.25	1.4	1.5

It must be recognized that with larger separation between the planes, the dose between the planes is decreased; thus the dose uniformity is inferior.

Special Cases. A single plane of needles or seeds can satisfactorily treat a slice of tissue 1.0 to 1.25 cm thick in which the radium plane is the center. When a thicker slice of tissue must be treated, two planes will be necessary. A two-plane implant can satisfactorily treat a block of tissue 2.5 cm thick. From Fig. 15.12 and Table 15.6, it is obvious that the dose between the planes is decreased if the separation of the planes is increased.

Table 15.6   Dose Calculation for a Two-Plane Implant

Distance, mgh/1000 cGy	Plane C, 0.5 cm, 618	Plane D, 1 cm, 967	Plane E, 1.5 cm, 1392
Dose for 600 mgh in plane A	971 cGy	620 cGy	431 cGy
Dose for 600 mgh in plane B	431 cGy	620 cGy	971 cGy
Dose for 1200 mgh in planes A and B	1402 cGy	1240 cGy	1402 cGy

Table 15.7 Surface Applicators and Planar Implants [a,b]

Area, cm²	Treatment Distance, cm									
	0.5	1.0	1.5	2.0	2.5	3.0	3.5	4.0	4.5	5.0
0	32	127	285	506	792	1139	1551	2026	2566	3166
1	72	182	343	571	856	1204	1625	2100	2636	3295
2	103	227	399	632	920	1274	1697	2172	2708	3349
3	128	263	448	689	978	1331	1760	2241	2772	3383
4	150	296	492	743	1032	1388	1823	2307	2835	3450
5	170	326	531	787	1083	1436	1881	2369	2896	3513
6	188	354	570	832	1134	1495	1938	2432	2956	3575
7	204	382	603	870	1182	1547	1993	2490	3011	3634
8	219	409	637	910	1229	1596	2047	2548	3067	3694
9	235	434	667	946	1272	1645	2099	2605	3123	3752
10	250	461	697	982	1314	1692	2149	2660	3178	3809
12	278	511	755	1053	1396	1780	2247	2769	3284	3917
14	306	557	813	1120	1475	1865	2341	2870	3389	4027
16	335	602	866	1184	1553	1947	2429	2968	3490	4131
18	364	644	918	1245	1622	2027	2514	3063	3585	4240
20	392	682	968	1303	1690	2106	2601	3155	3682	4341
22	418	717	1021	1362	1755	2180	2683	3242	3777	4441
24	444	752	1072	1420	1821	2252	2764	3326	3872	4540
26	470	784	1122	1477	1881	2328	2841	3405	3962	4634
28	496	816	1170	1530	1943	2398	2917	3484	4047	4730
30	521	846	1215	1582	2000	2468	2997	3562	4131	4824
32	546	876	1261	1635	2060	2532	3073	3639	4220	4915
34	571	909	1305	1688	2119	2598	3145	3713	4306	5000
36	594	935	1349	1743	2179	2662	3215	3787	4389	5089
38	618	967	1392	1793	2234	2726	3285	3859	4466	5174
40	642	994	1432	1843	2290	2787	3351	3931	4546	5258
42	664	1024	1472	1894	2344	2848	3421	4003	4626	5341
44	685	1053	1511	1942	2399	2908	3484	4071	4706	5422
46	708	1080	1550	1990	2452	2966	3548	4139	4781	5505
48	729	1110	1585	2037	2504	3025	3612	4207	4857	5586
50	750	1141	1619	2083	2556	3082	3676	4275	4929	5668
60	851	1283	1790	2319	2815	3362	3974	4605	5288	6054
70	947	1426	1944	2532	3059	3628	4257	4913	5632	6419
80	1044	1567	2092	2726	3301	3891	4532	5213	5958	6756

Filtration (mmPt)			0.3		0.5	0.6		0.8	1.0	1.5
Correction to mgh			−4%		0	+2%		+6%	+10%	+20%

[a] The table gives the R_A, the number of mgh required to deliver 1000 cGy to muscle tissue for different areas and treatment distances. Filtration 0.5 mmPt. The table may be used for planar implants by using a treatment distance of 0.5 cm.
[b] This table was prepared from the original by Meredith[25] by multiplying his values by C = 1.064. (From Johns HE, Cunningham JR: *The Physics of Radiology,* 4th ed., 1983. Courtesy of Charles C. Thomas, Publisher, Springfield, Illinois.)

In this example, the area of each plane is 38 cm² and the planes are separated by 2 cm. The dose is calculated using Table 15.7. The dose from implant plane A (600 mgh) along plane C (0.5 cm away) is 971 cGy. From Table 15.7, we find that 618 mgh delivers 1000 cGy at 0.5 cm distance, so 600 mgh delivers the following:

$$\frac{600 \text{ mgh} \times 1000 \text{ cGy}}{618 \text{ mgh}} = 971 \text{ cGy}$$

The dose on plane D will be the same from the two implant planes, that is, 620 cGy each. The dose on planes C and E will be the same, but C will receive a higher dose from implant plane A than from implant plane B because of the shorter distance. As the implant planes are separated farther, the dose on plane D will decrease.

Figure 15.13 shows three radioactive sources indicating the 10 cGy/h line from each source. The combined dose along lines B and C is the same, but it is higher than along lines A and D because they are closer to the center of the implant. The doses along lines E and G are the same, but they are lower than along line F, which crosses the implant at the center. The intersection of lines B and F, for example, lies within all three 10-cGy/h lines, while the intersection of lines A and E lies within only one 10-cGy/h

line. This illustrates the higher dose at the center of an implant when the activity is uniformly distributed.

Example 1. In this example, we will calculate the amount of radium required to deliver 3000 cGy in 48 h at 1 cm from the center of a 4 × 6 cm (24 cm²) planar implant. From Table 15.7, which gives the number of milligram hours required to deliver 1000 cGy at various distances from surface applicators and planar implants, 752 mgh are required for a uniform dose (± 10%) of 1000 cGy over the entire treated area. The original values of required milligram hours to deliver 1000 R given by Meredith[25] have been multiplied by 1.064 to describe the required number of milligram hours to deliver 1000 Gy in tissue rather than 1000 R in air.

The number of milligram hours required for 3000 cGy is

$$\frac{752 \text{ mgh} \times 3000 \text{ cGy}}{1000 \text{ cGy}} = 2256 \text{ mgh}$$

The number of milligrams of radium required is as follows:

$$\frac{2256 \text{ mgh}}{48 \text{ h}} = 47 \text{ mg}$$

Example 2. Using Table 15.7, calculate the amount of radium required to deliver 2000 cGy 0.5 cm from the center of a 6 × 6 cm implant in 40 h. From Table 15.7, we find that 594 mgh is required to deliver 1000 cGy at 0.5 cm from the center of the implant. The number of milligram hours required for 2000 cGy is therefore

$$\frac{594 \text{ mgh} \times 2000 \text{ cGy}}{1000 \text{ cGy}} = 1188 \text{ mgh}$$

Since 40 h are available, the number of milligrams of radium required is

$$\frac{1188 \text{ mgh}}{40 \text{ h}} = 29.7 \text{ mg}$$

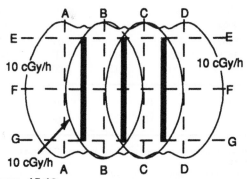

Figure 15.13 Three sources (solid black bars) and the 10-cGy/h line from each source. The sum of these dose-rate lines shows lower dose toward the ends of the sources and also in the periphery. The dose is highest in the center.

Elongated rectangular implants result in lower dose rates requiring increased milligram hours. The

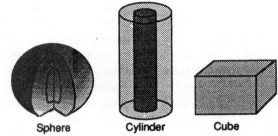

Sphere Cylinder Cube

Figure 15.14 Diagrams illustrating different geometric shapes of implants.

reasons for this lower dose is somewhat similar to that for the elongation effect in rectangular external fields described in Chap. 5. The elongation rules given by Paterson and Parker are as follows:

Length/width = 2; increase milligram hours by 5 percent

Length/width = 3; increase milligram hours by 9 percent

Length/width = 4; increase milligram hours by 12 percent

For example, an implant that is 10×5 cm has a length/width ratio (elongation factor) of 2 (10/5), so the milligram hours should be increased by 5 percent.

Volume implants are used when the three dimensions—length, width, and height—are approximately the same. The original distribution rules by Paterson and Parker for volume implants were limited to geometric forms such as cylinder, sphere, or cuboid (brick) forms (Fig. 15.14). The spherical form can really be obtained only by using seeds. The cuboid shape is obtained using multiplanar implant rules rather than volume rules.

Distribution rules for volume implants and the number of milligram hours necessary to deliver 1000 cGy to the volume are given in Table 15.8.

In this example, we will calculate the number of milligram hours required to deliver 2000 cGy in 48 h

Table 15.8 Volume Implant

Volume, cm³	R$_V$, mgh[a]	Distribution Rules
5	106	Volume should be considered as a surface with 75%
10	168	activity and core with 25%
15	220	
20	267	
30	350	Rules for cylinders:
40	425	Belt—50% activity with minimum 8 needles
50	493	Ends—12.5% of activity on each end
60	556	Core—25% with minimum of 4 needles
80	673	For each uncrossed end, reduce volume by 7.5%
100	782	
140	979	
180	1156	
220	1322	Length/diameter: 1.5 2.0 2.5 3.0
260	1479	Increase mgh: 3% 6% 10% 15%
300	1627	
340	1768	
380	1902	

[a] R$_V$ = mgh to give 1000 cGy to volume implant; radium equivalent for filtration of 0.5 mmPt.
Source: This table was prepared from the original by Meredith[25] by multiplying his values by C = 1.064. (From Johns HE, Cunningham JR: *The Physics of Radiology,* 4th ed., 1983. Courtesy of Charles C Thomas, Publisher, Springfield, Illinois.)

in a $3 \times 5 \times 6$ cm implant (90 cm^3). From Table 15.8, 728 mgh are required to deliver 1000 cGy. The number of milligram hours required to deliver 2000 cGy is therefore

$$\frac{728 \text{ mgh} \times 2000 \text{ cGy}}{1000 \text{ cGy}} = 1456 \text{ mgh}$$

Since 48 h are available, the number of mg Ra required is

$$\frac{1456 \text{ mgh}}{48 \text{ h}} = 30.3 \text{ mg Ra}$$

distributed according to the volume implant rules in Table 15.8.

Here we will use Table 15.8 to calculate the dose rate from a $6 \times 5 \times 3$ cm (90 cm^3) volume implant. The implant is designed according to the rules in Table 15.8 and contains 30 mg radium. From Table 15.8, we find that 728 mgh deliver 1000 cGy. The dose rate is

$$\frac{1000 \text{ cGy} \times 30 \text{ mg}}{728 \text{ mgh}} = 41.2 \text{ cGy/h}$$

The number of hours required to deliver 2000 cGy is therefore

$$\frac{2000 \text{ cGy}}{41.2 \text{ cGy/h}} = 48.5$$

The Paris System. Like the Quimby system, the Paris system, developed in the 1920s,[16] utilizes uniform distribution of the radioactivity, and the rules can be applied to volumes of any shape. The spacing of the sources ranges from 5 to 10 mm for small volumes to 15 to 22 mm for large volumes. The longer the sources are, the higher the dose around each source will be, thus allowing greater spacing. The tolerance of the irradiated tissues must also be considered in choosing the spacing. The high-dose volume in the immediate neighborhood of the radioactive source should never exceed 1 cm in diameter.

The uniform spacing of sources in the Paris system, as in the Quimby system, causes the dose to be higher in the center of the implant than in the periphery. This increased central dose is greater with larger implants. While in the Manchester system the treated volume is decreased by 10 percent when uncrossed ends are used, in the Paris system, 15 percent of the length is considered untreated at each end of the radioactive length. The radioactivity should therefore extend 15 percent beyond the target volume in each direction. When the target volume involves the skin or mucosa, the use of loops, or "hairpins" (U-shaped needles), is recommended. The loop, or the transverse section of the hairpin, acts as a substitute for a crossed end.

In the Paris system, the reference dose, as represented by the isodose line corresponding with the treated volume (minimum tumor dose), is 85 percent of what is called the basal dose. The basal dose is determined by finding the average dose at several low-dose points inside the perimeter formed by the most exterior sources of an implant (Fig. 15.15). The high-dose volume in the immediate neighborhood of each radioactive source is the volume enclosed by an isodose surface along which the dose is twice the reference value.

PERMANENT IMPLANTS

In the calculations described above, the radioactivity was removed when the prescribed dose was delivered. In many implants, however, removal is impossible and the sources are therefore left permanently to decay. In permanent implants, radioactive isotopes with relatively short half-lives are used, allowing the patient to be discharged from the hospital within a short time without posing a threat to the surrounding environment (family members and the general public). Dose calculations for permanent implants differ from those for the removed implants, first because they involve the concept of average life (T_{avg}) of the radioactive isotope and second because they obviously do not involve calculation of time. The average life (not to be confused with half-life) for the purpose of dose calculation is the time it takes for the isotope to decay completely, assuming that the decay is constant and occurs at the initial rate. In

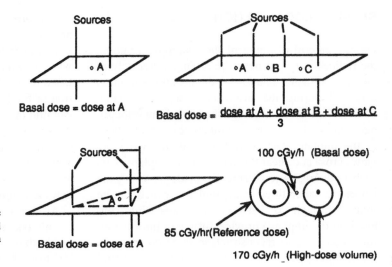

Figure 15.15 Determination of basal dose in the Paris system. Diagram illustrating basal dose, reference dose, and high-dose volume in a two-ribbon implant *(lower right)*.

actuality, the rate of decay (that is, the activity) decreases as time goes on; but if it continued at its original rate, the isotope would "last" at its original activity for a time (T_{avg}) and would then stop emitting. The average life of a nuclide is 1.44 times the half-life of the nuclide or

$$T_{avg} = 1.44 \, T_{1/2} \qquad (15.2)$$

Note that the average life is less than the half-life.

Calculation of the number of millicuries needed in permanent implants requires knowledge of the isotope to be used, the volume over which the activity will be distributed, and the prescribed dose. The goal of the calculation is to determine the number of millicuries needed to deliver the prescribed dose over the lifetime of the isotope. The number of millicurie hours is determined as described for temporary implants (i.e., the appropriate table is used to find the millicurie hours required to deliver 1000 cGy for a specified tumor size.

In the following example, 2000 cGy is to be delivered at 0.5 cm from a 5-cm² area using ^{198}Au seeds distributed on a single plane. From Table 15.7 we find that it requires 170 mgh to deliver 1000 cGy at

0.5 cm if we used ^{226}Ra. So to deliver 2000 cGy, we would need the following:

$$\frac{170 \text{ mgh} \times 2000 \text{ cGy}}{1000 \text{ cGy}} = 340 \text{ mgh}$$

Gold 198, which has a half-life of 2.7 days, has an average life of

$$T_{avg} = 1.44 \times 2.7 \text{ days} \times 24 \text{ h} = 93.3 \text{ h}$$

The exposure rate constant for ^{198}Au, however, is only 2.34, compared with 8.25 for radium, meaning that 1 mCi of ^{198}Au delivers 2.34 R/h at 1 cm from the source. Therefore, to deliver 2000 cGy at 0.5 cm using ^{198}Au, we need

$$\frac{2.34}{8.25} \times 93.3 \text{ mgh} = 26.46 \text{ mgh}$$

The number of millicuries of gold 198 needed is therefore

$$\frac{340}{26.46} = 12.85 \text{ mCi}$$

SOURCE LOCALIZATION

Despite careful planning of the source distribution, the radioactivity can never be arranged precisely as planned, so determination of the actual distribution achieved during the insertion is necessary (Fig. 15.16). This can be accomplished by taking orthogonal radiographs (that is, at right angles to each other) of the implant. The central axes of the two x-ray views cross at or near the center of the implant. Two such radiographs (conveniently made by using the isocentric capabilities of a simulator, which can be rotated through 90° between exposures while centered on the implant) provide sufficient information for a computer to reconstruct, in three dimensions, the geometry of the implant. Placement of metal clips to mark tumor margins is recommended to allow the relationship between the dose distribution and the tumor to be evaluated.

The orthogonal radiographs, of which examples are shown in Fig. 15.16, are enlarged views of the implant as well as the patient. A magnification ring with known dimensions and placed at the same distance in the beam as the implant facilitates calculation of the true size. When a simulator is used, one can find the magnification factor by setting a known field size (conveniently 10 × 10 cm) at the isocenter. For example, if the distance to the isocenter is 100 cm and the field size is 10 × 10 cm, the appearance of a 14 × 14 cm field on the radiograph means that the magnification is 1.4 (140/100 = 1.4).

An anterior radiograph and a lateral radiograph are usually taken, but the films do not have to be vertical and horizontal. Provided that they are orthogonal (at 90° to each other), they can be taken at *any* angles separated by 90°. In entering the three-dimensional source locations into treatment-planning computers, a coordinate system must be used. The conventional

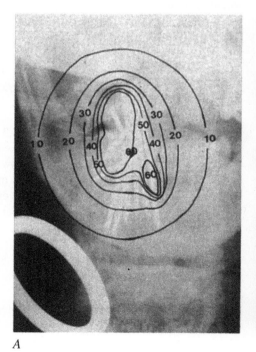
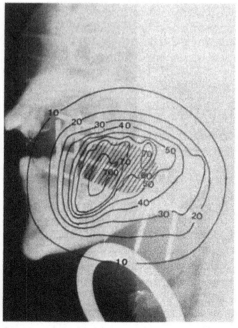

A   *B*

Figure 15.16   *A* and *B*. Radium needles implanted in a carcinoma of the tongue. The radioactivity is not always arranged precisely as planned. A magnification ring is used to facilitate calculation of actual dimensions.

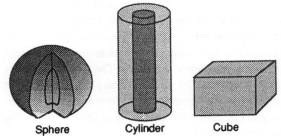

Figure 15.14 Diagrams illustrating different geometric shapes of implants.

reasons for this lower dose is somewhat similar to that for the elongation effect in rectangular external fields described in Chap. 5. The elongation rules given by Paterson and Parker are as follows:

Length/width = 2; increase milligram hours by 5 percent

Length/width = 3; increase milligram hours by 9 percent

Length/width = 4; increase milligram hours by 12 percent

For example, an implant that is 10×5 cm has a length/width ratio (elongation factor) of 2 (10/5), so the milligram hours should be increased by 5 percent.

Volume implants are used when the three dimensions—length, width, and height—are approximately the same. The original distribution rules by Paterson and Parker for volume implants were limited to geometric forms such as cylinder, sphere, or cuboid (brick) forms (Fig. 15.14). The spherical form can really be obtained only by using seeds. The cuboid shape is obtained using multiplanar implant rules rather than volume rules.

Distribution rules for volume implants and the number of milligram hours necessary to deliver 1000 cGy to the volume are given in Table 15.8.

In this example, we will calculate the number of milligram hours required to deliver 2000 cGy in 48 h

Table 15.8   Volume Implant

Volume, cm³	R_V, mgh[a]	Distribution Rules
5	106	Volume should be considered as a surface with 75%
10	168	activity and core with 25%
15	220	
20	267	
30	350	Rules for cylinders:
40	425	Belt—50% activity with minimum 8 needles
50	493	Ends—12.5% of activity on each end
60	556	Core—25% with minimum of 4 needles
80	673	For each uncrossed end, reduce volume by 7.5%
100	782	
140	979	
180	1156	
220	1322	Length/diameter: 1.5 2.0 2.5 3.0
260	1479	Increase mgh: 3% 6% 10% 15%
300	1627	
340	1768	
380	1902	

[a] R_V = mgh to give 1000 cGy to volume implant; radium equivalent for filtration of 0.5 mmPt.
Source: This table was prepared from the original by Meredith[25] by multiplying his values by C = 1.064. (From Johns HE, Cunningham JR: *The Physics of Radiology,* 4th ed., 1983. Courtesy of Charles C Thomas, Publisher, Springfield, Illinois.)

A more complex method of determining source location, which does not involve orthogonal radiographs, is the stereo-shift technique, in which the patient or the x-ray tube is shifted horizontally a certain distance between two exposures (Fig. 15.18). The x and y coordinates can be found on either of the two images, and the z coordinate can be derived from the known geometry of the two radiographs.[26] This method is useful in implants where sources cannot be identified by orthogonal films—for example, when a large number of seeds are used or when some sources are obscured by bone or lead shielding.[27,28]

COMPUTER DOSE CALCULATION

Dose calculations using tables give a very good guide to the required amount of radioactivity and the number of hours the implant must be left in place to deliver the treatment. This, however, does not provide information about the uniformity of the dose distribution. For information about the dose distribution surrounding an implant, computer calculations in multiple planes or in three-dimensional displays are necessary.

Computer calculation of dose distributions consists of summing the dose contributed by each source at grid points arranged in a three-dimensional lattice pattern and by connecting points receiving the same dose rate (centigray per hour). The dose-rate distributions can then be viewed in any plane within the implant. To perform the dose summing, it is necessary to input the source position in three dimensions, as just described.

In a uniformly implanted volume, dose-rate distributions calculated on three planes (between the implant planes, across them, and along the implanted needles or rows of seeds) is often sufficient for the evaluation of the dose distribution (Fig. 15.19), while in a nonuniform implant, additional planes may be necessary.

The dose-rate distributions calculated on planes parallel to the films can be enlarged and superimposed on the radiographs; however, caution should be used in interpreting the dose distribution with respect to the tumor volume when this method is used. This is because the dose distribution in any one plane represents only a very narrow segment of the implant, and the distribution can be quite different at a slightly different plane.

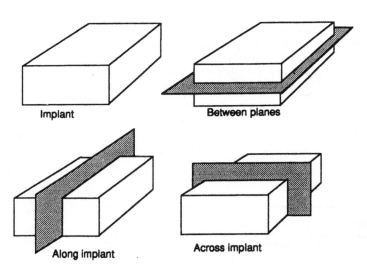

Figure 15.19 Dose-rate distributions are usually calculated along, across, and between two planes in a rectangular implant.

DOSE SPECIFICATION

One of the shortcomings of most computer programs is the failure to allow the user to outline the target volume or the anatomic structures within or near the implant. Dose specification in brachytherapy is therefore, in most cases, complicated by the inability to localize the target volume precisely with respect to the dose distribution. The very steep dose gradient near the implant and the very hot spots near each source also complicate the dose specification. Most physicians prescribe the treatment to the dose-rate line that adequately encompasses the target volume as viewed in multiple planes. There are obviously areas of significantly higher dose within that volume.

The significance of the rate at which brachytherapy treatment (which is continuous rather than fractional, as in teletherapy) is delivered has been discussed in the literature by several authors.[29-31] Experience of delivering continuous irradiation at dose rates on the order of 25 to 100 cGy/h to a total dose of 6000 to 7000 cGy in a large number of patients has been described by Pierquin and co-workers.[30,31] More recently, remote afterloading apparatus, described in Chap. 16, has been used to deliver brachytherapy treatments at very high dose rates (on the order of several hundred centigrays per hour). The biological effect of such a high-dose rate on tumors and normal tissues is not fully known.[32] Inconsistencies in dose specification, dose determination, and treatment techniques among treatment centers using high-dose-rate methods makes the interpretation of results very difficult.

Dose specification in intraluminal brachytherapy has been the subject of some discussion in recent literature.[33] Marinello *et al.* propose a terminology to define dosimetric guidelines for single ribbon implants. Here the dose is specified on the central plane perpendicular to the source and passing through the center of the implant. The treated volume is the volume encompassed by the reference isodose. They then describe a "hyperdose sleeve" as being the volume receiving equal to or greater than twice the reference dose. They also recommend reporting of the thickness of the tissues covered by the reference isodose line and the thickness of the tissue included in the hyperdose sleeve.

PROBLEMS

15-1 The half-life of an isotope is
  (*a*) The thickness of a given material necessary to reduce the intensity by half of the original value
  (*b*) The time required for a nuclide to divide in half
  (*c*) The time required for a nuclide to lose half of its original activity

15-2 Match the nuclides in the left-hand column with the half-lives in the right-hand column

	Isotope	Half-life
_____	^{60}Co	a. 30 years
_____	^{198}Au	b. 28 years
_____	^{192}Ir	c. 74 days
_____	^{137}Cs	d. 59.6 days
_____	^{125}I	e. 2.7 days
_____	^{90}Sr	f. 5.26 years

15-3   The exposure-rate constant for radium is defined as
   (*a*) The exposure rate at a point 1 cm away from 1 mCi of unfiltered radium
   (*b*) The exposure rate at a point 1 cm away from 1 mg of radium filtered by 0.5 mm of platinum
   (*c*) The exposure rate at a point 1 cm away from 1 curie of radium filtered by 0.5 mm of platinum

15-4   A half-strength radium needle has a linear activity of
   (*a*) 0.66 (mg Ra)/cm
   (*b*) 0.33 (mg Ra)/cm
   (*c*) 0.1 (mg Ra)/cm

15-5   The Manchester and the Quimby dosage systems
   (*a*) Use the same distribution rules for the radioactivity but differ in the prescription point
   (*b*) Use the same dosage tables but differ in the distribution rules for the radioactivity
   (*c*) Use different tables and different distribution rules for the radioactivity

15-6   Calculate the time necessary to deliver 2000 cGy at 0.5 cm from a surface mold that is constructed to treat a 2×3 cm area. The mold contains a total of 20 mg Ra eq of ^{192}Ir, which is uniformly distributed (use Table 15.4).

15-7   Calculate the mg Ra eq required to deliver 3000 cGy in 48 h in a $2 \times 2.5 \times 3$ cm volume implant (use Table 15.5).

15-8   Calculate the mg Ra eq required to deliver 3000 cGy in 42 h at 0.5 cm from a 6×6 cm single-plane implant where the radioactivity is distributed according to the Manchester system (use Table 15.7).

15-9   Calculate the time required to deliver 2000 cGy in a $4 \times 4 \times 5$ cm volume implant containing 20 mg Ra eq distributed according to the Manchester system (use Table 15.8).

15-10 In the Paris system
   (*a*) The reference dose is 85 percent of the high-dose volume
   (*b*) The reference dose is determined by finding the average dose rate at several points inside the implant
   (*c*) The reference dose is 85 percent of the basal dose

15-11 Calculate the number of mCi of ^{125}I needed to deliver 2000 cGy at 0.5 cm in a 4×4 cm single-plane permanent implant.

REFERENCES

1. Johns HE, Bates LM, Watson TA: 1,000 curie cobalt units for radiation therapy: 1. The Saskatchewan cobalt-60 unit. *Br J Radiol* 25:296, 1952.
2. Krishnaswamy V: Dose distribution around an I-125 seed source in tissue. *Radiology* 126:489, 1978.
3. Ling CC: Interstitial implant of I-125 seeds—Absolute activity calibration and angular distribution measurement with an Si (Li) detector (abstr). 4th International Conference on Medical Physics, Ottawa, Canada 1976. *Phys Can* 32:9, 1976.
4. Ling CC, Anderson LL, Shipley WU: Dose inhomogeneity in interstitial implants using I-125 seeds. *Int J Radiat Oncol Biol Phys* 5:419, 1979.
5. Ling CC, Yorke ED, Spiro IJ, et al. Physical dosimetry of I-125 seeds of a new design for interstitial implant. *Int J Radiat Oncol Biol Phys* 9:1747, 1983.

6. Nath R, Maigooni AS, Muench P, Melillo A: Anisotropy functions for ^{103}Pd, ^{125}I, and 192Ir interstitial brachytherapy sources. *Med Phys* 20:1465, 1993.
7. Nath R, Melillo A: Dosimetric characteristics of a double wall ^{125}I source for interstitial brachytherapy. *Med Phys* 20:1475, 1993.
8. Johns HE, Cunningham JR: *The Physics of Radiology,* 4th ed. Springfield, IL: Charles C Thomas, 1983.
9. Strauss L, Sturm V, George P, et al. Radioisotope therapy of cystic craniopharyngiomas. *Int J Radiat Oncol Biol Phys* 8:1581, 1982.
10. Wheldon TE, O'Donoghue JA, Barrett A, Michalowski AS: The curability of tumours of differing size by targeted radiotherapy using ^{131}I and ^{90}Y. *Radiother Oncol* 21:91, 1991.
11. Kumar PP, Good RR, Skultety FM, et al. Retreatment of recurrent cystic craniopharyngioma with Chromic P 32. *J Nat Med Assoc* 78:542, 1986.
12. Sievert RM: Die Intensitätsverteilung der primären Gamma-Strahlung in der Nähe medizinischer Radiumpräparate. *Acta Radiol* 1:89, 1921.
13. Sievert RM: Die Gamma-Strahlungsintensität an der Oberfläche und in der nächsten Umgebung von Radiumnadeln. *Acta Radiol* 11:249, 1930.
14. Dutreix A, Marinello G, Wambersie A (eds): *Dosimetric du system de Paris, Dosimétrie en Curiethérapie.* Paris, France: Masson, 1982.
15. Dutreix A, Marinello G: The Paris system, in Pierquin B, Wilson JF, Chassagne D (eds): *Modern Brachytherapy.* New York: Masson, 1987.
16. Regaud C: Radium therapy for cancer at the Radium Institute. *Am J Roentgenol* 21:1, 1929.
17. Paterson R, Parker HM: A dosage system for interstitial radium therapy. *Br J Radiol* 11:252, 1938.
18. Meredith WJ (ed): *Radium Dosage: The Manchester System.* Baltimore, Williams & Wilkins, 1949.
19. Glasser O, Quimby EH, Taylor LS, et al. *Physical Foundations of Radiology,* 3d ed. New York: Harper & Row, 1961.
20. Quimby EH: Dosage tables for linear radium sources. *Radiology* 43:572, 1944.
21. Dutreix A: Can we compare systems for interstitial therapy? *Radiother Oncol* 13:127, 1988.
22. Hendee WR: *Radiation Therapy Physics,* Chicago, IL, Year Book Medical Publishers, Inc., 1981.
23. Greenfield M, Richman M, Norman A: Dosage tables for linear radium sources filtered by 0.5 and 1.0 mm of platinum. *Radiology* 73:418, 1959.
24. Goodwin PN, Quimby EH, Morgan RH: *Physical Foundations of Radiology,* 4th ed. New York, NY, Harper & Row, 1970.
25. Meredith WJ (ed): *Radium Dosage: The Manchester System.* 2nd ed. Edinburg and London, UK. Livingstone, Ltd., 1967.
26. Khan FM: *The Physics of Radiation Therapy,* 2d ed. Baltimore, MD, Williams & Wilkins, 1994.
27. Anderson LL: Dosimetry of interstitial radiation therapy. *Handbook of Interstitial Brachytherapy,* Hilaris BS (ed) Acton, MA. Publishing Sciences Group, 1975.
28. Sharma SC, Willamson JF, Cytacki E: Dosimetric analysis of stereo and orthogonal reconstruction of interstitial implants. *Int J Radiat Oncol Biol Phys* 8:1803, 1982.
29. Hall EJ, Bedford JS: Dose rate: Its effect on the survival of He La cells irradiated with gamma rays. *Radiat. Res.* 22:305, 1964.
30. Pierquin B, Chassagne D, Baillet F, Paine CH: Clinical observations on the time factor in interstitial radiotherapy using iridium-192. *Clin Radiol* 24:506, 1973.
31. Pierquin B: The destiny of brachytherapy in oncology. *Am J Roentgenol* 127:495, 1976.
33. Marinello G, Pierquin B, Grimard L, Barret C: Dosimetry of intraluminal brachytherapy. *Radiother Oncol* 23:213, 1992.

16

Practical Application
of Brachytherapy Techniques

The development of artificial isotopes, afterloading techniques, and automatic devices with remote control has stimulated renewed interest in brachytherapy and also brought about the almost complete replacement of interstitial radium needles, which therefore are not discussed further in this text. Brachytherapy can be carried out using either external surface molds, intracavitary, interstitial, or intraluminal techniques, or, in some situations, a combination of these methods.

AFTERLOADING

Insertion into the tumor or cavities adjacent to the tumor of hollow applicators that are later loaded with the radioactive sources is referred to as an *afterloading technique.* This technique, originally developed for the purpose of reducing exposure to personnel,[1] has also made it possible to plan (1) an implant and prepare needed apparatus in advance and (2) facilitate the optimal loading of an implant after the apparatus is inserted but before the radioactivity is actually loaded.

Tumors of unusual shape or that are located adjacent to radiosensitive tissue benefit particularly from advance planning. Tumor size and shape, as well as outlines of anatomic structures, are established by the use of computed tomography (CT), magnetic resonance imaging (MRI), and orthogonal radiographs. The optimal source strengths and distribution of the radioactivity are then calculated with the aid of a treatment-planning computer. Some computer software has optimization capabilities in which the computer can calculate these variables once the tumor volume is entered and dose constraints (minimum, maximum, etc.) have been set by the user. Many of the implants described in this chapter were planned in advance and then an appliance (mold or template) was built to hold the radioactivity in place.

Idealized plans can be calculated in advance but often cannot be implemented in practice. However, in a short time, computers can calculate dose-rate distributions in three dimensions around the actual implant before the loading of the radioactivity takes place. The activity and spacing of sources are calculated from localization films taken with the apparatus in place. In gynecologic implants using cesium 137 or other isotopes in the shape of tubes, the dose distribution can be altered by changing the spacing and the activity of the sources within the already inserted apparatus. Sources can also be removed early in the case of a hot spot, but this practice is not recommended except in extreme situations. In many situations, however, adding a tube or source is not possible. In the case of seed ribbons with fixed seed activity, spacing, and length, which are usually purchased in advance, optimization is limited by the availability of seeds at the time of the loading. However, the dose deposited by the seeds in a ribbon can be modified by leaving the ribbon in place for a different length of time.

PREPARATION OF SURFACE MOLDS AND CUSTOMIZED APPLICATORS

Surface molds, which were briefly mentioned previously, are used when well-circumscribed surface lesions must be treated to high doses. Surface molds can be prepared to fig snugly over the surface of the lesion and the adjacent region. Pathways for radioactive ribbons are embedded in the mold at a distance from the lesion and spaced so that when the implant is loaded, an acceptable dose distribution is achieved. Lead shielding can be added in the mold to reduce total body dose to patient and personnel. Straps and hooks can also be built into the mold for anchoring the mold to the patient. Surface and intracavitary applicators, which conform to body surfaces or cavities and contain built-in pathways for afterloaded radioactive ribbons, can be constructed to fit practically any shape.

The procedure for making afterloadable surface applicators is very similar to that used for making the custom-designed intracavitary applicators, described later in this chapter. Before a suitable applicator can be fabricated, a detailed replica of the surface anatomy or cavity must be made. A model of the cavity alone is sufficient for lesions lying entirely within a cavity and distal to the exterior surface (Fig. 16.1). In those situations where the lesion extends to the margins of the cavity, it is appropriate to include a generous area of the exterior surface to which the applicator can be attached. The model should always encompass an area larger than that requiring treatment. Details of the anatomy must be precisely mirrored in the replica for a snug and comfortable fit of the applicator (Fig. 16.2). Irregular surfaces and recesses also increase stability and adhesiveness while the applicator is in place. Precise details of the tumor are helpful in the assessment of the area to be treated and for determination of necessary margins around the tumor.

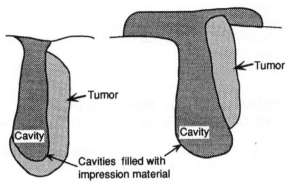

Figure 16.1   An impression of the cavity alone is sufficient when the lesion lies entirely within the cavity *(left)*. When the lesion extends outside the cavity, the impression must also include a generous area of the exterior surface.

An impression of the area or cavity under consideration is made with dental impression alginate.* This consists of a powder which when mixed with water becomes a creamy mixture and sets in 2 min to an elastic rubbery consistency. Unfortunately, this material shrinks and deteriorates rapidly and is therefore not itself suitable for use as final mold material. Impressions made of the entire face require that provision be made for breathing. A syringe barrel at least 1 cm in diameter provides an excellent airway when placed in the patient's mouth (Fig. 16.3).

The negative impression is filled with plaster or dental stone to form a replica (Figs. 16.2 and 16.3). The dental stone consists of a powder that is mixed with water until it becomes creamy. This mixture sets and becomes rock-hard in about 2 to 3 h. When possible, the tumor should be marked on the patient before the impression material is poured onto the surface. This allows tumor markings to be transferred onto the impression material and subsequently onto the replica of the patient. The impression material gives a very detailed surface, including that of a raised tumor. Tumor dimensions and position with respect to the subsequently constructed applicator are determined either via the transposed marks, the raised replica of the tumor, or—in the case of a body

* Jeltrate®, registered trade name of the L. D. Caulk Co., Milford, DE.

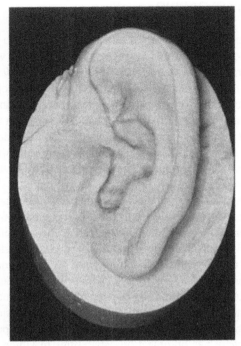

Figure 16.2   A detailed replica of the anatomy is necessary for a snug yet comfortable fit of customized applicators.

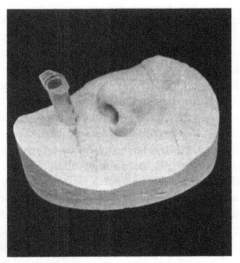

Figure 16.3   A syringe barrel in the patient's mouth provides adequate airway when impressions of the entire face are necessary. In this replica, the syringe remained as part of the impression of the patient's face.

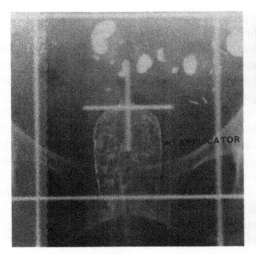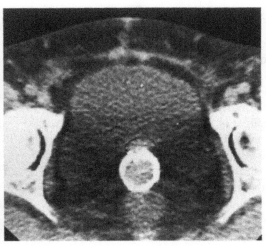

Figure 16.4 Radiographic examination with a customized vaginal applicator in place.

cavity—via radiographic examination with the applicator in place (Fig. 16.4). The source distribution and activity necessary to deliver the desired treatment can be planned from this information. The plastic tubes, which will provide pathways for the afterloaded radioactive ribbons, are arranged within the cavity that is obtained when another negative impression of the replica is made. Transparent acrylic is then poured into this cavity, leaving the hollow plastic tubes in place.

The pathways provided in molds for afterloading radioactive ribbons must obviously have a caliber larger than that of the ribbons. Plastic needles or other plastic tubing can be used. The plastic needles,

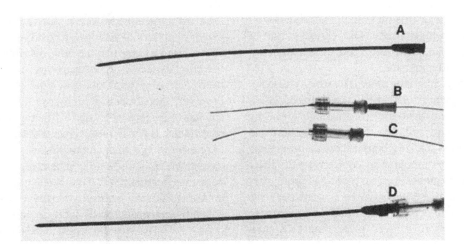

Figure 16.5 A Luer lock glued onto a plastic needle (A). A hypodermic needle is pushed through the rubber top of a heparin lock to facilitate pushing the radioactive ribbon through to the desired length (B). The needle is then withdrawn, leaving the radioactive ribbon secured in the heparin lock (C). The heparin lock is secured in the Luer lock (D). The rubber top of the heparin lock prevents the radioactive ribbon from sliding in or out.

also referred to as Flexiguides®™,* have the advantage of having very strong, sharp points, making it possible to insert them directly into tissue.

In some customized applicators, pathways are built to facilitate the insertion of the plastic needles beyond the mold and into the adjacent tissue. The pathways must then be large enough to accept the larger caliber of the plastic needles. The radioactive ribbons must be anchored securely inside the plastic needles. To do this, a Luer lock (Fig. 16.5) can be glued onto the open end of the plastic needle.[2] The radioactive ribbon is then threaded through a heparin lock to the desired length. The guiding needle is withdrawn and the rubber top prevents the ribbon from sliding out (Fig. 16.5). The radioactive ribbon is then inserted into the plastic needle and the heparin lock is secured onto the Luer lock.

INTRACAVITARY BRACHYTHERAPY OF GYNECOLOGIC MALIGNANCIES

Brachytherapy has been used as a treatment modality in the management of gynecologic malignancies since its beneficial effects on tumors were first discovered.[3,4] Insertion of radioactive sources into body cavities adjacent to tumors allows delivery of large doses in the tumor while minimizing adverse effects on regional normal tissue. The careless use of brachytherapy can, however, lead to irreversible injury in practically any site.

Intracavitary apparatus used in treatment of gynecologic malignancies is fairly standardized. In instances where the anatomy, sometimes distorted by surgery or tumor, precludes the use of standardized apparatus, individualized applicators, as previously described, can be prepared to conform to the body cavity to be treated. Various types of applicators holding the radioactivity have been used over the years. The inventors or the institutions at which these applicators were first used have often lent their names to such devices. Many of the older types of applicators did not facilitate afterloading techniques.

Some of the first gynecologic applicators were de-

signed to conform to the individual patient's anatomy. The arrangement of the radioactive sources was therefore unpredictable and could result in unsatisfactory dose distributions. Large, bulky tumors, for example, would cause the flexible apparatus to be pushed away from the tumor, resulting in underdosage. Later models of gynecologic applicators have been designed to be rigid and thus, to some extent, make the anatomy conform to the applicator yet provide some degree of choice of source arrangement within the apparatus.

Afterloading is a technique whereby the radioactivity is loaded after proper placement of the apparatus has been confirmed. Confirmation of placement of the apparatus is usually determined with "dummies" in place. Dummies are radiopaque markers that are identical to the radioactive sources in size and shape but have no radioactivity. Insertion of the apparatus usually takes place in the operating room, while the insertion of the radioactive sources takes place later, ideally in the patient's room, thus reducing unnecessary exposure to personnel, patients, and hospital visitors.

TANDEM AND OVOIDS

Gynecologic malignancies are usually treated using standard apparatus; however, due to unusual tumor extent or abnormal anatomy, a customized apparatus can be used to improve the dose distribution. Traditionally, gynecologic intracavitary irradiation has been delivered via low-dose-rate brachytherapy; however, more recently high-dose-rate brachytherapy has come into wide use.[5-7] The radiation therapy community is not in total agreement as to the merits of one versus the other technique, but several authors have made an attempt to compare high-versus low-dose-rate treatment.[8-10] The increasing use of high-dose-rate sources in brachytherapy has also raised concern about a potential increase in complication rates.[5,7,9-11] The initially reported high complication rates, however, have gradually decreased and are now comparable with those of low-dose-rate systems.

A system consisting of a tandem and a pair of ovoids (Fig. 16.6) is the most frequently used afterloading apparatus in the treatment of carcinoma of

---

* Registered trade name of Nuclear Associates, Inc., Carle Place, NY.

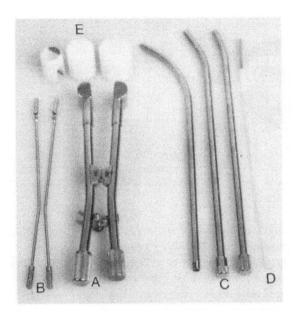

Figure 16.6   A set of Fletcher-Suit-Delclos intracavitary apparatus. A, a pair of ovoids (colpostats); B, source carriers for the ovoids; C, three tandems with different curvatures; D, an insert for afterloading of tandem sources; and E, three nylon caps for the ovoids. The shielding is seen on the smallest cap on the left.

the uterine cervix.[12,13] Tandem and ovoid systems described by Fletcher and Suit are rigid but yet flexible enough to be used in most situations. Tandems are designed to fit inside the uterine canal and extending out through the vagina when properly inserted. The tandem is a long, narrow, hollow tube with one end sealed to prevent sources from falling out inside the patient. Tandems are usually made of stainless steel and are approximately 12 in. long, with an outer diameter of approximately 1/4 in. The internal diameter is made so that the plastic tube holding the radioactive sources can be inserted without resistance. In most patients, the uterus is tilted anteriorly, causing an angle between the vagina and the uterus. Tandems are therefore curved to conform to this anatomy and because the degree of curvature varies from patient to patient, tandems with different curvature are available (Fig. 16.6).

The insertion of a tandem into the uterine canal is preceded by a sounding of the canal. The purpose of the sounding is to dilate the cervical os to allow passage of the tandem and establish the depth of the uterine canal. This is necessary in order to determine

the length of the tandem that will be within the uterus when it is fully inserted. When the tandem is properly inserted in the uterine canal, a keel is secured to the tandem at a distance equaling the sounded depth of the uterus. The keel will then be at the cervical os when the tandem is fully inserted into the uterus. The keel serves a marker of the external cervical os when the reference points used in the dose calculations are determined, and it also prevents the tandem from inadvertently being pushed farther into the uterus, possibly causing a perforation.

Ovoids (Fig. 16.6) are, as the name implies, roughly oval-shaped and are approximately 30 mm long and 20 mm in diameter. The hollow ovoid, also usually made of stainless steel, is attached to a hollow handle through which the radioactive source is inserted. When fully inserted, the handle will protrude outside the vagina. A set of ovoids consists of two slightly different pieces; one for insertion in the right fornix of the vagina and another, which is a mirror image, for insertion into the left fornix. When both ovoids are inserted, they are held together with a screw so that by pressing the distal end of the two handles together, one can force the ovoids laterally. This separation results in a higher dose in the parametria and also helps prevent a "hot spot" near the tandem. Spreading the ovoids too much may cause them to slip inferiorly, resulting in an unsatisfactory dose distribution. The long axis of the ovoids lies roughly perpendicular to the tandem, causing the tungsten shields, built in to the medial aspects at the ends of the ovoids (Fig. 16.7), to reduce the dose in the bladder and rectum.[12] Following successful insertion of the tandem and ovoids, the vagina is carefully packed with sterile gauze to prevent shifting of the application during the 2- to 3-day duration of the implant.

The apparatus just described is made of stainless steel, making it clearly visible on radiographs; however, dose calculations based on CT are desirable[14–17] because the location of radiosensitive organs (rectum, bladder, and small bowel) with respect to the sources can be better appreciated on CT. The artifacts on the CT image caused by the stainless steel prevent determination of the location of the sources and the critical organs. Recently, CT-compatible tandems and ovoids have been developed.[18,19]

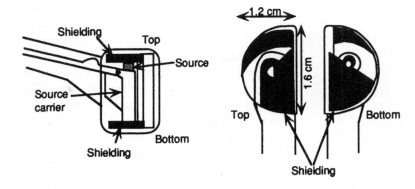

Figure 16.7 Tungsten shielding is built into the ovoids medially at each end to reduce dose to the bladder and rectum.

Apparatus of this kind is typically inserted in the operating room under general anesthesia. Orthogonal radiographs are obtained, usually in the operating room, to confirm satisfactory geometry and evaluate the position with respect to the bladder and the rectum. Although source strengths used in this type of application are very much standard given that the geometry of the application is good, radioactive sources are customarily not inserted until the optimal strengths have been determined by calculating the dose at various reference points as well as in the bladder and rectum. This type of apparatus is usually loaded when the patient has been returned to the hospital bed, thus reducing exposure to personnel in the operating room, recovery room, and during transfer between these areas.

Dose Calculation. In a typical tandem and ovoid application, only the segment of the tandem lying within the uterine canal should be loaded. The mucosa of the vaginal vault, uterus, and cervix can tolerate very high doses (10,000 to 12,000 cGy); however, a source protruding beyond the external os can cause the dose to be very high in the proximal vagina. The mucosa of the rectum and bladder may also lie closer to a source protruding into the vagina than to the uterine sources, where the thicker uterine wall causes the distance to be longer. The length of the uterine canal is approximately 6 to 7 cm, and since each radioactive tube is 2 cm long, three sources will usually fit. The keel on the tandem will indicate where the external cervical os is located and on a lateral radiograph one can measure the length of the tandem lying within the uterus. The distal source

should extend to but not beyond the keel, and if this requires more than three sources, nylon spacers of appropriate size can be added either at the proximal end of the tandem or between the sources. The desired dose distribution is approximately pear-shaped in the anterior view, with the widest part near the cervix (Fig. 16.8). Typically, the tandem is loaded with a 15-mg source at the proximal end, a 12-mg source in the center, and a 10-mg source in the distal end, which is in the cervix. The lower activity closer to the ovoid crossover is selected due to the added contribution from the ovoids and the proximity of the bladder and rectum.

Selection of source strength in the ovoids depends on their diameter and the separation between them. This separation also has some bearing on source-strength selection for the lowest source within the tandem. Large separation between the ovoids would create a cold area in the cervix between the two ovoids. This can be eliminated by placing a stronger source in the lower aspect of the tandem within the cervical canal. The dose contributed to the bladder and rectum might, however, limit the strength of this source. The standard ovoid is 20 mm in diameter, but in some patients with narrow vaginal vaults, a smaller miniovoid may be used, while in patients with large vaginal vaults, larger ovoids may be used. The diameter of an ovoid is increased by slipping a nylon cap over the stainless steel ovoid, thus increasing the distance from the source to the mucosa. Medium and large caps are 25 and 30 mm in diameter, respectively. Typical source strengths are 10 mg in miniovoids and 15, 20, and 25 mg in small, medium, and large ovoids respectively. This increase in

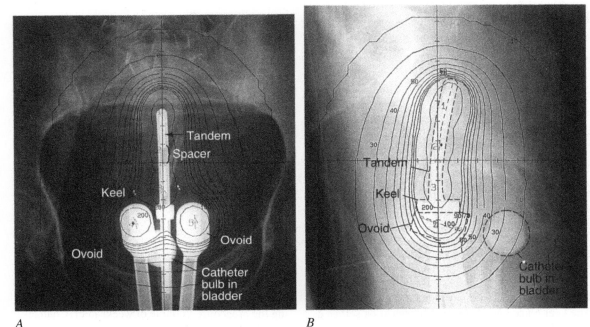

A   *B*

Figure 16.8   *A* and *B*. An anterior and a lateral radiograph of a typical tandem and ovoid intracavitary application. Note the spacers between dummy sources in the tandem. Three ^{137}Cs sources were used in the tandem without any spacers. Typical dose-rate distributions from a tandem and ovoid intracavitary application. (The number on each isodose line represents the dose per hour.)

source strength with larger-diameter ovoids compensates for the increased distance and roughly delivers the same dose rate in the mucosa at the ovoid surface (Chap. 15). Although the distance from the source to the lateral aspect of the miniovoid is the same as in the small ovoid, the medial distance is much less, causing a high dose rate on the mucosal surface of the cervix. Some miniovoids lack bladder and rectal shielding, which is also cause for concern in selecting source strength.

The crude statement of milligram hours as if it were a measure of dose has, through much accumulated experience, attained some meaning in this site; however, it can be misleading and should not be used. Expressing the dose in centigrays, however, is associated here with such complex factors that a special dosage system for this type of treatment has been developed.

The difficulties are primarily a result of great variations in shape, size, and type of tumor to be treated.

In an attempt to solve the problem of dose prescription, some points, at a distance where the dose is not highly sensitive to small and clinically unimportant alterations in the source position, have been chosen for dose prescription. Such points must be anatomically comparable from patient to patient and should be so placed as to allow correlation of dose with clinical effects. Thus, points A and B have been designated.

Point A has been selected to represent the paracervical triangle and is defined as a point 2 cm lateral to the center of the cervical canal and 2 cm from the mucous membrane of the lateral fornix in the plane of the uterus (Fig. 16.9). Another definition of point A is 2 cm cephalad from the external cervical os and 2 cm lateral in a plane perpendicular to the uterine canal (tandem). Although point A is defined in relation to important anatomic structures, these cannot be visualized on a radiograph; it is therefore necessary to establish some convention by which the posi-

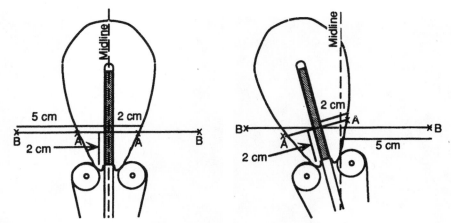

Figure 16.9 Diagram illustrating the position of points A and B in an ideal situation *(left)*. Frequently, the uterus is tilted toward one side *(right)*. Points A shift with the uterus, while points B, defined with respect to the patient's midline, remain unchanged.

tion of point A can be determined on a radiograph. The keel placed at the external cervical os serves as an important reference point because it can be visualized on a radiograph.

Point B is defined as a point 2 cm up (cephalad) from the external cervical os and 5 cm lateral of the patient's midline. In some cases, the uterus may be tilted to one side. In such situations, it is assumed that the tissues represented by point A are carried with the uterus, whereas point B, near the pelvic side wall, is located in tissues that are not dependent on the position of the uterus. It therefore has a fixed position relative to the bony pelvis.

Since the position of the apparatus may vary from patient to patient, no generalization can be made as to the doses delivered to points A and B; each case must be considered individually. Another solution to the problem of dose specification is standardization of the design and loading of applicators that will deliver the same dose rate to point A.

It often takes several days to deliver the desired dose through intracavitary implants; therefore it is delivered in two implants separated by approximately 2 weeks. This reduces the risks of circulatory and respiratory complications, since the patients must lie essentially motionless in bed for the duration of the implant.[20] Other complications from delivering very high doses to the tumor and to normal

organs in the region may also be reduced by repeating the procedure a couple of weeks later. Changes in relationship between anatomic reference points and the implant apparatus occurring between the first and second implant have been studied.[21] It is also important to bear in mind that the dose calculation of an implant represent only the situation at the time that the localization radiographs were taken. Moving the patient from the bed to a stretcher or turning the patient in bed can easily change the relative position of the radioactive sources and the adjacent organs, such as the bladder and rectum. Variations in the fullness of these organs can also change the distance between the sources and the bladder and rectal walls.[16] To minimize the variation in the fullness of the bladder, a catheter is left in place for the duration of the implant.

HEYMAN CAPSULES

Carcinoma of the endometrium is usually treated by hysterectomy. In inoperable cases, however, packing of the uterine cavity with stainless steel capsules — referred to as *Heyman capsules* — is occasionally done for intracavitary treatment following external beam irradiation. These capsules are slightly longer than the 20-mm source that fits inside and have an outer diameter of approximately 10 mm. Each capsule is loaded with a cesium-137 tube (10 mg Ra eq). The distal end of each capsule can be unscrewed to allow loading of the radioactive source. The original Heyman capsules were inserted into the uterus while they were "hot"; however, other, newer capsules that can be afterloaded are available. Heyman capsules are inserted by attaching a special long-handled instrument to an eyelet in the distal end of the capsule. When the capsule is in place in the uterus, the instrument is withdrawn. A metal wire used in removal is attached to the eyelet. At the end of the wire is a metal plate with an engraved number. When inserted into the uterus, the metal wires will protrude from the vagina; the numbers are for identifying the order in which the capsules were inserted so they can be removed in reverse order.

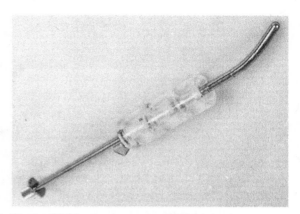

Figure 16.10   Delclos uterine-vaginal afterloading system.

VAGINAL CYLINDERS

Treatment of vaginal lesions requires a wide range of apparatus, often customized, to facilitate treatment of a vaginal lesion without delivering excessive radiation to the adjacent bladder and rectum. A typical standard set of applicators is the Burnett vaginal cylinders. These applicators are of different lengths and have various outer diameters, giving a range of choices in the selection of the applicator that best treats the individual situation. A blind canal inside the applicator facilitates afterloading of several radioactive tubes placed into a plastic insert and arranged in a fashion similar to that of a tandem. The sources are locked inside the applicator by a screw cap and the cylinder is sutured to the vulva to prevent it from falling out.

The Delclos uterine-vaginal afterloading system is designed for simultaneous treatment of the uterine cavity, cervix, and vaginal walls. This system consists of a tandem and six sets of segmented plastic cylinders with various diameters ranging from 2 to 4 cm (Fig. 16.10). The uterine tandem fits inside the vaginal cylinder and extends into the uterus. The length of the segment to be loaded and the strength of each source are determined prior to the actual loading of radioactive sources on the basis of the position of the tumor with respect to the apparatus and thick-

ness of the tumor. Linear sources are afterloaded via a plastic insert that fits inside the tandem. One disadvantage of this system of linear source arrangement is the increased dose to the bladder and rectum.

Other types of vaginal cylinders are constructed to facilitate simultaneous use of iridium ribbons and cesium tubes.[22] The pathways that hold the iridium ribbons are distributed lengthwise in two concentric rings, with a larger central canal in which cesium tubes can be placed (Fig. 16.11). The length and the pattern into which the sources must be loaded are determined from orthogonal radiographs. Metal clips marking the lesion are useful in this determination. Figure 16.12 shows a localization film of a patient with such a cylinder in place and with the dose-rate distribution superimposed.

Case Presentation.

A 63-year-old patient was referred for radiation therapy of recurrent squamous cell carcinoma of the cervix following a total hysterectomy. She was found to have a very small lesion in the lateral aspect of the superior portion of the left vaginal wall. She was also noted to have a 2- to 3-cm-diameter mass in the anterior aspect of the vaginal apex.

She received 4500 cGy to the whole pelvis via external-beam irradiation, which was followed by an intracavitary application using a vaginal cylinder. The cylinder was loaded with two 4.2 mg Ra eq ^{137}Cs sources in the apex surrounded by fourteen 6-cm-long ribbons

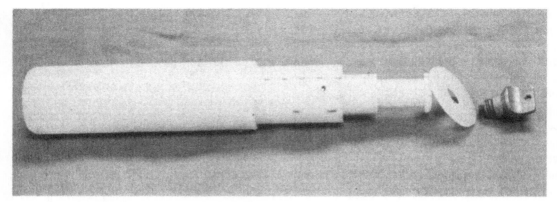

Figure 16.11   Vaginal cylinder that can hold several ^{137}Cs tubes and 14 ribbons of ^{192}Ir.

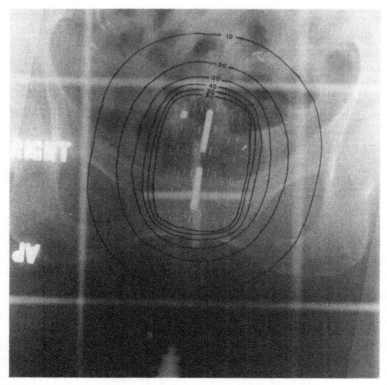

Figure 16.12   Dose-rate distribution superimposed on the localization film of the vaginal cylinder shown in Fig. 16.11. Two ^{137}Cs sources were also in this implant.

of ^{192}Ir arranged in two cylinder-shaped patterns (Fig. 16.12). The outer circle was 2 mm inside the outer surface of the apparatus and the inner circle was 1.2 cm from the surface. This delivered 50 cGy/h at 0.5 cm depth in tissue and remained in place for 30 h, delivering 1500 cGy.

Patients with recurrences in the cervical stump or with bulky tumors in the apex of the vagina often cannot be adequately treated with conventional apparatus.[23] The presence of bulky tumor and prior surgery distorts the normal anatomy of the vagina. A customized applicator that will allow adequate source position and also conforms to the anatomy can then be utilized. Figure 16.13 illustrates some customized applicators.

Case Presentation

The vaginal cylinder labeled A in Fig. 16.13 was used to treat an elderly women who, 38 years prior to this illness, had had a total hysterectomy followed by whole-pelvic irradiation using orthovoltage equipment. She was referred for consideration of radiation therapy for squamous cell carcinoma in the vaginal apex.

A vaginal applicator containing 14 iridium ribbons was custom-made for her treatment. The applicator was formed from an impression made of the vagina and the necessary configuration of iridium seeds was planned to achieve optimal coverage of the tumor (Fig. 16.14). The applicator was left in place for 50 h delivering 3000 cGy at 0.5-cm depth in tissue. The procedure was repeated 5 weeks later.

Case Presentation

This 68-year-old patient had undergone a total hysterectomy for papillary adenocarcinoma of the endometrium approximately 18 months prior to the discovery of a recurrence in the vaginal apex. Surgical resection was not possible due to tumor attachment to the bladder. The patient received 4000 cGy to the whole pelvis via external-beam irradiation, followed by a vaginal intracavitary application. A dummy applicator was made from a vaginal impression. The vaginal cylinder labeled B in Fig. 16.13 was constructed to provide a means of having the plastic needles, containing ^{192}Ir ribbons, extend beyond the mold into the tumor deep to the vaginal vault, thus combining intracavitary and interstitial treatment methods.

During the treatment-planning process, orthogonal radiographs were obtained and a CT examination was carried out with the custom-made dummy applicator in place. The tumor volume was marked with respect to the applicator and, following planning of optimal source configuration, the final cylinder was made. Eleven open pathways were built in so that the needles could extend beyond the applicators. The tumor extended cephalad of and anterior to the vaginal apex.

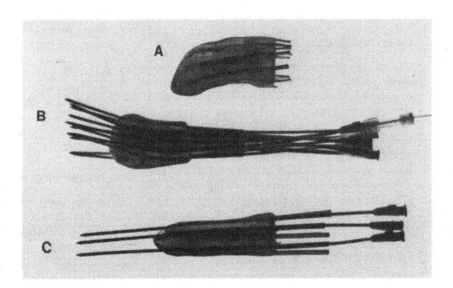

Figure 16.13 Three customized vaginal applicators. The cylinder labeled A was inserted without anesthesia, while B and C, having plastic needles extending beyond the cylinder, were inserted under general anesthesia. Note the heparin lock with a dummy ribbon in place in B.

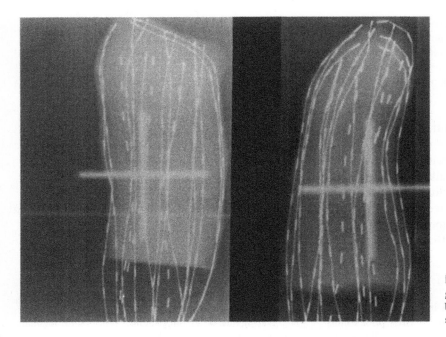

Figure 16.14 Orthogonal radiographs of the vaginal applicator labeled A in Fig. 16.13. Dummy seeds show the built-in source pathways.

Some of the pathways were therefore built with a curve to force the plastic needles to continue in an anterior direction beyond the cylinder. This apparatus was inserted under general anesthesia and was afterloaded with 11 ribbons of 8 iridium seeds each.

A cesium-137 (12.6 mg Ra eq) source was also inserted near the apex via a central blind canal within the applicator. The implant remained in place for 29 h delivering a minimum tumor dose of 2030 cGy.

Case Presentation

The vaginal cylinder labeled C in Fig. 16.13 was also constructed to allow the plastic needles to extend beyond the mold into the tissue. It was custom-built for a patient with recurrent adenocarcinoma in the apex of the vagina. The vaginal canal was narrow and could facilitate only seven pathways. The applicator was inserted under general anesthesia and was afterloaded with seven ribbons containing seven seeds each of [192]Ir. The implant remained in place for 31 h delivering 1550 cGy. The patient had received 4500 cGy to the whole pelvis via external-beam irradiation prior to the procedure.

Case Presentation

Figure 16.15 shows another vaginal applicator used for the treatment of a clear cell adenocarcinoma of the pos-

terior vaginal wall in a 26-year-old woman. Following resection of the lesion, a vaginal impression was made and a customized vaginal cylinder fabricated. Preservation of fertility was of concern to the patient and since the lesion was on the posterior wall of the vagina, the anterior half of the mold was filled with a low-melting-point alloy to provide shielding. In addition to four pathways for ^{192}Ir ribbons inside the applicator, a collar with evenly spaced holes facilitated the insertion of plastic needles into the rectovaginal septum. The applicator was inserted under general anesthesia and five plastic needles were introduced in a semicircular pattern 1 cm posterior to the embedded tubes inside the applicator, thus "sandwiching" the lesion between the planes. Nine ^{192}Ir ribbons containing six seeds each were afterloaded and remained in place 75 h delivering 4500 cGy to the posterior vaginal wall.

BLADDER AND RECTUM COMPLICATIONS

The uncertainty of dose determination of gynecologic intracavitary implants is high.[24] Numerous attempts at determining the dose in the bladder and rectum during intracavitary treatments have been made, either with thermoluminescent dosimeters (TLDs) or an ionization chamber in the rectum or by calculating the dose using orthogonal films.[25-27] The

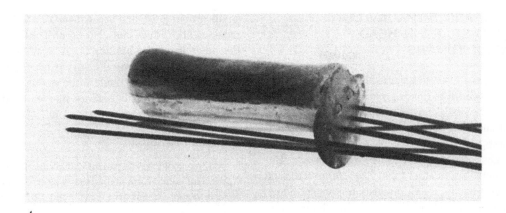

A

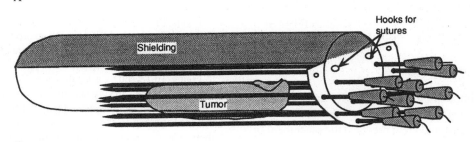

B

Figure 16.15   *A.* Customized vaginal cylinder used in combination with several interstitial needles "sandwiching" a tumor in the posterior vaginal wall.   *B.* Lead shielding was added in the anterior half of the applicator.

dosimetry of high-dose-rate intracavitary implants has been studied using orthogonal films, TLDs, and CT-assisted techniques.[14]

Many authors[28-40] have attempted to correlate the dose with the incidence of bladder and rectum injuries.

Contrast in the bladder and the rectum, used in radiographic localization to identify the position of these organs with respect to the implant, probably alters the distance between the radioactive sources and the walls of these organs when the contrast is evacuated and the walls collapse. Due to the very rapid fall-off of dose in brachytherapy, very small shifts of the anatomy can result in large differences in dose. When we also consider the changes in the relationship between the sources and the bladder and rectum—which occur during a 48- to 72-h period due to small changes in the patient's position, fecal

and gas accumulations, etc.—the uncertainties of dose delivered to these organs are further increased. If complication probabilities are to be assessed, it is not appropriate to relate these to the dose at some fixed point in the pelvis, such as point A, or to the number of milligram hours used, but rather to the dose actually received at the site of the injury.

Factors other than the dose may affect the complication rate in these organs. Previous surgery, poor nutritional status, anemia, age, and perhaps the dose rate at which the treatment is given are some of these predisposing factors. Technical factors such as the type of apparatus used in the intracavitary treatment, the arrangement of the sources, and the geometry of the application may also have a role in the incidence of complications and must therefore be carefully considered in attempts to reduce the dose delivered to the bladder and rectum.

SURFACE AND INTRACAVITARY BRACHYTHERAPY IN HEAD AND NECK TUMORS

Although less conventional, custom-built applicators holding radioactive ribbons can be used to boost small volumes of persistent or recurrent disease in the head and neck region, the placement of applicators holding radioactive sources directly on the lesion makes invasive procedures unnecessary. Because such applicators can be removed and repositioned easily, they may also, in some patients, be placed on the lesion during daytime hours only, thus obviating hospitalization. This text describes only some cases showing a variety of applications. Similar techniques have been described previously.[41]

ORAL CAVITY

Interstitial implants in the oral cavity are limited to sites where soft tissue surrounds the lesion. The presence of bone and teeth prevents the placement of interstitial implants in sites such as the hard palate and alveolar ridge. Instead, surface applicators can be used to boost the dose to small, shallow lesions following external-beam irradiation. Anchoring of surface applicators in the oral cavity is possible with small amounts of denture adhesive, and numerous recesses and ridges can also be utilized to maintain the position of the applicator. A very detailed impression of the entire oral cavity is necessary so that the appliance can be made large enough to include some of the irregular surfaces that will aid repositioning and anchoring.

Case Presentation

A 62-year-old female patient with a superficial lesion of the hard palate 2 cm in diameter was referred for radiation therapy. She received 5000 cGy through external-beam irradiation followed by an intraoral surface application.

Figure 16.16 shows a surface applicator fabricated to fit snugly against the hard palate. Tubes providing pathways for radioactive iridium ribbons were built into the appliance. Figure 16.17 shows the appliance in place.

Figure 16.18 shows a localization film with the applicator in place carrying six ribbons with a total of 47 ^{192}Ir seeds. The ribbons were separated by 0.5 cm and the seed spacing in the ribbons was also 0.5 cm, thus there was one seed in each 0.5 cm^2 of the area. The distribution of the seeds was similar to that for planar implants with one ribbon crossing the proximal end near the lesion. Two metal clips indicated the location of the lesion. The implant remained in place for 50 h, delivering 1500 cGy at the 30-cGy/h line.

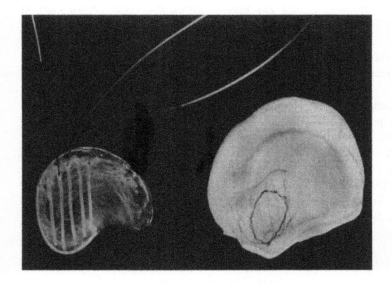

Figure 16.16 A replica of the hard palate with the tumor marked in black *(right)*. The surface applicator with some dummy ribbons inserted in the pathways *(left)*.

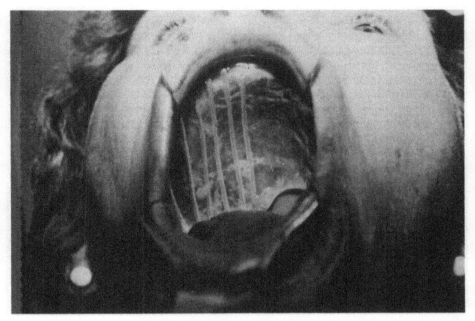

Figure 16.17   The appliance was held in place against the hard palate by the application of dental adhesive.

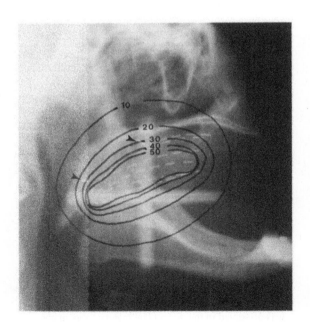

Figure 16.18   The dose-rate distribution superimposed on the lateral radiograph of the hard palate surface applicator shown in Figs. 16.16 and 16.17. Arrowheads indicate seeds marking the tumor.

NASAL CAVITY

Surface applicators to boost the dose to small lesions in the nasal cavity, vestibule, and the nasal alae are ideal.[42–45] Such surface applicators can be removed overnight, and the patient would not require hospitalization. Where the lesion is too thick for a surface applicator, a second plane of radioactive ribbons can be implanted interstitially. This would obviously require general anesthesia and hospitalization. A very detailed impression of the nose, particularly the nostrils, is necessary for a snug fit.

Case Presentation

A 63-year-old male patient was found to have a basal-cell carcinoma of the left nasal cavity. He underwent local resection of the tumor with a skin graft in the nasal septum. The surgical specimen showed tumor cells at the deep margins. The patient then received 3000 cGy via external beam irradiation using a three-field technique with a wax compensator over the nose. This vas followed by a treatment using an intracavitary applicator holding ^{192}Ir seeds. The applicator covered the left ala (Fig. 16.19) and had a cone-shaped segment holding

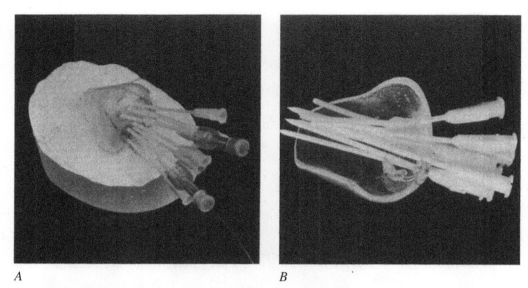

A   *B*

Figure 16.19 *A* and *B*. An intracavitary applicator used in an implant in the nasal cavity. Two dummy ribbons are shown inserted in pathways in the applicator. The metal spring was used to clamp the applicator in place.

five ribbons with four iridium seeds each (two seeds per centimeter), which fitted snugly into the left nostril. A springlike wire, embedded in the acrylic mold, was curved under the septum and into the right nostril, where a small soft pad (similar to that used in eyeglasses) clamped the applicator in place. A small opening in the cone-shaped segment in the left nostril facilitated airflow through the mold, making breathing more comfortable. This implant remained in place 25 h delivering 2500 cGy minimum surface dose to the nasal septum.

Figure 16.20 shows another nasal applicator that was used along with several interstitial plastic needles inserted in the nasal septum, thus combining intracavitary and interstitial techniques.

ORBITAL CAVITY

Tumors recurring subsequent to orbital exenteration can be treated via intracavitary applications. The bony boundaries of the orbit prevent local treatment with interstitial techniques.

Case Presentation

A 10-year-old girl had a left orbital exenteration for embryonal cell rhabdomyosarcoma followed by chemotherapy. Approximately 1 year later she presented with a mass in the upper medial region of the left orbit. The mass was removed and she received 5000 cGy to the left orbit via external-beam treatment. She presented again with a recurrence in the same location approximately 6 months later. She received 3000 cGy via external-beam treatment, which was followed by placement in the left orbit of an intracavitary applicator holding 11 ribbons of ^{192}Ir seeds (Fig. 16.21).

The applicator was removed intermittently, as she wanted to participate in activities with other children in the hospital. It remained in place a total of 60 h, delivering 3000 cGy. The applicator was made of a tissue-equivalent material consisting of water, gelatin, and glycerin. These ingredients were boiled after the gelatin was dissolved in the water. The material sets in approximately 2 h and has a rubbery consistency. It is not as durable as dental acrylic material but does not deteriorate like the alginate previously mentioned. The rubbery mold was comfortable for the patient and could be

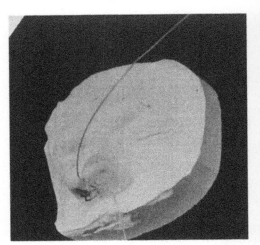

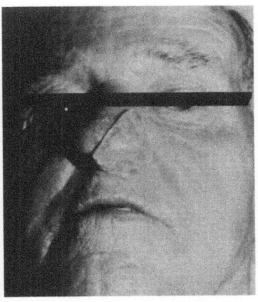

A   B

Figure 16.20   A replica of the patient *(A)* from which the nasal applicator *(B)* was made. Several interstitial needles were used.

inserted and removed from the already sore orbit without much manipulation or discomfort.

Retinoblastoma is often treated via external-beam irradiation. In cases where the tumors recur, cryotherapy, chemotherapy, enucleation, and additional radiation therapy may be tried. Delivering additional external-beam radiation therapy is difficult due to the proximity of the brain, which of necessity would have already been irradiated in the initial fields. If the patient has a solitary lesion and the eye is intact, a radioactive plaque may be used. Where there is recurrence following enucleation, an intracavitary implant may be feasible.[46]

Case Presentation

A 32-month-old child presented with a large calcified mass in the left eye and was staged with a group IV unilateral retinoblastoma. The patient received 4500 cGy via external-beam radiation therapy using anterior and lateral fields with only 20 percent of the dose delivered through the anterior field. A wedge and a hanging

lens shield was used in the anterior field. Approximately 8 months later, the tumor recurred and was treated with cryotherapy. The tumor continued to grow and enucleation was performed. Eleven months following enucleation, a protrusion of the prosthesis was noted and a biopsy confirmed recurrent retinoblastoma. The tumor was firmly adherent to the periosteum and could therefore not be totally resected. Staging studies were performed and revealed only the localized tumor recurrence.

The patient was referred for additional external-beam radiation therapy. There was concern that the patient might be at risk for dissemination of the tumor into the central nervous system. Combined-modality treatment, consisting of chemotherapy and radiation therapy, was undertaken. The patient received 1800 cGy to the left orbit and whole brain followed by an intracavitary implant. The purpose of the implant was to sterilize the entire orbit while sparing the adjacent brain tissues.

The patient was brought to the operating room for an examination under anesthesia and to obtain an impression of the empty orbit for construction of a seed-carrying mold. During the examination, it was determined that the use of a conventional methylmethacrylate con-

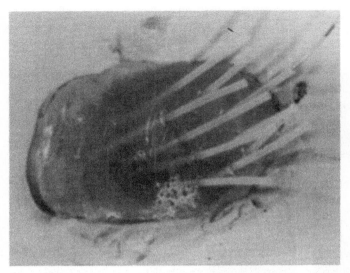

A

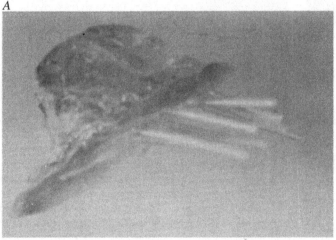

B

Figure 16.21 A direct view *(A)* and a lateral view *(B)* of an intraorbital applicator used in the treatment of a recurrent rhabdomyosarcoma.

former as a seed carrier would produce a superior dose distribution with much less difficulty. A canal was drilled into the center of a 16-mm-diameter eye sphere and a high-activity (44.4-mCi) ^{125}I seed was inserted. Approximately 5 weeks following completion of the external beam treatments, the conformer holding the seed was inserted into the orbit and the eyelids were sutured closed. The implant remained in place for 44.8 h delivering 4260 cGy on the surface of the sphere and 2640 cGy at 2-mm depth in the orbital tissues.

Iodine 125 was chosen over iridium 192 in this treat-

ment because of its low energy and because the efficacy of the bone as a protective barrier is substantially greater for ^{125}I than for ^{192}Ir. The doses in the optic chiasm and in the retina of the remaining eye was estimated, assuming that the intervening tissues were equivalent to water, and were found to be 290 and 166 cGy respectively. The doses actually delivered in these tissues were negligible when a correction for attenuation by bone was applied.

The child remains disease-free 5 years following the implant.

EXTERNAL AUDITORY CANAL

Although rare, tumors occurring in the external auditory canal can be treated via a customized applicator. The anatomy of the ear provides many structures that increase the stability and fit of the applicator (Fig. 16.22).

Case Presentation

A 52-year-old male patient presented with a basal cell carcinoma of the lower aspect of the external auditory canal. The lesion was resected but the deep margins were positive for tumor. The patient had a history of multiple basal-cell carcinomas treated surgically over several years. An acrylic applicator, containing four tubes for ^{192}Ir ribbons, was fabricated (Fig. 16.22). The appliance was made to include a semicircle over the preauricular area. Six holes were drilled through this collar 1 cm apart and 1 cm from the segment in the auditory canal. Six interstitial needles were planned in this semicircle to achieve a two-plane implant. Planning

of four ribbons with four seeds each in the mold and three seeds in each interstitial needle with a seed spacing of 0.5 cm indicated too high a dose in the external auditory canal. It was elected to load only three of the four ribbons in the auditory canal to reduce the hot spot.

The appliance, which was made with an anchoring loop around the ear (similar to those used for eyeglasses), was placed in the ear, and the needles were inserted under local anesthesia only 1 cm deep in the preauricular area. The implant remained in place for 48 h, delivering an estimated minimum tumor dose of 1470 cGy. A second procedure included only the four ribbons in the auditory canal. This implant was left in place for 96 h, delivering 4800 cGy, thus giving a total dose of 6270 cGy.

NASOPHARYNGEAL CAVITY

Treatment of recurrent tumors in the nasopharynx following curative doses of irradiation must be lim-

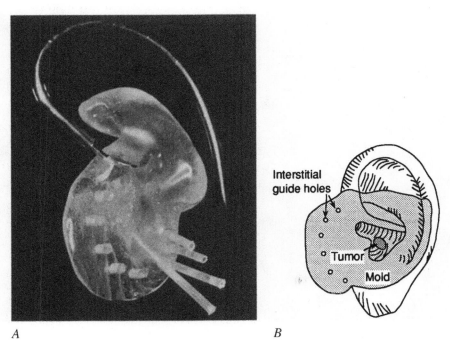

A   *B*

Figure 16.22   *A.* An acrylic applicator used to treat a lesion in the auditory canal (the replica of the ear is shown in Fig. 16.2). The metal loop, which fits around the external ear, was used to stabilize the position. Six holes drilled through the applicator in the preauricular area were used to guide interstitial needles *(B).*

ited to small volumes because of the proximity of vital organs. Consideration must be given to the dose in, for example, the spinal cord, brain, lens of the eye, and the optic chiasm. Interstitial implants are not possible due to the inaccessible location. Intra-

cavitary placement of radioactive sources, usually cesium 137, has been used by several authors.[47-50]

A cesium 137 tube secured inside a small (< 2 cm in diameter) Manchester ovoid can be pulled via a nasogastric tube into the nasopharyngeal cavity. The

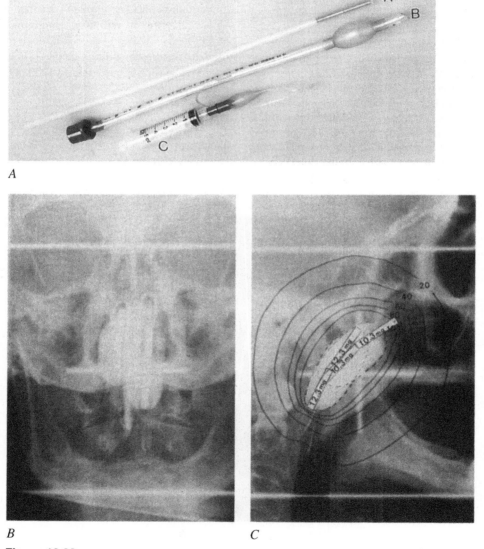

Figure 16.23 *A.* An endotracheal tube used for afterloading nasopharynx implant. A tandem source carrier is inserted through the tube until the sources are inside the balloon. A, source carrier; B, endotracheal tube with the balloon expanded, and C, syringe for injection of contrast in balloon. *B* and *C*. Orthogonal radiographs of an afterloaded nasopharyngeal implant.

diameter of the ovoid is important in maintaining an adequate distance between the radioactive source and the mucosa. If the source were placed directly on the mucosa, the dose rate would be very high and would fall off very rapidly within the first couple of millimeters. Increasing the distance to the mucosa results in a lower dose rate on the surface, but the fall-off is then less rapid. The disadvantage with this technique is the necessity of hot loading (with the radioactive sources in place).

An alternative technique is to insert two endotracheal tubes (pediatric #5) into the nasopharynx through the nostrils (Fig. 16.23). The balloon near the tip of an endotracheal tube is filled with contrast (diluted Renografin™*). Following radiographic verification, using dummy sources, that the endotracheal tubes are successfully positioned, the tubes are secured to the patient's nose. The needed source activity is determined from precalculated dose distributions. A plastic tube, identical to the tubes used to afterload tandems in gynecologic implants, is loaded with the cesium-137 sources and is introduced through each of the endotracheal tubes. Following radiographic verification of the position, the plastic tubes holding the sources are secured to the endotracheal tube. The contrast remains in the bulb during the implant to help in maintaining the distance between the radioactivity and the mucosa. This afterloading technique allows one to verify the position prior to loading and reduces exposure to personnel.

Case Presentation

An 81-year-old man was referred for consideration of radiation therapy of a recurrent squamous-cell carcinoma in the nasopharynx. Fifteen years prior to the referral he had received 6000 cGy via external-beam treatment to the nasopharynx and bilateral cervical lymph nodes. Valium was administered orally 45 min prior to the procedure. A 2% cocaine spray was used as a vasoconstrictor in each nostril at the beginning of the procedure.

An endotracheal tube was inserted through each nostril. The position of the endotracheal tubes was confirmed by inserting dummy sources. The bulb of each endotracheal tube was then filled with 5 cc diluted Renografin. Two ^{137}Cs sources were loaded into each tube.

Dose distributions calculated prior to the procedure showed that higher-activity sources were needed in the left tube, where the lesion extended to a greater depth. Two 12.3 mg Ra eq sources were inserted on the left side and two 10.3 mg Ra eq sources were inserted on the right side. These sources were left in place 36 h, delivering 3000 cGy minimal dose to the tumor. The procedure was repeated approximately 5 weeks later, delivering a minimum tumor dose of 6000 cGy.

REMOVABLE INTERSTITIAL IMPLANTS USING OPEN-ENDED PLASTIC TUBING

In anatomic regions where there is no body cavity or orifice to accept radioactive sources, it is necessary to place the radioactivity directly into the tissue. Such removable interstitial implants can be used only in areas that are accessible to direct instrumentation. Insertion of hot needles directly into tumors has largely been replaced by insertion of hollow steel needles or plastic tubing, which are threaded through the tumor or tumor bed for subsequent loading of radioactivity.[51] Several different techniques can be employed, depending on the size and the location of the tumor. Only some of these techniques are summarized in this text.

In soft tissues, hollow stainless steel needles can be pushed through the tumor at the desired spacing so that both ends are accessible (Fig. 16.24). A hollow plastic tube with an inner caliber that can accommodate the seed ribbon is then pushed through each needle. The stainless steel needles are removed, leaving the hollow plastic tubing in the tissues. A button is loosely fastened to the plastic tube on each side of the implanted tissues to prevent it from shifting. This procedure is usually performed in the operating room under general anesthesia. Following the patient's recovery, orthogonal radiographs are obtained to determine the position of each tube. Since the rigid stainless steel needles have been removed, the flexible plastic tubes tend to curve and change position slightly. Nonradioactive "dummy" ribbons are inserted into each plastic tube to (1) make it possible to visualize the tubes on a radiograph and (2) determine the number of seeds needed in each tube. When the implant is loaded, all seeds should be in the portion of the tubes that is inside the tissues. No

* Renografin™, Squibb Diagnostics, Princeton, NJ.

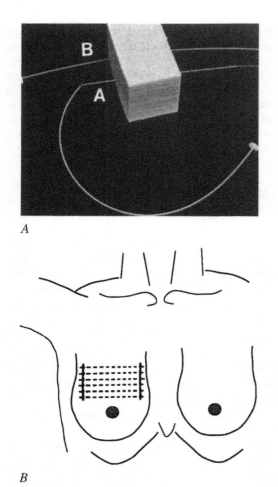

A

B

Figure 16.24   *A.* Stainless-steel needles are pushed through the tissues (a block of Styrofoam is used in this illustration) until both ends are visible *(above)*. Plastic tubes are pulled through the needles (A), which are then removed, leaving the plastic tubes in the tissue (B).   *B.* Diagram of a breast implant using the open-ended tubing technique.

seed should be nearer than 0.5 cm to the skin surface so as to reduce the risks of poor cosmesis. Following the localization procedure, the dummy ribbons are removed and replaced with the radioactive ribbons. Both ends of each plastic tube are then sealed by either soldering the plastic tube and the ''tail'' of the seed ribbon together or by tightly crimping buttons onto both ends of each tube, fixing the seed ribbons and plastic tubes together to prevent shifting. Although more comfortable for the patient, this flexible system gives rise to a somewhat less uniform dose distribution than the older system using rigid radium needles. This type of implant is particularly useful in treatment of tumors of the breast and head and neck region.[52]

BREAST IMPLANTS

The conservative management of early carcinoma of the breast with tumor excision (tylectomy) and breast irradiation is becoming increasingly accepted as an alternative to radical mastectomy.[53-56] Radiation therapy typically follows the excisional biopsy and usually consists of 4500 to 5000 cGy delivered via external-beam irradiation and a boost of 1500 to 2000 cGy to the tumor bed using an electron beam or an ^{192}Ir interstitial implant.[57] The value of boosting the dose to the tumor bed has been presented by several investigators.[58,59] Typically, the sequence of the radiation therapy is that the interstitial implant follows the external-beam irradiation. However, because the status of the axillary nodes plays an important role in the management of this disease, an axillary dissection is often carried out prior to any radiation therapy. If the axillary nodes are microscopically negative, an interstitial implant is sometimes used to boost the tumor area. Since both the axillary node dissection and the interstitial implant require general anesthesia, the two procedures can be carried out at the same time, followed later by external-beam irradiation.

An increasingly popular method of interstitial implantation for breast carcinoma is a Quimby-like implant using ^{192}Ir seeds. The seeds are uniformly distributed throughout the target volume, resulting in higher dose in the center of the implant and lower dose in the periphery, with very rapid fall-off outside the implanted volume.[60] In the Manchester (Paterson-Parker) system, crossing sources are recommended to achieve dose uniformity within 10 percent at a distance of 0.5 cm from the implant plane (see Chap. 15). This is usually not possible in breast implants because of the presence of the nipple and areolar region near the implant. In the absence of crossing ribbons, several authors recommend that the source lengths be considerably longer than the target length.[61-65] The use of extended source length in breast implants, however, is not always possible because it may result in the placement of radioactive seeds in proximity to the skin.

Ideally, the nylon ribbons containing the seeds are spaced 1 cm apart and are parallel with one another. In each ribbon, the seeds are spaced 1 cm apart (center to center); thus there is one seed per cm³ of tissue. Alternatively, continuous ^{192}Ir wires rather than discrete seeds can be used. These deliver a more uniform dose along the tubes.[66] With an activity of 0.33 mg Ra eq per seed, the dose-rate line encompassing the implanted volume is approximately 40 cGy/h. The dose rate near each seed is considerably higher, but it falls off very rapidly with distance from the seed. The tubing into which the nylon ribbons holding the seeds are loaded creates some distance between the radioactive seed and the tissue, thus reducing the hot spots considerably.

Several afterloading techniques have been described,[2,57] but a typical implant uses the open-ended plastic tubing technique described above. The stainless steel needles are pushed through the breast tissue until each needle exits on the opposite side. When the plastic tubing is pulled through and the rigid steel needles are removed, the flexible plastic tubes tend to follow the curvature of the breast tissue (Fig. 16.25). With dummy seeds in place, the implant is now verified radiographically to facilitate dose calculation. The depth of each tube is measured using dummy ribbons and the radioactive ribbons are cut to appropriate length. The seeds must be well within the breast tissue to prevent very high doses to the skin surface, where the plastic tubes enter and exit the breast. The buttons holding the tubes in place are crimped when the loading is completed so as to prevent the ribbons from shifting during the implant. The loading of the radioactivity can take place in the patient's room or, alternatively, in the simulation room. The latter permits verification films to be taken of the actual sources in place, but it means a few additional minutes of exposure for the simulator technologist. The transport of the patient to the room also means additional exposure to personnel, but both can be minimized with good planning and experienced staff.

Case Presentation

A 58-year-old woman noted a lump in the lower outer quadrant of her right breast. A mammogram confirmed the presence of a lesion suspicious for carcinoma. A needle aspirate confirmed the diagnosis of adenocarcinoma and she underwent local excision of a mass 2 cm in diameter. Approximately 1 week later she underwent an axillary dissection and an interstitial implant. Twenty-one lymph nodes removed during the dissection were all negative for malignancy. The implant consisted of two planes with six ribbons in each plane. Ten ribbons had seven seeds each and the remaining two had six seeds each. A higher dose is sometimes observed in areas of the implant where, due to the curvature of the implant, the calculation plane is closer to one of the implant planes (Fig. 16.26). Small areas of high dose rate (80 to 90 cGy/h), representing points where the calculation plane intersects or is near a seed, can also be observed. The implant remained in place 38 h, delivering 1900 cGy at the 50-cGy/h line. This was followed by a course of external-beam irradiation consisting of 4600 cGy to the right breast delivered via parallel opposed tangential photon beams.

HEAD AND NECK IMPLANTS

The management of head and neck malignancies often includes brachytherapy. Delivering canceroci-

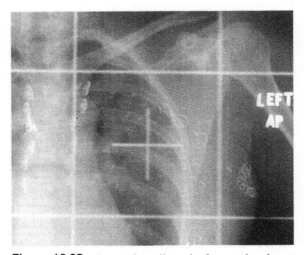

Figure 16.25 An anterior radiograph of a two-plane breast implant.

dal doses of radiation in these sites is often difficult and is limited by the tolerance of adjacent normal tissue. Interstitial implants using radium needles have been used in the management of persistent or recurrent tumors for many years.[12] More recently, nylon ribbons containing ^{192}Ir seeds have been used. Several techniques, some of which are described below, have been investigated.[67,68]

Open-ended plastic-tube techniques, described above for breast implants, are also used in persistent neck nodes or lip tumors.

Case Presentation

A 72-year-old male patient with a 2-year history of progressive exophytic growth on the lower lip was referred for radiation therapy when a biopsy revealed well-differentiated squamous-cell carcinoma. Previous biopsies had shown actinic cheilitis. On examination, the patient was found to have an exophytic lesion covering the entire lower lip. The lesion infiltrated the entire thickness of the lip but did not extend into the labiogingival sulcus. The oral cavity and neck were free of disease. The patient received 3000 cGy via external-beam irradiation followed by an interstitial implant using four ribbons with six ^{192}Ir seeds each. The technique used

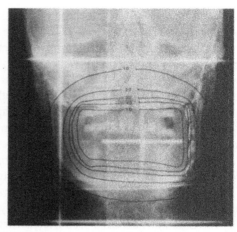

Figure 16.27   An anterior radiograph of a lower-lip implant with the resulting dose-rate distribution superimposed.

was the same as that described for the breast treatment. Following insertion of the plastic tubing, dummy seeds were inserted and orthogonal films to facilitate dose calculation were obtained. The implant remained in place 50 h, delivering 3500 cGy at the 70-cGy/h line (Fig. 16.27).

TEMPLATE-GUIDED INTERSTITIAL IMPLANTS

BLIND-NEEDLE TECHNIQUES

In anatomic sites where the open-ended plastic-tube technique cannot be used, a blind needle (sealed at the pointed end) can be inserted through the tumor and the radioactive ribbons loaded directly into the needles. The spacing and direction of these needles is difficult to control unless some kind of template is used. These difficulties have led to the development of templates that can either be customized or bought commercially. Because template techniques are practically always used with blind needles, the descriptions of these techniques are combined in this text.

TRANSPERINEAL TEMPLATE IMPLANTS

Templates, developed to guide the spacing and parallelism of interstitial needles, are popular in trans-

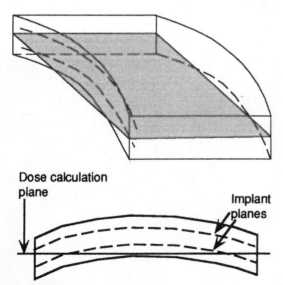

Dose calculation plane

Implant planes

Figure 16.26   The calculation plane cannot follow a curved implant, so the dose rates are higher where the plane is closer to a row of seeds.

perineal implants.[52,67,69–73] The Syed-Neblett "butterfly" template is probably the most commonly used type. It consists of a removable vaginal obturator and an acrylic perineal plate. The vaginal obturator has a central canal which facilitates the insertion of a tandem. Holes drilled through the plate in a predetermined pattern serve as guides for the spacing of the stainless steel or plastic needles that are inserted in five concentric cylinders around the lateral plane of the vagina. The needles are afterloaded with ^{192}Ir seeds in nylon ribbons, and intrauterine cesium tubes can be inserted in the tandem. More recent models are made to facilitate other patterns of needle distribution. The perineal plate in the newer models is made of softer silicone material, which is more comfortable for the patient. The removable obturator in the center of the template is inserted into the vagina to stabilize the template. For rectal, prostatic, and urethral lesions, the template is stabilized by threading it over a rectal tube or a catheter in the bladder. Once confirmation of placement is obtained, dose calculations are completed and radioactive ribbons are inserted into the needles.

Transperineal templates can also be customized[74] to suit a particular situation (Fig. 16.28). Such customized templates are superior to standard models because they can be designed with a needle pattern that, when loaded, results in a uniform dose distribution conforming to the shape of the target (Fig. 16.29A). The extent of the tumor in the "template's eye-view" is determined from a series of CT images with an obturator in the vagina as a reference marker. The tumor outline in each image is then superimposed, using the obturator as the reference (Fig. 16.29B). The composite of these tumor outlines represents the extremes of the tumor in the template's-eye view. Based on this area, the pattern of the seed ribbons is calculated so that when the ribbons are in place, an acceptable dose distribution results. The template is then made, with holes for the guide needles in the predetermined pattern along with a hole for the vaginal obturator, as well as holes to facilitate suturing of the device to the perineum.

The pattern of guide holes actually used in each implant and the depth to which the radioactivity is inserted can, to a limited degree, be tailored to match the target volume. This, of course, requires very detailed characterization of the target in terms of its size, shape, and location with respect to the obturator or other reference point. For smaller target volumes, smaller templates can be used. Rectal and prostatic templates have been developed to treat single sites, providing a much smaller and thus more comfortable appliance.[75–79] The combination of an intracavitary tandem containing cesium sources with interstitial iridium seeds in treatment of locally advanced pelvic disease has been described by multiple authors.[69,70,72,80]

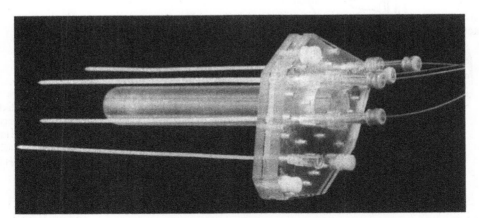

Figure 16.28 A customized template used for guiding needles in a perineal implant. The pattern of holes drilled for insertion of needles is tailored for treatment of a lesion in the lower pelvis.

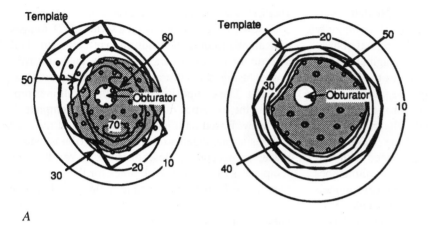

A

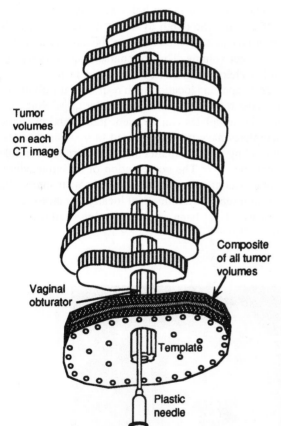

B

Figure 16.29 *A.* With standard templates *(left),* the needle pattern is predetermined and can result in hot spots and lack of target coverage, while customized templates *(right)* can be designed to provide optimal dose uniformity and target coverage. *B.* The tumor extent in each CT image is "stacked" with respect to the vaginal obturator. The shape of the tumor in the "template's-eye view" is then determined.

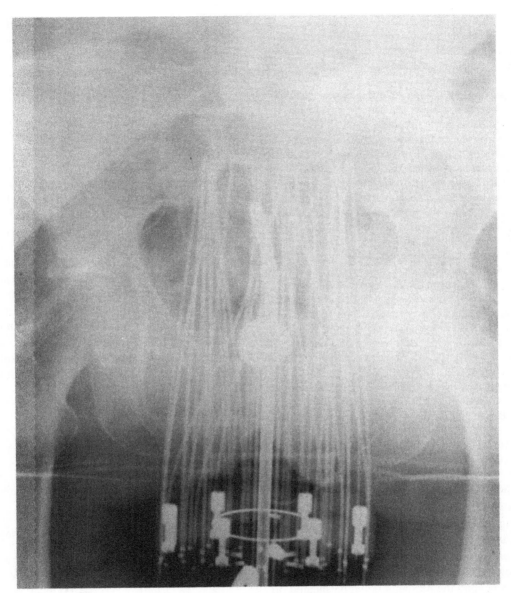

Figure 16.30 Radiograph of perineal template using steel needles and a uterine tandem. As with all larger transperineal implants, the needles often change path as they encounter bone or a hard tumor mass and are thus deflected.

Case Presentation

A 76-year-old woman was referred for consideration of radiation therapy for a squamous cell carcinoma of the uterine cervix, stage IIIA. On examination, she was found to have a friable tumor mass involving the cervix and extending onto the walls of the vaginal canal down to the introitus. There was bilateral medial parametrial involvement. The patient had undergone a supracervical hysterectomy 36 years prior to the diagnosis of malignant disease. Metastatic workup revealed no rectal or bladder involvement and no extension beyond the pelvis. The patient received 5040 cGy to the whole pelvis via external-beam irradiation. At the completion of the course of external-beam treatment, there was essentially complete regression of the tumor mass in the cervix and vaginal walls.

Approximately 3 weeks following the completion of external-beam irradiation, the patient was admitted for an interstitial template implant.

Based on the configuration of the disease, it was elected to load only 27 of the 44 guide holes in the transperineal butterfly template. The guide holes in the most lateral aspects of the template were each loaded with ten ^{192}Ir seeds, but only in the deepest segment of the needles to provide coverage of the parametrial region. Difficulty was encountered in the insertion of some of these needles, due to the intersecting bone, which forced the needles to curve medially. The centrally located guide holes were loaded with ten ^{192}Ir seeds each, but only in the lower region surrounding the vagina. The central guide holes anterior and posterior to the vaginal obturator were not loaded in an attempt to reduce the dose to the bladder and rectum. An intracavitary tandem, loaded with two cesium sources (14.4 and 10.5 mg Ra eq), was inserted into the remaining cervical canal (Fig. 16.30).

The sources remained in place for 22 h, delivering an estimated dose of 3080 cGy to point A, 1540 cGy to point B, and 1100 cGy at 0.5 cm depth in the vaginal mucosa. The maximum dose to the bladder was estimated to be 1500 cGy, and to the rectum approximately 1200 cGy.

The insertion of an interstitial template implant requires general anesthesia, while it can be removed following administration of oral analgesics. The needles used in perineal templates must have blind ends to prevent the radioactive ribbons from projecting beyond the tips of the needles. If a loaded ribbon protrudes beyond the needle, it could be sheared off during removal, causing sources to be left behind unintentionally.

OTHER TEMPLATE IMPLANTS

Improved spacing and parallelism could be achieved in a breast implant if, for example, a template similar to that described for transperineal implants were used. Hollow tubes such as nasogastric tubes can also be used. The tubes are secured on the breast

surface in the entrance and exit region. Holes are made at the desired spacing and stainless steel needles are pushed through the breast to the opposite side. Corresponding holes are made in the nasogastric tubes placed in the exit region and the exiting needles are pushed through these holes as well. The plastic tubing is inserted through the needle and the needle is then withdrawn, leaving the plastic tubing in place, as previously described. The implant is then loaded in conventional fashion.

Small rectal lesions can be implanted using a similar technique. A nasogastric tube with stainless steel needles pushed through the walls at equal spacing can be curved to form a semicircle (or, alternatively, a circle) and placed overlying the lesion adjacent to the anal canal (Fig. 16.31). The nasogastric tube is secured by suturing it to the skin. The blind stainless steel (or, alternatively, plastic) needles are pushed in through the lesion (Fig. 16.32). A second plane of needles can be inserted in a similar fashion outside the first. Figure 7.32 illustrates such a two-plane rectal implant; it uses blind stainless steel needles, but plastic needles would probably make the procedure

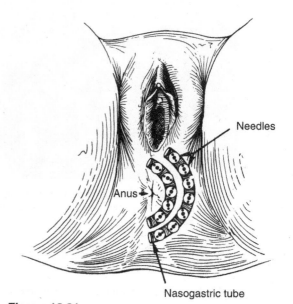

Figure 16.31 An individualized template can be made of nasogastric tubing, which is used to guide the spacing of the needles.

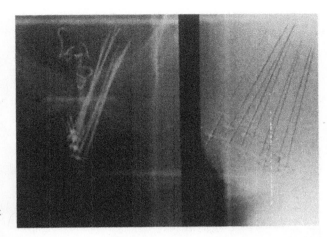

Figure 16.32   Orthogonal radiographs of a rectal implant using two semicircles, as shown in Fig. 16.31.

more comfortable for the patient. The length of the needles is determined by the depth of the lesion. A similar technique can be used for implants of urethral or paravaginal lesions.

Case Presentation

A 48-year-old female patient presented with a lesion 2 cm in diameter on the left lateral wall of the rectum 4 to 5 cm above the anal verge. A biopsy showed adenocarcinoma, and the patient was diagnosed as having adenocarcinoma of the rectum, stage A. She underwent a wide local excision followed by 4500 cGy to the whole pelvis via external-beam irradiation. This was followed approximately 2 weeks later by a two-plane semicircular iridium implant. The inner semicircle contained four blind needles with eight ^{192}Ir seeds each, and the outer semicircle, placed 1 cm farther out from the anus, contained five needles with eight ^{192}Ir seeds each. The seeds were spaced 1 cm apart in the ribbon and the needles were spaced 1 cm from each other. Figure 16.32 shows the anterior and lateral localization films obtained for dose-calculation purposes. The implant remained in place 21.5 h, delivering a minimum target-volume dose of 1500 cGy.

Case Presentation

A 72-year-old female patient was referred for postoperative irradiation of a periurethral lesion. She underwent a radical hysterectomy 8 years prior to the referral for stage 1B carcinoma of the cervix. She did well until 2 years prior to her referral, when she was found to have squamous cell carcinoma of the vagina. This was thought to be a new primary tumor. The lesion was excised, but 1 year following the excision, she was found to have a periurethral nodule just inside the introitus. This was also excised, leaving practically no vaginal canal, and she was referred for postoperative irradiation. Physical examination was unremarkable with the exception of the pelvic exam, which revealed absence of the vagina and some induration in the right periurethral area. The patient was diagnosed as having squamous-cell carcinoma of the vagina, recurrent post-local excision. She received 3000 cGy to the lesion via external-beam irradiation using two anterior oblique wedged fields. This was followed approximately 2 weeks later by an interstitial iridium implant.

The implant technique was similar to the one described for the rectal lesion. She had two planes forming two parallel semicircles from approximately 1 to 5 o'clock. There were four needles in the inner and five in the outer semicircle. Each needle was loaded with four ^{192}Ir seeds spaced 1 cm apart (Fig. 16.33). The implant remained in place for 44 h, delivering 3520 cGy to the volume encompassed by the 80-cGy/h line.

These two cases were treated using the same technique, although both the anatomy and the location of the tumor were very different. They are included to illustrate how one technique can easily be adapted to other situations.

A note of caution must be added regarding the

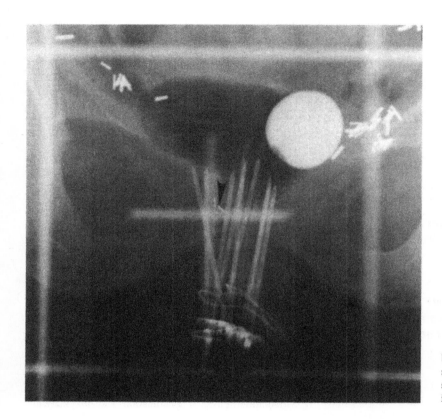

Figure 16.33 A periurethral lesion implanted using a custom-designed template technique. Arrowhead indicates tumor-marking seeds.

removal of this kind of implant. Blind needles must be used to prevent the radioactive ribbons from exiting the deep end of an open needle and entering the tissue. During removal, the segment extending outside the needle can easily be sheared off and thus become lodged in the tissues, as previously indicated. When this happens, surgical removal is the only option; this is difficult, hazardous, and embarrassing.

OTHER IMPLANT TECHNIQUES

GOLD-BUTTON TECHNIQUES

A gold-button technique is sometimes used for implants of head and neck lesions. Hollow stainless steel needles are inserted into the neck through the tumor until they extend into the oral cavity. With one end of the needle projecting through the oral mucosa and the other end presenting on the skin surface, plastic tubes with a gold button attached to the already sealed intraoral end, and with a silk thread tied under the button, are threaded through the needles, starting at the intraoral end of the needle (Fig. 16.34). The stainless steel needles are then removed and the plastic tubes are left in place. Steel buttons are lightly crimped onto the tubes close to the skin surface. When all plastic tubes are fixed in place, all silk threads are brought through a Penrose drain, which is taped to the patient's cheek. The loading of radioactive ribbons through the tubes is practically the same as described above for other techniques.

The gold-button technique serves a dual role: it spaces and retains the plastic tubes in place and protects overlying tissues against unnecessary irradiation and friction caused by the needles. This technique is most useful for interstitial therapy of oral and oropharyngeal tumors.

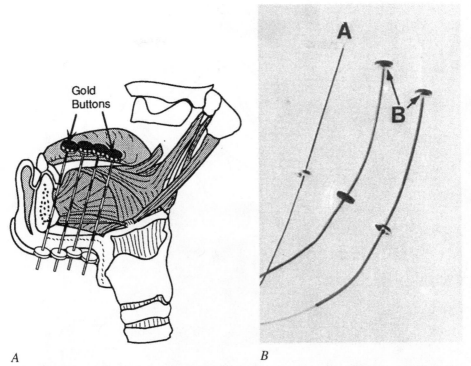

Figure 16.34 *A.* Diagram of a gold-button implant in the tongue. *B.* A blind needle (A) and two gold-button ribbons (B).

Case Presentation

A 52-year-old female patient presented with squamous-cell carcinoma of the posterior tongue. She received 5000 cGy via external-beam irradiation followed by an interstitial implant using the gold-button technique previously described. Seven ribbons, each containing ^{192}Ir seeds, were inserted (Fig. 16.35). The first two seeds at the end nearest the gold button were spaced only 0.5 cm apart; in the remainder of the ribbons, the seeds were spaced 1 cm apart. The intention was to substitute higher loading near the end of the implant for the crossing needle.

LOOP TECHNIQUES

Alternatively, a loop technique can be used for implants in the oral cavity. This technique utilizes pairs of hollow steel needles that are inserted through the neck on either side of the mandible throughout the tumor volume. The needles protrude through the oral mucosa, with the other end presenting on the skin surface. Open-ended plastic tubing, previously described, is threaded through each pair of needles so that the result is an inverted "U." The steel needles are removed and the plastic tubes are left in place (Fig. 16.36). The fixation, localization, dose calculation, and loading procedures are essentially the same as previously described.

REMOVAL OF INTERSTITIAL IMPLANTS

Removal of temporary interstitial implants requires care and skill, or seeds may accidentally be left in the patient. For the removal of implants using open-ended plastic tubing, such as shown for breast im-

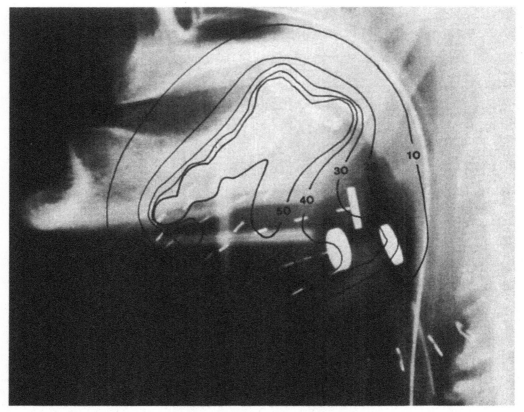

Figure 16.35   Dose-rate distribution superimposed on a radiograph of an implant in the posterior third of the tongue using a gold-button technique.

plants above, a special wire cutter, adjusted to clip only the outer plastic tube and spare the seed ribbon, is used in the removal. The plastic tube should be cut between the skin surface and the button, revealing the radioactive ribbon, which is then removed and the seeds counted before being placed in an appropriately shielded container. Following assurances that all seeds have been removed, including a negative radiation survey of the patient, the plastic tube is cut near the skin on the opposite side and the remaining portion is pulled out. Radioactive sources must always be removed before the plastic tube is pulled out so that, in the rare event that a source (seed) is left behind, a pathway for its retrieval remains intact.

REMOVABLE INTERSTITIAL BRAIN IMPLANTS

The use of removable implants in the management of certain brain tumors is becoming increasingly popular. Some solitary brain tumors can be cured by surgery and radiation therapy. Delivery of cancerocidal doses to large brain fields via external-beam irradiation is often prevented by the radiation toxicity in the surrounding normal brain tissue. External-beam irradiation can therefore be followed by a boost (higher dose to a smaller volume) via an interstitial implant using ^{192}Ir or another radionuclide. Interstitial implants, using low-energy, high-activity ^{125}I seeds, can be used to treat recurrent brain tumors in patients

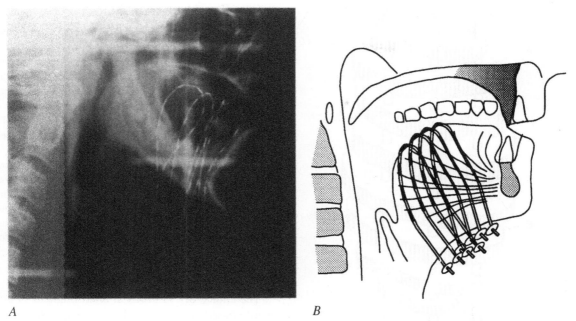

A

B

Figure 16.36   Radiograph *(A)* and a diagram *(B)* of a loop implant in the tongue. The implant consisted of four loops each holding eleven ^{192}Ir seeds.

who have already received high-dose irradiation and in whom it is therefore critical to tailor the dose distribution to the shape of the tumor. The relatively low energy of ^{125}I and rapid dose fall-off away from the seeds makes it more suitable for such tailoring than most other radionuclides.

Although not practiced extensively, interstitial brachytherapy has been used to treat brain tumors since the early 1900s.[81] In the last several decades, stereotactic implantation of radioisotopes, primarily to treat low-grade gliomas, has been practiced, particularly in Europe.[82-87] The integration of stereotactic systems with computed tomography scanners, with which tumor targets can be visualized and implants precisely placed, as well as the availability of possibly more effective isotopes, are some factors that make the continued use and refinement of brachytherapy attractive in the treatment of malignant brain tumors.[88,89]

The procedure is very labor-intensive and requires special equipment and computers for use in treatment planning. Very high activity ^{125}I seeds (ap-

proximately 40 mCi/seed) are typically used, although other isotopes can also be employed. This requires special ordering of seeds several days prior to the procedure. Efforts to minimize the number of seeds in order to limit the cost of the procedure are made by optimized planning of seed placement. Three-dimensional viewing of the target volume is possible with some treatment-planning computer software, but a manual three-dimensional reconstruction, although a time-consuming procedure, can be made (Fig. 16.37). Prior to the actual insertion of the catheters, a stereotactic frame is attached to the patient's cranium.[90-92] A contrast-enhanced CT study is then obtained throughout the tumor volume (Fig. 16.38).

Placement of the catheters or tubes holding the radioactive seeds is chosen from at least two CT images. The points selected for a given catheter, with respect to reference points of the frame, are entered into the computer that drives the stereotactic device. The computer calculates the coordinates, angle, and depth necessary for precise placement of each cath-

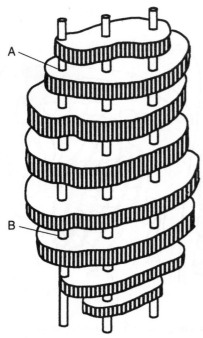

Figure 16.37 Three-dimensional representation of a brain tumor and the planned catheter placement. A point through which the catheter must pass is selected on each of two images (*A* and *B*). These points must be selected so that the catheter also pass through the tumor at the desired locations on all other images.

eter. After these parameters are set on the stereotactic device, the location of the entry point is indicated on the scalp. A hole is then drilled through the cranium at this point and at the angle indicated by the computer. The catheter is then pushed through the tumor to the depth indicated by the computer. When the catheter is in place, it is sutured to the scalp to prevent motion. This procedure is carried out in the operating room under light sedation and local anesthesia.

Following the patient's recovery, the position of the catheters is verified radiographically. Dose distributions are calculated using dummy seeds inserted in afterloading tubes that fit inside the catheters. When the placement of the dummy seeds is acceptable, they are replaced by identical inserts carrying the active seeds, which remain in place for several days until the desired dose is delivered.

Case Presentation

A 32-year-old female patient was referred for consideration of stereotactic brain implant of a recurrent astrocytoma. Three years prior to the referral she underwent resection of a grade I–II malignant astrocytoma. This was followed by 5900 cGy via external-beam irradiation. Approximately 2 years later, she presented with a recurrence, which was resected and showed grade III–IV astrocytoma. She was subsequently given seven cycles of chemotherapy, but failed again.

Three stereotactically controlled catheters were inserted into the tumor in the operating room. She was then brought to the simulator room, where orthogonal radiographs (Fig. 16.39), using dummy seeds, were obtained. Two high-intensity (40 mCi) ^{125}I seeds were inserted in each catheter. The implant was left in place for 144 h, delivering 8640 cGy at the 60-cGy/h line, which enclosed the lesion and a 0.5 cm margin.

The choice of ^{125}I seeds in brain implants is primarily based on its relatively low energy, which results in accentuated sparing of surrounding normal tissue. The cranium functions as a shield during the implant, and radiation that does have sufficient energy to penetrate the bone can effectively be stopped by a lead-shielded helmet. Personnel are easily protected by lead aprons, which are virtually useless for protection against commonly used isotopes other than ^{125}I.

The use of a stereotactic frame has been extended to include localization of the target in an external-beam treatment technique referred to as stereotactic radiosurgery. In this technique, also discussed in Chap. 10, a very high dose (1000 to 3000 cGy) is delivered in a single fraction to small brain tumors or arteriovenous malformations (AVM), a benign condition. Precise tailoring of the dose to the target is critical in these treatments due to the very high single-fraction dose.

OPHTHALMIC PLAQUE TREATMENT

Treatment of ocular malignancies using ^{222}Ru seeds was described many years ago.[93] More recently, plaques using ^{60}Co, ^{106}Ru, ^{192}Ir, or ^{125}I have been used for the treatment of ocular melanomas.[94–102]

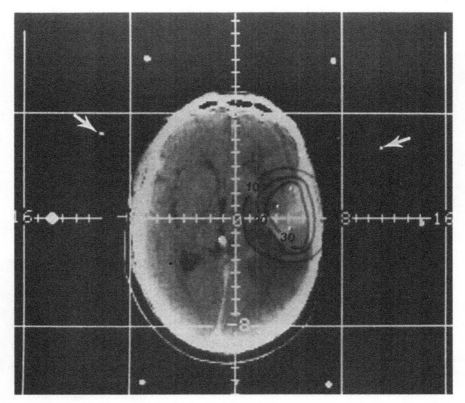

Figure 16.38 A contrast-enhanced CT obtained with the stereotactic frame in place immediately prior to a brain implant. The bars of the frame (seen as light spots in the periphery of the skull) are used as reference points.

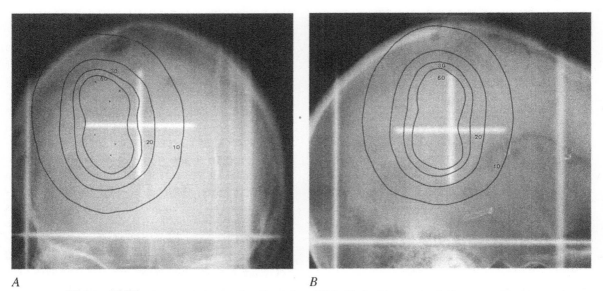

A   *B*

Figure 16.39 Orthogonal localization films of an ^{125}I implant of a recurrent brain tumor with the dose-rate distribution superimposed. The dose in this patient was calculated to the 30 cGy/h line as seen in the dose distribution.

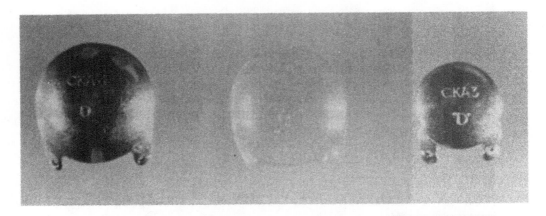

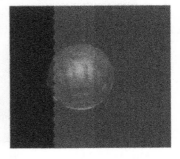

Figure 16.40   Cobalt-60 eye plaques (10 and 15 mm in diameter) with an acrylic dummy *(above)*. Iodine-125 eye plaque with the seed carrier loaded and in place inside the gold shield *(right)*. (Also see Fig. 15.4, Chap 15.)

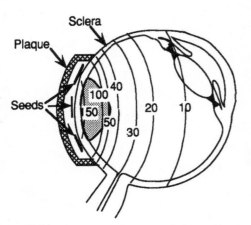

Figure 16.41   Dose-rate distribution (cGy/h) resulting from a ^{125}I loading with 13 seeds containing 1 mCi/seed.

Cobalt-60 plaques can be purchased in standard sizes and shapes, while plaques with a seed-carrier insert can be individually made to fit a given lesion (Fig. 16.40). The desired dose rate and dose pattern are calculated prior to the purchase of the seeds.[103] The seeds are then loaded into the seed carrier in the planned pattern. The plaques have at least two suturing eyelets, so that they can be anchored to the eye over the lesion. Figure 16.41 shows dose rates from a 16-mm-diameter ^{125}I plaque and a schematic representation of an ophthalmic implant. The dimensions of the lesion are determined via ultrasound. The treatment is usually prescribed at the apex of the lesion and doses on the order of 8000 to 10,000 cGy are typically delivered over several days. The maximum dose is obviously at the base of the lesion, which is nearest the surface of the plaque.

The dose to the sclera exceeds 40,000 cGy in some cases.

These plaques are inserted and removed in the operating room in a procedure that requires mild sedation and local anesthesia. The tumor margins, visualized when a light source is placed on the opposite side, are marked on the sclera. The dose to the operating surgeon is limited by the use of a transparent dummy plaque, with suture eyelets identical to those of the hot plaque. The dummy is sutured to the sclera over the tumor in such a way that it can be removed while the sutures remain in the tissues. A second transillumination procedure, verifying that the tumor shadow lies within the boundaries of the transparent plaque, is carried out before the dummy plaque is removed. The dummy plaque is replaced by the hot plaque, which is quickly anchored to the eye by threading the already existing sutures through the matching eyelets. This type of plaque treatment has also been described for the treatment of retinoblastoma.[104,105]

A strontium-90 ophthalmic applicator, primarily used for treatment of pterygium, a benign condition of the cornea, is described in Chap. 15.

PERMANENT INTERSTITIAL IMPLANTS

The advantage of permanent implants is that the seeds can be placed in inaccessible tumors where removal would be impractical or impossible. An example of this would be a deep pelvic or abdominal tumor where the radioactive sources can be im-

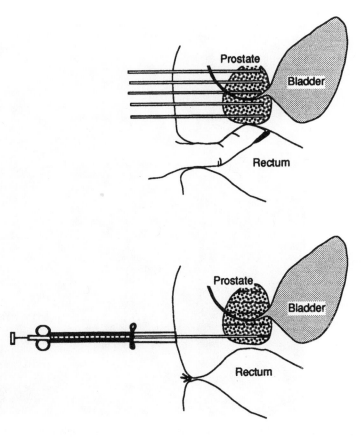

Figure 16.42 Permanent implant of ^{125}I seeds in the prostate. Digital palpation is employed to prevent puncture of the rectal wall and to guide the needles in the prostate *(top)*. A gun-type device is then used to deposit the seeds with uniform spacing as each needle is withdrawn *(bottom)*.

planted during a surgical procedure. Removal would require another surgical procedure within a few days, which the patient's condition may not permit.

Radioisotopes with relatively short half-lives are best suited for permanent implants because most of the dose is deposited early on, before the seeds have a chance to become displaced. Iodine 125, which also has relatively low energy, is beneficial in implants of tumors near radiosensitive organs, where a very rapid fall-off of dose is desired. Low-activity ^{125}I seeds implanted in the prostate (Fig. 16.42), where the proximity of the rectum prevents high doses from being delivered via external-beam treatment, are sometimes used.[106–109] Permanent implants of ^{125}I seeds in other pelvic, abdominal, or lung tumors can also be used.[110]

Since devices such as those used to insert and maintain seed spacing in the removable implants previously described cannot be used in permanent implants, other devices built to insert and guide the spacing of permanently implanted seeds have been developed.[111–113]

A gun-type applicator is used to insert seeds in a uniform pattern in deep-seated tumors. The seeds are loaded into a cartridge that fits onto the applicator. Hollow stainless steel needles are inserted into the tumor to the desired depth and with uniform spacing. The applicator is attached to one needle at a time. One seed is pushed through the needle into the tissues, using a plunger. The stainless steel needle is withdrawn 1 cm (for 1-cm spacing) and another seed is deposited at the tip of the needle. This procedure is repeated until the desired length has been implanted, after which the needle is removed. The remaining needles are then loaded in a similar fashion until all needles have been removed. This technique is par-

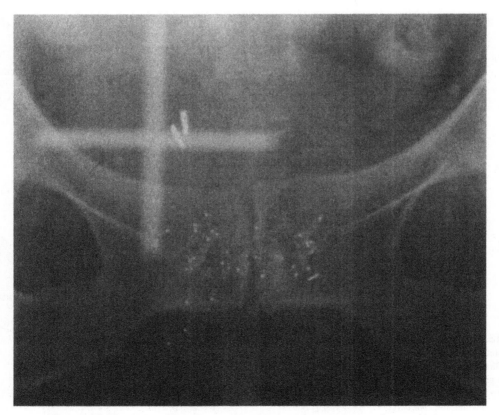

Figure 16.43   Iodine-125 seeds permanently implanted in a recurrent periurethral lesion.

ticularly useful for deep-seated tumors in the pelvis and abdomen.

PERMANENT IMPLANTS IN THE PELVIS

Case Presentation

A 60-year-old female patient was referred for radiation therapy of a periurethral recurrence of a squamous cell carcinoma of the cervix. She underwent a full course of radiation therapy to the whole pelvis via external-beam treatment and two intracavitary ^{137}Cs insertions 9 years prior to the presentation. An earlier recurrence was treated by a radical hysterectomy.

Under general anesthesia, 17 steel needles were placed in the tumor in a cylindrical fashion. These were afterloaded with ^{125}I seeds using the gun-type applicator previously described. A total of 64 seeds were inserted. The average activity was 0.62 mCi per seed (Fig. 16.43), which delivered 4000 cGy to the implanted volume. The patient was instructed to collect and submit all urine for survey to detect radioactive seeds that could possibly have been excreted in the urine.

Dose calculation for a large number of seeds is very complicated, and the ^{125}I seeds are also very difficult to visualize on a radiograph, even under optimal conditions. A technique referred to as the dimension-averaging technique has been developed and used for many years in permanent implants.[114,115] In this technique, the total activity, in mCi, of ^{125}I is taken to be five times the average of three mutually perpendicular dimensions, in centimeters of a treatment region encompassing the tumor. In a 4 × 5 × 2 cm tumor, the average dimension is 3.66 cm; therefore, 18.3 (3.66 × 5) mCi I-125 is needed. The number of seeds required is given by dividing the total activity needed by the available seed strength. The seed activity is usually between 0.4 and 0.6 mCi/seed. Prescription for the spacing of the seeds can be obtained from an ^{125}I spacing nomograph.[114]

PERMANENT IMPLANTS IN THE LUNG

Gold (Au 198) seeds are also suitable for permanent implants due to their very short half-life (2.7 days from Table 15.1). Although the use of ^{125}I seeds in implants of bronchial lesions appears more popular[116-122], gold seeds are also used. Serious difficulty is sometimes encountered in the precise placement of the seeds in lung implants due to the long distance over which one must manipulate the instrument and the seeds. Optimized distribution rules for gold implants have been studied.[123]

Case Presentation

A 56-year-old male patient was referred for consideration of a bronchial implant of a recurrent squamous cell carcinoma of the lung. The patient received 5500 cGy to the primary lesion in the right upper lobe via external-beam irradiation approximately 1 year prior to the consultation. Bronchoscopy revealed a mass growing into the right side of the trachea approximately 1 cm above the branching off of the right main stem bronchus. Further external-beam irradiation was precluded because the normal-tissue tolerance in this region had been reached.

The patient was taken to the operating room where eight ^{198}Au seeds were inserted via a bronchoscope. A long steel needle, especially designed for this type of implant, was used. Each seed contained 5.8 mCi at the time of the procedure. The implant delivered a minimum tumor dose of 3000 cGy (Fig. 16.44). This procedure was carried out in an attempt to palliate symptoms of bleeding and coughing.

PERMANENT IMPLANTS IN THE HEAD AND NECK

Gold seeds, permanently implanted, can be effective in the treatment of very small lesions in the oral cavity, particularly as an alternative to a more invasive procedure in patients who cannot undergo general anesthesia.[124]

Case Presentation

An 88-year-old female patient was referred for radiation therapy of a recurrent squamous cell carcinoma of the floor of the mouth. She had received 6000 cGy via external-beam irradiation 8 years prior to this recurrence. The patient had a history of congestive heart failure, so an implant requiring general anesthesia was precluded. Examination of the oral cavity revealed a 2.5 × 3.5 cm lesion on the left oral tongue with extension into the buccal gingival sulcus. Under local anesthesia, six ^{198}Au seeds were inserted in the lesion (Fig. 16.45). Each seed had an activity of 2.8 mCi at the time

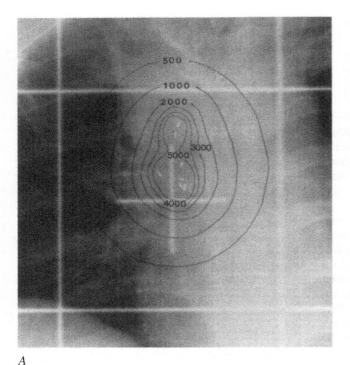

A

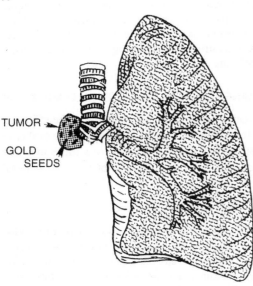

B

Figure 16.44 *A*. Eight [198]Au seeds implanted in a recurrent lesion in the trachea just above the branching off of the right main stem bronchus. The numbers along the lines of the superimposed dose distribution on this lateral radiograph represent the total dose delivered, in centigray. A diagram *(B)* shows the tumor location.

of the insertion and dose calculations showed that the minimum tumor dose from the implant was 4000 cGy. The patient tolerated the procedure very well despite her age and was able to return home the same day without requiring hospitalization.

PERMANENT IMPLANTS USING ABSORBABLE SUTURES

Another technique for permanent seed implantation that has been described consists of inserting absorb-

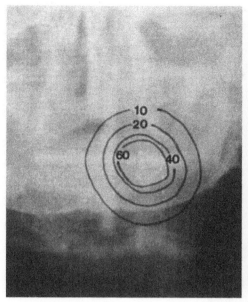 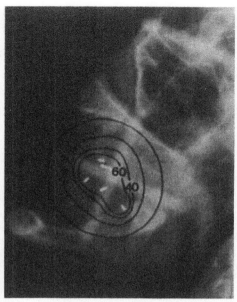

Figure 16.45   Six ^{198}Au seeds permanently implanted in a recurrent lesion in the floor of the mouth of an 88-year-old female patient. The numbers along the lines in the superimposed dose distribution represent the total dose in grays delivered to the tumor.

able sutures with ^{125}I seeds interspaced at 1-cm distances.[125–128] This method is primarily used for relatively flat tumors of the bladder, chest wall, and so on. A technique utilizing ^{125}I seeds embedded in absorbable Gelfoam which is sewn in place with an absorbable Vicryl mesh* has also been described.[129]

A similar technique using an absorbable mesh for the treatment of chest wall tumors has been described.[130] In this technique, the gross tumor is surgically resected and a layer of absorbable Vicryl mesh is sutured to the tumor bed. Afterloading catheters, separated by 1.5 cm, are sewn into the mesh using absorbable chromium sutures. The ends of the catheters extend outside the chest cavity and a second layer of Vicryl mesh is sutured on top of the afterloading catheters and to adjacent fixed tissues. The catheters are sutured to the skin to prevent motion and wire cables are placed inside the catheters to keep them patent until loading of the ^{192}Ir seed ribbons takes place. At the completion of the implant, the radioactive seed ribbons are removed and, since the catheters were secured by using absorbable su-

tures, they can also be pulled out if enough time has elapsed for the sutures to disintegrate. The mesh dissolves over a period of time and leaves no residue. This procedure has been used to treat both lung tumors and chest wall lesions.

INTRALUMINAL IMPLANTS

A plastic tube holding radioactive sources and inserted into the lumen of a tube-shaped organ such as the biliary tract, bronchus, or the esophagus is referred to as an intraluminal implant.[131–140]

Obstructing lesions in the bile duct require high radiation doses to a very limited volume. Insertion of ^{192}Ir seed ribbons into a percutaneously placed intracholangial catheter (Fig. 16.46) can be used in the treatment of such lesions.[131,133,135,138,139] The radioactive ribbon is inserted under fluoroscopic guidance. Contrast is introduced to determine the dimensions of the bile duct for dose calculation purposes. The implant remains in place until approximately 5000 cGy is delivered at 5 mm from the center of the catheter. The rapid fall-off of dose allows high mu-

* Ethicon, Sommerville, NJ.

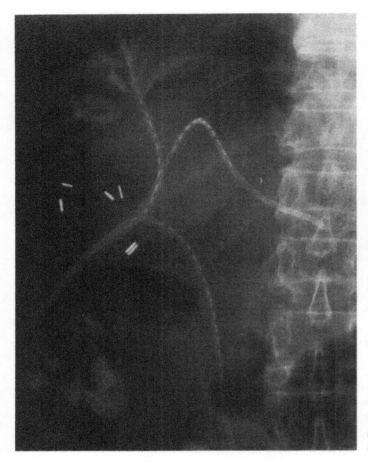

Figure 16.46   Intraluminal ^{192}Ir treatment of obstructive biliary duct tumor. The radioactive ribbons are inserted via an intracholangial catheter.

cosal dose to be delivered without adverse effects. When external-beam and intraluminal irradiation are combined, the dose is modified. The authors of a study in which the two modalities were combined conclude that 4000 cGy via external beam and 2000 cGy delivered in five high-dose-rate fractions was appropriate and was well tolerated.[133]

Insertion of radioactive sources in the bronchus or trachea to treat obstructing bronchial tumors was first described by Yankauer using radium[141] and more recently by other authors using iridium.[142–144] An afterloading tube is inserted under fiberoptic bronchoscopic guidance. A lead marker in the leading end of the tube indicates the depth of insertion on radiographs. Following radiographic verification of

location and determination of the length of the radioactive ribbon using dummy seeds, the ^{192}Ir seed ribbon is inserted (Fig. 16.47). The dose is usually calculated at 0.5 cm from the center of the seed ribbon and a dose of 3000 cGy is delivered in approximately 2 days.

Placement of radioactive sources in the esophagus to boost the dose in small esophageal lesions or for palliation of symptoms in patients with recurrent tumors is sometimes used in desperate attempts to prolong the survival of patients with a dismal prognosis (Fig. 16.48). Syed *et al.* reported 37 patients with primary esophageal carcinoma treated with external-beam irradiation to 45 to 50 Gy followed by intraluminal irradiation delivering 25 to 35 Gy in

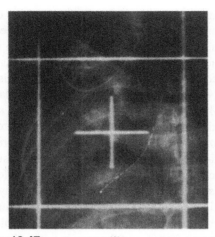

Figure 16.47 A bronchial ^{192}Ir seed ribbon containing 23 seeds spaced 0.5 cm apart is placed inside an afterloading tube. Note the leading lead marker. This ribbon was left in place for 48 h, delivering 3000 cGy at 0.5 cm from the center of the seed ribbon.

two applications and 10 patients with recurrent esophageal carcinoma treated only with two intraluminal applications delivering 50 to 60 Gy. The dose was calculated at 0.5 cm from the outer surface of the applicator. Both groups also received 5-flourouracil infusion. Eighty-one percent (38/47) of these patients had excellent palliation of symptoms and were able to swallow until they died of metastatic disease.[140] Caspers *et al.* reported on 35 patients receiving 50 to 60 Gy via external-beam irradiation followed by a boost using a low-dose-rate intraluminal implant delivering 15 to 20 Gy. The acute toxicity was minor. Six weeks posttreatment, 32 of 35 patients were able to eat solid food. The median survival, however, was 11 months, with a 1- and 2-year survival of 42 and 10 percent, respectively. Late complications were seen in 17 percent of the patients, but these were severe in only one instance and were probably treatment-related.[145] Hishikawa *et al.* have reported on the use of high-dose-rate intraluminal implants in esophageal carcinoma[146] and have also reported on autopsy findings of patients treated using external-beam irradiation alone or in combination with high-dose-rate intraluminal irradiation.[147]

REMOTE-CONTROLLED AFTERLOADING DEVICES AND TECHNIQUES

All afterloading techniques described in the previous sections require handling of radioactive sources during the preparation and actual loading of the sources into the previously inserted apparatus. Direct handling of the radioactivity is eliminated by using a remote-controlled afterloading technique. Such equipment, developed during the early 1960s, has gained increased popularity in recent years. These units were first designed for use in gynecologic brachytherapy,[7,148-153] but more recent models can be used for other sites as well.

Modern remote-controlled afterloading units consist of a lead-shielded storage area for radioactive sources, several channels for source transport, a remote loading and unloading system, and a variety of applicators that are inserted into the patient in the usual fashion. Following radiographic verification of their position using dummy sources, the optimal source configuration and dose distribution are determined and the desired loading is programmed on a microcomputer. The sources, shaped as pellets or

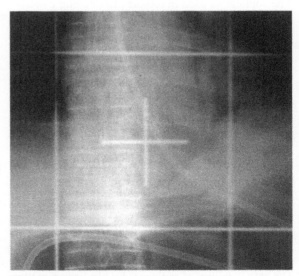

Figure 16.48 Intraluminal implant to treat an esophageal tumor.

tubes, are automatically arranged as programmed within each channel, with inactive spacers between the active pellets to achieve the desired spacing. Each transport tube is coupled to each receptor of the apparatus in the patient, who remains in an adjoining room during the treatment. After all personnel have left the treatment room and the door is closed, the treatment is initiated from a remote-controlled switch. The sources and spacers are transported via a pneumatic transport system into the applicator within a few seconds. The unloading of the sources is also accomplished via remote control and requires only a few seconds. Sedation is seldom needed, and multiple treatments are given usually on an outpatient basis.

Other remote-controlled afterloading units use one high-activity linear source, which is inserted into apparatus previously placed in or adjacent to the tumor. The computer of the afterloading unit is programmed so that the source will oscillate within each channel of the applicator[154,155] and so that it remains longer at a segment requiring a higher dose than at segments requiring a lower dose.

Remote-controlled afterloading systems can be used with various types of applicators, not only those designed for gynecologic intracavitary brachytherapy but also those used in interstitial brachytherapy. The applicators used in remote afterloading gynecologic brachytherapy are similar in design to the conventional tandem-and-ovoid system. Remote afterloading eliminates any contact with the radioactive material for the clinical staff. The ease with which the sources are loaded and unloaded makes it possible to return them to the shielded system while personnel work near the patient, thus minimizing staff exposure.[1] Remote afterloading systems are not totally problem-free and must be operated by trained and experienced personnel who exercise extreme caution and follow all safety procedures.

QUALITY ASSURANCE AND RADIATION SAFETY

The safe handling of radioactivity has been a matter of concern in hospitals for many years. The generally very small, innocuous-looking sources can cause considerable harm to uninformed and unsuspecting persons, but they present little danger when strict regulations with respect to handling and storage are enforced and proper facilities are provided. It is particularly necessary to have a carefully planned source-handling room (often called a *radium room*, although radium is rarely used any longer) in order to minimize exposure to personnel.[156] A comprehensive quality-assurance program specifically designed for brachytherapy procedures should be in effect in all radiation oncology departments with brachytherapy facilities.[157] Such protocols should be in compliance with the regulations of the Nuclear Regulatory Commission (NRC) and the state in which the institution is located. The aim of these procedures should be to minimize exposure to personnel, patients, and visitors. The exposure to personnel can be reduced by minimizing the time during which the radioactive sources are being transferred between their storage place and the patient. Using tools with long handles increases the distance between the source and the hands of the user; thus exposure is reduced. Finally, standing behind a shield when the sources are handled further reduces exposure to the body of the user. Adequate equipment, in addition to well-trained personnel, is also necessary for the safe handling of radioactive sources. Consideration should be given to limiting the number of staff persons in the room where radioactive sources are being loaded or removed from either the afterloading carriers or the patient. In teaching institutions, where it is necessary to teach others proper handling procedures, the trainees should be as far away as possible while still being able to observe.

An adequate inventory of sources and source activities must always be maintained for gynecologic implants. The sources should be stored in a locked room in an inaccessible area. A shielded "safe" with several drawers, of which only one is opened at a time, will minimize exposure to personnel who must open the safe for loading and unloading. Each drawer should contain approximately the same amount of activity to minimize exposure while it is opened for source removal or return. The location of each individual tube, identified by an engraved serial number, and its current activity should be carefully documented on a map located near the storage safe. Color coding of the sources simplifies identification, thus reducing the exposure time and the risks for errors. Only the color-coded end should be visible when the drawer is opened, and the remainder of the source should be behind sufficient lead to prevent unnecessary exposure. Long-handled instruments must also be used to maintain the greatest possible distance between the source and the operator.

A lead-shielded work space immediately adjacent to the safe is necessary so that the person loading the sources into the apparatus can stand behind the shield while manipulating the sources with long-handled instruments. The shield should be high enough to protect the person up to the shoulders. A lead glass window placed above this allows visualization of the work area and also provides some shielding of the face and head. A lamp with a magnifying glass attached is very useful when serial numbers on the sources must be verified. A clamp to hold the tubes or apparatus when the sources are being loaded is a practical way of reducing the number of persons needed during the loading.

It is a good practice to limit the number of persons with access to the safe. An inventory log book is necessary to maintain strict control of where the sources are at any given time. Routine checks of the inventory must be made to verify that all sources are in the correct location.

Sources or seeds with short half-lives that are purchased for a certain implant are handled somewhat differently. Iridium seeds, for example, are purchased in nylon ribbons, while ^{125}I and ^{198}Au seeds are usually shipped individually. Immediately upon arrival, all seeds should be counted to ensure that nothing has been lost during transport. Shipping documents will indicate activity per seed on a certain date, as determined by the supplier. However, it is recommended that the user also determine the activity of each source before use. The seeds must be kept in a shielded and locked cabinet until they are returned to the supplier or are otherwise disposed of except, of course, when they are in the patient.

The number of seeds, the activity, and the container identification must be part of the record keeping. When the seeds are inserted into the patient, the number of seeds used, the time of the insertion, and the patient's name are noted along with the physician's name. The same information is noted at the time of removal. After the removed seeds are counted, the patient must be surveyed by means of a sensitive survey meter to verify that no radioactivity is left behind. This negative survey must be noted in the patient's chart.

As soon as possible following removal from the patient, the sources should be returned to the supplier or otherwise be disposed of. ^{198}Au and ^{125}I seeds, which are not usually returnable, should be removed from the active area and placed in a shielded and locked place to decay and prevent mixup with current seeds.

The time taken in preparing the sources and loading them into the patient must be kept to a minimum. Specially designed loading mechanisms can be built to minimize the exposure. Mirrors can be used to allow source preparation to be carried out behind lead shields via indirect visualization. All radioactive sources and seeds must be handled very carefully to avoid scratching, bending, or breaking them. Utmost care must be taken not to cut through a seed during these procedures. Some radioactive eye plaques, for example, must not be handled by any other part than by the suture eyelets, so as to avoid scratching the very thin platinum shell over the radioactive material. Wipe tests of such eye plaques, to verify that no leakage has occurred, are necessary before each implantation. Any leakage would result in radioactive deposits on the eye. A wipe test consists of careful wiping of the source with a moist cotton ball and then testing for the presence of radioactivity on the cotton ball, using a sensitive counter. These tests should be performed by a radiation safety officer or physicist, depending on the organization in the institution, and the results kept in a log.

Quality-control procedures must also be followed in the prescription and dose calculation of brachytherapy implants. It is particularly important that each computer-calculated dose distribution be verified by a hand calculation using standard tables. Tremendous errors can occur if, for example, a decimal point is wrongly placed when entering the source activity or if the magnification factors on the localization films are in error. A thorough review of the dose calculation is not always possible prior to loading of the sources, but it should be made as soon as possible, so that an error in the required duration of the implant can be discovered and corrected by either removing the entire implant or some source(s) prematurely or leaving them in longer. Dose distributions in several planes are necessary, particularly through areas where hot spots may be found. Omission of sources in that location, loading a lower activity source, or premature removal of sources in that area may be considered.

PROBLEMS

16.1 Afterloading techniques were developed primarily to reduce
   (a) The possibilities of errors in loading
   (b) The time required for the implant
   (c) Exposure to personnel

16.2 Radioactive sources frequently used in tandems and ovoids are in the shape of
   (a) Tubes
   (b) Seeds
   (c) Needles

16.3 Radioactive isotopes used in tandems and ovoids are usually
   (a) Iridium 192
   (b) Cobalt 60
   (c) Cesium 137
   (d) Strontium 90

16.4 Point A is defined in gynecologic implants to be a point located
   (a) 2 cm cephalad of the external cervical os and 5 cm lateral to the patient's midline
   (b) 2 cm cephalad of the external cervical os and 2 cm lateral to the patient's midline
   (c) 2 cm cephalad of the external cervical os and 5 cm lateral to the uterine tandem
   (d) 2 cm cephalad of the external cervical os and 2 cm lateral to the uterine tandem

16.5 In which of the following situations is the use of a tandem and ovoid *least* useful?
   (a) In a patient with a large exophytic lesion in the cervix extending into the vaginal apex
   (b) In a patient who has undergone a radical hysterectomy for squamous cell carcinoma of the cervix and now has a recurrence in the vaginal apex
   (c) In a patient who has undergone a supracervical hysterectomy and now has a recurrence in the cervical stump

16.6 Open-ended plastic tubing can be inserted and loaded
   (a) In implants where the tube can exit the tissue on the opposite side
   (b) In transperineal implants where there is no exit on the opposite side
   (c) In a brain implant where there is no exit on the opposite side

16.7 Ophthalmic plaques can be constructed for use with
   (a) Cobalt 60
   (b) Iodine 125
   (c) Ruthenium 106

      (*d*) Iridium 192

      (*e*) All of the above

16.8   High-activity iodine 125 seeds (40 mCi/seed) are frequently used in

      (*a*) Ophthalmic plaques

      (*b*) Brain implants

      (*c*) Lung implants

      (*d*) Esophageal implants

16.9   Isotopes used in permanent implants are most frequently

      (*a*) Iodine 125 and gold 198

      (*b*) Iridium 192 and gold 198

      (*c*) Cesium 137 and iridium 192

      (*d*) Radium 226 and iodine 125

16.10   Isotopes used in permanent implants are selected primarily because of their

      (*a*) Specific activity

      (*b*) Half-value thickness

      (*c*) Half-life

      (*d*) Durability

16.11   Customized transperineal templates are superior to standard templates because

      (*a*) They are easier to load

      (*b*) They are more comfortable for the patient

      (*c*) They can be designed to cover the target and loaded to deliver better dose uniformity

      (*d*) They can be designed to better cover the target and spare more normal tissue

16.12   Surface molds can be used to treat all of the following tumors *except*

      (*a*) A deep-seated tumor in the pelvic side wall

      (*b*) A lesion on the hard palate

      (*c*) A lesion in an exenterated orbit

      (*d*) A 1-cm-deep lesion in the preauricular region

16.13   Remote afterloading apparatus was first designed for

      (*a*) High-dose-rate treatment in any site

      (*b*) Gynecologic implants

      (*c*) Intraoperative use

      (*d*) Low-dose-rate treatment in any implant

16.14   To produce approximately the same dose rate on the surface of an ovoid, the source activity must

      (*a*) Be decreased as the ovoid diameter increases

      (*b*) Be increased as the ovoid diameter decreases

      (*c*) Be increased as the ovoid diameter increases

      (*d*) Not be changed

16.15   In ophthalmic plaque treatment of ocular melanoma, the scleral dose may exceed

      (*a*) 80,000 cGy

      (*b*) 60,000 cGy

(c) 40,000 cGy

(d) 100,000 cGy

16.16   In handling radioactive sources, long-handled instruments must be used to

(a) Reduce the time spent loading

(b) Reduce the exposure to the hands of the loader

(c) Increase the distance to the patient and thus reduce exposure to the patient

(d) Improve the accuracy of loading

16.17   Which of the following statements *best* describes the proper removal of an implant?

(a) The radioactive sources and apparatus holding the sources are all removed simultaneously

(b) The radioactive sources are removed first and then the apparatus holding the sources

(c) The apparatus holding the radioactive sources is not removed until all radioactive sources are accounted for and a negative survey has been obtained

(d) The order in which the implant sources and apparatus are removed is not important as long as the patient does not experience any pain

16.18   The use of intraluminal implants has been described for various sites except for the

(a) Esophagus

(b) Duodenum

(c) Biliary duct

(d) Bronchus

16.19   The isotope most frequently used in nasopharyngeal implants is

(a) Cesium 137

(b) Gold 198

(c) Iodine 125

(d) Strontium 90

16.20   The use of radium is rapidly being abandoned because

(a) There is none available to purchase

(b) It is especially hazardous

(c) The half-life is too long

(d) It is too expensive

REFERENCES

1. Grigsby PW, Perez CA, Eichling J, et al: Reduction in radiation exposure to nursing personnel with the use of remote afterloading brachytherapy devices. *Int J Radiat Oncol Biol Phys* 20:627, 1991.

2. Boyer AL, Wang CC, Gitterman M: A Luer lock afterloading device for iridium 192 brachytherapy. *Int J Radiat Oncol Biol Phys* 6:511, 1980.

3. Béclère A. La radiothérapie des fibromes utérins. in *Trans Int Cong Med* London: 1914.

4. Forssell G: Radium behandling av maligna tumörer i kvinnliga genitalia. *Hygien* 74:445, 1912.

5. Shu-Mo C, Xiang W, Qi W: High-dose after-loading in the treatment of cervical cancer of the uterus. *Int J Radiat Oncol Biol Phys* 16:335, 1989.

6. Teshima T, Chatani M, Hata K, Inoue T: High-dose rate intracavitary therapy for carcinoma of the uterine cervix: General figures of survival and complication. *Int J Radiat Oncol Biol Phys* 13:1035, 1987.

7. Utley JF, von Essen CF, Horn RA, Moeller JH: High dose rate afterloading brachytherapy in carcinoma of the uterine cervix. *Int J Radiat Oncol Biol Phys* 10:2259, 1984.

8. Fu KK, Phillips TL: High-dose-rate versus low-dose-rate intracavitary brachytherapy for carcinoma of the cervix. *Int J Radiat Oncol Biol Phys* 19:791, 1990.

9. Inoue T, Hori S, Miyata Y, et al. High versus low dose

rate intracavitary irradiation of carcinoma of the uterine cervix: A preliminary report. *Acta Radiol Oncol* 17:277, 1978.

10. Taina E: High versus low-dose rate intracavitary radiotherapy in the treatment of carcinoma of the uterus. *Acta Obstet Gynecol Scand* 103:1, 1981.

11. Shigematsu Y, Nishiyama K, Masaki N, et al: Treatment of the uterine cervix by remotely controlled afterloading intracavitary radiotherapy with high-dose rate: A comparative study with a low-dose rate system. *Int J Radiat Oncol Biol Phys* 9:351, 1983.

12. Fletcher GH: *Textbook of Radiology,* 3d ed. Philadelphia: Lea & Febiger, 1980.

13. Suit HD, Moore EB, Fletcher GH, Worsnop B: Modification of Fletcher ovoid system for afterloading using standard size radium tubes (milligram and microgram). *Radiology* 81:126, 1963.

14. Kapp KS, Stuecklschweiger GF, Kapp DS, Hackl AG: Dosimetry of intracavitary placements for uterine and cervical carcinoma: Results of ortogonal film, TLD, and CT-assisted techniques. *Radiother Oncol* 24:137, 1992.

15. Ling CC, Schell MC, Working KR, et al: CT-assisted assessment of bladder and rectum dose in gynecologic implants. *Int J Radiat Oncol Biol Phys* 13:1577, 1987.

16. Pilepich MV, Prasad S, Madoc-Jones H, Bedwinek JM: Effect of bladder distension on dosimetry in gynecological implants. *Radiology* 140:516, 1981.

17. Yu WS, Sagerman RH, Chung CT, et al: Anatomical relationships in intracavitary irradiation demonstrated by computed tomography. *Radiology* 143:357, 1982.

18. Schoppel SL, LaVigne ML, Martel MK, et al: Three-dimensional treatment planning of intracavitary gynecologic implants: Analysis of ten cases and implications for dose specifications. *Int J Radiat Oncol Biol Phys* 28:277, 1993.

19. Weeks KJ, Montana GS, Bentel GC: Design of a plastic minicolpostat applicator with shields. *Int J Radiat Oncol Biol Phys* 21:1045, 1991.

20. Lanciano R, Corn B, Martin E, et al: Perioperative morbidity of intracavitary gynecologic brachytherapy. *Int J Radiat Oncol Biol Phys* 29:969, 1994.

21. Grigsby PW, Georgiou A, Williamson JF, Perez CA: Anatomic variation of gynecologic brachytherapy prescription points. *Int J Radiat Oncol Biol Phys* 27:725, 1993.

22. Scott WP: Cervicovaginal irradiator—A triple applicator. *Am J Roentgenol* 96:52, 1966.

23. Lichter AS, Dillon MB, Rosenshein NB, Order SE: The use of custom molds for intracavitary treatment of carcinoma of the cervix. *Int J Radiat Oncol Biol Phys* 4:874, 1978.

24. Chow H, Lane RG, Rosen II: Uncertainty in dose estimation for gynecologic implants. *Int J Radiat Oncol Biol Phys* 19:1555, 1990.

25. Cunningham DE, Stryker JA, Velkley DE, Chung CK: Routine clinical estimation of rectal, rectosigmoidal, and bladder doses from intracavitary brachytherapy in the treatment of carcinoma of the cervix. *Int J Radiat Oncol Biol Phys* 7:653, 1981.

26. Million RR, Mauderli W, Bruno FP: Modification of technique for bladder and rectal measurements in carcinoma of the cervix. *Radiology* 60:921, 1966.

27. Roswit B, Malsky SJ, Reid CB, Amato CG, Gobels R: *In vivo* radiation dosimetry: Review of a 12 year experience. *Radiology* 97:413, 1970.

28. Fletcher GH, Brown TC, Rutledge FN: Clinical significance of rectal and bladder dose measurements in radium therapy of cancer of the uterine cervix. *Am J Roentgenol* 79:421, 1958.

29. Gray MJ, Kottmeier HL: Rectal and bladder injuries following therapy for carcinoma of the cervix at the Radiumhemmet. *Am J Obstet Gynecol* 74:1294, 1957.

30. Hamberger AD, Unal A, Gershenson DM, Fletcher GH: Analysis of the severe complications of irradiation of carcinoma of the cervix: Whole pelvis irradiation and intracavitary radium. *Int J Radiat Oncol Biol Phys* 9:367, 1983.

31. Lee KH, Kagan AR, Nussbaum H, et al: Analysis of dose, dose-rate and treatment time in the production of injuries by radium treatment for cancer of the uterine cervix. *Br J Radiol* 49:430, 1976.

32. Montana GS, Fowler WC, Varia MA, et al: Carcinoma of the cervix stage IB: Results of treatment with radiation therapy. *Int J Radiat Oncol Biol Phys* 9:45, 1983.

33. Montana GS, Fowler WC, Varia MA: Analysis of results of radiation therapy for stage II carcinoma of the cervix. *Cancer* 56:956, 1985.

34. Montana GS, Fowler WC, Varia MA, et al: Carcinoma of the cervix stage III: Results of radiation therapy. *Cancer* 57:148, 1986.

35. Orton CG, Wolf-Rosenblum S: Dose dependence of complication rates in cervix cancer radiotherapy. *Int J Radiat Oncol Biol Phys* 12:37, 1986.

36. Perez CA, Breaux S, Bedwinek JM, et al: Radiation therapy alone in the treatment of carcinoma of the uterine cervix II: Analysis of complications. *Cancer* 54:235, 1984.

37. Pitts HC, Waterman GW: Report of results of radium treatment of carcinoma of cervix. *Am J Obstet Gynecol* 29:607, 1930.

38. Pourquier H, Dubois JB, Delard R: Cancer of the uterine cervix: Dosimetric guidelines for prevention of late rectal and rectosigmoid complications as a result of radiotherapeutic treatment. *Int J Radiat Oncol Biol Phys* 8:1887, 1982.

39. Strockbine MF, Hancock JE, Fletcher GH: Complications in 831 patients with squamous cell carcinoma of the intact uterine cervix treated with 3000 rad or more whole pelvis radiation. *Am J Roentgenol* 58:293, 1970.

40. Villasanta U: Complications of radiotherapy for carci-

noma of the uterine cervix. *Am J Obstet Gynecol* 114:717, 1972.

41. Karolis C, Reay-Young PS, Walsh W, Velautham G: Silicone plesiotherapy molds. *Int J Radiat Oncol Biol Phys* 9:569, 1983.

42. Ang KK, Jiang GL, Frankenthaler RA, Kaanders JHAM: Cacinomas of the nasal cavity. *Radiother Oncol* 24:163, 1992.

43. Pop LAM, Kaanders JHAM, Heinerman ECM: High dose rate intracavitary brachytherapy of early and superficial carcinoma of the nasal vestibule as an alternative to low dose rate interstitial radiation therapy. *Radiother Oncol* 27:69, 1993.

44. Chassagne D, Wilson JF: Brachytherapy of carcinomas of the nasal vestibule (editorial). *Int J Radiat Oncol Biol Phys* 10:761, 1984.

45. Ibrahim E, Chassagne D, Cachin Y, Haie C: Les epithélioma du seuil narinaire: A propos de 36 cas traités à l'Institute Gustave-Roussy de 1961 a 1975. *Les Cahiers D'ORL* 17:109, 1982.

46. Bentel GC, Halperin EC, Buckley EG: ^{125}I embedded in an orbital prosthesis for retreatment of recurrent retinoblastoma. *Med Dosim* 18:1, 1993.

47. Fu KK, Newman H, Phillips TL: Treatment of locally recurrent carcinoma of the nasopharynx. *Radiology* 117:425, 1975.

48. Smith HS, Lapinski MV, Barr CE: A simplified method for intracavitary radiation for recurrent nasopharyngeal carcinoma. *Radiology* 131:534, 1979.

49. Wang CC, Schulz MD: Management of locally recurrent carcinoma of the nasopharynx. *Radiology* 86:900, 1966.

50. Wang CC, Busse J, Gitterman M: A simple afterloading applicator for intracavitary irradiation for carcinoma of the nasopharynx. *Radiology* 115:737, 1975.

51. Henschke UK, Hilaris BS, Mahan GD: Afterloading in interstitial and intracavitary radiation therapy. *Am J Roentgenol* 90:386, 1963.

52. Syed AMN, Feder BH: Technique of afterloading interstitial implants. *Radiol Clin* 46:458, 1977.

53. Calle R, Pilleron JP, Schlienger P, Vilcoq JR: Conservative management of operable breast cancer: Ten years' experience at the Foundation Curie. *Cancer* 42:2045, 1978.

54. Fisher B, Montague E, Redmond C, and other NSABP investigators: Comparison of radical mastectomy with alternative treatments of primary breast cancer: A first report of results from a prospective randomized clinical trial. *Cancer* 39:2827, 1977.

55. Pierquin B, Owen R, Maylin C, et al: Radical radiation therapy of breast cancer. *Int J Radiat Oncol Biol Phys* 6:17, 1980.

56. Prosnitz LR, Goldenburg IS, Packard RA, et al: Radiation therapy as initial treatment for early stage cancer of the breast without mastectomy. *Cancer* 39:917, 1977.

57. Zwicker RD, Schmidt-Ullrich R, Schiller B: Planning of

Ir-192 seed implants for boost irradiation of the breast. *Int J Radiat Oncol Biol Phys* 11:2163, 1985.

58. Harris JR, Botnick L, Bloomer WD, et al: Primary radiation therapy for early breast cancer: The experience of the Joint Center for Radiation Therapy. *Int J Radiat Oncol Biol Phys* 7:1549, 1981.

59. Levene MB: Interstitial therapy of breast cancer. *Int J Radiat Oncol Biol Phys* 2:1157, 1977.

60. Kwan DK, Kagan AR, Olch AJ, et al: Single and double plane iridium-192 interstitial implants: Implantation guidelines and dosimetry. *Med Phys* 10:456, 1983.

61. Anderson LL, Wagner LK, Schauber TH: Memorial Hospital methods of dose calculations for 192-Ir, in George FW III (ed): *Modern Interstitial and Intracavitary Radiation Cancer Management.* New York: Masson, 1981.

62. Anderson LL, Hilaris BS, Wagner LK: A nomograph for planar implant planning. *Endocuriether Hyperther Oncol* 1:9, 1985.

63. Gillin MT, Kline RW, Wilson JF, Cox JD: Single and double plane implants: A comparison of the Manchester system with the Paris system. *Int J Radiat Oncol Biol Phys* 10:921, 1984.

64. Pierquin B, Dutreix A, Paine CH, et al: The Paris system in interstitial radiation therapy. *Acta Radiol Oncol* 17:33, 1978.

65. Pierquin B, Chassagne DJ, Chahbazian CM, Wilson JF: *Brachytherapy.* St. Louis, MO: Warren H. Green, 1979.

66. Marinello G, Valero M, Leung S, Pierquin B: Comparative dosimetry between iridium wires and seed ribbons. *Int J Radiat Oncol Biol Phys* 11:1733, 1985.

67. Syed AMN, Puthawala A, Neblett D, et al: Primary treatment of carcinoma of the lower rectum and anal canal by combination of external irradiation and interstitial implant. *Radiology* 128:199, 1978.

68. Vora N, Forell B, Desai K, Bradley W: Technique to maintain separation of mandibular loops in interstitial implantation of head and neck tumors. *Int J Radiat Oncol Biol Phys* 9:261, 1983.

69. Ampuero F, Doss LL, Khan M, et al: The Syed-Neblett interstitial template in locally advanced gynecologic malignancies. *Int J Radiat Oncol Biol Phys* 9:1897, 1983.

70. Feder BH, Syed AMN, Neblett D: Treatment of extensive carcinoma of the cervix with the "transperineal parametrial butterfly": A preliminary report on the revival of Waterman's approach. *Int J Radiat Oncol Biol Phys* 4:735, 1978.

71. Flemming P, Syed AMN, Neblett D, et al: Description of an afterloading Ir-192 interstitial-intercavitary technique in the treatment of carcinoma of the vagina. *Obstet Gynecol* 55:525, 1980.

72. Martinez A, Cox RS, Edmundson GK: A multiple-site perineal applicator (MUPIT) for treatment of prostatic, anorectal, and gynecologic malignancies. *Int J Radiat Oncol Biol Phys* 10:297, 1984.

73. Syed AMN, Puthawala A, Tansey LA, et al: Temporary

iridium-192 implantation in the management of carcinoma of the prostate, in Hilaris B, Batata M (eds): *Brachytherapy Oncology*. New York: New York Memorial Sloan-Kettering Cancer Center, 1983.

74. Bentel GC, Oleson JR, Clarke-Pearson D, et al: Transperineal templates for brachytherapy treatment of pelvic malignancies — A comparison of standard and customized templates. *Int J Radiat Oncol Biol Phys* 19:751, 1990.

75. Nori D, Donath D, Hilaris BS, et al: Precision transperineal brachytherapy in the treatment of early prostate cancer. *Endocuriether Hyperther Oncol* 6:119, 1990.

76. Osian AD, Anderson LL, Linares LA, et al: Treatment planning for permanent and temporary percutaneous implants with custom made templates. *Int J Radiat Oncol Biol Phys* 16:219, 1989.

77. Roy JN, Wallner KE, Chiu-Tsao S, et al: CT-based optimized planning for transperineal prostate implant with customized template. *Int J Radiat Oncol Biol Phys* 21:483, 1991.

78. Wallner KE, Chiu-Tsao S, Roy J, et al: An improved method for transperineal prostate implants. *J Urol* 146:90, 1991.

79. Wallner K, Roy J, Zelefsky M, et al: Fluoroscopic visualization of the prostatic urethra to guide transperineal prostate implantation. *Int J Radiat Oncol Biol Phys* 29:863, 1994.

80. Martinez A, Edmundson GK, Cox RS, et al: Combination of external beam irradiation and the multiple-site perineal applicator (MUPIT) for treatment of locally advanced or recurrent prostatic, anorectal and gynecologic malignancies. *Int J Radiat Oncol Biol Phys* 11:391, 1985.

81. Bernstein M, Gutin PH: Interstitial irradiation of brain tumors: A review. *Neurosurgery* 9:741, 1981.

82. Mundinger F: Langzeitergebnisse der stereotaktischen Radio-Isotopenbestrahlung von Hypophysentumoren. *Strahlentherapie* 116:523, 1961.

83. Mundinger F: Die interstitielle Radioisotopen-Bestrahlung von Hirntumoren mit vergleichenden Langzeitergebnissen zur Röntgentiefentherapie. *Acta Neurochir* 11:89, 1963.

84. Mundinger F: Dynamics of technetium 99m in normal and pathological CSF-spaces with digital autofluoroscope (Gammacamera), in *Meeting of the British and German Neurological Societies*. London: 1968.

85. Mundinger F: The treatment of brain tumors with interstitially applied radioactive isotopes, radionuclide applications in neurology and neurosurgery, in Wang Y, Paoletti P (eds): *Radionuclide Applications in Neurology and Neurosurgery*. Springfield, IL: Charles C Thomas, 1970, p 199.

86. Szikla G: *Stereotactic Cerebral Irradiation*. Amsterdam: Elsevier/North Holland, 1979.

87. Talairach J, Ruggiero G, Aboulker J, David M: A new method of treatment of inoperable brain tumours by stereotaxic implantation of radioactive gold — A preliminary report. *Br J Radiol* 28:62, 1955.

88. MacKay AR, Gutin PH, Hosobuchi Y, Norman D: Computed tomography-directed stereotaxy for biopsy and interstitial irradiation of brain tumors (technical note). *Neurosurgery* 11:38, 1982.

89. Mundinger F, Birg W, Ostertag CB: Treatment of small cerebral gliomas with CT aided stereotaxic curie therapy. *Neuroradiology* 16:564, 1978.

90. Gutin PH, Phillips TL, Hosobuchi Y: Permanent and removable implants for brachytherapy of brain tumors. *Int J Radiat Oncol Biol Phys* 7:1371, 1981.

91. Gutin PH, Phillips TL, Hosobuchi Y: Local treatment of malignant brain tumors by removable stereotactically implanted radioactive isotopes, in Karcher KH, Kogelnik HD, Reinartz G (eds): *Progress in Radio-Oncology II*. New York: Raven Press, 1982.

92. Gutin PH, Phillips TL, Wara WM, et al: Brachytherapy of recurrent malignant brain tumors with removable high activity iodine-125 sources. *J Neurosurg* 60:61, 1984.

93. Moore RF: Choroidal sarcoma treated by the intraocular insertion of radon seeds. *Br J Ophthalmol* 14:145, 1930.

94. Bedford MA: The use and abuse of cobalt plaques in the treatment of choroidal malignant melanomata. *Trans Ophthalmol Soc UK* 93:139, 1973.

95. Brady LW, Shields JA, Augsburger JJ, et al: Posterior uveal melanomas, in Phillips TL, Pistenmaa DA (eds): *Radiation Oncology Annual*. New York: Raven Press, 1984.

96. Lommatzsch P: Treatment of choroidal melanomas with Ru-106, Rh-106 beta ray applicators. *Surg Ophthalmol* 19:85, 1974.

97. Lommatzsch PK: Results after β-irradiation (^{106}Ku/^{106}Rh) of choroidal melanomas: 20 years experience. *Br J Ophthalmol* 70:844, 1986.

98. Packer S, Rotman M: Radiotherapy of choroidal melanoma with iodine-125. *Ophthalmology* 87:582, 1980.

99. Packer S, Rotman M, Fairchild RG, et al: Irradiation of choroidal melanoma with iodine-125 ophthalmic plaque. *Arch Ophthalmol* 98:1453, 1980.

100. Petrovich Z, Luxton G, Langholz B, et al: Episcleral plaque radiotherapy in the treatment of uveal melanomas. *Int J Radiat Oncol Biol Phys* 24:247, 1992.

101. Sealy R, le Roux PLM, Rapley F, et al: The treatment of ophthalmic tumours with low energy sources. *Br J Radiol* 49:551, 1976.

102. Stallard HB: Malignant melanoblastoma of the choroid. *Mod Prob Ophthalmol* 7:18, 1968.

103. Astrahan MA, Luxton G, Jozsef G, et al: An interactive treatment planning system for ophthalmic plaque therapy. *Int J Radiat Oncol Biol Phys* 18:679, 1990.

104. Ellsworth RM: The practical management of retinoblastoma. *Trans Am Ophthalmol Soc* 67:462, 1969.

105. Stallard HB: Radiotherapy of malignant intraocular neoplasms. *Br J Ophthalmol* 32:618, 1948.

106. Hilaris BS: *Handbook of Interstitial Brachytherapy*. Boston: Publishing Science Group, 1975.

107. Kumar PP, Good RR, Rainbolt C, et al: Low morbidity following transperineal percutaneous template technique for permanent iodine-125 endocurie therapy of prostate cancer. *Endocuriether Hyperther Oncol* 2:119, 1986.

108. Shipley WU, Kopelson G, Novack DJ, et al: Preoperative irradiation, lymphadenectomy, and I-125 implant for selected patients with localized prostatic carcinoma: A correlation of implant dosimetry with clinical results. *J Urol* 24:639, 1981.

109. Whitmore WF, Hilaris BS, Grabstald H: Retropubic implantation of I-125 in the treatment of prostatic cancer. *J Urol* 108:918, 1972.

110. Shipley WU, Nardi GL, Cohen AM, Ling CC: Iodine-125 implant as boost therapy in patient irradiated for localized pancreatic carcinoma: A comparative study to surgical resection. *Cancer* 45:709, 1980.

111. Hawliczek R, Neubauer J, Schmidt WFO, et al: A new device for interstitial [125]iodine seed implantation. *Int J Radiat Oncol Biol Phys* 20:621, 1991.

112. Scott WP: A spacer/injector needle for I-125 and other radioactive sources in permanent seed implant. *Radiology* 122:832, 1977.

113. Schulz V, Bush M: Ein neuer Applikator zur interstitiellen Therapie mit Au-198 und I-125 seeds. *Strahlentherapie* 157:104, 1981.

114. Anderson LL: Spacing nomograph for interstitial implants of I-125 seeds. *Med Phys* 3:48, 1976.

115. Henschke UK, Cevc P: Dimension averaging, a simple method for dosimetry of interstitial implants. *Radiobiol Radiother* 9:287, 1968.

116. Hilaris BS, Luomanen RK, Beattie EJ: Integrated irradiation and surgery in the treatment of apical lung cancer. *Cancer* 27:1369, 1971.

117. Hilaris BS, Martini N, Batata MA, Beattie EJ: Interstitial irradiation for unresectable carcinoma of the lung. *Ann Thorac Surg* 20:491, 1975.

118. Hilaris BS, Martini N, Loumanen RK: Endobronchial interstitial implantation. *Clin Bull* 9:17, 1979.

119. Hilaris BS, Martini N, Nori D, Beattie EJ Jr: The place for radiotherapy in the treatment of lung cancer. *World J Surg* 5:675, 1981.

120. Hilaris BS, Nori D, Beattie EJ, Martini N: Value of perioperative brachytherapy in the management of non-oat cell carcinoma of the lung. *Int J Radiat Oncol Biol Phys* 9:1161, 1983.

121. Hilaris BS, Gomez J, Nori D, et al: Combined surgery, intraoperative brachytherapy, and postoperative external beam radiation in stage III non-small cell lung cancer. *Cancer* 55:1226, 1985.

122. Scott WP: Simplified interstitial therapy technique (Vicryl I-125) for unresectable lung cancer. *Radiology* 117:734, 1975.

123. Dale RG: Calculation by computer of dose-distributions for superficial gold-198 implants and the derivation of optimized distribution rules. *Br J Radiol* 49:533, 1976.

124. Horiuchi J, Takeda M, Shibuya H, et al: Usefulness of [198]Au grain implants in the treatment of oral and oropharyngeal cancer. *Radiother Oncol* 21:29, 1991.

125. Goode R, Fee W, Goffinet D, Martinez A: Radioactive suture in the treatment of head and neck cancer. *Laryngoscope* 89:349, 1979.

126. Harter DJ, Delclos L: Sealed sources in synthetic absorbable suture. *Radiology* 116:721, 1975.

127. Palos BB, Pooler BA, Goffinet DR, Martinez A: A method for inserting I-125 seeds into absorbable sutures for permanent implantation in tissue. *Int J Radiat Oncol Biol Phys* 6:381, 1980.

128. Scott WP: Interstitial therapy, using non-absorbable (iridium-192 nylon ribbon) and absorbable (I-125 "Vicryl") suturing techniques. *Am J Roentgenol Radiat Ther Nucl Med* 124:560, 1975.

129. Marchese MJ, Nori D, Anderson LL, Hilaris BS: A versatile permanent planar implant technique utilizing iodine-125 seeds imbedded in Gelfoam. *Int J Radiat Oncol Biol Phys* 10:747, 1984.

130. Pisch J, Berson AM, Harvey JC, Mishra S, Beattie EJ: Absorbable mesh in placement of temporary implants. *Int J Radiat Oncol Biol Phys* 28:719, 1994.

131. Conroy RM, Shahbazian AA, Edwards KC, et al: A new method for treating carcinomatous biliary obstruction with intracatheter radium. *Cancer* 49:1321, 1982.

132. Fletcher MS, Dawson JL, Wheeler PG, et al: Treatment of high bile duct carcinoma by internal radiotherapy with Ir-192 wire. *Lancet* 2:172, 1981.

133. Fritz P, Brambs HJ, Schraube P, et al: Combined external beam radiotherapy and intraluminal high dose rate brachytherapy on bile duct carcinomas. *Int J Radiat Oncol Biol Phys* 29:855, 1994.

134. Gonzàlez D, Gerard JP, Maners AW, et al: Results of radiation therapy in carcinoma of the proximal bile duct (Klatskin tumor). *Semin Liver Dis* 10:131, 1990.

135. Herskovic A, Heaston D, Engler MJ, et al: Irradiation of biliary carcinoma. *Radiology* 139:219, 1981.

136. Ikeda H, Kuroda C, Uchida H, et al: Intraluminal irradiation with iridium-192 wires for extrahepatic bile duct carcinoma: A preliminary report. *Nippon Igaku Hoshasen Gakkai Zasshi* 39:1356, 1979.

137. Jager JJ, Pannebakker M, Rijken J, et al: Palliation in esophageal cancer with a single session of intraluminal irradiation. *Radiother Oncol* 25:134, 1992.

138. Johnson DW, Safai C, Goffinet DR: Malignant obstructive jaundice: Treatment with external beam and intracavitary radiotherapy. *Int J Radiat Oncol Biol Phys* 11:411, 1985.

139. Mahe M, Romestaing P, Talon B, et al: Radiation therapy in extrahepatic bile duct carcinoma. *Radiother Oncol* 21:121, 1991.

140. Syed AMN, Puthawala AA, Severance SR, Zamost BJ:

Intraluminal irradiation in the treatment of esophageal cancer. *Endocuriether Hyperther Oncol* 3:105, 1987.

141. Yankauer S: Two cases of lung tumor treated bronchoscopically. *NY Med J Med Rec* 115:741, 1922.

142. Gauwitz M, Ellerbroek N, Komaki R, et al: High dose endobronchial irradiation in recurrent bronchogenic carcinoma. *Int J Radiat Oncol Biol Phys* 23:397, 1992.

143. Lo TCM, Beamis JF Jr, Weinstein RS, et al: Intraluminal low-dose rate brachytherapy for malignant endobronchial obstruction. *Radiother Oncol* 23:16, 1992.

144. Schray MF, McDougall JC, Martinez A, et al: Management of malignant airway obstruction: Clinical and dosimetric considerations using an iridium 192 afterloading technique in conjunction with the neodymium laser. *Int J Radiat Oncol Biol Phys* 11:403, 1985.

145. Caspers RJL, Zwinderman AH, Griffioen G, et al: Combined external beam and low dose rate intraluminal radiotherapy in oesophageal cancer. *Radiother Oncol* 27:7, 1993.

146. Hishikawa Y, Kurisu K, Taniguchi M, et al: High-dose-rate intraluminal brachytherapy for esophageal cancer: 10 years experience in Hyogo College of Medicine. *Radiother Oncol* 21:107, 1991.

147. Hishikawa Y, Taniguchi M, Kamikonya N, et al: External beam radiotherapy alone or combined with high-dose-rate intracavitary irradiation in the treatment of cancer of the esophagus: Autopsy findings in 35 cases. *Radiother Oncol* 11:223, 1988.

148. Henschke UK, Hilaris BS, Mahan GD: Remote afterloading with intracavitary applicators. *Radiology* 83:344, 1964.

149. Howard N: Cathetron: High intensity cobalt. *Int J Radiat Oncol Biol Phys* 5:1885, 1979.

150. Liversage WE, Martin-Smith P, Ramsey NW: The treatment of uterine carcinoma using the cathetron. *Br J Radiol* 40:887, 1976.

151. O'Connell D, Howard N, Joslin CAF, et al: A new remotely controlled unit for the treatment of uterine carcinoma. *Lancet* 2:570, 1965.

152. O'Connell D, Howard N, Joslin CAF, et al: The treatment of uterine carcinoma using the cathetron. *Br J Radiol* 40:882, 1967.

153. Goldson AL, Niphanupudy JR: Guidelines for comprehensive quality assurance in brachytherapy. *Int J Radiat Oncol Biol Phys* 10(suppl 1):111, 1984.

Answers to the Problems

CHAPTER 1

1–1	*(b)*
1–2	*(d)*
1–3	*(b)*
1–4	*(b)*
1–5	*(a)*
1–6	*(c)*
1–7	*(a)*
1–8	*(c)*
1–9	*(b)*
1–10	*(c)*
1–11	*(a)*
1–12	*(d)*

CHAPTER 2

2–1	*(d)*
2–2	*(c)*
2–3	*(b)*
2–4	*(a)*
2–5	*(c)*
2–6	*(b)*
2–7	*(b)*
2–8	*(a)*
2–9	*(a)*
2–10	*(b)*
2–11	*(b)*
2–12	*(b)*
2–13	*(c)*
2–14	*(b)*
2–15	*(c)*
2–16	*(b)*
2–17	*(a)*
2–18	*(c)*
2–19	*(a)*
2–20	*(b)*

CHAPTER 3

3–1	*(c)*
3–2	*(b)*
3–3	*(d)*
3–4	*(c)*
3–5	*(b)*
3–6	*(c)*
3–7	*(d)*
3–8	*(c)*
3–9	*(2)*
3–10	*(b)*
3–11	*(c)*
3–12	*(a)*
3–13	*(c)*
3–14	*(b)*
3–15	*(d)*
3–16	*(c)*

CHAPTER 4

4–1	4 min, 41 s
4–2	344 MU
4–3	1 min, 45 s
4–4	193 MU
4–5	6 min, 28 s
4–6	303 MU
4–7	2 min, 7 s
4–8	118 MU
4–9	1 min, 7 s/field
4–10	164 MU
4–11	Midplane dose:147 cGy
	D_{max} dose:163 cGy
4–12	*(a)* 220 cGy
	(b) 203 cGy
	(c) 286 cGy
4–13	Right side: 1 min, 18 s
	Left side: 39 s
4–14	*(a)* Unwedged field:
	91 MU
	(b) Wedged fields:
	113 MU/field
4–15	246 MU
4–16	57 s
4–17	115 MU
4–18	216 MU
4–19	A&B: 65 MU
	C&D: 87 MU
4–20	*(a)* Field A: 146 MU
	Field B: 114 MU
	(b) D_{max}, field A: 210 cGy,
	D_{max}, field B: 210 cGy

CHAPTER 5

5–1	*(a)*
5–2	*(a)*
5–3	12 cm^2
5–4	*(d)*
5–5	*(b)*
5–6	*(b)*
5–7	255 cGy
5–8	0.046
5–9	14 cGy
5–10	2 min, 29 s
5–11	144.8°/min

CHAPTER 6

6–1	*(c)*
6–2	*(d)*
6–3	*(a)*
6–4	*(b)*
6–5	*(d)*
6–6	*(b)*
6–7	*(a)*
6–8	*(c)*
6–9	*(a)*
6–10	*(b)*
6–11	*(a)*
6–12	*(b)*
6–13	*(c)*
6–14	*(a)*

6−15 *(d)*
6−16 *(d)*
6−17 *(b)*
6−18 *(a)*
6−19 *(c)*
6−20 *(b)*

CHAPTER 7

7−1 *(c)*
7−2 *(a)*
7−3 *(d)*
7−4 *(b)*
7−5 *(d)*
7−6 *(a)*
7−7 *(c)*
7−8 *(a)*
7−9 *(b)*
7−10 *(c)*
7−11 *(c)*
7−12 *(d)*
7−13 *(b)*
7−14 *(a)*
7−15 *(b)*
7−16 *(c)*
7−17 *(b)*
7−18 *(d)*
7−19 *(a)*
7−20 *(c)*

CHAPTER 8

8−1 *(d)*
8−2 *(b)*
8−3 *(a)*
8−4 *(b)*
8−5 *(a)*
8−6 *(d)*
8−7 *(c)*
8−8 *(c)*
8−9 *(b)*
8−10 *(a)*
8−11 *(d)*
8−12 *(c)*
8−13 *(a)*

8−14 *(b)*
8−15 *(c)*
8−16 *(b)*
8−17 *(b)*
8−18 *(d)*
8−19 *(a)*
8−20 *(b)*

CHAPTER 9

9−1 *(d)*
9−2 *(b)*
9−3 *(d)*
9−4 *(b)*
9−5 *(b)*
9−6 *(a)*
9−7 *(d)*
9−8 *(c)*
9−9 *(a)*
9−10 *(b)*
9−11 *(c)*
9−12 *(b)*
9−13 *(c)*
9−14 *(b)*
9−15 *(a)*
9−16 *(b)*
9−17 *(d)*
9−18 *(a)*
9−19 *(c)*
9−20 *(d)*

CHAPTER 10

10−1 *(d)*
10−2 *(b)*
10−3 *(d)*
10−4 *(b)*
10−5 *(c)*
10−6 *(b)*
10−7 *(c)*
10−8 *(b)*
10−9 *(c)*
10−10 *(c)*
10−11 *(a)*
10−12 *(d)*

10−13 *(b)*
10−14 *(b)*
10−15 *(a)*
10−16 *(c)*
10−17 *(a)*
10−18 *(d)*
10−19 *(b)*
10−20 *(d)*

CHAPTER 11

11−1 *(b)*
11−2 *(b)*
11−3 *(c)*
11−4 *(d)*
11−5 *(c)*
11−6 *(c)*
11−7 *(b)*
11−8 *(c)*
11−9 *(a)*
11−10 *(a)*
11−11 *(d)*
11−12 *(b)*
11−13 *(a)*
11−14 *(d)*
11−15 *(a)*
11−16 *(b)*
11−17 *(b)*
11−18 *(d)*
11−19 *(a)*
11−20 *(b)*

CHAPTER 12

12−1 *(c)*
12−2 *(d)*
12−3 *(b)*
12−4 *(a)*
12−5 *(c)*
12−6 *(d)*
12−7 *(b)*
12−8 *(c)*
12−9 *(a)*
12−10 *(c)*
12−11 *(a)*

12–12   *(c)*
12–13   *(b)*
12–14   *(c)*
12–15   *(b)*

CHAPTER 13

13–1   *(b)*
13–2   *(c)*
13–3   *(c)*
13–4   *(a)*
13–5   *(d)*
13–6   *(c)*
13–7   *(b)*
13–8   *(a)*
13–9   *(c)*
13–10   *(a)*
13–11   *(d)*
13–12   *(b)*
13–13   *(c)*
13–14   *(b)*
13–15   *(d)*
13–16   *(a)*
13–17   *(b)*
13–18   *(c)*
13–19   *(a)*
13–20   *(c)*

CHAPTER 14

14–1   *(c)*
14–2   *(b)*
14–3   *(a)*
14–4   *(b)*
14–5   *(d)*
14–6   *(b)*
14–7   *(b)*
14–8   *(d)*
14–9   *(d)*
14–10   *(b)*
14–11   *(d)*
14–12   *(b)*
14–13   *(a)*
14–14   *(d)*
14–15   *(b)*
14–16   *(d)*
14–17   *(a)*
14–18   *(c)*
14–19   *(a)*
14–20   *(c)*

CHAPTER 15

15–1   *(c)*
15–2   cobalt 60, f
        gold 198, e
        iridium 192, c
        cesium 137, a
        iodine 125, d
        strontium 90, b
15–3   *(b)*
15–4   *(b)*
15–5   *(c)*
15–6   11 h
15–7   35.9 mg Ra eq
15–8   42.4 mg
15–9   67.3 h
15–10   *(c)*
15–11   1.62 mCi

CHAPTER 16

16–1   *(c)*
16–2   *(a)*
16–3   *(c)*
16–4   *(d)*
16–5   *(b)*
16–6   *(a)*
16–7   *(e)*
16–8   *(b)*
16–9   *(a)*
16–10   *(c)*
16–11   *(c)*
16–12   *(a)*
16–13   *(b)*
16–14   *(c)*
16–15   *(c)*
16–16   *(b)*
16–17   *(c)*
16–18   *(b)*
16–19   *(a)*
16–20   *(b)*

Appendix

Table A.1. Percent Depth Dose Data for Cobalt 60, SSD 80 CM

Depth, cm	Field Size, Side of Square Field, cm						
	5.0	8.0	10.0	12.0	15.0	18.0	20.0
0.5	100.0	100.0	100.0	100.0	100.0	100.0	100.0
1.0	97.0	97.8	98.1	98.3	98.4	98.4	98.4
2.0	91.3	92.7	93.2	93.6	93.8	93.9	94.0
3.0	85.6	87.6	88.3	88.7	89.2	89.5	89.6
4.0	80.2	82.5	83.3	83.9	84.6	85.0	85.2
5.0	74.8	77.4	78.4	79.2	80.0	80.5	80.9
6.0	69.5	72.3	73.5	74.3	75.3	76.0	76.5
7.0	64.4	67.5	68.7	69.7	70.7	71.6	72.2
8.0	59.4	62.7	64.0	65.1	66.4	67.4	68.1
9.0	55.0	58.2	59.6	60.7	62.1	63.3	64.2
10.0	50.7	54.0	55.5	56.8	58.3	59.5	60.4
11.0	46.9	50.1	51.7	53.0	54.6	55.9	56.9
12.0	43.2	46.4	48.0	49.4	51.0	52.5	53.5
13.0	40.0	43.2	44.8	46.2	47.8	49.3	50.3
14.0	36.8	40.1	41.7	43.1	44.8	46.3	47.3
15.0	34.1	37.2	38.9	40.2	41.9	43.5	44.5
16.0	31.5	34.5	36.1	37.5	39.2	40.8	41.9
17.0	29.3	32.2	33.8	35.1	36.8	38.4	39.5
18.0	27.1	29.9	31.5	32.8	34.5	36.2	37.3
19.0	25.1	27.8	29.3	30.6	32.3	34.0	35.2
20.0	23.1	25.7	27.2	28.5	30.2	32.0	33.1
25.0	16.3	18.4	19.7	20.9	22.4	23.9	25.0
30.0	10.6	12.3	13.4	14.4	15.7	17.1	18.0

Table A.2.   Percent Depth Dose Data for 4-MV Photons, SSD 80 cm

Depth, cm	Field Size, Side of Square Field, cm						
	5.0	8.0	10.0	12.0	15.0	18.0	20.0
1.0	100.0	100.0	100.0	100.0	100.0	100.0	100.0
2.0	96.4	97.0	97.2	97.3	97.5	97.6	97.7
3.0	91.2	92.2	92.5	92.7	93.0	93.3	93.5
4.0	95.5	86.9	87.4	87.8	88.4	88.9	89.2
5.0	80.0	81.8	82.4	82.8	83.2	83.8	84.1
6.0	74.4	76.8	77.7	78.2	78.7	79.3	79.6
7.0	69.3	72.0	73.0	73.7	74.4	74.9	75.3
3.0	64.7	67.6	68.6	69.3	70.0	70.8	71.3
9.0	60.2	63.3	64.3	65.1	66.0	66.9	67.6
10.0	56.4	59.3	60.5	61.4	62.4	63.3	63.9
11.0	52.5	55.5	56.7	57.6	58.7	59.7	60.3
12.0	48.7	51.8	53.1	54.1	55.2	56.2	56.9
13.0	45.4	48.4	49.8	50.8	51.9	53.0	53.7
14.0	42.3	45.3	46.7	47.7	48.8	49.9	50.6
15.0	39.5	42.3	43.7	44.7	45.9	47.0	47.7
16.0	36.8	39.5	40.8	41.8	43.0	44.2	45.0
17.0	34.4	37.0	38.3	39.3	40.6	41.8	42.6
18.0	32.1	34.6	35.9	37.0	38.2	39.4	40.2
19.0	29.8	32.4	33.7	34.7	36.0	37.1	37.9
20.0	27.7	30.1	31.5	32.5	33.8	35.0	35.8
25.0	19.8	21.8	22.9	23.9	25.0	26.0	26.7
30.0	13.9	15.6	16.5	17.3	18.4	19.4	20.1

Table A.3. Tissue-Air Ratios for Cobalt 60

Depth, cm	Field Size, Side of Square Field, cm									
	0.0	5.0	8.0	10.0	12.0	15.0	18.0	20.0	30.0	35.0
0.5	1.000	1.012	1.022	1.030	1.039	1.049	1.056	1.060	1.080	1.090
1.0	0.966	0.994	1.012	1.023	1.033	1.044	1.052	1.056	1.076	1.086
2.0	0.904	0.957	0.982	0.995	1.007	1.020	1.028	1.033	1.056	1.067
3.0	0.845	0.919	0.949	0.964	0.977	0.993	1.002	1.008	1.035	1.049
4.0	0.792	0.880	0.914	0.931	0.946	0.963	0.974	0.981	1.013	1.029
5.0	0.741	0.839	0.877	0.895	0.912	0.931	0.944	0.951	0.988	1.007
6.0	0.694	0.797	0.838	0.857	0.875	0.895	0.910	0.919	0.963	0.985
7.0	0.649	0.753	0.798	0.818	0.837	0.859	0.875	0.885	0.935	0.960
8.0	0.608	0.710	0.757	0.778	0.798	0.822	0.841	0.852	0.907	0.935
9.0	0.570	0.670	0.716	0.739	0.759	0.785	0.805	0.818	0.880	0.911
10.0	0.534	0.631	0.678	0.701	0.723	0.750	0.771	0.784	0.849	0.881
11.0	0.501	0.595	0.642	0.665	0.687	0.716	0.738	0.752	0.820	0.854
12.0	0.469	0.559	0.606	0.629	0.652	0.681	0.705	0.719	0.791	0.827
13.0	0.440	0.527	0.574	0.598	0.620	0.650	0.674	0.689	0.762	0.798
14.0	0.412	0.495	0.541	0.566	0.589	0.619	0.643	0.658	0.733	0.770
15.0	0.387	0.467	0.512	0.536	0.559	0.589	0.614	0.629	0.705	0.743
20.0	0.278	0.345	0.383	0.405	0.427	0.457	0.483	0.500	0.584	0.626
25.0	0.211	0.265	0.296	0.316	0.335	0.362	0.386	0.402	0.479	0.517
30.0	0.144	0.185	0.209	0.226	0.244	0.268	0.290	0.304	0.374	0.409

Table A.4. Tissue-Air Ratios for 4-MV Photons

Depth, cm	Field Size, Side of Square Field, cm								
	0.0	5.0	8.0	10.0	11.0	12.0	15.0	17.0	20.0
1.0	0.999	1.017	1.029	1.036	1.039	1.042	1.051	1.055	1.061
2.0	0.973	1.004	1.022	1.031	1.035	1.039	1.049	1.055	1.061
3.0	0.928	0.972	0.994	1.004	1.009	1.014	1.025	1.031	1.040
4.0	0.881	0.933	0.959	0.971	0.977	0.982	0.996	1.004	1.015
5.0	0.835	0.892	0.923	0.936	0.942	0.947	0.960	0.967	0.978
6.0	0.780	0.848	0.885	0.902	0.909	0.915	0.928	0.936	0.947
7.0	0.734	0.807	0.847	0.866	0.874	0.880	0.896	0.905	0.915
8.0	0.690	0.769	0.812	0.831	0.839	0.846	0.862	0.871	0.884
9.0	0.655	0.731	0.775	0.795	0.803	0.810	0.828	0.839	0.854
10.0	0.612	0.697	0.743	0.763	0.771	0.779	0.799	0.810	0.825
11.0	0.582	0.663	0.707	0.729	0.738	0.747	0.767	0.779	0.794
12.0	0.552	0.628	0.672	0.695	0.705	0.714	0.736	0.747	0.763
13.0	0.521	0.597	0.641	0.664	0.675	0.684	0.706	0.717	0.733
14.0	0.490	0.566	0.610	0.634	0.644	0.653	0.676	0.688	0.704
15.0	0.462	0.538	0.581	0.604	0.615	0.623	0.646	0.659	0.676
16.0	0.435	0.510	0.553	0.575	0.585	0.593	0.617	0.630	0.643
17.0	0.413	0.486	0.527	0.549	0.559	0.568	0.592	0.605	0.623
18.0	0.392	0.462	0.501	0.524	0.534	0.543	0.567	0.580	0.598
19.0	0.370	0.437	0.476	0.498	0.509	0.518	0.542	0.555	0.573
20.0	0.348	0.413	0.450	0.473	0.483	0.492	0.517	0.530	0.548
21.0	0.332	0.394	0.430	0.452	0.462	0.471	0.495	0.509	0.526
22.0	0.315	0.375	0.410	0.431	0.441	0.450	0.474	0.487	0.504
23.0	0.299	0.356	0.389	0.410	0.420	0.428	0.453	0.466	0.483
24.0	0.282	0.337	0.369	0.389	0.398	0.407	0.431	0.444	0.461
25.0	0.269	0.322	0.353	0.372	0.381	0.390	0.413	0.426	0.443
26.0	0.255	0.306	0.336	0.355	0.364	0.372	0.395	0.408	0.424
27.0	0.242	0.291	0.320	0.338	0.347	0.355	0.377	0.390	0.406
28.0	0.228	0.275	0.304	0.322	0.330	0.338	0.359	0.372	0.388
29.0	0.214	0.260	0.287	0.305	0.313	0.320	0.341	0.354	0.370
30.0	0.201	0.244	0.271	0.288	0.296	0.303	0.323	0.336	0.352

Table A.5.   Tissue-Maximum Ratios for 10-MV Photons

Depth, cm	Field Size, Side of Square Field, cm										
	0.0	5.0	6.0	8.0	10.0	12.0	15.0	17.0	20.0	25.0	30.0
1.0	0.835	0.859	0.864	0.874	0.884	0.888	0.893	0.896	0.903	0.913	0.922
2.0	0.956	0.968	0.970	0.971	0.972	0.975	0.980	0.981	0.982	0.985	0.985
2.5	1.000	1.000	1.000	1.000	1.000	1.000	1.000	1.000	1.000	1.000	1.000
3.0	0.983	1.000	1.000	1.000	1.000	1.000	1.000	1.000	1.000	1.000	1.000
4.0	0.955	0.992	0.992	0.993	0.993	0.993	0.993	0.993	0.993	0.994	0.994
5.0	0.914	0.962	0.963	0.965	0.966	0.967	0.968	0.970	0.971	0.972	0.973
6.0	0.885	0.929	0.933	0.935	0.938	0.940	0.944	0.947	0.949	0.950	0.951
7.0	0.856	0.899	0.905	0.910	0.913	0.916	0.920	0.921	0.924	0.928	0.931
8.0	0.826	0.868	0.878	0.884	0.888	0.891	0.895	0.900	0.906	0.908	0.910
9.0	0.800	0.840	0.850	0.858	0.862	0.865	0.872	0.876	0.883	0.885	0.889
10.0	0.772	0.812	0.823	0.830	0.836	0.842	0.850	0.856	0.864	0.862	0.869
11.0	0.746	0.785	0.798	0.807	0.814	0.818	0.825	0.828	0.843	0.845	0.849
12.0	0.722	0.760	0.771	0.781	0.791	0.797	0.803	0.813	0.821	0.823	0.829
13.0	0.696	0.735	0.749	0.759	0.768	0.772	0.783	0.788	0.801	0.803	0.809
14.0	0.674	0.708	0.725	0.736	0.745	0.752	0.762	0.767	0.774	0.783	0.790
15.0	0.651	0.685	0.700	0.712	0.720	0.730	0.740	0.746	0.755	0.765	0.771
16.0	0.630	0.665	0.676	0.690	0.701	0.710	0.720	0.727	0.734	0.744	0.751
17.0	0.608	0.640	0.656	0.669	0.680	0.689	0.700	0.708	0.714	0.726	0.735
18.0	0.586	0.616	0.634	0.648	0.659	0.669	0.680	0.690	0.695	0.707	0.717
19.0	0.568	0.595	0.613	0.628	0.639	0.649	0.661	0.670	0.676	0.689	0.699
20.0	0.550	0.574	0.593	0.609	0.620	0.632	0.642	0.651	0.658	0.670	0.680
21.0	0.531	0.552	0.573	0.580	0.601	0.611	0.622	0.626	0.640	0.653	0.662
22.0	0.512	0.531	0.552	0.570	0.581	0.591	0.603	0.606	0.621	0.637	0.645
23.0	0.494	0.514	0.535	0.550	0.565	0.574	0.587	0.595	0.608	0.619	0.632
24.0	0.477	0.494	0.515	0.532	0.545	0.555	0.570	0.578	0.589	0.601	0.615
25.0	0.456	0.477	0.498	0.516	0.530	0.539	0.553	0.560	0.570	0.583	0.598
30.0	0.380	0.395	0.416	0.434	0.448	0.558	0.474	0.482	0.494	0.510	0.522

Table A.6. Equivalent Squares of Rectangular Fields

Short Axis, cm

Long Axis, cm	1	2	3	4	5	6	7	8	9	10	11	12	13	14	15	16	17	18	19	20	22	24	26	28	30
1	1.0																								
2	1.4	2.0																							
3	1.6	2.4	3.0																						
4	1.7	2.7	3.4	4.0																					
5	1.8	3.0	3.8	4.5	5.0																				
6	1.9	3.1	4.1	4.8	5.5	6.0																			
7	2.0	3.3	4.3	5.1	5.8	6.5	7.0																		
8	2.1	3.4	4.5	5.4	6.2	6.9	7.5	8.0																	
9	2.1	3.5	4.6	5.6	6.5	7.2	7.9	8.5	9.0																
10	2.2	3.6	4.8	5.8	6.7	7.5	8.2	8.9	9.5	10.0															
11	2.2	3.7	4.9	5.9	6.9	7.8	8.6	9.3	9.9	10.5	11.0														
12	2.2	3.7	5.0	6.1	7.1	8.0	8.8	9.6	10.3	10.9	11.5	12.0													
13	2.2	3.8	5.1	6.2	7.2	8.2	9.1	9.9	10.6	11.3	11.9	12.5	13.0												
14	2.3	3.8	5.1	6.3	7.4	8.4	9.3	10.1	10.9	11.6	12.3	12.9	13.5	14.0											
15	2.3	3.9	5.2	6.4	7.5	8.5	9.5	10.3	11.2	11.9	12.6	13.3	13.9	14.5	15.0										
16	2.3	3.9	5.2	6.5	7.6	8.6	9.6	10.5	11.4	12.2	13.0	13.7	14.3	14.9	15.5	16.0									
17	2.3	3.9	5.3	6.5	7.7	8.8	9.8	10.7	11.6	12.4	13.2	14.0	14.7	15.3	15.9	16.5	17.0								
18	2.3	4.0	5.3	6.6	7.8	8.9	9.9	10.8	11.8	12.7	13.5	14.3	15.0	15.7	16.3	16.9	17.5	18.0							
19	2.3	4.0	5.4	6.6	7.8	8.9	10.0	11.0	11.9	12.8	13.7	14.5	15.3	16.0	16.7	17.3	17.9	18.5	19.0						
20	2.3	4.0	5.4	6.7	7.9	9.0	10.1	11.1	12.1	13.0	13.9	14.7	15.5	16.3	17.0	17.7	18.3	18.9	19.5	20.0					
22	2.3	4.0	5.5	6.8	8.0	9.1	10.3	11.3	12.3	13.3	14.2	15.1	16.0	16.8	17.6	18.3	19.0	19.7	20.3	20.9	22.0				
24	2.4	4.1	5.5	6.8	8.1	9.2	10.4	11.5	12.5	13.5	14.5	15.4	16.3	17.2	18.0	18.8	19.6	20.3	21.0	21.7	22.9	24.0			
26	2.4	4.1	5.5	6.9	8.1	9.3	10.5	11.6	12.6	13.7	14.7	15.7	16.6	17.5	18.4	19.2	20.1	20.9	21.6	22.4	23.7	24.9	25.0		
29	2.4	4.1	5.6	6.9	8.2	9.4	10.5	11.7	12.8	13.8	14.8	15.9	16.8	17.8	18.7	19.6	20.5	21.3	22.1	22.9	24.4	25.7	27.0	28.0	
30	2.4	4.1	5.6	6.9	8.2	9.4	10.6	11.7	12.8	13.9	15.0	16.0	17.0	18.0	18.9	19.9	20.8	21.7	22.5	23.3	24.9	26.4	27.7	29.0	30.0

Source: Reproduced with permission from Cohen M, Jones A, Green D (eds): Central axis depth dose data for use in radiotherapy. *Br J Radiol* (suppl 11), page 99, 1972. Copyright 1972 by the British Institute of Radiology, London, England.

Table A.7. Scatter-Air Ratios (SAR): Cobalt 60

r, Field Radius in Centimeters at Depth d

Depth d, cm	1.0	2.0	3.0	4.0	5.0	6.0	7.0	8.0	9.0	10.0	11.0	12.0	13.0	14.0	15.0	16.0	17.0	18.0	19.0	20.0	21.0	22.0	23.0	24.0
0.5	0.007	0.014	0.019	0.026	0.032	0.037	0.043	0.048	0.054	0.058	0.063	0.067	0.070	0.073	0.076	0.078	0.080	0.082	0.084	0.085	0.086	0.087	0.088	0.088
1	0.013	0.025	0.037	0.048	0.058	0.066	0.073	0.078	0.084	0.089	0.094	0.098	0.101	0.104	0.107	0.109	0.112	0.114	0.116	0.118	0.119	0.120	0.121	0.122
2	0.023	0.045	0.064	0.080	0.091	0.102	0.110	0.116	0.122	0.127	0.133	0.139	0.142	0.146	0.149	0.152	0.154	0.156	0.158	0.160	0.161	0.162	0.164	0.166
3	0.032	0.061	0.084	0.103	0.118	0.130	0.139	0.147	0.154	0.161	0.166	0.172	0.176	0.180	0.184	0.187	0.190	0.193	0.195	0.198	0.200	0.202	0.203	0.204
4	0.038	0.071	0.099	0.121	0.137	0.151	0.162	0.170	0.179	0.186	0.191	0.197	0.201	0.205	0.210	0.215	0.218	0.222	0.225	0.228	0.231	0.233	0.235	0.237
5	0.041	0.076	0.107	0.134	0.152	0.166	0.178	0.189	0.198	0.206	0.212	0.218	0.224	0.229	0.235	0.240	0.245	0.248	0.252	0.255	0.258	0.261	0.263	0.264
6	0.042	0.080	0.114	0.141	0.160	0.176	0.190	0.201	0.211	0.219	0.226	0.234	0.241	0.246	0.252	0.257	0.262	0.265	0.269	0.272	0.275	0.278	0.280	0.282
7	0.042	0.081	0.115	0.143	0.164	0.181	0.196	0.209	0.220	0.229	0.239	0.246	0.254	0.260	0.267	0.273	0.278	0.282	0.287	0.290	0.294	0.296	0.299	0.302
8	0.041	0.080	0.114	0.142	0.165	0.185	0.199	0.214	0.225	0.236	0.246	0.254	0.263	0.271	0.278	0.285	0.289	0.294	0.298	0.301	0.305	0.309	0.311	0.313
9	0.040	0.078	0.112	0.140	0.164	0.183	0.200	0.216	0.228	0.240	0.251	0.260	0.269	0.277	0.284	0.292	0.298	0.303	0.308	0.312	0.316	0.319	0.322	0.324
10	0.038	0.075	0.109	0.136	0.161	0.181	0.199	0.215	0.229	0.242	0.252	0.262	0.271	0.279	0.288	0.295	0.302	0.308	0.314	0.318	0.324	0.327	0.331	0.333
11	0.036	0.071	0.104	0.132	0.157	0.178	0.197	0.213	0.227	0.241	0.252	0.262	0.272	0.280	0.289	0.296	0.304	0.311	0.316	0.322	0.328	0.331	0.334	0.337
12	0.035	0.069	0.099	0.128	0.153	0.174	0.194	0.210	0.225	0.239	0.251	0.261	0.272	0.281	0.290	0.297	0.305	0.312	0.318	0.324	0.330	0.333	0.337	0.340
13	0.034	0.066	0.095	0.124	0.149	0.170	0.190	0.207	0.223	0.237	0.249	0.260	0.270	0.280	0.290	0.298	0.306	0.313	0.319	0.325	0.332	0.335	0.340	0.342
14	0.032	0.063	0.063	0.092	0.120	0.168	0.186	0.204	0.220	0.235	0.247	0.258	0.268	0.279	0.288	0.297	0.305	0.313	0.320	0.326	0.333	0.337	0.341	0.344
15	0.031	0.060	0.089	0.116	0.140	0.162	0.182	0.200	0.216	0.231	0.244	0.255	0.266	0.277	0.286	0.295	0.303	0.311	0.318	0.325	0.331	0.336	0.340	0.344

Source: Reproduced with permission from Saylor WL and Ames TE: Dosage Calculation in Radiation Therapy. Baltimore, MD: Williams & Wilkins, copyright 1979.

Table A.8.   Scatter-Air Ratios (SAR): Varian Clinac 4-MV X-Rays (Lead Flatness Filter)

r, Field Radius at Depth d, cm

Depth, cm	1	2	3	4	5	6	7	8	9	10	11	12	13	14	15	16	20	25
1.2	0.007	0.013	0.020	0.026	0.033	0.039	0.046	0.052	0.058	0.062	0.066	0.068	0.070	0.072	0.073	0.075	0.077	0.079
2.0	0.020	0.035	0.047	0.055	0.064	0.073	0.080	0.088	0.093	0.098	0.103	0.105	0.107	0.108	0.110	0.112	0.115	0.118
3.0	0.027	0.048	0.067	0.081	0.093	0.102	0.111	0.118	0.125	0.130	0.134	0.137	0.140	0.141	0.143	0.146	0.150	0.154
4.0	0.032	0.058	0.079	0.097	0.112	0.125	0.136	0.145	0.152	0.157	0.161	0.164	0.168	0.171	0.174	0.180	0.188	0.195
5.0	0.034	0.063	0.089	0.110	0.127	0.141	0.154	0.165	0.173	0.179	0.185	0.189	0.193	0.197	0.200	0.206	0.214	0.222
6.0	0.035	0.067	0.095	0.119	0.137	0.155	0.170	0.181	0.190	0.196	0.202	0.207	0.212	0.216	0.220	0.228	0.237	0.246
7.0	0.035	0.068	0.098	0.125	0.146	0.163	0.180	0.193	0.203	0.211	0.217	0.223	0.228	0.233	0.237	0.246	0.257	0.268
8.0	0.035	0.069	0.101	0.128	0.152	0.170	0.187	0.201	0.213	0.222	0.230	0.236	0.242	0.247	0.252	0.261	0.272	0.283
9.0	0.035	0.069	0.102	0.131	0.156	0.174	0.192	0.207	0.220	0.230	0.239	0.246	0.252	0.258	0.263	0.273	0.283	0.296
10.0	0.034	0.068	0.102	0.132	0.158	0.177	0.195	0.210	0.224	0.236	0.246	0.253	0.259	0.265	0.271	0.282	0.291	0.303
11.0	0.034	0.067	0.101	0.131	0.158	0.178	0.196	0.213	0.227	0.240	0.252	0.258	0.266	0.272	0.278	0.289	0.300	0.315
12.0	0.034	0.066	0.100	0.130	0.157	0.178	0.197	0.215	0.229	0.242	0.255	0.263	0.271	0.277	0.283	0.295	0.308	0.318
13.0	0.033	0.065	0.098	0.128	0.155	0.177	0.196	0.214	0.230	0.243	0.256	0.266	0.274	0.281	0.288	0.299	0.314	0.325
14.0	0.033	0.063	0.095	0.125	0.152	0.175	0.195	0.212	0.229	0.243	0.256	0.267	0.275	0.283	0.289	0.302	0.316	0.330
15.0	0.032	0.062	0.093	0.122	0.148	0.171	0.192	0.210	0.226	0.241	0.255	0.266	0.275	0.283	0.290	0.302	0.316	0.330
16.0	0.031	0.060	0.090	0.118	0.144	0.168	0.188	0.206	0.223	0.239	0.252	0.264	0.273	0.282	0.289	0.302	0.316	0.325
17.0	0.030	0.059	0.087	0.114	0.140	0.163	0.184	0.202	0.220	0.235	0.249	0.261	0.270	0.279	0.287	0.301	0.314	0.323
18.0	0.030	0.057	0.084	0.110	0.135	0.159	0.179	0.197	0.215	0.230	0.245	0.257	0.267	0.276	0.284	0.300	0.312	0.320
19.0	0.029	0.056	0.081	0.107	0.132	0.154	0.175	0.193	0.211	0.226	0.240	0.252	0.262	0.272	0.281	0.297	0.310	0.318
20.0	0.028	0.054	0.079	0.104	0.128	0.150	0.170	0.188	0.206	0.221	0.235	0.247	0.257	0.267	0.276	0.293	0.306	0.314

Source: Reproduced with permission from Saylor WL and Ames TE: *Dosage Calculation in Radiation Therapy.* Baltimore, MD: Williams & Wilkins, copyright 1979.

INDEX

INDEX

Note: Page numbers in italics refer to figures; page numbers followed by t indicate tables.

ISBN 0-07-005115-1

9 780070 051157

BENTEL-U.S.